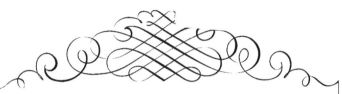
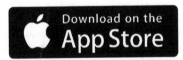
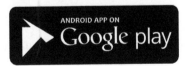

ISBN 978-0-265-70741-8
PIBN 10982687

1 MONTH OF
FREE
READING

at
www.ForgottenBooks.com

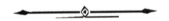

By purchasing this book you are eligible for one month membership to ForgottenBooks.com, giving you unlimited access to our entire collection of over 700,000 titles via our web site and mobile apps.

To claim your free month visit:
www.forgottenbooks.com/free982687

ANNALS

OF

SURGERY

A MONTHLY REVIEW OF SURGICAL SCIENCE AND PRACTICE

EDITED BY

LEWIS STEPHEN PILCHER, M.D., LL.D.,

OF NEW YORK

WITH THE COLLABORATION OF

Sɪʀ WILLIAM MACEWEN, M.D., LL.D., | Sɪʀ W. WATSON CHEYNE, C.B., F.R.S.,
OF GLASGOW, | OF LONDON,
Professor of Surgery in the University | Professor of Surgery in King's College.
of Glasgow.

VOLUME LXXII

JULY—DECEMBER, 1920

PHILADELPHIA

J. B. LIPPINCOTT COMPANY

1920

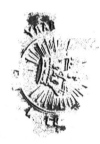

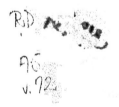

CONTRIBUTORS TO VOLUME LXXII

ADAIR, FRANK, M.D., of New York, N. Y.

ASHHURST, ASTLEY P. C., M.D., of Philadelphia, Pa.

BLOODGOOD, JOSEPH COLT, M.D., of Baltimore, Md.

BOHMANSSON, G., M.D., of Orebro, Sweden.

BOORSTEIN, SAMUEL W., M.D., of New York, N. Y.

BREWER, GEORGE EMERSON, M.D., of New York, N. Y.

BROWN, ALFRED J., M.D., of Omaha, Neb.

BUNTS, FRANK E., M.D., of Cleveland, Ohio.

CHURCHMAN, JOHN W., M.D., of New York, N. Y.

COLBY, WILLIAM B., M.D., of New York, N. Y.

CORNISH, PERCY G., JR., M.D., of Buffalo, N. Y.

COTTON, FREDERIC J., M.D., of Boston, Mass.

CRILE, GEORGE W., M.D., of Cleveland, Ohio.

CROSSAN, EDWARD T., M.D., of Philadelphia, Pa.

DAVIS, JOHN STAIGE, M.D., of Baltimore, Md.

DAVIS, LINCOLN, M.D., of Boston, Mass.

DINEGAR, ROBERT HENRY FALES, M.D., of New York, N. Y.

DOWD, CHARLES N., M.D., of New York, N. Y.

DUFFY, WILLIAM C., M.D., of New Haven, Conn.

EGGERS, CARL, M.D., of New York, N. Y.

ELIOT, ELLSWORTH, JR., M.D., of New York, N. Y.

FARR, CHARLES E., M.D., of New York, N. Y.

FAUNTLEROY, A. M., M.D., U. S. Navy.

FRAZIER, CHARLES H., M.D., of Philadelphia, Pa.

FREEMAN, LEONARD, M.D., of Denver, Colo.

GIBSON, CHARLES L., M.D., of New York, N. Y.

HARRIGAN, ANTHONY H., M.D., of New York, N. Y.

HARTWELL, JOHN A., M.D., of New York, N. Y.

HEDBLOM, CARL A., M.D., of Rochester, Minn.

HEUER, GEORGE J., M.D., of Baltimore, Md.

HEYD, CHAS. GORDON, M.D., of New York, N. Y.

HOGUET, J. PIERRE, M.D., of New York, N. Y.

HUFFMAN, LYMAN FOSTER, M.D., of Cleveland, Ohio.

IMBODEN, H. M., M.D., of New York, N. Y.

JACKSON, JABEZ N., M.D., of Kansas City, Mo.

JOHNSON, T. M., M.D., of Philadelphia, Pa.

JUDD, EDWARD STARR, M.D., of Rochester, Minn.

CONTRIBUTORS TO VOLUME LXXII

iv

ANNALS of SURGERY

| Vol. LXXII | JULY, 1920 | No. 1. |

THE DUTIES AND RESPONSIBILITIES OF THE CIVIL SURGEON WHEN CALLED TO ACTIVE MILITARY SERVICE *

By George Emerson Brewer, M.D.
of New York, N. Y.

It has always been the custom of the American Surgical Association to allow the president a large measure of latitude in selecting the subject of his inaugural address; and while in the majority of instances the subjects presented have been strictly professional, in that they have dealt with some live surgical problem, on not a few occasions the topics chosen have been of historic or biographic interest, or have presented thoughts on medical education, professional ethics, public health, or military preparedness.

That the interest of the surgical profession, here and elsewhere, has been acutely centred, during the past few years, upon the various military phases of our art, is evidenced by the large number of communications presented at our last meeting which dealt with the treatment of battle casualties, and with their associated infections; or the new and improved methods employed in the care of those who had been injured by the novel and cruelly destructive agencies of modern warfare, which by their diabolical ingenuity, have far outclassed in their mutilating effects anything which the world has ever known; and if it were not for the fact that in our present session a part of our program is made up of papers dealing with these same topics, I feel that I might have yielded to the strong impulse to present to you on this occasion some personal observations and experiences in front area work.

I have, however, elected to speak this morning upon two matters not strictly germane to either the scientific or practical aspects of our professional work, but which I venture to hope may be of interest. The first is a report on the activities of the Fellows of this Association in war work, and the other the duties and responsibilities of the civil practitioner in time of war, or perhaps, to state it more definitely, the relationship between the Army Medical Corps and the trained civil surgeon when called to active military service.

When we consider that our Association embraces in its membership the great majority of the recognized leaders of surgery in America, that owing to the conditions of fellowship over 90 per cent. of its active members are well above the military age, and were under no moral obligation

* President's Address before the American Surgical Association, May 3, 1920.

to enter the Government service, it is a matter of genuine pride and satisfaction to know that over 85 per cent. of our Fellows promptly volunteered and gave generously of their time and effort to the cause. I know of no other body of men of equal standing in the community who gave so much and at a greater sacrifice of personal interests.

It is fitting, therefore, that some record of their activities be preserved and made a part of our Association Archives, not only to record the historic facts, but to furnish an example to those who may follow, in the event of another and similar national emergency.

I have, therefore, attempted to collect all available data as to the service rendered by members of this Association, and will give you a brief summary of the result.

The total number of Fellows, active and senior, who offered their services to the Government or engaged in actual war work was 154, the average age of these was fifty-six and one-half years. It is worthy of note that of the 33 senior Fellows, 25 volunteered or engaged in active service, the average age of this group being seventy.

Number holding commissions in the U. S. Army, including two contract surgeons.. 96
Number holding commissions in the British Army 4
Number holding commissions in the Canadian Army 6
Number holding commissions in the French Army 1
Members of the Reserve Corps, who volunteered but were not called to active duty
    or were rejected on account of age or physical disability 6
Volunteer surgeons serving with the British Army previous to 1917 5
Volunteer surgeons serving with the French Army previous to 1917 13
Commissioned officers in the U. S. Navy 9
Fellows serving in the Red Cross Society 13
Fellows serving in the Medical Advisory Committee of the Council of National
    Defense 9
Enrolled in the Volunteer Medical Service Corps 11
Serving in local military or examining boards, State organizations or detailed to
    give instruction in military surgery 36

Of the 107 who held commissions in our own or one of the Allied armies, there were:

> Brigadier-generals 1
> Colonels 25
> Lieutenant-colonels 37
> Majors 31
> Captains 7
> First lieutenants 4

In two instances the rank was not mentioned.

Of these, 57 served in France with the A. E. F., 48 in the United States, 11 in the French or British armies.

As a number of officers served at different times in two or more of the Allied armies, and in different organizations in our own army, the totals in this and the following groups obviously will not correspond to the exact number of commissioned officers.

THE CIVIL SURGEON IN ACTIVE MILITARY SERVICE

Number serving in base or general hospitals 55
Number serving in evacuation hospitals or casualty clearing stations 12
Number serving in mobile hospitals 3
Number serving in camp hospitals 6
Number serving as heads of surgical teams 19
Number serving as consultants 26
Number serving at Headquarters at Washington 8
Number serving at Headquarters, A. E. F. 2
American delegates to Interallied Surgical Conferences in Paris 6
Fellows receiving one or more promotions 77
Fellows receiving decorations 22
Fellows receiving citations 10
Fellows mentioned in dispatches 4
Fellows serving in front area during one or more of the great battles 47

This is but a brief and incomplete statement of the actual service rendered by our members, and is introduced here, merely to give a general idea of the important and responsible positions they held during the World War. I have prepared a fuller record of the services rendered by each of the Fellows, which will be appended to this address and published in the transactions.

Let us now consider my second topic, *The duties and responsibilities of the trained civil surgeon when called to active military service.*

That he has a definite responsibility can not be questioned when we consider that in time of war or active mobilization, the Medical Corps of the Army is of necessity greatly augmented by the enlistment of men from the reserve corps and from civil practice. To illustrate the extent of this augmentation, allow me to call attention to the fact that at the time of our declaration of war, the Medical Corps of our Army consisted of less than 500 medical officers. At the time of the armistice the number of commissioned medical officers was considerably over 30,000, which indicates that at that time more than 59/60, or 98.3 per cent., of the medical service of the Army was rendered by civilian practitioners, including surgeons, internists, sanitary experts, laboratory workers, and other specialists.

The chief function of the Medical Corps of an army is to render the best possible sanitary service to the troops, to keep them in the best physical condition, and to provide individual care and skilled professional attention for the sick and injured.

During peace this is not difficult, the number of sick and injured is small, the skill and experience of the officers are well known, and they easily can be assigned to duties which they are qualified to assume. In time of war or active mobilization, however, the problem is far more difficult, for it necessitates a complete reorganization of the corps, the assimilation of thousands of new men who are ignorant of army routine, and whose professional qualifications are to a large extent unknown.

When we consider the magnitude of the problem and the difficulties under which the Surgeon General labored during our recent mobilization, the marvel is that so much in the way of efficient organization was accomplished.

3

GEORGE EMERSON BREWER

Laying aside for the moment the activities of the medical, sanitary, laboratory, and special departments, what was the chief surgical problem to be solved? I take it you will all agree with me that it was to render prompt and skilled surgical care to the man wounded in battle. The man who has the courage, patriotism, and determination to go into battle and give every ounce of energy and strength which he possesses to defeat the enemy, who cheerfully faces death and the chance of mutilating and disabling injury, is certainly entitled, when wounded, to the best surgical skill which his Government is able to provide. If he receives anything less than this, he is not being treated fairly, or, to use a commonplace expression, he is not getting a square deal.

How best can this be accomplished? To what extent was this accomplished in our own army during its participation in the great war? In answering the first question, I believe that one of the most important factors is to avoid misfits. By that I mean men who are assigned to duties they are not qualified to fulfill, or retained in such positions after their unfitness has been demonstrated. To obtain the best results only men of adequate surgical training and of large experience should be selected as operating surgeons in advanced hospitals where the wounded receive their first surgical treatment; and the work of these men should under no circumstances be hampered or interfered with by men of higher rank, but without skill, training, or experience in modern surgical procedures. Likewise in the base hospitals to which the wounded are quickly transferred from the front area, there should be a sufficient number of trained surgeons to oversee and direct the work of a larger number of junior officers, younger men, who have had at least some preliminary training in modern surgical technic.

That this ideal arrangement has not generally been carried out in the past will be evident to any one who will take pains to read the medical and surgical histories of any of the great wars of modern times. In the majority of instances these failures have been due, not to indifference on the part of a Government to the fate of its wounded soldiers, but to misfits in the professional personnel; expert surgeons who are assigned to purely executive duties, medical men who are assigned to responsible surgical posts, oculists, aurists, dermatologists, and X-ray operators who are obliged to work in medical or surgical wards, or in some specialty not their own, when their skill is urgently needed elsewhere; men well trained in laboratory methods but without experience in clinical work, obliged to give their entire attention to clinical problems.

All of these misfits I have personally observed in innumerable instances, have watched their bungling unproductive work, and have listened to a recital of their many efforts made through various channels to be given work which they felt themselves competent to carry out. I am not now speaking alone of our army, but of experience gathered while serving with the French or British forces; and I think it only fair to state

4

that, while numerous examples could be pointed out of such misfits in our own organization, my observations lead me to believe that there were fewer such instances in the A. E. F. than in the other Allied forces, and that it was far easier with us to effect satisfactory transfers, largely through the cordial relations which existed between our Chief Surgeon and the commanding officers of our sanitary groups.

One of the causes of this difficulty in the past has been due to the fact that ranking officials in the administrative bureaus, while perhaps possessing expert ability in executive matters, fail to recognize how highly specialized medicine has become during the past half century, to realize that the battle casualties of modern warfare present, in perhaps the majority of instances, the gravest of surgical problems, or to appreciate how utterly futile it is to expect these problems to be successfully met by men without or with but limited training or experience. As one British officer stated, "The men at Headquarters feel that every man possessing a medical diploma is capable of any and all kinds of professional work."

Another and perhaps the chief cause of misfits is the appointment of men to positions of grave professional responsibility on account of rank or previous service rather than professional qualifications. But the question is asked, How could this be otherwise without demoralizing the morale of the corps? The Army is an organization into which men enlist for life. They begin at the bottom and gradually work their way to the higher ranks by years of painstaking conscientious work, and when a man of mature age, after fifteen or twenty years of faithful service, reaches the rank of major, lieutenant-colonel, or colonel, is he not qualified to accept grave responsibility, and in the event of war, is it fair that he should be cast aside and replaced by a civilian who has never served in the Regular Army, and knows nothing of military routine?

Let us meet the issue squarely, and consider it from every angle, bearing in mind the paramount duty of the Government, which is to render to the wounded soldier the best possible surgical skill.

In the Regular Army the medical officer at the time of his enlistment is a highly qualified man, but with limited experience. During the first eight or ten years of his service, he is assigned to one or several military posts, where he has the care of a limited number of physically fit men, and the families of the officers. Between these assignments he may be stationed at a military hospital where he may have purely administrative duties, or may serve in medical or surgical wards. At other times he may have bureau work at Washington or at some divisional headquarters. As he advances in rank, he is given more responsible duties of an administrative character with a progressive diminution in actual professional work. As one major expressed it to the writer, "I have been seventeen years in the service. During my first six years my work was largely professional, during the next four or five years it was about equally divided between professional and administrative duties; and for the past seven years I have had practically no professional responsibility."

Certainly the army in peace time is not an ideal school for the training of surgeons, and while there are, of course, notable exceptions, of men who have had long periods of service in hospitals on account of special aptitude for medical, surgical, or special work, the opportunities for intensive surgical training are few, and the majority of army surgeons who have served perhaps fifteen or more years, and have reached the rank of major or lieutenant-colonel, while they may be expert administrative officials, can not be regarded as highly qualified modern surgeons. Such an experience can not qualify even the most gifted man to meet the emergencies or assume the grave responsibilities of treating battle casualties.

With the recent civilian graduate who has chosen surgery as his special life work, it is entirely different. From the time he leaves the medical school his energy is directed in a single channel. He passes through the positions of surgical interne, house surgeon, or resident surgeon, out-patient surgeon, assistant surgeon to the wards, associate or junior surgeon; and at the age when our military surgeon reaches the rank of major or colonel, the civilian practitioner if capable and industrious has reached the goal of his ambition, is an attending surgeon to some hospital, a position gained by fifteen or twenty years of continuous intensive surgical training.

If in the necessary reorganization of the army medical corps in time of war, the general policy were followed of selecting highly qualified civilian surgeons, but without army experience, to positions of purely professional responsibility, where a knowledge of army administrative methods is not essential; and of the highly qualified members of the regular corps to positions of high administrative command, where their knowledge and experience are most needed, it would provide promotion and dignified positions for all the capable ranking men of the service, and would in no way tend to demoralize the morale of the department. It would also prevent in a large measure the misfits to which I have alluded, and would be the greatest factor in providing for the wounded soldier the highest type of surgical skill. This was the general policy in our army during the recent war; but with a less enlightened and broad-minded Surgeon General it might not be the policy in a future war. Moreover, the line was never definitely drawn between administrative and professional control, and most of us who served in France saw examples of men of high rank holding executive positions, issuing orders which if carried out to the letter would have sadly interfered with the orderly carrying on of modern surgical procedures.

This brings me to the second factor in accomplishing the highest degree of professional service to the wounded man; and that is the plan of dual control in all hospitals and all organizations in which the medical department has important activities. I realize that the term dual control of any military formation will be said to be a blow at the very foundation of military discipline. Yet I venture to approve the plan for the reason that I believe it to be fundamentally sound, that it was first suggested and put into operation by our own Surgeon General, and also for the reason that I think it can be shown that by a reasonable interpretation it will not affect or interfere with military discipline in the slightest degree.

It will be recalled that long before we entered the war the Surgeon General authorized the organization of fifty Red Cross Base Hospitals, with the understanding that in case of war they would be taken over by the War Department and made an integral part of the army. The plan of organization was to supply for each a commanding officer appointed from the Medical Corps of the Regular Army, who would have complete administrative and disciplinary control of the unit; and a director who would be responsible for the actual care of the patients. By this plan these hospitals were placed on the same basis as our own best civil hospitals in which the Board of Trustees or administrative department is entirely separate from the professional, and in no way interferes with or attempts to dictate the scientific activities of the professional staff; but at all times is in absolute control, as they have the power of appointment and removal.

The success of the plan was, I think, generally admitted. In the unit to which I was attached and in a number of others in which there was a reasonable coöperation between the commanding officer and director, there was not the slightest friction, and no question of authority was ever raised; the director recognized that the commanding officer was his superior officer, and the commanding officer recognized the professioual responsibilities of the director and never interfered with the clinical work of the unit.

In the late autumn of 1917 orders were sent from Washington to the A. E. F. to organize a group of professional consultants, to take over the responsibility of the care of patients in the various divisions as they became ready for active duty. Without going into detail in regard to the organization of this group, with which you doubtless are all familiar, I may briefly state that there was a chief consultant in surgery, a chief consultant in medicine, and a chief consultant in the laboratory specialties. Under each of these departments there were a number of subdivisions, those in surgery being: General surgery, orthopedics, urology, otology and laryngology, ophthalmology, facio-maxillary surgery, neurological surgery, and experimental surgery.

Special divisional consultants were first appointed in general surgery, orthopedic surgery, and urology. Later consultants in medicine, neurology, and some of the other specialties were appointed to divisional, corps, and army headquarters. At a still later period, surgical consultants were sent to a number of the large base hospital centres, where they would direct and supervise the professional work in the various hospital units.

7

Shortly after the creation of the Consulting Board, the Chief Surgeon of the A. E. F. authorized the chief consultant in surgery to organize surgical teams for active service at the front, relying upon his judgment in the selection of the officers to head each team. More than one hundred such teams, representing the best surgical talent in the overseas army, were organized and sent to the evacuation and advanced hospitals in the three or four great battles in the summer and autumn of 1918. During this active period the chief consultant arranged frequent conferences at which a number of the front area divisional or corps consultants took part, and at these meetings general rules regarding the surgical care and operative treatment of the various types of battle casualties were freely discussed and adopted, and instructions issued to all consultants to be transmitted to the heads of the surgical teams. These instructions in general conformed with the suggestions issued by the Inter-Allied Surgical Conference, modified to some extent by the experience of our own men. While few of our operating surgeons heading surgical teams had had any experience in the treatment of battle casualties, they were nearly all men of experience, with adequate surgical training, and in not a few instances had had opportunities to observe the best type of military surgical procedure in some of the best French, English, and Belgian hospitals, as well as in our own Evacuation Hospitals Nos. 1 and 2, which were organized early, in quiet sectors, and in which some of our most experienced men were operating and giving instruction in the technic of modern military surgery. This and the fact that nearly all of our consultants in the front area had had previous experience in the British, French, or Belgian armies, made it possible for our advanced hospitals to render such excellent service during the periods of great activity.

While I would not have you believe that this advanced service in any way approached perfection, I think I can truthfully say that, taken as a whole, it was better than I had previously observed in any sector of the same size during a period of active military operations. When failure or disaster occurred, it was not the result of lack of skillful operative measures, but was rather due to overcrowding, delayed transportation and absence of forethought in providing adequate hospital accommodations, teams, nurses, and supplies. In other words, it was due to administrative rather than professional errors.

From this brief statement regarding the general plan of dual control, I feel that you will all agree that it represented a wise and honest attempt on the part of our Surgeon General to improve the quality of the service rendered to our wounded men. That it was not more satisfactory in its operation was due to a number of circumstances.

In the first place the plan should have been carefully considered and its organization thoroughly effected before we entered the war.

Specific regulations should have been adopted defining the duties of the administrative and professional chiefs, so that there should be no conflict of authority.

Copies of these regulations should have been sent to all commanding officers and to chief divisional, corps, and army surgeons, well in advance of assigning consultants to duty.

The official orders to consultants should have been uniform, explicit, and delivered at the time of appointment.

Had this been done, the status of the consultant would have been established. As it was, the arrival of the consultant at divisional headquarters was often the first intimation the chief divisional surgeon had that such a position had been created; and if, as frequently happened, the consultant's orders were not explicit, his presence was resented and looked upon as an attempt to destroy the prestige and undermine the authority of the divisional chief. In a few instances this resulted in open hostility and complete lack of coöperation, rendering the consultant's position extremely trying, and greatly interfering with his usefulness.

Lack of uniformity or great delay in issuing orders was a frequent source of misunderstanding. On more than one occasion I was sent to various parts of the line without any written orders. At other times my orders would read, " Will proceed to this or that headquarters and report to the divisional or corps surgeon." On other occasions my orders would be explicit and state, " Will proceed to Division ———, will supervise and direct the surgical work in all divisional hospitals, and all evacuation hospitals assigned to or situated in that sector; operate himself when deemed advisable; and in general carry out the orders of the Chief Surgeon, A. E. F., and chief consultant in surgery," thus clearly indicating that in professional authority he was responsible only to the chief consultant or the chief surgeon of the expeditionary force.

When we consider that the plan was an entirely new one, was not mentioned in the manual, was hastily considered in Washington, and transmitted to the A. E. F. without definite instructions, that no definite and uniform rules were established for its operation, that orders were not uniform, were frequently vague, and often greatly delayed, and that the line officers were generally left in complete ignorance of the plan and the status and authority of the consultants; it is a marvel that it succeeded as well as it did. In my opinion, its limited success was due to the vision and broad-minded attitude of General Ireland and his able assistants at the Chaumont Headquarters, to the honest efforts of the consultants themselves, and the hearty and intelligent coöperation of the majority of the regular officers.

I am thoroughly convinced that had the war lasted another six months, and had General Ireland's wise policy been continued in the A. E. F., after his promotion to the position of surgeon general, all obstacles would have been overcome, and the American system of professional control would have been declared an unqualified success.

In these few remarks I have attempted to answer briefly the two questions propounded in the opening paragraphs of this part of my address, but there is now another and more important question to be considered, and that is, what in the light of our past experience can be done now to insure better treatment for our wounded men in the event of another war, or to provide better care of our mobilized men if laws should be enacted authorizing universal military training.

In answer to this question permit me to say that, in my opinion, we can not do better than to adopt in principle the plan of dual control proposed by our surgeon general.

I sincerely believe, as stated above, that it is fundamentally sound, and the only plan that will insure to the wounded the highest degree of professional service.

That it was far from perfect in its operation during the late war, we will admit; but its imperfections and disadvantages were trivial in comparison to the advantages it presented, and easily could be remedied by more perfect organization. While doubtless it would be desirable to modify to some extent the regulations in force during the war, the plan should be essentially the same, and should embody the appointment of a chief consulting surgeon, a man of the broadest experience chosen from the civilian profession, possessing the highest qualities of surgical judgment and technical skill, who has had previous military experience, and who is also possessed of organizing ability. His headquarters should be in the office of the surgeon general, and to him all questions dealing with the actual surgical care of patients should be referred for his expert advice. That this chief consultant should have a number of deputies or assistant chief consultants, also men of conspicuous surgical ability and large experience. One of these to be assigned to headquarters of each army to coöperate with the administrative chief of the medical service. Under this deputy chief consultant there should be an adequate number of active consultants who could be assigned to corps or divisional areas in charge of the surgical work of the various hospital units, and who would be responsible through the army and chief consultant to the surgeon general for the carrying out of the most approved modern surgical methods in the treatment of the wounded men. This plan would obviously include a similar organization of the departments of internal medicine and sanitary service, with as many subdivisions of each as would be found to be necessary.

This, I beg you to bear in mind, is but the expression of my own personal view. I do not suggest it as a plan to be blindly followed or adopted without the fullest and freest discussion, in a conference composed of regular army officials and civilian practitioners who have had actual military experience; but I think that the time is now ripe for such a conference and interchange of views, and that now in time of peace some plan should be worked out to give to the American Army the best professional service which it is possible to organize, which will insure to the sick and injured soldier the same degree of professional skill that he could receive in the best organized and equipped civil hospital in the country.

While such a plan would be an emergency measure, and while the consulting staffs would be members of the reserve corps, and not on duty in peace time, it should be organized now, down to the last detail, so that in the event of our country facing another military crisis, it would not be necessary to devise ways and means to meet the emergency in haste, during a period of stress, excitement, anxiety, and feverish activity.

I do not feel that we as an association of civilian surgeons should apologize for considering this problem, or should hesitate to offer to the military authorities our suggestions on a subject which so deeply concerns us. If in time of war we are to bear such a large proportion of the burden of responsibility, we are certainly entitled to a voice in the making of plans and regulations under which we are to assume it. It is for this reason that I have brought this matter to your attention. I have been so overwhelmingly impressed with the importance of this subject, that it seems to me it would be a gross neglect of duty if I were to have chosen for this address another and perhaps more conventional topic.

My message comes from the heart of one who has been an eye witness to the monstrous and cruel toll in mortality and wrecked lives which war inflicts upon the flower of the youth and promising manhood of a nation; and I urge upon you, as members of the most distinguished group of surgeons in America, to be prepared, if the opportunity is offered, to co-operate with our Government officials in proposing some enlightened plan which will raise the standard of our military medical service to a plane never before reached in the world's history.

OBSERVATIONS ON EMPYEMA *

By Astley P. C. Ashhurst, M.D.

of Philadelphia, Pa.

surgeon to the episcopal hospital, associate in surgery in the university of pennsylvania

At the meeting of the American Surgical Association, twenty-six years ago, my father opened the discussion on empyema. He laid down the following six propositions for discussion:

1. No operation is justifiable
    (a) Unless the presence of pus is certain.
    (b) Unless thorough treatment by medicinal agents, blisters, etc., has failed.
    (c) Or unless the symptoms, dyspnœa, etc., are so urgent as to demand imme-
        diate relief.
2. The first operation should consist of simple aspiration with antiseptic precautions.
3. That when the fluid has partially reaccumulated, as it almost certainly will do if
    purulent, incision and drainage should be practiced
4. That drainage is best effected by making two openings, one at the lowest available
    point, and carrying a large drainage tube through the cavity from one opening
    to the other.
5. That drainage should be supplemented by washing out the cavity with mild anti-
    septic fluids. When the lung has expanded and discharge has nearly ceased, the
    tube should be shortened, the upper opening being allowed to heal and the tube
    being then gradually withdrawn through the lower opening.
6. That when the lung is so bound down by adhesions that it cannot expand, resection
    of one or more ribs should be practiced (Estlander's operation, so called), in order
    to allow collapse of the chest wall and to promote healing by bringing the costal
    and visceral layers of the pleura into contact. The more extensive operations of
    Schede and Tillmans, while probably justifiable in exceptional cases, are not to be
    recommended for general employment.

The mortality following operation for empyema at that time averaged from 20 to 30 per cent., and such it still remained in the hands of the average surgeon during the generation which has elapsed since 1894. It is true that in most of the fatal cases the operation is not to blame for the fatality, but merely fails to save life; and that death is due to the under-lying disease—empyema.

It is my object in this discussion to see, if possible, in what ways we have made an advance over the teachings and practices of a generation ago.

In the first place, I call attention to the *first proposition,* "That no operation is justifiable except under one of these conditions," *viz., (a)* that the presence of pus is certain, (*b*) that medical treatment has failed, (*c*) or that the symptoms are very urgent. Is any one at present ready to go beyond this, and adopt operation under any other circumstances? Do we not always receive our patients from the physician, whose treat-

---

* Read before the American Surgical Association, May 3, 1920.

ment has failed? True it is that the physician almost invariably has made one or more punctures of the chest, with or without success in locating pus, before he calls the surgeon into consultation; and that similarly even when pus has been found he is often loath to turn the patient over to the surgeon until he finds that the pus does reaccumulate; and even under the latter circumstances he may persist in the attempt to cure the patient without surgical assistance, by means of antiseptic injections into the pleural cavity. So eminent and able a surgeon as John B. Murphy, it will not be forgotten, advocated and practised injections of a 2 per cent. solution of formalin in glycerine for the cure of empyema; but no statistics of this treatment, showing its results, have ever been .

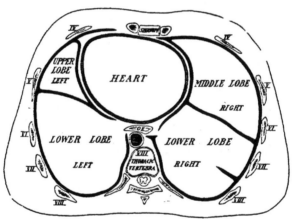

FIG. 1.—Cross-section of thorax at level of eighth thoracic vertebra. Pleural cavities outlined in black.

published, so far as I am aware. Nor has the treatment been generally accepted; though it must be acknowledged that in perhaps 2 or 3 per cent. of cases in which the first aspiration shows only sero-pus, not frank pus, it is possible that a cure may be secured either by repeated aspiration alone, or by aspiration followed by injection of formalin-glycerine solution, flavine, etc. So much, therefore, for the contingency which renders operation proper when medical treatment has failed.

Now if the symptoms are very urgent, that is, if there is extreme dyspnœa, cyanosis, bulging interspaces, etc., every one admits the propriety of aspirating the chest whether or not it is certain beforehand that pus, not serum, is the cause of the symptoms. Finally, if the presence of pus is certain, comparatively few surgeons deny the propriety of attempting to evacuate it.

But one may rejoin, how is it possible to be certain that pus is

13

present except by aspiration? Are the clinical history, the physical signs, the X-ray findings, and the symptoms always sufficient to render a diagnosis certain? To this I think we must reply in the negative; but I submit we must at the same time recognize that there are cases where the presence of pus is so nearly certain, even when it cannot be located by puncture, that it is not only justifiable but imperative for the surgeon to open the thorax, search for the encapsulated empyema, and effect its evacuation and drainage.

Some years ago, before the Section on General Medicine of the College of Physicians of Philadelphia, I presented[1] a plea for exploratory

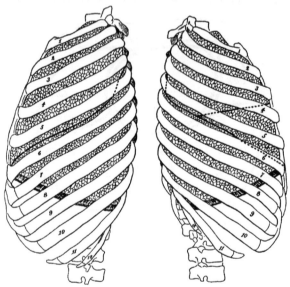

FIGS. 2 AND 3.—Interlobar fissures and their relation to the ribs.

thoracotomy in just such cases of encysted empyema as these—cases where repeated puncture failed to locate pus; where the physical signs were suggestive; and where the symptoms were urgent. Realizing that the patients would die of their empyema unless the pus were drained, it seemed better to me to run the risk of failure to relieve them by exploration, rather than to fold my surgical hands together in impotence, and reiterate to the physicians who called me as consultant, what I know they

---

[1] "Surgical Experiences with Encapsulated Empyema and Abscess of the Lung; a Plea for Exploratory Thoracotomy"; Medical and Surgical Reports of the Episcopal Hospital, Philadelphia, 1916, iv, 226.

had heard before in similar circumstances from other surgeons, a request
to the physician to find the pus, with the statement that then, and then
only, would the surgeon undertake to drain it! Some surgeons, I may add,
are even more conservative than this, and even though pus has been
found by puncture by the physician, refuse to undertake any operation
unless they themselves succeed in finding pus by a puncture made on the
operating table. To my mind, pus is pus, whether found by the physician
or surgeon; and I believe if it is found within the pleura the chances that
it will be absorbed and cause no further trouble are so very remote that

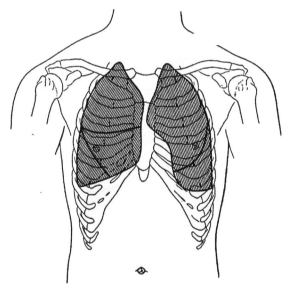

FIG. 4.—Fissures of the lungs viewed from the front.

unnecessary delay in resorting to operation is unjustifiable. In some
cases, of course, it is possible that an undrained interlobar empyema will
drain itself by rupture into a bronchus; but it has yet to be shown that
this event improves the patient's chance of recovery. Of two cases in my
series (Cases VIII and XIII) only one recovered.

In the report to which allusion has already been made, I recorded:

1. A case of empyema encapsulated between the upper and middle
lobes of right lung, discharging through the bronchus; punctures negative; empyema found on exploratory operation; death from exhaustion
and sepsis (Case VIII of the present series).

2. A case of empyema encysted between the upper and middle lobes of

15

the right lung. Numerous punctures negative; empyema not located at exploratory operation, but later burst into drainage tract; ultimate recovery (Case XVIII of the present series).

3. A case of empyema encysted between the left lung and the diaphragm. Punctures negative; empyema found on exploratory operation; recovery (Case XXIV).

4. A case of empyema encapsulated between the upper and middle lobes of the right lung. Puncture negative; empyema found on exploration; recovery (Case XXV).

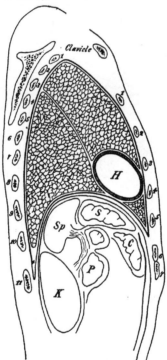

FIG. 5.—Sagittal section of thorax through middle of left clavicle.

5. A case of empyema encapsulated between the left lung and pericardium. Punctures negative; empyema not found at exploratory operation; death eight days later from continuing sepsis (Case XXVI).

Now I think it is worthy of note that in the last mentioned case, had an X-ray examination been available before operation, it is extremely

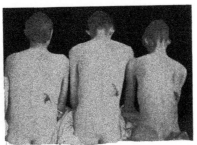

FIG. 6.—The site of election for draining an empyema; ninth, tenth or eleventh ribs posteriorly. The ages of the patients are given above, and the interval since operation below.

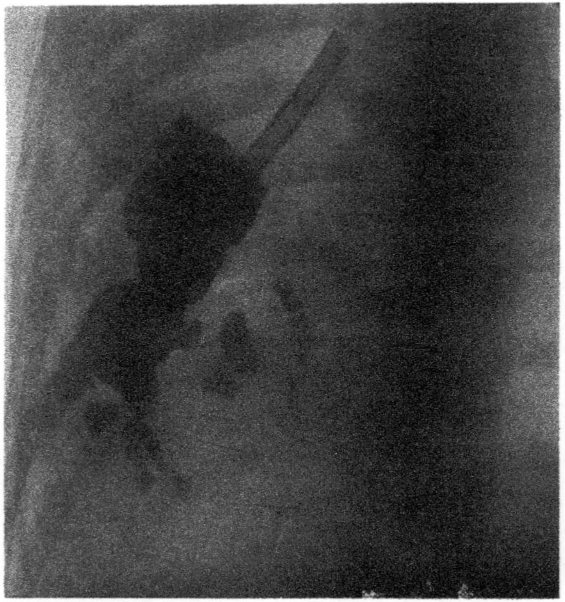

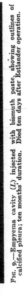

FIG. 8.—Rubber tube lost in empyema cavity for three months. Bismuth injections unavailing. Sinus healed permanently three weeks after removal of tube and Estlander operation.

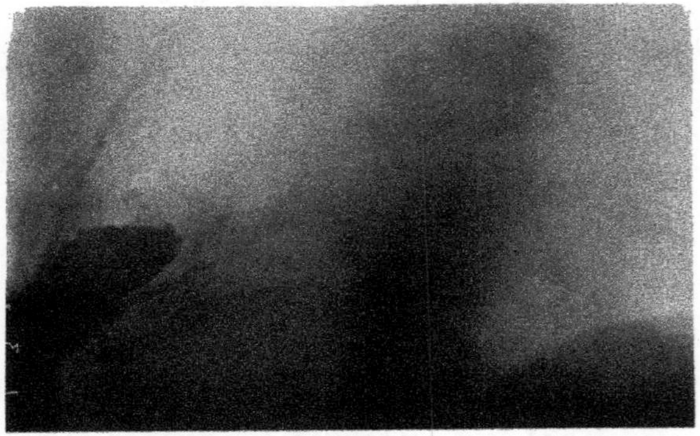

FIG. 9.—Empyema cavity (L) injected with bismuth paste, showing outlines of calcified pleura; ten months' duration. Died ten days after Estlander operation.

probable that the empyema might have been located when the chest was opened; since X-ray examination subsequent to operation (after necessary repairs to the X-ray plant) showed distinctly the outlines of the abscess cavity, and since autopsy showed that the interlobar dissection made at the time of the operation almost had reached the abscess.

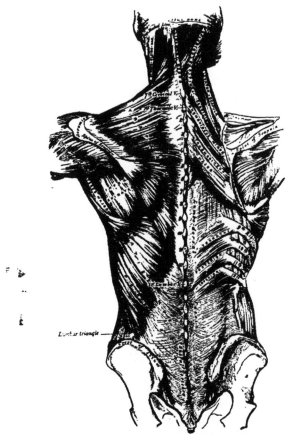

Fig. 7.—The ninth, tenth, eleventh and twelfth ribs exposed on the right side by removal of the latissimus dorsi. Note that the eighth and higher ribs are overlapped by the scapula. (From Gray's Anatomy.) Courtesy of Messrs Lea and Febinger.

So that, with regard to the *first and second propositions* laid down twenty-six years ago, I think we must understand them as permitting and encouraging at the present time, *exploratory thoracotomy*, when symp-

2   17

toms are urgent, medical measures have failed, repeated punctures are negative, and yet the presence of pus seems certain. Under these circumstances I have opened the thorax for exploration on six occasions (Cases VIII, XVIII, XXIV, XXV, XXVI, XXX), and except in the two cases just mentioned (Cases XVIII and XXVI) succeeded in finding and draining the empyema every time; and while only three of these patients recovered, I am sure more patients would have died if I had not been willing to explore the thorax; and if I had been allowed to do exploratory thoracotomy sooner in Case VIII, it is possible his life also might have been saved.

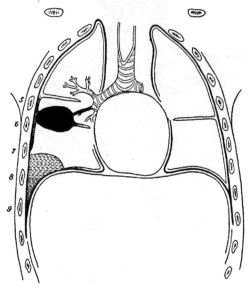

FIG. 10.—Case VIII. Interlobar empyema ruptured into a bronchus (pleural vomica). Note pleural effusion in costo-phrenic sinus.

I must, however, put on record the following case, in which I opened the thorax after negative puncture and found no pus, the patient subsequently dying from pneumonia.

Mildred C., three years. December 16, 1919: Admitted to the Episcopal Hospital, service of Doctor Carson, referred from Medical Dispensary by Dr. R. S. Hooker, with diagnosis of pneumonia. Has had a cold for three weeks with cough and expectoration; not confined to bed. Is fretful and unable to breathe properly at night. On admission: Temperature 101° F. (by rectum); anæmic, rachitic child, with Harrison's groove and rachitic rosary pronounced. Res-

18

pirations very short and rapid. Expansion of chest very asymmetrical. Apex beat of heart in midaxillary line about sixth interspace; marked pulsation over entire left chest. Rate rapid and sounds of good quality, no thrills or murmurs. Breath sounds rather harsh and many moist râles are heard over entire chest; no evidence of consolidation on percussion. Abdomen is distended, liver enlarged; no dullness in flanks. Extremities negative.

December 17th: Slight cough, no expectoration. Throat is clear. Not restless.

December 21st: Improving. Temperature 98° to 100° F.

December 30th: Temperature steady at 99° for last two days. Much improved. Sent home.

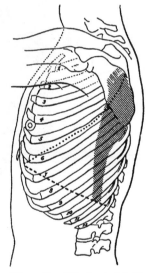

FIG. 11.—Case XV. Large, but distinctly encapsulated empyema.

January 6, 1920: Brought to Medical Dispensary and again seen by Doctor Hooker. Since being home the cough has continued and the child's general condition has been poor. Diagnosis of left-sided empyema was made by Doctor Hooker from dullness and diminished breath sounds. Sent into hospital and seen in Receiving Ward by Doctor Ashhurst.

Puncture of left chest over area of impaired resonance is negative. Under local anæsthesia 2 cm. of tenth left rib is resected, in midscapular line. Few adhesions between lung and diaphragm and between lobes of lung, but no pus found. Rubber tube inserted in

19

expectation that pus will later rupture into drainage tract. Time of operation twenty minutes.

January 7th: Condition poor. Lips cyanotic; respirations rapid and labored. No pus from tube. High-pitched bronchial breathing at left apex.

January 8th: Condition worse. Patient died at 5.15 P.M. Exploration of wound with finger after death could detect no adhesions between lobes and no evidence of empyema. Death from lobar pneumonia.

Technic of Exploratory Thoracotomy.—Let me here repeat what I understand by exploratory thoracotomy:

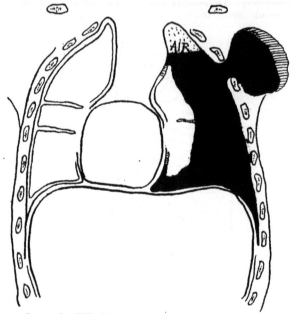

Fɪɢ. 12.—Case XVII. Pulsating empyema necessitatis=pyo-pneumo-thorax.

The patient is given, about thirty minutes before the commencement of the operation, a hypodermic injection of morphine (0.010 gm.) and atropin (0.00045 gm.); these doses may be larger in robust adults and smaller in children.

The patient is placed *prone* on the table, is made comfortable with pillows, and his head is turned away from the side on which operation is to be done. The arms are placed above the head. Care is necessary to see that the patient lies flat on his abdomen and thorax, and is *not turned on the healthy side,* as this will hinder respiration.

The proposed skin incision, over the eighth or ninth rib, back of the angle of the scapula, is then infiltrated with the local anæsthetic,[2] and the intercostal nerves above and below the rib to be resected are blocked with an injection of about 2 c.c. each of the anæsthetic fluid. These nerves are located by making the point of the needle impinge upon the rib above the nerve, and then prodding the rib with the point of the needle until the lower border of the rib is found, when, after pushing the needle about 0.5 cm. further into the intercostal structures the injection is made. This should be at a point 8 to 10 cm. from the spinous processes. When the anæsthetic has been properly injected the incision of the soft parts and the resection

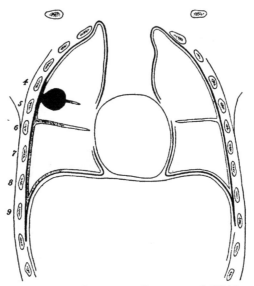

Fig. 13.—Case XVIII. Empyema encysted between upper and middle lobes of right lung; not found at operation. Later ruptured into drainage tract.

of the rib may be done absolutely painlessly. If, after the pleura has been opened and explored, more room is desired, it is perfectly easy to resect the rib next above or below by (1) infiltrating the skin parallel to the spinal column upward or downward from the posterior end of the primary incision; (2) blocking a third intercostal nerve as already indicated; (3) raising the soft parts in a flap; and (4) resecting (subperiosteally) as much as is required of the next rib. Usually it is not necessary

[2] I prefer novocain, 1:400; but when this was not available have used eucain, 1:100; to every 30 c.c. of the solution is added one drop of adrenalin chloride solution (1:10,000). This quantity (30 c.c.) usually is sufficient.

to divide the intercostal structures between the ribs resected, since when the ribs have been removed the intervening soft parts may be drawn aside by retractors. The length of rib to be resected depends on the size of the thorax and the extent of the intrathoracic exploration. As a rule, from 8 to 10 cm. is sufficient.

The pleura is opened between forceps, as the peritoneum is treated. Usually in cases of suspected empyema there is no collapse of the lung, which is adherent to the costal or diaphragmatic pleura. Even if the lung is not adherent it seldom collapses to less than half its bulk, when the

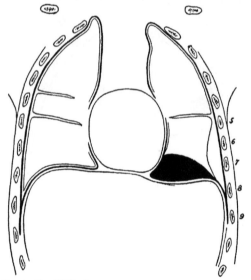

FIG. 14.—Case XXIV. Empyema encysted between left lung and diaphragm. Case XXXVI was quite similar, but on the right side.

patient is lying prone, and there is comparatively little respiratory disturbance. Wide opening of the pleura causes less dyspnœa than a small and valve-like opening which favors the development of a tension pneumothorax.

After opening the pleura and before conducting any exploration for an encysted empyema, the structures should be inspected. The lung may be so closely adherent to the diaphragm that it will be very difficult to recognize the line of junction. After ocular inspection, which may give a clue as to the first place to be searched for the abscess, the remainder of the pleural cavity should be walled off with hot moist gauze. Then with fingers, dissecting forceps, or even knife and scissors (according to the density of the adhesions), the lung should be gently released.

Usually it is well to clear the diaphragm first. If no pus is found here, the packs are rearranged so as to protect the lower part of the pleural cavity, and a search is begun in the fissures of the lung. If the lung is not readily accessible, its lower lobe is caught in two or three pairs of volsella forceps, and maintained within reach. A single pair of volsella forceps is more apt to tear out and so damage the lung than are two or three simultaneously applied. Fixing the lung in the wound steadies the mediastinum, enables the diaphragm to resume its piston action, and thus ventilates the other lung. The lung is absolutely insensitive to these

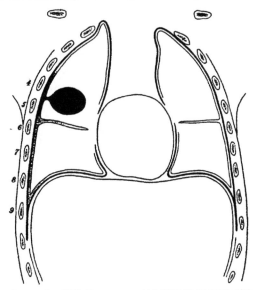

FIG. 15.—Case XXV. Empyema encapsulated between upper and middle lobes of right lung. Evacuated by thoracotomy. Compare Fig. 13 (Case XVIII).

manipulations. Often it is not necessary to fix the lung in this way, and the surgeon proceeds at once to separate the lobes from each other. Usually where the adhesions are densest, pus will be found.

When pus is finally located, and has been evacuated, a rubber tube (with a lumen at least of 1 cm.) surrounded with loose iodoform gauze is placed in the abscess cavity, the isolating packs are removed, and the wound is closed in layers, but not too tightly, around the drainage tract—the pleura and intercostal structures in one layer, then the skin.

The frequency of encapsulated empyema I am sure is not recognized. In my experience it has been present in no less than one-fourth of the cases. It is true, of course, that every empyema is, in a sense, encapsu-

23

lated; in other words, that it does not involve the entire pleural cavity. Pleuritis is in a way analogous to peritonitis: only so long as the effused fluid is sero-pus is it unconfined by adhesions. By the time frank pus has formed, in every case, whether in the peritoneum or the pleura, adhesions set certain limits, large or circumscribed, to the cavity in which pus is found. The only " free pus " that can exist in a body cavity such as the pleura or peritoneum is pus which is suddenly effused in overwhelming quantities into previously normal pleura or peritoneum, by the rupture of a localized abscess (appendicular or pelvic abscess, empyema of

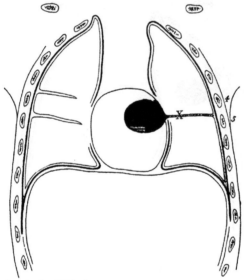

FIG. 16.—Case XXVI. Empyema encapsulated between fissure of left lung and pericardium. X indicates the point reached at operation.

the gall-bladder, abscess of the liver or spleen, encysted empyema, etc.). But what I understand by encapsulated empyema is either one which comes into contact with the costal pleura at no point (Cases XVIII, XXIV, XXV, XXVI, XXVII, XXXVI) or over so small an area that it is difficult, if not impossible, to locate pus until after the thorax has been opened (Cases VII, VIII, XXVIII, XXIX, XXXV), or until an empyema necessitatis has formed. It should be recognized also that there may be more than one distinctly encapsulated empyema in the same patient (Cases XVI, XXIX, XXXV); and that occasionally an hour-glass empyema may exist, the channel of communication being large (as in Cases XXXVII and XLIII), or so small that drainage of one loculus is ineffective in producing cure of the other (as in Case XXXVIII). It is on account of the occurrence of cases such as these that 1 urge that, if the condition of the patient permits, exploration should be adequate to ensure that no such encapsulated foci are overlooked. (I am not prepared, however, to adopt Lilienthal's "Major thoracotomy" under general anæsthesia, so long as I continue to find a medium thoracotomy under local anæsthesia satisfactory.) In all cases with massive empyema, of course,

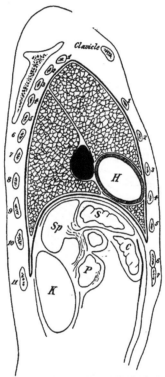

FIG. 17.—Case XXVI. Diagram of sagittal section through middle of left clavicle, indicating site at which pus was found at autopsy.

removal of a large amount of the pus by aspiration should precede by one or two days the formal operation of thoracotomy; and in no case where the fluid can be removed by aspiration need drainage by thoracotomy be regarded as an emergency operation (*third proposition*).

Let me revert now to the *fourth proposition* I have quoted at the beginning of this discussion, namely, " that drainage is best effected by making two openings, one at the lowest available point, and carrying a

large drainage tube through the cavity from one opening to the other."
It seems to me that the doctrine of through-and-through drainage merely
follows as a corollary in cases where the primary opening has been made
too high; in other words, that if the primary opening is made at the site
of election, which I regard as the ninth or tenth (occasionally the eleventh
or twelfth) ribs near their angles (Figs. 6 and 7) ; it is unnecessary to make
a counter-opening, as one is already at the "lowest available point." I repeat, that in cases of exploratory thoracotomy as well as in cases of
massive empyema, I practise and recommend that the opening should

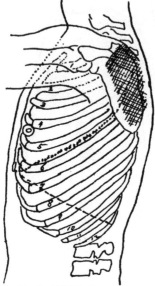

Fig. 19.—Case XXVIII. Empyema encapsulated over posterior end of left interlobar
fissure.

be made at the site mentioned, even if the needle has shown pus in the
sixth or seventh interspace. It is so nearly invariably the rule that the
empyema cavity extends down to the diaphragm, and it is so easy after
opening the pleura low down to drain an empyema which may extend
already to within a few centimetres of the opening, by breaking through
its limiting adhesions at their most dependent portion; and a higher opening unless supplemented by a counter-opening at the lowest available
point gives rise to so very prolonged a convalescence, that I believe there
are exceedingly few cases in which it is desirable to be limited in selecting
the site for drainage by the location at which pus was found on puncture.
Only once since I adopted this rule have I encountered an empyema

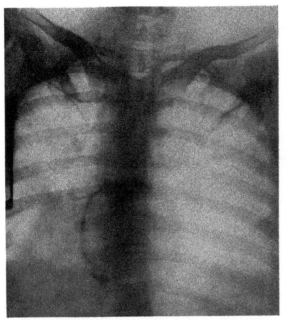

Fig. 18.—Case XXVI. Encysted empyema three days after operation, at which no pus was found. Note distinct outlines of abscess cavity overlying shadows of sixth, seventh and eighth thoracic vertebræ, mostly to left of midline.

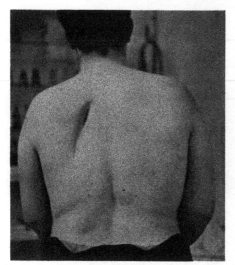
FIG. 20.—Case XXVIII. Resection of fourth and fifth ribs. Three years and a half after operation.

situated so very high and with the lower portion of the thorax so certainly intact, as to induce me to make a higher opening: in this patient (Case XXVIII) the empyema appears to have formed between the lobes of the left lung and to have finally come into contact with the parietal pleura between the vertebral column and the scapula at the level of the spine of the latter bone; and yet the drainage tract at this site, though it was nearly at the lowest level of the empyema cavity, nevertheless required over four months for healing.

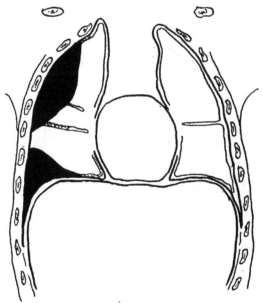

Fig. 21.—Case XXXV. Two distinct encapsulated empyemata.

Resection of a rib I regard as important in all cases. Intercostal incision alone does not afford adequate drainage, and frequently secondary operations are required. I have employed it only once (Case IV) in a baby six months old; a month later it was necessary to resect a rib to improve the drainage, but two months after the first operation the patient died with unhealed sinus, probably from sepsis arising in the inefficiently drained pleura. In another case which came later under my care (Case XIII), intercostal incision was employed by another surgeon, but this healed upon an infected cavity, and the empyema not being drained externally ruptured into a bronchus; finally, the original operative sinus opened again, and eventually I had to resect the eighth and ninth ribs;

definitive healing then occurred in eight weeks. I have never seen necrosis of the rib ends, and cannot believe the possibility of such an occurrence is to be regarded as contra-indicating rib resection.

Next we come to the *fifth proposition,* "that drainage should be supplemented by washing out the cavity with mild antiseptic fluids. When the lung has expanded and discharge has nearly ceased the tube should be shortened . . . and gradually withdrawn." With the very gradual shortening and withdrawal of the tube I am in entire accord, but I do not see that anything is gained by irrigations in the ordinary

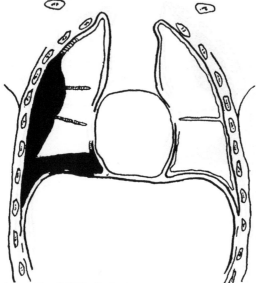

FIG. 22.—Case XXXVII. Massive hour-glass empyema. Case XLIII was quite similar.

case of empyema. I suspect that the main function they served in my father's day was to keep the lumen of the through-and-through drainage tube open, and that the fluid injected at one end of the tube almost immediately escaped by the other end, without making a very extensive journey into the empyema cavity. And I am quite sure that in some cases injudicious irrigations are productive of harm. It is quite evident, I believe, that death in two of my patients (Cases XXX and XXXI) some weeks after they passed from under my care, is directly attributable to sepsis arising in the wound in the thoracic wall, not in the empyema cavity, and that this sepsis was produced by irrigation, and probably aided in Case XXXI by too tight closure of the wound of the second operation.

That irrigations with Dakin's hypochlorite solution, by the Carrel technic, are of no value in any cases, I am not prepared to admit. But I am quite thoroughly convinced that in the vast majority of cases of empyema they are quite unnecessary, and that except in cases of very long standing, with much thickened pleura and non-expansile lung, healing will occur quite as promptly, as pleasantly, and as definitively by means of large and dependent drainage. I do not think it can be denied that in many patients of the class of cases just mentioned the irrigations with

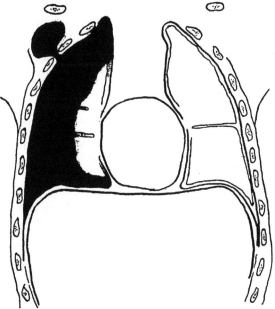

FIG. 23.—Case XXXVIII. Massive empyema necessitatis, pointing beneath right pectoral muscles. With metastatic abscess between left scapula and chest wall.

Dakin's solution will eat away the inflammatory lymph deposited on the visceral pleura and that the lung will thereafter expand sooner and more completely than if such irrigations had not been employed. Nor can it be denied that it is possible to sterilize an empyema cavity by this means, at least temporarily, and then to permit the thoracic wound to close upon the sterile pneumothorax; but I also know that the same event may take place simply as the result of efficient drainage without any irrigations, at any time (Cases XIV and XXXV). Speaking for myself, I may say that I have never employed the Carrel-Dakin treatment for empyema, and that I should be surprised to encounter a recent case in which I thought it indicated.

The *sixth proposition,* which has to do with unhealed empyema cavities, I am sure must undergo great modification in view of advances in surgery since it was formulated. I am convinced that unhealed empyema is infrequent compared to its incidence a generation ago, largely due to the earlier recognition and more efficient treatment of the acute cases. Indeed, it is probably true that if any surgeon conscientiously follows up the treatment the occurrence of an unhealed case will be extremely rare. One patient (Case VI) on whom I operated in 1909 is known to have had his sinus still unhealed nine months after operation; but among the remainder of my patients the longest period of healing was seven months, and in not one of those who remained under my care was a second operation required. One patient (Case XXXI) who passed from my care two weeks after the operation, and from whom the tube was removed too early, was reoperated on later for an accumulation of pus and eventually died of sepsis arising in the thoracic wound of the second operation. Another patient (Case XXXV) who was tuberculous and whose thoracic wound healed within seven weeks upon a pneumothorax, five months later had a little discharge from the sinus which healed again in three weeks; twenty-two months after my operation another empyema developed and was drained; seven months after this second operation the patient moved to Colorado, and since that time (September, 1919) he has had one slight reaccumulation which was opened and healed at the end of six weeks. He writes (March, 1920) that he is now apparently in perfect health.

I should like to say a good word for bismuth injections in the treatment of unhealed sinuses, as advocated by Ochsner. In one patient (Case XXXVI) (the only one in whom I began to despair of seeing the sinus close spontaneously) and in whom removal of the tube was followed on several occasions by rise of temperature, I had just about determined on reopening the wound (twelve weeks after operation) and injected it with 10 per cent. bismuth paste to ascertain the outlines of the cavity by skiagraphy: the next day the sinus was found healed, with the paste retained, and the wound remained healed when the patient was last seen five months later.

Unhealed empyema must be rare in Philadelphia, as I have had occasion to operate on not more than two patients.

In the *first patient,* John K., sixteen years of age, operation had been done by another surgeon April 19, 1911, for a left-sided empyema five weeks after the onset of pneumonia. On June 11th the tube was not found when the wound was dressed, and on June 17th the patient was discharged with unhealed sinus. Soon after this he came under my care in the Episcopal Hospital, and was treated with bismuth injections. The sinus sometimes would close for a few days but always reopened. Finally, an X-ray picture was taken and showed the tube lying in the pleural cavity (Fig. 8).

September 15, 1911 (three months after the first operation) : Under ether, I resected about 6 cm. each of the seventh, eighth, and ninth ribs (the eighth, which had been excised at the former operation, was of cartilaginous consistency). The drainage tube and large masses of bismuth paste were removed, and a fair amount of pus was evacuated. All the lymph adherent to the visceral pleura that could be detached was removed, all the adhesions of the lung to the parietal pleura were broken through, and the cavity thoroughly wiped with iodoform gauze. One long and wide strip of iodoform gauze was left in for drainage.

In two weeks the wound was practically closed, and was firmly healed by October 7, 1911, twenty-two days after operation.

In the *second patient*, James K., fifty-one years of age, there was a history of some severe injury to the chest twenty-eight years previously. He had had many attacks of " pleurisy " following occasioual attacks of rheumatism.

May 24, 1913: Admitted to the Episcopal Hospital, Doctor Mutschler's service. About fifteen months previously he had developed a heavy cough followed by swelling in left thorax, diagnosed by family physician as tumor. The family physician incised this swelling and quite a large quantity of pus was removed. The sinus healed up after a long time. There had been no discharge for the past four or five months. About ten days ago he began coughing again and the sinus opened and discharged pus. Has been having night sweats. Does not spit any blood.

On admission : Sinus in left thorax between sixth and seventh ribs, in nipple line, from which a small amount of pus is oozing. Two scars of healed sinuses. Temperature 101°. Large-framed man, thorax well developed, expansion limited on left which is dull front and back below fourth rib, with distant breath sounds and harsh crepitant râles.

May 26, 1913: X-ray 6442—heart displaced to right by pus in left pleura up to sixth rib.

May 27th: Operation by Doctor Mutschler (ether) : Sixth left rib excised in anterior axillary line and much pus discharged (pneumococci).

May 30th: Temperature normal.

June 28th: Still free discharge. Temperature hectic since last note. 98°-101°. X-ray 6640—heart still to right, some collapse of left lung.

July 25th: Still same amount of discharge. Temperature 98°-100°.

August 1st: Service taken over by Doctor Ashhurst. The patient walks about and does not complain of anything; general condition about same. Dressings always saturated over night. Coughs a little.

August 8th: X-ray 7213 (bismuth) shows large cavity extending from eleventh rib to upper thorax (Fig. 9).

August 23d: Discharge no less. Temperature 98°-100°.

31

August 29th: Operation—ether (Ashhurst). Patient prone. Incision 12 cm. long made over sinus of previous operation (over sixth left rib in anterior axillary line), and about 10 cm. each of the sixth, seventh, eighth, and ninth ribs resected, from their angles forward. This uncovered very dense parietal pleura, which was found to be lined by a calcareous deposit about 5 mm. thick, as were also the exposed surfaces of the lung and diaphragm. The rigid walled cavity extended as high as the finger could reach through the wound. The calcareous lining was peeled off the parietal pleura, the diaphragm, and the lung, except at the apex of the cavity where a few plates had to be left, as it was impossible to remove them without tearing the lung. The lung was found still to be bound down by dense pleura, beneath the calcareous deposit, but the condition of the patient did not warrant continuing the operation by decortication or discission of the pleura. The lung moved a little more in respiration than before the calcareous plates were removed, but it was evident that only by collapse of the soft parts could the cavity be obliterated; and though complete obliteration was not hoped for, it was thought the marked reduction in size of the cavity would considerably reduce the discharge and promote the patient's comfort. Drainage was provided by iodoform gauze and a large rubber tube. The wound was closed in layers about the drainage.

August 31st: Dressed, dressings soiled but not saturated, as before operation. No calcareous matter could be felt by finger introduced through wound.

September 6th: Temperature fell after last dressing to normal and has not varied more than one-half degree since. To-day rose to 100°. Seems irrational, no cough.

September 7th: Restless, on gradual decline. Pulse weak, rapid (150). Temperature 101°. Respiration 34.

September 8th: Died 6 A.M. Temperature having risen rapidly to 104°. No post-mortem, but by opening wound calcareous matter found only around apex of cavity. Lung and diaphragm covered with gray lymph, phlegmonous in type.

It is a question in my mind whether in this latter patient the condition of his pleura did not date from his original injury twenty-eight years previously. Certainly it would be very unusual for such dense calcareous deposits to have occurred between the time of the two operations done in the Episcopal Hospital only three months apart; but the presence of a hemorrhagic pleural effusion many years ago, which remained unabsorbed, will account for the patient's repeated attacks of pleurisy as well as for the densely calcareous deposit. In this connection the appearance of the X-ray in Case XXVI (Fig. 17) is suggestive that here also a cavity containing sterile fluid may have persisted for over four years, this patient having been under treatment in another hospital for supposed empyema, which could not be located, that length of time before she came under my care with recurrence of similar symptoms.

CONCLUSIONS

From this discussion it seems to me that the propositions laid down twenty-six years ago must be modified in the following particulars:

1. Cases of pleural effusion suspected of being purulent should be punctured (with hollow needle attached to air-tight syringe); and if the effusion is massive most of it should be removed by aspiration one or two days before thoracotomy is undertaken.

2. If the fluid found on puncture is serous, or sero-purulent, thoracotomy usually may be postponed, until frank pus has formed, as this delay will permit the formation of firmer adhesions and thus prevent complete collapse of the lung when the empyema is opened. Cures of such sero-purulent effusions, however, have so rarely occurred without final resort to thoracotomy that attempts to cure them by injection of antiseptic fluids into the unopened pleura are usually detrimental to the patient.

3. If in a case of suspected empyema the symptoms are urgent, but pus cannot be found by puncture, exploratory thoracotomy should be undertaken in an effort to locate and drain the pus.

4. The operation of thoracotomy for empyema should provide free and dependent drainage, secured by resection of a rib, usually the ninth, tenth, or eleventh, in front of its angle. This operation may be done with perfect satisfaction to both patient and surgeon *under local anæsthesia,* and in most cases this is preferable to a general anæsthetic. (I have used local anæsthesia with satisfaction in 27 patients, including one baby sixteen months of age; and have employed it in every one of my last 20 patients, some of them requiring rather extensive intrathoracic manipulations. It is interesting and perhaps significant to note that only two patients in the entire series (Cases III and XI) developed pneumonia of the opposite lung after operation, and that both these patients had taken ether.)

5. Post-operative irrigations are unnecessary, unless after several months the lung shows no tendency to expand; when the use of Dakin's fluid may prove beneficial. In selected cases (those with small cavity) injections of bismuth paste may procure closure of the sinus.

6. If the cavity cannot be made to heal by these means, the surgeon should do a major thoracotomy, combined with decortication of the lung and discission of the pleura, and in some cases resection of a number of ribs to permit the chest wall to collapse in part and meet the expanding lung.

In closing, I may be permitted to give a summary of my own cases, few in number, perhaps, but studied with such attention as was possible. Among 42 patients there have been 9 deaths, a general mortality of 20.9 per cent. Among the first 9 of these patients there were 5 deaths, three of which were in babies less than a year of age. But if there are included only the last 34 patients operated on since adopting the system of wide and de-

3   33

pendent drainage,[*] there were in this number only 4 deaths, a mortality of less than 12 per cent. Moreover, of these four fatal cases:

(a) In the first (Case XXII) the child also had extensive gangrenous stomatitis (noma) and died from this.

(b) In the second (Case XXVI) the empyema (which was encapsulated against the pericardium) was not found at operation, and the patient died eight days after operation unrelieved.

(c, d) In the third and fourth cases (Cases XXX and XXXI) death occurred some weeks after the patients passed from my care; and as the result not of their empyema, but from sepsis arising in the thoracic wound and brought on by irrigations.

From which facts I conclude that the mortality of empyema, if promptly and efficiently treated, need not exceed 10 per cent.

The *average time required for firm healing of the thoracic wound,* in 24 cases in which this is known, was just over nine weeks, the shortest being three and the longest thirty weeks. In those patients (18 in number) who remained under my personal supervision, the average time until firm healing was just over seven weeks, the shortest time being three and the longest twelve weeks.

In 5 cases (Cases XXX, XXXI, XXXVI, XXXIX and XL) (2 of these patients (Cases XXXVI and XXXIX) being still under my personal care at the time) there was more or less interruption to the progress of wound healing by pocketing of pus, due to too early withdrawal of drainage; and in 2 of my early cases (Cases IV and V) where dependent drainage was not secured at the first operation, secondary operation was required some time after they passed from my care. With the exception of Case V, a patient who passed from under my care after the operation, there were no cases unhealed at last note, and in none had an Estlander or similar operation been required to secure closure of the empyema cavity.

Certain cases in the subjoined list deserve more than passing attention.

Cases of encapsulated empyema, with limited contact with parietal pleura (Cases VII, VIII, IX, XV, XVI, XXI, XXVIII).

Cases of encapsulated empyema, without any contact with parietal pleura (Cases XVIII, XXIV, XXV, XXVI, XXVII, XXXVI).

Cases of two distinctly encapsulated empyemata within same pleural cavity (Cases XVI, XXIX, XXXV).

Cases of hour-glass empyema (Cases XXXVII, XXXVIII).

Cases of empyema necessitatis, Cases VI, XVII (pulsating), XXI, XXXVIII.

Cases of empyema as part of a general septicæmia, Cases XIV (peritonitis and abscess), XXIV (streptococci in blood), XXXIII (jaundiced), XXXIV (pericarditis, endocarditis), XXXVIII (metastatic abscess and pyæmia).

[*] It is proper that I should give due credit to T. Turner Thomas, whose studies in 1913 turned my attention particularly toward the value of dependent drainage.

OBSERVATIONS ON EMPYEMA

Cases of encapsulated empyema rupturing through a bronchus, Cases VIII, XIII.

Cases of tuberculous empyema, Cases XII, XVII, XXXV.

Case in which drainage tube fell into empyema cavity, Case XVI.

Case complicated by noma (gangrenous stomatitis), Case XXII.

Case complicated by independent pleural effusion on same side, Case XXI.

The subjoined table gives the salient features in all the cases encountered, and, in accordance with the motto "*Ars medica tota est in observationibus*" abstracts of the case histories are appended.

CASE REPORTS

CASE I.—Empyema, right. Recovery. John C., aged five years.

September 22, 1906, admitted to the Children's Hospital, Dr. Hutchinson's service. Ill for six weeks with pneumonia at Atlantic City; then in Children's Hospital (Dr. Charles H. Weber's service) for the last three weeks. Empyema suspected, but Doctor Weber had four dry taps. Last night pus was found (diagnosed as interlobar in position by Doctor Weber).

September 22, 1906: Operation (Doctor Ashhurst)—ether. Excised 2.5 cm. right eighth rib in mid-axillary line. Pleura thickened (50 to 60 mm.); incised, and incision dilated with hæmostat. Pus oozed out with little force, then as child began to cry on coming out of ether (ammonia substituted for ether after opening pleura), pus was ejected with much force, creamy, pale yellow, sour. Pus appeared to extend from diaphragm up, not interlobar (only). Before operation respirations were 60, fell to 40 immediately after and to 22–24 after two hours. Pus gave a pure culture of pneumococci.

November 8, 1906: Tube out.

July 27, 1907: Seen at Country Branch of Children's Hospital, in excellent health; wound closed.

CASE II.—Empyema, left. Died, one week (enteritis). Joseph S., five months.

July 26, 1907: Admitted to the Children's Hospital, Dr. E. B. Hodge's service. Had been ill three weeks with pneumonia. Doctor Hand aspirated (July 25, 1907) about 50 c.c. of pus (diplococcus, biscuit-shaped).

July 26, 1907: Operation (Doctor Ashhurst)—ether. Resected 2.5 cm. of eighth left rib, about 100 c.c. thick inodorous pus. Time—six minutes. Child very ill. Temperature normal after operation and did well for four or five days, then got severe enteritis, with high fever. Lungs clear, wound clean.

August 2, 1907: Died, one week after operation, from enteritis.

CASE III.—Empyema, left. Died, two weeks (pneumonia of other lung). Edward W., aged eleven and a half months.

July 25, 1908: Admitted to the Children's Hospital, Dr. E. B. Hodge's service. Has been in hospital about two weeks with pneumonia; temperature came to normal, but rose again on July 22d and July 23d. Doctor Hand aspirated July 24th and got 25 c.c. pus.

Examination.—No dyspnœa lying down; lessened expansion, dulness, absence of breath sounds at left base. Mucous râles at apex.

July 25, 1908: Operation (Doctor Ashhurst)—ether. Excised 2 cm. rib (about eighth) below angle of scapula, patient on back. About 100 c.c. thick creamy pus, slight odor (staphylococci and few diplococci). Rubber tube.

July 28, 1908: Since operation almost no discharge of pus.

July 29, 1908: Temperature up, cyanosis, dull over lower part upper lobe.

July 30, 1908: Doctor Hand suggested collection of pus.

July 31, 1908: Sinus explored with finger, only firm adhesions found, lung expands well. No pus by needle inserted in the dull area. Bronchial breathing above empyema cavity.

August 4, 1908: Pneumonia in right lung discovered.

August 8, 1908: Died of pneumonia of right lung.

CASE IV.—Empyema, left. Died, two months (sepsis from pleura?). Katharine P., aged six months.

July 22, 1909: Admitted to the Children's Hospital, Dr. E. B. Hodge's service. Pneumonia four weeks ago. Aspirated (Doctor Ashhurst) and 100 c.c. pus (pneumococci) evacuated. Did well until July 24, when dyspnœa returned.

July 24, 1909: Operation (Doctor Ashhurst)—ether. Intercostal (seventh to eighth?) incision, left; about 500 c.c. of pus evacuated, and tube inserted.

July 27, 1909: Doing well.

August 2, 1909: Has had rapid respiration, 72–84; pulse, 160–170. Temperature, 101° to 102° for last few days. Wound doing well. Eats well; bowels normal.

August 4, 1909: After taking ammonium carbonate, syrup of senega, respirations are only 60–70. Pulse 140–150. Temperature 99°. Still miserable.

August 14, 1909: Much improved.

August 19, 1909: No more improvement.

Later in August, Doctor Hodge resected a rib to secure better drainage. In September the child was taken home, taking a milk mixture. Death towards the end of September, two months after operation, perhaps from sepsis from the pleura, the wound not having healed.

CASE V.—Empyema, left. Recovery. Joseph T., aged six years.

July 24, 1909: Admitted to the Children's Hospital, Dr. E. B. Hodge's service. Had pneumonia five weeks ago. Aspirated ten days ago at home, one litre of pus obtained. On admission, the apex beat of heart is to right of sternum. Marked orthopnœa. After aspiration of 100 c.c. no more pus would run.

Operation (Doctor Ashhurst)—ether; resection of 2 cm. of eighth rib in left anterior axillary line, and evacuation of about a litre of pus and flocculent lymph.

July 27, 1909: Pulse still weak, no fever. Lying down for first time since operation. Bloody pus discharging.

July 29, 1909: Tube removed, only blood-stained serum discharged and smaller tube replaced.

August 3, 1909: Tube left out; nothing in sinus. Slight discharge.

September, 1909: Doctor Hodge resected another rib, for better drainage. Doing well in end of month.

March 9, 1910: Readmitted and record shows only use of bismuth paste. Discharged April 23, 1910. "Discharge disappearing rapidly." Cannot be traced.

CASE VI.—Empyema, left. Recovery. Elias R., aged three years.

July 29, 1909: Admitted to the Children's Hospital, Dr. E. B. Hodge's service. Pneumonia five weeks ago. Developed deformity of chest which family physician called "post-pneumonic pigeon-breast." On admission had empyema necessitatis (left), apex beat in second interspace right. Whole left thorax tense, with fluid between ribs and skin and muscles. Aspirated by resident, large quantity of creamy pus.

July 29, 1909: Operation (Doctor Ashhurst)—ether. Resected 2 cm. of sixth or seventh rib in anterior axillary line and evacuated over a pint or less creamy pus.

July 30, 1909: Sitting up and playing around bed.

August 4, 1909: Uneventful recovery after this date.

CASE VII.—Empyema, left. Recovery. Sam S., aged five years.

July 22, 1909: Admitted to the Children's Hospital, Doctor Hand's service. Illness began July 18th with chill and fever. Has had temperature of 103° since. Pneumonia in left lung. Empyema suspected yesterday, but two punctures by Doctor Hand drew no pus. Transferred to Doctor Hodge's service July 29th.

July 29, 1909: Doctor Ashhurst punctured twice in anterior axillary line, left, where auscultation and percussion indicated pus, but found nothing. Then punctured in seventh interspace in posterior axillary line, where was most tenderness and very slight œdema, but no auscultatory signs, and drew very foul pus from considerable depth. Expectoration slight but very foul, like pulmonary abscess (mixed growth).

Operation.—Ether. Resected 3 cm. of eighth left rib in posterior axillary line, without injuring pleura, suspected pulmonary abscess, but on incising pleura quantity of thin turbid pus (colon smell) squirted; later some coagula of lymph. Drainage tube.

July 30, 1909: Temperature normal, little discharge.

August 5, 1909: Temperature normal ever since operation.

August 25, 1909: Temperature up for one or two days, two weeks ago, and again yesterday and to-day. Uneventful recovery therafter.

CASE VIII.—Empyema, right, discharging through bronchus. Died third day. Pleural vomica. Sepsis. William L., aged fifty-two years.

July 26, 1912: Admitted to the Episcopal Hospital; under Dr. E. J. Morris's care until August 1, 1912, then on Doctor Robertson's service.

Family History.—Father, grandmother and brother died of tuberculosis.

Past History.—Pertussis as child. Tobacco and beer to excess.

Present Illness.—Began ten days ago as sudden sharp pain in right side, after lying on that side on grass for an evening. Pain gradually subsided after few days. Then got short of breath. Family physician gave medicine without effect. Walked to dispensary and sent to ward.

Examination on Admission.—Large, full-blooded, dyspnœic; constant cough and expectoration. Breath very fœtid. Right chest: flat below fourth rib, with hyperresonance above. Left apex: impaired resonance. Râles and harsh breathing at right apex and below fourth rib. Absent breath sounds and fremitus. Expectorates 500 c.c. daily of very foul smelling pus. Temperature, 99°–100°.

July 27, 1912: Constant cough. Cannot sleep, cannot speak above a whisper. White blood count, 16,680. No tubercle bacilli found in sputum in five separate examinations; elastic tissue absent.

August 6, 1912: Seen by Doctor Eves for aphonia; examination negative except for acute laryngitis.

August 18, 1912: Growing weaker. Temperature ranges from 99° to 102° F.

September 3, 1912: Aspiration negative on right, below angle of scapula (Doctor Robertson). Still septic.

September 7, 1912: Tapped by Doctor Robertson (negative) below angle of right scapula. Oxygen introduced into pleura until dyspnœa was produced and entire area of dulness became tympanitic. Dyspnœa soon disappeared and patient became comfortable.

September 9, 1912: Dulness as before over right chest.

September 10, 1912: Oxygen again introduced by Doctor Robertson. Patient nearly died, was unconscious for fifteen minutes; pulse 150.

September 11, 1912: Improved, dyspnœa disappeared. Temperature 99°–103° F.

September 13, 1912: Transferred to Doctor Frazier's surgical service. Seen by Doctor Ashhurst, who thought it to be an encapsulated empyema rupturing through bronchus. Patient is very dyspnœic and coughs frequently until expectoration of very foul greenish material. Pulse fairly strong, 92–96. Respiration, 28–32. Temperature, 100°; no pain. Whole right chest is flat from middle of scapula down; breath sounds weak, many crackling râles. Breath sounds amphoric below angle of scapula for distance of two ribs. Repeated punctures have located no pus.

September 14, 1912: Operation (Doctor Ashhurst)—eucain 2 per cent. in intercostal nerves of eighth and ninth ribs, and by infiltration also. Incision in eighth interspace

37

posterior axillary line, patient lying on face. Excised 5 cm. of ninth rib and 6 cm. of eighth rib. Ligated both intercostals front and back. Patient complained of pain *in abdomen.* This exposed diaphragm. Bloody serum evacuated on opening pleural cavity; lung stripped easily from ribs except beneath scapula (sixth to eighth ribs, in front of angles). Here it was densely adherent. Packed remainder of pleural space. Lung densely adherent to dome of diaphragm and to posterior parietal pleura beneath scapula. Burrowed with finger among these adhesions beneath scapula, and ruptured into abscess, which discharged with a gush 30 c.c. or more of same pus as is expectorated. (Aromatic ammonia to stifle fœtid stench.) This cavity was beneath sixth and seventh ribs in posterior axillary line, about 7 by 5 cm.; though finger could not reach upper limits (Fig. 10). Inserted rubber tube (1.25 cm. in diameter) and iodoform gauze around tube. Time, one-half hour. Patient asked for his supper as soon as he was turned over on his back, and was given it on return to ward.

September 15, 1912: Very dyspnœic, pulse very rapid and weak. Tube to lung drains large amount of greenish pus. Dressed wound.

September 16, 1912. Died 4:30 P.M.

CASE IX.—Empyema (encysted), left. Died, six days (sepsis). Minnie Y., aged fifty-nine years.

December 10, 1912: Admitted to Episcopal Hospital, Doctor Piersol's service. Ill for four days, with pain in left chest. Examination showed pneumonia of left lower lobe.

December 15, 1912: Temperature fell by crisis (ninth day).

December 20, 1912: Empyema suspected—dulness persists, impaired fremitus. Very ill.

December 24, 1912: Temperature suddenly rose to 104.3°. More toxic. Tapped, thick greenish pus from left pleura, base of lung (culture, pneumococcus).

December 25, 1912: Transferred to Doctor Frazier's surgical service. Patient appears to be insane. Very emaciated and weak, bed-sore, etc.

Operation (Doctor Ashhurst).—Cocain, 2 per cent. Patient prone. Injected intercostal nerves at and below eleventh rib at angle. Then waited five minutes. Skin not anæsthetized yet, so infiltrated it (15 minims of 2 per cent. cocain). Same amount had been used for each of two nerves). Then entire operation (resection of one and a half inches of eleventh rib) was done absolutely painlessly. After removing rib, found pleura unruptured. Opened this (as peritoneum) with scalpel, and found lung lightly adherent, and showing no tendency to collapse. Packed pleural cavity off above with one strip of gauze, then burrowed in region of densest adhesions (just anterior to opening) and thick (semi-solid) pus welled up with each respiration. Inserted one-half inch rubber tube (about two and a half inches inside thorax), packed it around with iodoform gauze; withdrew isolating gauze; dressed wound, and turned her on her back.

December 27, 1912: Doing well. Temperature fell to normal after operation and remained there..

December 29, 1912: Temperature 96°.

December 30, 1912: Temperature 103°. Lungs negative. Drains well. Bed-sore slough removed.

December 31, 1912: Died from exhaustion and sepsis from bed sore.

CASE X.—Empyema, left. Recovery. Mary O'B., aged five years.

January 10, 1913: Admitted to the Episcopal Hospital, Dr. Piersol's service. Ill three days with pneumonia of left lower lobe. Temperature reached normal by lysis on January 17, 1913.

January 20, 1913: Temperature 101°–104°. Aspiration in ninth left interspace gave a large amount of pus (diplococcus pneumococcus).

January 22, 1913: Transferred to surgical service. Temperature still high.

Operation (Doctor Ashhurst).—Ether. Patient prone. Resected 3 cm. of ninth rib, in front of its angle; gush of yellow curdy pus (about 250 c.c.). Drain. Rubber tube.

February 18, 1913: Tube discontinued.

March 10, 1913: Out of bed.

March 21, 1913: Discharged. Wound healed.

September 28, 1916: Social Service Department reports; has moved and cannot be found.

CASE XI.—Empyema, left. Recovered. James F., aged seven years.

February 10, 1913: Admitted to Episcopal Hospital, Doctor Piersol's service. Ill three weeks at home, feverish and coughing. Effusion in left lower chest. Needle gave thick, greenish pus. Culture, pure pneumococci. Temperature, 102°. Delirious.

February 12, 1913: Temperature normal. Flat all over left chest, posteriorly.

February 14, 1913: Operation (Doctor Ashhurst)—ether. Patient prone. Excised 3 cm. of eleventh rib at angle. Gush of pus when periosteum was torn through, before fragment of rib was excised. No hæmostats required. About 500 c.c. of yellow inodorous creamy pus, with large amounts of lymph. Lung not much bound down by adhesions, and expanded well after removal of pus. Drain tube 1 cm. lumen, inserted about 5 cm., so as to be above level of diaphragm when this rose.

February 17, 1913: Pneumonia at right apex. Delirious, very weak. Temperature since operation, 99°–102° F.

February 21, 1913: Temperature normal.

February 27, 1913: Bed-sore over sacrum.

March 11, 1913: Slowly improving.

March 21, 1913: Tube replaced.

April 3, 1913: Bed-sore healed.

April 11, 1913: Tube removed.

April 20, 1913: Tube replaced.

April 28, 1913: Tube removed. Out of bed.

May 10, 1913: Discharged. Sinus gives slight discharge.

September 13, 1916: Healed three or four weeks after leaving hospital. No deformity; rib has reformed. Impaired resonance and a little distant breath sounds. Well and hearty.

CASE XII.—Empyema, left. Recovered. Walter H., aged fifteen years.

August 21, 1913: Admitted to Episcopal Hospital, Doctor Frazier's service.

Family History.—No tuberculosis.

Past History.—Pneumonia at five years; well since. School-boy.

Present Illness.—In October, 1912, noticed some swelling on left side, dull pain. Broke open in one month and discharged a little pus. Dressed twice daily since. Slight cough, frequent night sweats. Very little expectoration.

Examination.—Right apex impaired resonance. Left is fair. Right apex bronchial breathing and pectoriloquy. After each five or six beats of heart a very loud friction rub is heard, evidently pericardial, and systolic in time. From sixth rib to base on left is dull front and back. Scars of two healed sinuses, anteriorly in seventh interspace. Sinus below angle of scapula discharges whitish inodorous pus. Probe enters four inches and detects bare carious rib.

August 23, 1913: White blood count, 18,320.

August 26, 1913: Operation (Doctor Ashhurst)—eucain, 2 per cent. One and a half inches of tenth left rib removed; great amount of greenish pus exuded. (Smear: few micrococci; culture: negative.) Tube.

August 28, 1913: Not much pus.

September 6, 1913: Discharge less, irrigated daily.

September 8, 1913: Blows Wolfe bottles.

September 12, 1913: Better expansion of left.

September 20, 1913: No discharge. Sent home. Temperature never above 99° after operation.

September 28, 1916: Three years after operation reported to have left the city.

CASE XIII.—Empyema, left. Recovered. Edna P., seven years.

June 25, 1913: Admitted to Episcopal Hospital, Doctor Mutschler's service. Had been ill for six weeks. Acute onset with meningeal symptoms. In bed since with pain in left side. Weakness and cough and yellowish expectoration. Whole left chest full of fluid.

June 27, 1913: Operation by Doctor Mutschler. Intercostal incision, sixth to seventh ribs, left; large amount pus evacuated.

July 1, 1913: Improved. Temperature irregular but not high.

July 20, 1913: Only small sinus remains.

July 29, 1913: Temperature rising.

August 1, 1913: Service transferred to Doctor Ashhurst. Temperature, 103°. Signs of fluid; two taps negative. Old sinus entirely healed.

August 2, 1913: White blood count, 26,000.

August 5, 1913: Temperature, 100°–102°. X-ray.

August 10, 1913: Coughed up some pus; sent to Laboratory. Negative for tubercle bacilli; diplococcus predominates.

August 13, 1913: Sinus ruptured during night. Temperature lower.

August 19 to August 24, 1913: No improvement. Patient feels ill. Temperature up.

August 25, 1913: Better; thick, yellowish expectoration. X-ray after bismuth injection shows cavity extending from fourth to eleventh ribs.

August 26, 1913: Temperature normal.

August 27, 1913: Operation (Doctor Ashhurst)—ether. Patient prone. Excised 3 cm. of ninth and eighth ribs, near angle, opening cavity in pleura (no communication with bronchi apparent); removed bismuth; broke up some adhesions. Drain tube and iodoform gauze. Large amount of bloody pus removed.

September 18, 1913: Tube removed.

October 22, 1913: Entirely healed, out of bed.

October 27, 1913: Discharged.

September 6, 1916: Very slight scoliosis convex to left. (Left ribs were resected.) Ribs reformed. No disability. Attends State Dispensary for Tuberculosis.

February 21, 1920: Nearly seven years since operation; patient now fourteen years of age. Grandfather, living in same house, died of phthisis soon after her return home from hospital. Examination shows expansion of chest limited at both apices, but the lungs are normal. There is no increase in the slight left convex scoliosis noted three and a half years ago, and no disability.

CASE XIV.—Empyema, left (pleuro-peritonitis). Recovered. Margaret P., aged twelve years.

October 27, 1914: Admitted to the Episcopal Hospital on Doctor Fussell's service, Had been ailing off and on for three weeks before onset of acute illness, but attended school daily. One week before admission had sudden violent pain in lower left abdomen. Began vomiting and has been vomiting ever since. Castor oil not effectual. Bowels not open for one week. No cough. Pains her to be moved and to take deep breath. Pains to urinate or make any motion with abdominal muscles.

Examination on admission by Dr. J. W. Moore: Temperature, 103°; pulse, 136–120. Well developed and well nourished, but anæmic. Lips red, face pale. Breathing rapid, but rather full respiration. No œdema or cyanosis. Not apathetic. Teeth good. Tonsils very large and red and pharynx red. White blood count, 30,000; polynuclears, 75 per cent.; hæmoglobin, 75 per cent.; red blood count, 4,220,000.

Chest: Expansion good and equal on both sides. No thrills or frictions. Tactile fremitus normal everywhere. Whole lung resonant to percussion except an area, size of quarter, under angle right scapula, which is dull, and an area in right midclavicular line fourth rib (anteriorly), which seems hyperresonant, almost tympanitic. Breath sounds vesicular *all over*, including dull area, but here is heard an occasional crackling râle. No bronchophony or whispered pectoriloquy.

Heart: Negative.

Abdomen: Very rigid and tender all over, especially in epigastrium, right and left iliac fossæ. Not scaphoid nor markedly distended. Spleen and liver not palpable because of rigidity, but spleen not enlarged to percussion and liver dulness present. Abdomen resonant throughout, no dulness in flanks. Active peristalsis all over abdomen.

Rectum: No masses or areas of exquisite tenderness.

October 28, 1914: Examination by Doctor Fussell.—Patient looks ill. Complains of pain in abdomen when moved. There is a red flush on right forehead. Constantly makes outcries because she states she has pain in her stomach. Slight crusted scar on lower right lip, may or may not be herpes. Slight glandular enlargement in both axillæ and both groins. Breathing rapid and rather quick. No dulness on left side in front or laterally. Dulness on right, beginning at fifth rib in mid-axilla and merging into liver dulness. No dulness on right side behind. No blowing breathing posteriorly on either side. During examination dulness in right axilla disappears. Liver dulness begins at fourth rib parasternal line and extends almost to edge of the ribs. Splenic dulness is apparently increased. In respiration the abdominal wall is absolutely fixed. On palpation there are no masses or any particularly tender points. There is a great deal of abdominal tenderness in addition to the rigidity. Halfway between xiphoid and umbilicus the respiratory murmurs are curiously well heard. There is no sign of peristalsis. (Treatment just after admission is not recorded.) Rectum is ballooned out, but there is no mass.

Transferred to Doctor Ashhurst's service (day after admission): Temperature 103°; pulse, 120-130; respiration, 38-40; white blood count, 31,000. Eyes bright, cheeks red, rapid costal breathing. Abdomen very rigid all over, a little distended below umbilicus. Three doctors had examined her by rectum and felt no mass. Doctor Ashhurst did not examine chest or rectum; he thought it a surgical case (peritonitis), but that child was too sick for operation. Transferred to surgical ward and enteroclysis given, *nothing* by mouth (still vomiting frequently, and has been having water in medical ward, but no enteroclysis) and continued head-high posture. Also camphor and digitalis hypodermically (not given in medical ward).

October 29, 1914: Got out of bed last night and managed to get a little water (delirious). White blood count, 23,840; polynuclears, 92 per cent. (Nothing by mouth, continued enteroclysis.) Abdomen distended, tympanitic to percussion everywhere, save in right iliac fossa, where a dull area can be made out. Right side more rigid than left. Has vomited only twice. Nose-bleed at 3.30 A.M.

October 30, 1914: Much weaker and more restless. Abdomen not so distended, but boardlike rigidity over entire abdomen. Does not vomit, has not passed any fiatus; paristalsis can be heard in upper abdomen; complains of great thirst. Still nothing by mouth, and enteroclysis. Temperature, 101°-103°. Pulse, 120; respiration, 26-30. Given digitalis and strychnin. No sign of localization of peritonitis.

October 31, 1914 (Saturday): Decidedly better. Upper abdomen just a little softer. Suspicious baggy feel by rectum (Doctor Ashhurst's first examination). Respiration still very rapid. Temperature, 99°. Pulse, 110-115. By noon, hot water given by mouth. By afternoon (Doctor Ashhurst's third visit this day), feels almost convalescent, she says. Complained of pain "around heart" and left lower chest at A.M. visit; P.M. temperature, 101°.

November 1, 1914 (Sunday): Temperature, 101° (steady); pulse, 108-120; respiration, 32-40. Respirations still very rapid. Left cheek flushed. Alæ nasi play violently. Abdomen rather rigid, no dulness, rectal examination negative. Chest

41

negative anteriorly. Doctor Ashhurst determined on thorough chest examination (his first), because of failure of abdominal abscess to appear. No evidence of subphrenic abscess (Hoover's sign). Right lung negative. Left dull from angle of scapula down, posteriorly and in axillary line, not anteriorly. Tender on pressure in intercostal spaces here. *Perhaps* slight bulging of these spaces. Breath sounds distant. *Needle* inserted in seventh interspace below angle of scapula drew pus (diplococci in chains). Doctor Fussell came in consultation and said subphrenic abscess, *no* evidence of empyema. Doctor Ashhurst maintained it was *empyema thoracis.*

Operation (Doctor Ashhurst).—Gas, 2.30 P.M. Resected eighth rib in anterior axillary line; 150 c.c. pus from pleura (streptococci). Tube. Liquids by mouth. At 10 P.M. abdomen less tender, lungs œdematous. Heart good. Given morphine and atropine. Temperature, 104°. Pulse, 120–140. Respiration, 40–48.

November 2, 1914: Profuse discharge of pus from pleura; heart displaced to right. Abdomen softer, normal bowel movement (first since enema October 29). White blood count, 47,760; polynuclears, 89 per cent.

November 3, 1914: Temperature falling. Continue morphin, atropin and stimulation. Three normal bowel movements (no purge).

November 4, 1914: Better, abdomen softer, no bowel movement.

November 5, 1914: Temperature gradually falling. Pulse, 120–130. Respiration, 30–38. Bowels open daily from now on. Examination by Doctor Fussell. Labored breathing. Heart: right border one and a half inches to right of sternum, sounds are very rapid and feeble. Right chest anteriorly and posteriorly many râles. Left chest: pneumothorax. Abdomen is tender, especially over McBurney's point.

November 6, 1914: Examination by Doctor Ashhurst. No rigidity of abdomen, no tenderness to a reasonable degree of pressure over appendix or any other part of abdomen. To all intents and purposes the abdomen is normal. Respirations are thoracic. Fair expansion on both sides of upper chest; below nipples expansion better on right than left. No breath sounds heard anteriorly on left; normal on right. Right chest posteriorly is normal, on left posteriorly—pneumothorax.

November 7, 1914: Herpes on lip and tongue.

November 8, 1914: Improved.

November 10, 1914: Profuse discharge from chest still.

November 14, 1914: Fluid suspected at right base, no puncture.

November 16, 1914: Tube shortened.

November 22, 1914: Tube removed. Heart in normal position. Left thumb opened for infection (pure staphylococcus).

December 5, 1914: Out of bed. Thumb badly infected. Furunculosis of back.

December 11, 1914: Convalescent for two weeks and in chair now and chest normal. Thin.

December 14, 1914: Chest healed.

December 17, 1914: Gained three pounds in last three days.

December 23, 1914: Severe cough. Examination by Doctor Piersol: Compensatory emphysema of upper and middle right lobes; slight fluid or thickened pleura at right base from seventh dorsal spine down. Consolidation or compression of upper left lobe; below effusion and air.

December 24, 1914: Feels fine. Examination by Doctor Ashhurst; dulness at right base, breath sounds distant, consolidation at left base; sounds diminished, pneumothorax. Abdomen negative.

December 25, 1914: This afternoon had attack of acute pain in abdomen, vomited once. Temperature, 100°. Abdomen tender throughout and some rigidity.

December 26, 1914: Temperature 99°–101°. Right lower quadrant rigid. Liquid diet.

December 30, 1914: Sequestrum removed from thumb.

December 31, 1914: Chest unchanged. Aspiration on right: no fluid.

January 3, 1915: Temperature, 99°–101°. Pulse, 104–120. Respiration, 28. Vomited this A.M.

January 4, 1915: No better. Slight pneumothorax anteriorly on left; empyema scar solid.

January 5, 1915: Examination by Doctor Frazier (rectal and abdominal), who found no abscess. Resident physician (Sproul) could not feel anything by rectum. Doctor Ashhurst examined patient again and found all abdomen below navel rigid and tender and dull, and in rectum a distinct bulging abscess. White blood count, 26,000 for last week. Polynuclears five days ago, 82 per cent.; yesterday, 72 per cent.

Diagnosis.—Pelvic abscess from appendix, relighted by Xmas dinner.

Operation.—Gas, 11:30 A.M. Incision right paramedian two inches, suprapubic. Transversalis fascia and peritoneum matted together and dense; at once on opening peritoneum white creamy pus welled out, about 50 c.c. in all. Finger inserted felt intestines matted together by adhesions; and burrowed to Douglas's pouch; rubber tube, and iodoform gauze. No sutures. Time, ten minutes. (Culture, streptococcus.)

January 6, 1915: Temperature normal; free discharge of pus; much better.

January 10, 1915: Bloody purulent expectoration. Sitting in chair.

January 13, 1915: Tube removed from abdomen.

January 15, 1915: Weight, fifty-four and a half pounds.

January 17, 1915: Slight discharge. Gaining weight.

January 23, 1915: Went home, weight fifty-nine pounds. Sinus closed.

October 4, 1915: Scar two inches. No hernia. No disability. Appendix has never been removed.

April, 1920. Family report patient in good health. Is a professional dancer.

CASE XV.—Empyema, right. Recovered. Hugh McI., aged forty-three years.

November 7, 1914: Admitted to the Episcopal Hospital to Doctor Frazier's service. Ailing all summer. Pneumonia four weeks ago, crisis three weeks ago, but did not get well, had fever, cough and marked expectoration. In bed all the time. Bed-sore beginning. Temperature, 101° F.; right lung from middle down gives absent breath sounds and fremitus, and is flat. Aspiration gives pus in seventh interspace posteriorly (pneumococcus).

November 8, 1915: Operation—eucain, 2 per cent. Patient prone. Resection of 3 cm. of ninth right rib in posterior axillary line. The sinus of empyema runs up posteriorly to the region of the third rib, where the cavity is larger. The lung is bound down tight by adhesions (Fig. 11).

November 9, 1914: Temperature normal.

November 18, 1914: Tube out.

November 23, 1914: Discharged.

September 28, 1915. Refuses to return for examination. Wife says he is in good health but has a cough.

CASE XVI.—Empyema, left. Recovered. Joseph R., aged nineteen years.

December 3, 1914: Admitted to Doctor Frazier's service, Episcopal Hospital. Pneumonia (left) three weeks ago; crisis two weeks ago, but did not get well. Fever developed with pain in left chest and dyspnœa. Cough and expectoration continued. Needle in seventh interspace shows pus. (Family physician.)

Examination on Admission.—Left base, absent breath sounds and fremitus with flatness. Hoover's sign positive. White blood count, 15,840. Temperature 103° F.

December 4, 1914: Operation—eucain, 2 per cent. Excised 2.5 cm. of eighth left rib posteriorly; 500 c.c. of pus (diplococci).

December 8, 1914: Tube lost in wound (was sutured to skin by No. 1 chromic gut). X-ray 3376a shows it inside chest.

December 11, 1914: Efforts yesterday failing to extract tube. Doctor Ashhurst to-day, (gas) resected 2.5 cm. more off same rib at anterior and then at posterior end of former section, and finally found tube in spinal gutter posteriorly. *Large pus pocket* opened and drained. Tube fastened with silkworm gut and safety pin. Temperature has been normal since operation last week.

December 14, 1914: Drainage has about stopped.

December 18, 1914: Out of bed.

December 22, 1914: Discharged.

September 28, 1916: Has moved to Wilkes-Barre, Pa.

CASE XVII.—Pulsating empyema necessitatis, left. Recovered. Gerald L., aged twenty-eight years.

December 10, 1914: Admitted to Doctor Frazier's service, Episcopal Hospital.

Past History.—Is tuberculous; has been ill off and on for seven years. In February, 1911, had left pneumonia, followed by pleural effusion (empyema); tapped, tube inserted (no rib resected). Acute illness lasted six months. Sinus ran nearly one and a half years. Recovered and resumed work about one and a half years ago (laborer).

Present Illness.—Ailing for one month, very ill for one week, high fever, bad cough, pain in chest; expectoration offensive and profuse.

Examination.—Extremely ill, delirious, cyanosed and dyspnœic. Empyema necessitatis over second left rib and in upper axilla. Former pulsates synchronously with heart. Above middle of scapula there is Skodaic resonance; below this flat, immobile (Hoover's sign very pronounced), breath sounds and fremitus absent. Over apex (L) breath sounds loud and blowing, almost amphoric. Right lung full of crepitant râles. White blood count, 50,000. Polynuclears, 91.3 per cent. Temperature, 99°. Pulse, 100–128.

Diagnosis.—Pyopneumothorax. Heart displaced 4 cm. to right of sternum. Thirty-eight ounces (well over one litre) of pus removed by aspiration in left eighth interspace posteriorly. Foul and fæcal smelling. (Long pale bacillus with streptococcus predominating.) After aspiration bulging area disappeared below clavicle, and this was sucked in with each respiration. Given morphin for cough (Fig. 12).

December 11, 1914: Still in poor condition, but much better than on admission.

Operation.—Eucain, 2 per cent. Excised 3¼ cm. of ninth rib (left). Patient lying prone. Pleura very thick (5 mm.) and prune juice looking pus evacuated after breaking up some adhesions. Exceedingly bad stink of H₂S gas. Long tube inserted.

December 12, 1914: Better; marked discharge. Temperature, 102°.

December 14, 1914: Temperature again normal.

December 18, 1914: Tube removed.

December 29, 1914: Went home against advice, but in very good condition, out of bed several days.

September 28, 1916: Has moved to Souderton, Pa.

CASE XVIII.—Empyema, right (encysted). Recovered. Tony V., two years.

·November 10, 1915: Admitted to Doctor Frazier's service at the Episcopal Hospital. Three weeks ago became ill and treated at home for pneumonia; seen to-day by Dr. R. S. Hooker at home and diagnosed as empyema. On admission, temperature, 102°; pulse, 108–148; respiration, 32–40; white blood count, 25,000. Poorly nourished, thin profuse nasal discharge. Pharynx unusually red. Thorax: resonance good, a few râles low in right axilla, and breath sounds are harsh around angle of both scapulæ.

November 11, 1915: Aspiration (numerous punctures) of right pleural cavity, no fluid obtained. Temperature down.

November 13, 1915: Temperature up.

November 15, 1915: Aspirated again in left axilla, no fluid obtained.

November 16, 1915: White blood count, 36,640. Lymphocytes, 40 per cent. Polynuclears, 46 per cent. Hæmoglobin, 59 per cent.

November 17, 1915: Temperature down.

November 18, 1915: Temperature up.

November 19 to 23, 1915: Temperature, 100°–103°, irregular. Seen in consultation

44

by Dr. W. E. Robertson, who diagnosed fluid under the sixth rib right. X-ray confirms this.

November 23, 1915: Operation (Doctor Ashhurst)—ether. Time, ten minutes. Patient prone; resection of 3 cm. of seventh right rib near angle of scapula. Pleura thick. Opened this, no pus. Finger introduced found lung lightly adherent to parietal pleura and diaphragm all over. No dense adhesions. No interlobar collection between middle and lower lobes found. Only blood. Culture, sterile. Drain, rubber tube.

November 26, 1915: Wound doing well.

November 29, 1915: Temperature has fallen gradually to normal.

December 1, 1915: Sudden profuse discharge of pus through wound. (Culture, streptococci and staphylococci.) Evidently an encysted empyema had broken into wound (Fig. 13). Temperature, 101° F.

December 3, 1919: Considerable drainage.

December 8, 1915: Discharge scanty.

December 12, 1915: Chest still draining but scanty.

February 5, 1915: Went home. Sinus healed dry.

September 6, 1916: No deformity, lung normal, rib reformed.

CASE XIX.—Empyema, right. Recovered. Joseph F., aged nine years.

November 17, 1915: Admitted to Doctor Stevens's service, Episcopal Hospital. About four days ago became sick, attributed to eating some cabbage two days before. Pain in abdomen and then vomited; pain was continuous. This morning pain seemed localized to upper right abdomen and patient then began to show rapid and shallow respirations and to dart his tongue in and out. Has eaten very little since illness began, but has not been constipated.

On admission, heart not enlarged, no murmurs. Lungs, anteriorly resonant throughout, breath sounds normal posteriorly, dulness and absent breath sounds over right lower lobe up to angle of scapula. Diminished resonance over left lower lobe (Grocco's sign). Few moist râles above area of dulness on right. Liver not enlarged, great tenderness and much rigidity in right upper quadrant, no marked tenderness in right iliac fossa.

November 18, 1915: White blood count, 25,200.

November 27, 1915: Diagnosis of empyema made and transferred to surgical service. Temperature has been 102°–103° ever since admission, growing more irregular (99°–104°) since November 23d.

November 28, 1915: 500 c.c. of colon smelling pus removed by aspiration. Dyspnœa much relieved. Culture of pleural fluid: mixed growth.

November 30, 1915: Operation (Doctor Ashhurst)—gas. Patient supine, right chest projecting over edge of table. Resected 4 cm. of ninth rib below angle of scapula, evacuating nearly 500 c.c. of colon pus; undoubtedly *not* subphrenic, but in pleural cavity. No perforation of diaphragm felt. Drainage tube. Temperature fell at once.

December 3, 1915: Drainage freely.

December 12, 1915: Drainage much less.

December 22, 1915: Out of bed, temperature still down.

January 3, 1916: Went home. Small tube still in sinus and some discharge.

August 29, 1916: Examination in dispensary. Very slight scoliosis; sinus healed by February 1, 1916. Lung sounds normal.

CASE XX.—Empyema, recurrent (right). Recovered. Francis P., aged eleven years.

October 13, 1915: Admitted to Doctor Deaver's service, Episcopal Hospital. Two and a half weeks ago developed pneumonia; for past five days excessive cough and profuse expectoration. On admission, temperature, 101°. Pulse, 112. Respiration, 36. Respiration shallow. Right chest more prominent and motionless on breathing. Flatness over whole right chest, feeble breath sounds, tubular on deep breathing. Left chest hyperresonant, few râles. Heart displaced to left: apex in fifth interspace, anterior axillary line. By aspiration, 5 c.c. foul, greenish pus—staphylococci, diplococci and streptococci.

October 14, 1915: Operation (Doctor Deaver)—ether. Resected 2.5 cm. of seventh rib left mid-axillary line; 200 c.c. of pus. Rubber tube.

October 24, 1915: Still profuse discharge. Temperature, 99°-103°.

October 29, 1915: White blood count, 14,640; lymphocytes, 44 per cent.

November 1, 1915: Transferred to Doctor Frazier's service. Dressings still require changing twice daily; tube still in. Temperature, 99°-101°.

November 8, 1915: Dressed once daily.

November 17, 1915: Drainage less.

November 26, 1915: Temperature up.

November 29, 1915: Temperature still up.

December 3, 1915: Second operation (Doctor Ashhurst)—ether. Old sinus excised by incision in long axis of patient's body. Excised 3 cm. of rib next above and 3 cm. more off anterior end of that formerly excised (almost closed). Burrowed between adherent lung and thoracic wall posteriorly, gush of fœtid thin pus. (Culture, streptococcus.) About 150 c.c. Rubber tube drain.

December 5, 1915: Foul discharge (B. pyocyaneus).

December 12, 1915: Improved.

December 13, 1915: Seen by Doctor Stevens, who diagnosed pus in extreme lower part of right pleural cavity. Circulation not very good.

January 14, 1916: Sinus is being exposed to sun daily.

January 24, 1916: Temperature much lower, drainage less.

February 1, 1916: Discharge very slight. Breath sounds good.

February 3, 1916: Discharged from hospital.

September 13, 1916: Robust and rosy. No deformity. Sinus healed solidly since March. Rib reformed. Thickened pleura, but lung normal. (Impaired resonance and fremitus and distant breath sounds.)

CASE XXI.—Empyema, left. Encapsulated, with separate pleural effusion. Recovered. Joseph B., aged thirty-four years.

December 8, 1915: Admitted to Doctor Piersol's service, Episcopal Hospital.

Present Illness.—Three weeks ago pain in left chest and cough. On admission, temperature, 100°. Pulse, 92. Respiration, 20-24. White blood count, 22,000. Polynuclears, 89 per cent. Pain in lower left chest, slight cough. Not toxic. Not dyspnœic. Bulging of left antero-lateral chest wall; dull red, extremely tender and resistant, from anterior axillary line into axilla. Respiratory excursions limited over left lower thorax; vocal fremitus absent, anteriorly below level of nipple, in left axilla below this level and posteriorly below angle of scapula. Skodaic resonance over upper left lung. Traube's semilunar space seems obliterated. Flatness over left chest below nipple, also absent vocal resonance and breath sounds inaudible.

Right lung: rough puerile breathing throughout and dry râles. Left chest tapped posteriorly, turbid straw-colored fluid, not true pus. (Laboratory report: gelatinous, 320 cells per cubic mm.; 80 per cent. polynuclears; 20 per cent. lymphocytes.) Blood Wassermann negative.

December 9, 1915: Seen in consultation by Doctor Ashhurst. Evidently an extrathoracic abscess over left antero-lateral chest, and inflammatory exudate in pleura. Transferred to surgical service.

Operation (Doctor Ashhurst).—Novocain, ¼ per cent. Resected two inches of left eleventh rib posteriorly—pleura opened—profuse discharge of slightly turbid fluid. No odor. (Laboratory report: negative.) Diaphragm comes up against wound in expiration, and fluid only discharges when diaphragm is pushed away. Finger introduced finds no adhesions except where diaphragm comes against ribs. Lung not felt. About 300-350 c.c. of turbid fluid evacuated and more drains while dressing wound.

46

Tube inserted up four inches and stream of turbid serum escaped through it. Tube sutured to skin, and ends of skin wound closed. Culture of serum.

Patient on back. Novocain. Incision over subcutaneous (left) phlegmon—thick, yellow, inodorous pus (culture, staphylococcus). This pus has spread over area 8 cm. in diameter superficial to ribs and discharged between seventh and eighth ribs through orifice admitting little finger, into walled-off cavity about 8 cm. in diameter—encapsulated empyema necessitatis. Iodoform gauze drain.

(Query: Is free pleural fluid tuberculous? Presumably it is analogous to that in pleura in subphrenic abscess, and to that in knee in osteomyelitis of tibia.)

December 10, 1915: Temperature, 98°–103° F.

December 15, 1915: Temperature steady, 98°–99°/₄°.

December 25, 1915: Tube out from posterior wound.

December 29, 1915: Out of bed.

January 7, 1916: No drainage. Went home at own request.

September 20, 1916: Examination: Returned to work two months after leaving hospital. No disability since. Both wounds solidly healed, lung normal on examination.

CASE XXII.—Empyema, right; necrosis of mandible (from noma). Died, two days (noma). Edward S., aged seven years.

December 11, 1915: Admitted to Doctor Frazier's service, Episcopal Hospital. Pneumonia at home for three weeks. December 7th refused to eat because of sore mouth, and for four days before admission was pulling out loose molar teeth with his fingers; had very foul breath. Entire alveolus of lower jaw (right and left), except under the three front teeth, is necrotic, and the noma extends on to cheeks. Right lung: dull, except over extreme apex, breathing tubular and fairly loud where dull, and fremitus increased. Left lung: numerous râles and tubular breathing at base.

1 P.M.—Red blood count, 2,800,000. Hæmoglobin, 35 per cent. White blood count, 15,800. Temperature, 101°/₄°. Condition very poor. Aspiration right chest—10 c.c. thick, yellowish pus.

2 P.M.—Child desperately ill from sepsis.

5 P.M.—Operation (Doctor Ashhurst)—gas. Resection of 3 cm. of eighth right rib in posterior axillary line, patient on back. Pleura not injured. On opening it (rather thick) a squirt of thick creamy yellow pus, no odor. (Culture, mixed growth.) About 300 c.c. evacuated. Cavity extends three ribs lower, to costophrenic space, and up as far as finger can reach toward apex. Respirations very bad. (Inhalation of ammonia.) Rubber tube drain. Then fuming nitric acid to mouth, and alveolus of mandible excised.

December 13, 1915: Died, 1 A.M.

CASE XXIII.—Empyema, left. Recovered. James C., aged three years.

January 4, 1916: Admitted to the Episcopal Hospital, Doctor Ashhurst's service. Three weeks ago became ill with cough, high temperature and pain in left side. On admission, respiration rapid, expansion absent on left. Fremitus is diminished and breath sounds almost absent; entire left chest is dull on percussion. Apex beat in mid-line. White blood count, 16,640. Polynuclears, 71 per cent. 500 c.c. pus drawn by aspirator. No dyspnœa before or after. Report from Laboratory, January 5th: Pneumococcus.

January 7, 1916: Operation (Doctor Ashhurst)—ether. Patient prone, resected tenth left rib in posterior axillary line; 250 c.c. of creamy pus evacuated, no masses of lymph. Loosened lung from diaphragm and from spinal gutter, whereupon it expanded 50 per cent.

January 17, 1916: Drainage much less.

January 22, 1916: Temperature up, slight cough.

January 26, 1916: Developed measles and sent to Philadelphia General Hospital.

February 3, 1916: Returned from Philadelphia Hospital. Temperature, 100°–101°.

February 6, 1916: Temperature, 104°. Draining freely.

47

February 15, 1916: Temperature falling.
February 26, 1916: Tube removed.
March 1, 1916: Tube replaced.
March 6, 1916: Tube removed. No drainage.
March 10, 1916: Discharged. Sinus healed.
September 6, 1916: No scoliosis, rib reformed, perfect result.
CASE XXIV.—Empyema, encysted left. Recovered. Philip G., aged fourteen years.
December 27, 1915: Admitted to Doctor Piersol's service at the Episcopal Hospital. Two weeks ago developed chill, headache, vomited several times and had generalized slight pain. After few days felt better and went out. Then right ear began to ache; and two days ago developed cough, and became constipated. Has now coryza, cough, slight dyspnœa and is constipated. No appetite since illness began.

On admission, fairly well built, slender, not emaciated, no adenopathy. Heart is not enlarged nor displaced, apex beat in usual location, no murmurs, sounds of fair quality. Lungs are negative, good breath sounds, good resonance throughout. Abdomen negative. White blood count, 11,040.

December 30, 1915: Marked diminution in breath sounds over left base posteriorly, few sonorous râles in lower left axilla. Sputum negative for tubercle bacilli.

January 2, 1916: Widal negative.

January 4, 1916: Marked bronchial breathing over right apex posteriorly.

January 6, 1916: Blood culture—short chain streptococcus. Malaria negative. White blood count, 19,960.

January 12, 1916: Dulness on percussion and great tenderness at left base posteriorly. Nothing obtained on exploratory puncture.

January 13, 1916: Examined by Doctor Ashhurst in consultation. Has been in medical ward over two weeks with septic temperature (100°-104°) and chills. Patient is extremely emaciated and anæmic. Left lung dull at base, all signs of empyema, but needle found no pus. Very tender in left costovertebral angle. Excursion of costal margin from midline (Hoover's test) not increased, no more tender in left than in right hypochondrium. X-ray (only properly interpreted after operation) shows dense shadow above left diaphragm, upper level horizontal (not domed) and higher than diaphragm on right. A diagnosis was made of encysted empyema and exploratory operation advised.

January 14, 1916: Operation (Doctor Ashhurst)—stovain, locally, for resection of rib; gas for intrathoracic explorations. Patient prone. Excised 5 cm. of tenth rib near angle. Then incised pleura. Lung did not collapse. Diaphragm exposed, soft; spleen easily palpated through diaphragm, no sign of subphrenic abscess, and on retracting upper ribs (now general anæsthetic) lung was seen to be plastered on to diaphragm. Extended incision up parallel to spine, excised 6 cm. more of rib at vertebral end. Dissected carefully with finger, raising lung from diaphragm: a flood of pus (500 c.c.) (culture, streptococci) from between lung and diaphragm (Fig. 14). Lung now collapsed. Drain, rubber tube and iodoform gauze between lung and diaphragm. Ends of incision (12.5 cm.) closed with silkworm-gut.

January 15, 1916: Given enteroclysis and liquids by mouth. Looks better, quiet, comfortable, but very weak and thin.

January 17, 1916: Temperature, 98°-100° ever since operation. Eating better. Looks better.

January 22, 1916: Tube shortened.
January 25, 1916: Tube removed. Rapidly improving.
January 31, 1916: Up in chair.
February 14, 1916: Able to walk.
February 26, 1916: Sent home.
August 9, 1916: In dispensary in good general health, sinus in wound just admits probe; has been dressed three times weekly by family physician since leaving hospital;

OBSERVATIONS ON EMPYEMA

tube was retained until last week, since when gauze has been employed. It was recommended that the packing be discontinued.

February 29, 1920: Sinus closed permanently a week after the gauze packing was
discontinued. The only symptom he complains of now is a pricking in the scar at
times, on exertion. He works as meatchopper, lifting heavy portions of the carcasses
without disability. There is no scoliosis and no deformity, except the very much
depressed scar. The lungs are normal, but the ribs below the scar do not move in
forced respiration as do those on the other side.

CASE XXV.—Empyema, encysted, right. Recovered. William B., aged thirty years.

December 22, 1915: Admitted to the Episcopal Hospital, Doctor Piersol's service.
Six weeks ago developed pain in back and slight dyspnœa; began to cough with slight
muco-purulent expectoration. Yesterday pain in right side at costal margin, cough,
some dyspnœa, rapidly becoming worse. On admission, temperature, 103°. Pulse,
104–108. Respiration, 32. White blood count, 10,000. Polynuclears, 91 per cent. Well
developed, dyspnœic, alæ of nose moving in each respiration. Lungs: impairment of
resonance over right side, most marked in middle and lower lobes; tactile and vocal
fremitus decreased, and bronchial breathing with moist râles over middle and lower
lobes. Few sonorous and crepitant râles over right upper lobe. Left lung negative.
Heart normal. Liver enlarged 5 cm. below costal margin.

December 26, 1915: Temperature fell by lysis to 100°.

December 30, 1915: General condition improved. Temperature, 100°–103°. Marked
bronchial breathing over middle of right lung posteriorly.

January 3 to 14, 1916: Temperature, 99°–101°–102°, irregular.

January 13, 1916: Seen by Doctor Ashhurst in consultation. In medical ward
(Piersol) some weeks with sepsis following pneumonia ("unresolved").

Examination.—Right chest dull (flat) from angle of scapula down, fremitus normal, breath sounds distant. A diagnosis of empyema was made from history and
condition of "unresolved pneumonia." Medical attendants could not locate pus.
Needle in eighth interspace drew only blood.

January 14, 1916: Transferred to surgical ward. Dulness over middle and lower
lobes right. Right base, however, transmits vocal fremitus, although voice and breath
sounds are diminished. X-ray shows haziness in upper and middle lobes.

Operation (Doctor Ashhurst).—Novocain, ¼ per cent. Patient prone. Incision
10 cm. over ninth rib, excised 8 cm. Diaphragm and lightly adherent lung presented
on opening pleura. Separated lung from diaphragm by finger far as could reach, no pus.
Surface of diaphragm rather sensitive, lung insensitive. Then burrowed between middle
and lower lobes, no pus; entirely insensitive. Then burrowed up along parietal pleura,
and found very dense adhesions up along fifth to sixth ribs, finally broke through,
when just about to abandon operation, and got a flood (perhaps 250 c.c.) of blood-
stained pus. (Culture, pneumococcus.) Evidently had been interlobar (upper and
middle lobes) and had worked out to parietal pleura (Fig. 15). Parietal pleura
rather sensitive. Slight coughing on evacuation of pus, and partial collapse of
lung. Drain: rubber tube up along parietal pleura for four inches.

January 15, 1916: Looks convalescent.

January 16, 1916: Drains freely.

January 20, 1916: Tube removed.

January 23, 1916: Temperature normal. Out of bed. Sputum negative for
tubercle bacilli.

January 31, 1916: Convalescent.

February 3, 1916: No discharge. Small granulating wound. Sent home.

August 9, 1916: Cannot be traced.

CASE XXVI.—Interlobar empyema, left (against pericardium). Died. Katherine
D., aged thirty-eight years.

August 3, 1916: Admitted to Doctor Ashhurst's service, Episcopal Hospital.

4   49

ASTLEY P. C. ASHHURST

Past History—Four and a half years ago had attack of pneumonia and pleurisy (left sided) and was in another hospital five months; had septic temperature and chills. Was aspirated, but no pus could be obtained.

Present Illness.—Has had no trouble since, until six weeks ago, when she had pain in left side for two days, severe pain for three-quarters of an hour, followed by chill. July 28th had temperature of 103°, pulse, 120, and sent for Doctor Shannon. Has had chills. August 1 went to bed complaining of weakness and fever and pain on left side. Last night (August 2d and 3d) had pain in right shoulder, relieved by hot-water compresses. Has had slight cough, but not much expectoration. Coughed more before taking to her bed.

On admittance, well nourished, no evidence of acute suffering. Breath foul. Temperature, 101°-105°. Pulse, 120-150. Respiration, 32-40. White blood count, 21,000. Chest: posteriorly inspection and palpation negative, except for slight restriction of expansion and decreased fremitus at base of left lung. Percussion note is impaired from seventh interspace in mid-axillary line to vertebral column and extending to base of left lung. Auscultation shows decreased breath sounds over this area. Right lung negative, breath sounds normal. Heart rapid (no murmurs), outline normal. Abdomen negative. Puncture in seventh interspace, anterior axillary line (record syringe) gave no fluid. After admittance had chill.

August 4, 1916: Another chill to-day. Temperature, 101°-104°. X-ray apparatus out of order and no röntgenological examination could be made.

August 5, 1916: Operation (Doctor Ashhurst)—novocain, ¼ per cent. Patient prone. Incision 10 cm. over left eighth rib, excised 8 cm. Opened pleura, lung lightly adherent throughout, but freely movable. Packed off above. Dissected lung from diaphragm. No pus. Felt inner border of spleen through diaphragm no subphrenic abscess. Packed over diaphragm, removed upper packing and separated lung from parietal pleura. Then extended skin incision, excised 3 cm. more of eighth rib and 10 cm. of seventh; dissected with two forceps in interlobar space for 5 or 6 cm., but found only dark blood. (Culture, sterile.) Iodoform gauze stuffed in this hole and wound closed in layers (Fig. 16). (Hoped pus would break into wound as in Case XVIII.)

August 7, 1916: Examination by Doctor Hooker. On left side down to angle of scapula there are normal breath sounds, resonance and fremitus. Unable to examine below on account of dressings. Heart: second aortic accentuated, no murmurs. Blood culture negative. One chill to-day. Temperature, 98.4°-104°.

August 9, 1916: Examination by Doctor Hooker. Heart: second aortic accentuated, roughening at mitral valve, presystolic. Entire right lung shows increased vocal resonance, many crepitant rales, impaired note on percussion, typical pneumonia (hypostatic in origin). Left lung same as last examination. Drainage removed and wound cleaned.

August 10, 1916: Expression is anxious, apathetic, listless, but rather restless. Heart sounds distant. Some evidence of pus on dressings, not present yesterday. Neck held very rigid, moves extremities when attempts are made to flex neck. White blood count, 19,000; polynuclears, 79 per cent.; hæmoglobin, 55 per cent. Temperature does not fall below 101° any more. X-ray shows shadow of abscess to left of mid-line of thorax, under sixth and seventh ribs (Fig. 18).

August 13, 1916: Died of sepsis. Had been moribund for last three days. Wound explored after death by Dr. H. S. Spruance (ward surgeon) after removal of two more ribs. He found gauze pack had been correctly placed in interlobar space, and by separating lobes farther (about 2.5 cm.) through dense adhesions he came on abscess (100 c.c.) in interlobar space and against pericardium. Pericardium·when opened was found to contain many recent fibrinous adhesions, but no pus (Fig. 17).

CASE XXVII.—Empyema, left, encysted above diaphragm. Recovered. James McG., aged thirty years.

OBSERVATIONS ON EMPYEMA

October 30, 1916: Admitted to the Episcopal Hospital, Doctor Robertson's service.

Present illness began October 19th with coryza. October 28th had chill and began expectorating; continuous pain in left chest. On admittance, signs of pneumonia at base of left lung.

November 5, 1916: Temperature falling by lysis.

November 11, 1916: Temperature has not reached normal. Puncture of chest negative.

November 12, 1916: Puncture again negative.

November 16, 1916: Third puncture reaches pus in eighth interspace, 40 c.c. of pus withdrawn. Smear and culture of fluid is negative.

November 17, 1916: Transferred to surgical ward (Doctor Ashhurst). Temperature, 99°–103° for the last week.

Operation (Doctor Ashhurst).—Eucain, 1 per cent. Excised 5 cm. of tenth rib, lung does not collapse, lightly adherent to costal pleura and densely to diaphragm. Separated costal adhesions, no pus within reach of opening. Separated lung from diaphragm as far as possible, no pus, but adhesions at limit of fingers were more dense. Excised 5 cm. of ninth rib, and after gauze pack above, dug lung away from diaphragm to dome, when about 60 c.c. of pus discharged. Drain: rubber tube wrapped in iodoform gauze.

November 18, 1916: Temperature still up.

November 22, 1916: Still draining freely. Temperature, 100°–103°.

December 1, 1916: Tube removed. Out of bed.

December 8, 1916: For continuing temperature and history of syphilis is given neosalvarsan.

December 12, 1916: Temperature normal.

December 18, 1916: No drainage; incision closing. Sent home.

January 16, 1917: Seen by Dr. Spruance, ward surgeon; healed firmly for about one month. In perfect health.

February 29, 1920: Examination; is police officer. In perfect health. Lungs normal. On palpation ribs seem to have reformed.

Case XXVIII.—Empyema, left, encysted, upper lobe. Recovered. William B., aged twenty years.

October 18, 1916: Admitted to the Episcopal Hospital, Doctor Robertson's service. Blind since illness with pneumonia at five years of age. Onset of present illness, October 16, with chilliness, during evening; awoke during night with pain in left chest. On admission, pneumonia over upper left lobe.

October 23, 1916: Temperature falling by lysis.

November 4, 1916: Temperature has not reached normal. Signs of fluid. Puncture below angle of scapula negative.

November 16, 1916: Signs of fluid still present now confined to upper lobe, left. Puncture between angle of scapula and spine gives 30 c.c. pus. Sent to laboratory. Previous punctures all over left chest had been negative.

November 17, 1916: Seen by Doctor Ashhurst in consultation. Has been in ward over four weeks with continued temperature following typical pneumonia (left upper lobe), which declined by lysis over three weeks ago. *Repeated* punctures negative until yesterday pus was found (30 c.c. easily drawn) in fourth interspace at spine of scapula. Transferred to surgical service (Doctor Ashhurst).

Operation.—Eucain, 1 per cent. (Patient blind since five years and neurotic.) Excised 4 cm. of fourth and fifth left ribs between scapula and spine, flood of curdy pus and great handfuls of coagulated lymph. Cavity extends to first rib and down only to sixth or seventh in mid-axillary line, evidently encapsulated over interlobar fissure. Drain: large rubber tube and iodoform gauze (Fig. 19).

November 18, 1916: Temperature falling, profuse drainage.

December 27, 1916: Up and about ward part of day.

51

December 30, 1916: 50,000,000 autogenous vaccins, given with idea of hastening closure of cavity.

January 8, 1917: 100,000,000 vaccins given.

January 16, 1917: Still in ward, not much discharge. Temperature normal for one week, until to-day, sudden rise.

January 26, 1917: Temperature about normal. Scarcely any discharge. Up all day.

January 27, 1917: Sent home. Scarcely any discharge.

February 21, 1920. Three years after leaving hospital, examination shows him fat and healthy (Fig. 20). The sinus did not heal entirely for nearly ten weeks after his discharge (over four months after the operation). Examination shows the lungs normal. He has full use of his left shoulder, in spite of section of trapezius and rhomboid muscles at time of operation. As far as can be felt the ribs have reformed. His only complaint is of a pricking feeling in the scar when he puts his hand to small of back.

CASE XXIX.—Empyema, left (two distinct encysted empyemas). Recovered. Johan L., aged twenty-three years.

December 28, 1916: Admitted to the surgical ward from medical ward with post-pneumonic empyema. Temperature, 102°. Originally admitted to Doctor Deaver's service, October 6, 1916, with diagnosis of syphilis, having contracted mixed chancre about one month previously, followed in two weeks by suppurative left inguinal adenitis, there being unhealed sinuses here on admission. November 6th, transferred to medical ward (Dr. A. A. Stevens) for constitutional treatment for syphilis, local lesions being under control.

December 4, 1916: Developed pneumonia at base of left lung.

December 15, 1916: Temperature falling by lysis.

December 18, 1916: Temperature has not reached normal. Signs of fluid; 100 c.c. of cloudy fluid at second puncture, at angle of scapula. (Culture, pneumococcus.)

December 21, 1916: Flatness extends almost to spine of scapula; heart displaced 2.5 cm. toward right.

December 23, 1916: On puncture a small amount of pus recovered from depth at left scapular angle. (Culture, diplococci.)

December 25, 1916: No improvement.

December 27, 1916: Temperature slightly higher (101°–103° since December 24th).

December 28, 1916: Transferred to surgical ward (Doctor Ashhurst) with diagnosis of empyema.

December 29, 1916: In medical ward many weeks with pneumonia, after this temperature reached normal, then rose again and for a couple of weeks has been high and irregular. Five recent punctures negative where signs indicated fluid. Yesterday puncture in eighth interspace below angle of scapula drew 40 c.c. pus (pneumococcus).

Operation.—Eucain, 1 per cent. Patient prone. Resected 5 cm. of eighth or ninth left rib and pus oozed before it was removed; pleura nevertheless thick (2 mm.); pus thick, creamy, many curds. Cavity about 8 to 10 cm. in diameter on diaphragm and against costal pleura. Burrowing in adhesions opened *another pocket of pus* above and against ribs. Cavity extended upward toward interlobar region. Lower lobe densely adherent to diaphragm at one point, loose all around. This piece of lung was dissected from diaphragm. Considerable complaint and coughing when costal pleura was rubbed in burrowings, but lung and diaphragm insentitive. Drain: rubber tube and iodoform gauze. No ligatures. No sutures.

January 15, 1917: Drainage lessening.

February 2, 1917: No discharge. Temperature normal. Wound granulating. Up and about ward.

February 9, 1917: Discharged.

52

OBSERVATIONS ON EMPYEMA

February, 1920: The Swedish Consul at Philadelphia reports that this patient was last seen by him about one year ago, apparently in good health.

CASE XXX.—Empyema, left. Died after five weeks (sepsis from thoracic wound). Robert S., aged seven years.

January 17, 1917: Admitted to the Episcopal Hospital, Doctor Ashhurst's service. Had had pains in left side and stomach for a week or ten days; January 5th took his bed; vomited; had cough, chills and high fever. Treated at home for twelve days for bronchopneumonia. Family physician diagnosed empyema following pneumonia.

January 17, 1917: On admission, an anæmic, poorly nourished boy. Has incomplete cleft of palate; had operation for harelip as infant. Expansion of left chest limited. Palpation negative, dulness and distant breath sounds. *Puncture negative.*

January 18, 1917: Operation (Doctor Ashhurst)—eucain, 1 per cent. Patient prone. Resected 4 cm. left eleventh rib, posteriorly. Opened pleura, flood of reddish brown pus (culture, diplococci). Tube passed upward four inches and held in by silkworm-gut suture. Lung could not be felt. Time, fifteen minutes.

January 23, 1917: Temperature normal until to-day. Tube removed. Out of bed.

January 25, 1917: Draining slightly. Temperature normal to 100° since removal of tube.

January 26, 1917: Up in chair all day, no discharge.

January 27, 1917: Wound healing well.

January 31, 1917: Temperature rose to 104° suddenly. Transferred to Doctor Mutschler's service.

February 2, 1917: Vomits, no drainage. Temperature, 100°–103°.

February 3, 1917: Wound explored with hæmostat and several ounces of pus obtained. Tube replaced. Temperature fell to normal.

February 5, 1917: Draining well.

February 7, 1917: In good general condition. Temperature normal. Slight drainage of purulent fluid from tube. Cavity irrigated with normal saline. This causes some pain. Fluid comes back clear. Temperature rose to 100°/₂°.

February 9, 1917: Appetite excellent, only slight discharge, but child is fretful and nervous. Daily irrigations.

February 12, 1917: Temperature, 98°–100°.

February 15, 1917: Temperature rose suddenly to 103° and continued hectic 100°–104° until death, February 23. Daily irrigations.

February 18, 1917: Septic temperature with sweats. No chills. Vomited. Unproductive cough. Small area of cellulitis around drainage tract with extreme tenderness. Chest negative, but no pus draining. Pulse rate now 120–140, formerly 80. Respiration, 28–32, formerly 20. Slightly impaired percussion note over left chest posteriorly, two punctures negative. Irrigations continued.

February 20, 1917: No drainage. Unable to sit up without support, will not eat. Vomits at intervals. A maculo-papular rash like measles over trunk and extremities. Throat negative. Irrigations continued.

February 21, 1917: Sweats, paroxysms of vomiting without other abdominal signs or symptoms, anorexia and increasing weakness continue.

February 22, 1917: Irrigated. Tract is open, but there is no drainage. Marked abdominal distention but no pain or rigidity. Rash still present. Temperature falling.

February 23, 1917: Died with acute dilatation of heart, 11:30 A.M. Temperature subnormal. Cause of death: Sepsis from wound of thoracic wall.

CASE XXXI.—Empyema, right. Died (sepsis from thoracic wound). Stanley K., aged nine years.

January 15, 1917: Admitted to the Episcopal Hospital, Doctor Ashhurst's service. Present illness began December 24, 1916, with chill, fever, vomiting and jaundice. Four days later, pain in right side radiating to shoulder and to left chest, finally localized to right costal margin. Short of breath and breathing pained him. Was treated for lobar pneumonia. Two days before admission mother noticed right chest was swollen, called doctor's attention to it, and he found pus on puncture.

On admission, right lower chest had interspaces obliterated, flat, absent breath sounds, apparently massive empyema, two punctures in axilla, negative, but pus found below angle of scapula (Doctor Spruance, ward surgeon); 200 c.c. pus removed by puncture. Smear and culture negative. Polynuclears, 55 per cent.; lymphocytes, 45 per cent.; temperature, 101²/₆° F.; pulse, 160; respiration, 42.

January 16, 1917: Operation (Doctor Ashhurst)—eucain, 1 per cent. Patient prone. Resected 4 cm. of eleventh right rib. Pleura opened just above its reflection on to diaphragm. No pus found here. Inserted finger and in adhesions above tenth rib, close to spine, got a gush of pus (culture, negative). Pus reddish brown, no curds. Cavity runs up spinal gutter as far and as wide as finger can reach. Inserted rubber tube upward 10 cm. and more pus then spurted when he coughed. (One litre in all.)

January 21, 1917: Draining considerably.

January 22, 1917: Tube removed.

January 25, 1917: Still draining. Out of bed on house diet. Temperature, 99°-100°.

January 26 to 31, 1917: Temperature, 99°-103°. Pus probably dammed up.

January 31, 1917: Transferred to Doctor Mutschler's service.

February 1, 1917: Wound closed. Temperature irregular.

February 1 to 5, 1917: Temperature, 99°-103° F.

February 7, 1917: Operation wound granulating, no discharge. On deep inspiration (which brings on coughing) there is limitation of expansion on right side above. Tactile fremitus absent and breath sounds distant in right scapular region. At right base many moist bubbling râles. Percussion note hyperresonant except in scapular region where it is flat.

February 6 to 8, 1917: Temperature, 99°-102°.

February 8, 1917: Finger inserted in old sinus (no anæsthetic) base of lung felt to crepitate and expand with inspiration. Adhesions bound an area from the ninth rib above, in front by posterior axillary line, below by diaphragm. These adhesions cannot be broken by gentle pressure and more is not attempted because of fear of pleural reflex. Temperature fell from 102° to 99°.

February 10, 1917: Dyspnœa increasing. Drenching sweats twice daily. Well-defined area of flatness extending from scapular spine to its angle and as far forward as mid-axilla. Puncture in sixth interspace at angle of scapula, and creamy purulent fluid is withdrawn about the consistency of molasses in March. A second futile attempt is made to drain this encysted collection of pus through the old incision.

February 9 to 12, 1917: Temperature, 99°-101° F.

February 12, 1917: General condition excellent.

February 13, 1917: Operation (Doctor Mutschler)—ether; 3 cm. of seventh right rib resected in mid-scapular line, and 2 oz. (60 c.c.) of creamy, purulent, viscid fluid evacuated. Pleural cavity is then irrigated with sterile water until latter comes away clear. Rubber tube inserted 6 cm., stitched to skin by silkworm gut. Incision is then closed with interrupted silkworm-gut sutures and dressing applied. On return to ward able to breathe comfortably in recumbent position.

February 14, 1917: Dressings soaked with purulent blood-stained discharge. Old tract has definitely closed. Pleural cavity is irrigated with warm normal saline solution, injected through rubber drain tube and again withdrawn.

February 15, 1917: Dressings and irrigation repeated. Unable to sit up without excruciating pain in right scapular region. The wound is draining well, but temperature continues elevated (100°-103°).

February 17, 1917: Drainage less. Well-defined area of induration, redness, tenderness, swelling and œdema around drainage tube. Irrigation is followed by a fit of coughing and fluid expelled is seen to contain small pieces of coagulated exudate.

OBSERVATIONS ON EMPYEMA

February 17 to 20, 1917: Temperature, 100°-104°, and so on until death, February 25.

February 19, 1917: Pulse feeble, rapid but regular. Vomited. Takes liquids sparingly, no food. Macular rash, coppery in color, over limbs and trunk. Is evidently exceedingly toxic, wound drains little. Rubber tube removed, irrigation performed. Percussion note is resonant to level of ninth rib, below this there is flatness, with distant breath sounds. Puncture in ninth interspace causes no pain, clear, colorless fluid, evidently residue of irrigating fluid, is withdrawn; contains small fragments of floating exudate.

February 20. Obviously very ill. No appetite, listless all day long. Area of cellulitis around tube is larger. Movements are painful, as if they involve the muscles in this area. Sutures removed.

February 24, 1917: Vomited large quantity of greenish material. Dyspnœic, toxic, dull and drowsy. Toward evening cyanotic.

February 25, 1917: Died, 3:30 A.M. Cause of death: Sepsis from wound in thoracic wall.

CASE XXXII.—Empyema, right. Recovered. Whitman L., aged forty-six years.

January 3, 1917: Admitted to the Episcopal Hospital, Doctor Stevens's service. Has had a cough for years. Last evening was taken with chills and sweats, vomiting and severe headache. This morning had general pains and pain on inspiration in right chest. Typical pneumonia at right base.

January 12, 1917: Signs of fluid at right base. Temperature has never reached normal (99°-101°).

January 14, 1917: Developed bilateral suppurative otitis media. Paracentesis of right chest negative.

January 17, 1917: Temperature rising (101°-103°). Still signs of fluid at right base. Is not septic.

January 22, 1917: Signs of fluid at right base, puncture gave pus (culture and smear, diplo-bacillus).

January 23, 1917: Puncture draws 250 c.c. creamy pus.

January 24, 1917: Transferred to surgical service (Doctor Ashhurst). Operation (Doctor Ashhurst)—eucain, 1 per cent. Patient prone. Resected 4 cm. of eleventh rib, found very much thickened pleura, cut through it and exposed fibres of diaphragm. Then cut higher in pleura (costo-phrenic sinus) and opened pleural cavity whence over 500 c.c. of pus was discharged, creamy, inodorous. (Culture, diplococcus and pneumococcus?) Diaphragm not sensitive, costal pleura very sensitive. Cavity extends up and back beyond reach of finger. Drain: large rubber tube up for 10-12 cm.

January 26, 1917: Drainage almost stopped. Sat up in chair awhile.

January 31, 1917: Still draining profusely. Temperature normal ever since operation.

February 10, 1917: Less drainage. Learning to walk.

February 12, 1917: Tube removed.

February 17, 1917: Went home.

February 29, 1920: Wound healed firmly four weeks after leaving hospital. No disability. Lungs normal.

CASE XXXIII.—Empyema, right. Recovered. John B.; aged twenty-six years.

January 10, 1917: Admitted to the Episcopal Hospital, Doctor Stevens's service. Illness began January 4th with chill and sweat, and pain in right side; has had sweat almost every night. On admission exceedingly toxic and sick, entire body deeply jaundiced. Cyanosis of finger tips. Pneumonia at base of right lung.

January 12, 1917: Has been markedly delirious. Strapped to bed. Temperature low, never up to 101°, evidently poor reaction.

January 16, 1917: Rational. Jaundice subsiding.

January 23, 1917: Signs of fluid at right base (apical pneumonia). Puncture gives pus. Temperature, 101°-103° since January 21st.

55

ASTLEY P. C. ASHHURST

January 24, 1917: Transferred to surgical ward (Doctor Ashhurst). Operation—eucain, 1 per cent. Patient prone. Resected 4 cm. of eleventh rib, pleura thickened, pus gushed on opening it. Finger introduced found opening at lowest limit of cavity, which extended up and back beyond reach of finger, limited in front and below by the attachments of diaphragm. About 1 litre of curdy yellow pus evacuated (culture, pneumococcus) and drains profusely when tube is inserted, up 10–12 cm. along spine.

January 26, 1917: Drainage almost stopped. Sat up in chair awhile.

January 31, 1917: Still draining profusely.

February 6, 1917: Sits up each day. Temperature, 98°–102°.

February 12, 1917: Tube removed, temperature having reached normal.

February 18, 1917: Discharged. Temperature normal since last note. Patient not traced.

CASE XXXIV.—Empyema, right. Recovered. William D., aged sixteen years.

January 9, 1917: Admitted to the Episcopal Hospital, Doctor Stevens's service. Chief complaint: pain in right chest worse on coughing and on deep inspiration. Temperature, 103°. Onset January 5th with chill and sweat; cough, blood-stained sputa; headache and weakness. Excessively ill with typical lobar pneumonia, right middle lobe.

January 11, 1917: Type II pneumococcus reported in sputum.

January 12, 1917: Pericardial friction sounds. Very toxic. Abdomen markedly distended. Temperature fell by crisis to 99°.

January 16, 1917: Temperature has gradually risen again to 103° F. Pneumonia at left base.

January 21, 1917: Still very ill. Temperature irregular, 100°–103°. Sweats at night. Signs suggestive of fluid at right base. Consolidation at left base.

January 25, 1917: 250 c.c. pus drawn by puncture in ninth interspace, posterior right side.

January 26, 1917: Transferred to surgical service (Doctor Ashhurst). Temperature fell to normal after puncture. Is blue, thin, anæmic. Right chest (lower) is flat, distant breath sounds, somewhat diminished fremitus.

Operation (Doctor Ashhurst).—Eucain, 1 per cent. (10 c.c. only). Patient prone. Resected 4 cm. of eleventh right rib, pus oozed before rib was resected. About 500 c.c. creamy yellow pus evacuated. (Culture, diplococcus, pneumococcus.) Finger introduced felt no lung or adhesions. Opening was at bottom of coto-phrenic sinus. Large rubber tube passed up 8–10 cm. and held to upper skin margin by silkworm-gut suture. Time, ten minutes.

January 27, 1917: Temperature normal.

January 31, 1917: Temperature irregular, 98°–102°.

February 3, 1917: Still draining freely.

February 6, 1917: Out of bed daily. Temperature still irregular.

February 12, 1917: Smaller tube inserted.

February 18, 1917: Temperature normal. Free drainage. Learning to walk.

February 19, 1917: Tube removed.

February 21, 1917: Wound closes between daily dressings, damming up a few drops of pus.

February 22, 1917: Small tube reinserted. Went home.

February 21, 1920: Three years after operation. Scar has remained healed since discharge from hospital. Then weight was eighty pounds. In four weeks it reached one hundred and fourteen pounds, and is now steady at one hundred and twenty pounds. Went to State Sanitorium for Tuberculosis on discharge and remained there for nearly a year. Lungs are normal on examination, except slightly distant breath sounds over right chest posteriorly. Chest expands normally. Well-developed chest. No deformity. Rib has reformed. Some evidence of old endocarditis audible, and gets out of breath easily, but able to do a man's work.

OBSERVATIONS ON EMPYEMA

CASE XXXV.—Empyema, right (two distinct encysted empyemas). Recovered. Edward H., aged thirty-two years.

April 7, 1917: Admitted to the Episcopal Hospital, Doctor Ashhurst's service. Referred by Dr. H. R. M. Landis. Taken ill ten weeks ago. Diagnosis: pneumonia, right. Sent to a hospital and after about seven weeks as he did not get well they said he was tuberculous (called it "unresolved pneumonia") and sent him to White Haven, Pa. Seen there March 17, 1917 (three weeks ago), by Doctor Landis, who drew off a quantity of *sterile* pus, and referred him to Doctor Ashhurst.

Examination.—Emaciated, free expectoration of muco-pus (not fœtid). Right chest dull over lower lobe and signs of fluid. Needle drew from eighth interspace in posterior axillary line, 350 c.c. of pus (92 per cent. polynuclears; smear, negative).

April 8, 1917: Operation (Doctor Ashhurst)—eucain, 1 per cent. Resected 5 cm. of ninth right rib. Patient prone. The pleura much thickened (2–3 cm.). Spurting intercostal artery tied by suture, caused much pain, checked by eucain injection. On opening pleura pus escaped, from *thoroughly walled off abscess between diaphragm and lung.* Diaphragm felt normal, soft, depressible; and smooth liver palpable beneath it. The upper margin of cavity was formed by lung, densely adherent at periphery to costal pleura, just above ninth rib. Diaphragm rose to tenth rib. Supraphrenic abscess extended four inches toward dome of diaphragm. With much difficulty but *without causing any pain*, adhesions of lung to costal pleura were broken through by the fingers, first far posteriorly, and then lung was peeled off the costal pleura all the way front (here it was painful, under anterior costal margin, eighth, seventh and sixth ribs) (Fig. 21).

It was noted that the needle puncture which drew pus in the eighth interspace was above the level where the lung was adherent to the chest wall. *On detaching the lung a perfect flood of pus (over 500 c.c.) came from above, from between the lung and ribs;* this cavity extended up as far as finger could reach. (Culture, diplococcus.)

Drain: rubber tube between lung and diaphragm and another (2 cm. lumen) between lung and costal pleura, running up toward apex 15 cm. Iodoform gauze stuffed in wound between these two tubes to hold margin of consolidated lung away from wound and convert the two abscess cavities into one. Wound not sutured (12.5 cm. incision). Time, thirty minutes.

May 27, 1917: Uneventful convalescence. Wound has been merely moist for last two weeks.

June 3, 1917: Went home. Wound now closed for a week with normal temperature, though up to then small tube entered six inches easily. Weight, one hundred and fifty pounds, gain of twenty-three pounds in eight weeks since operation. Breath sounds normal. No symptoms. Right chest moderately contracted in front.

July 6, 1917: Reports he will return to work in one week.

November, 1917: Sinus discharged but healed in three weeks.

February, 1919: Empyema formed again and another operation, 5 cm. above former operation, done by Doctor Schell at Northwestern General Hospital. Recovered. Weight, one hundred and seventy pounds.

September, 1919: Moved to Denver. Since then one reaccumulation was opened; healed in six weeks.

March, 1920: Weight, one hundred and seventy pounds. Excellent health, no symptoms of tuberculosis, working every day.

CASE XXXVI.—Empyema, right, encapsulated. Recovered. Oliver C., aged twenty-one years.

July 9, 1919: Admitted to the Episcopal Hospital, Doctor Robertson's service. Ill since July 7th, typical pneumonia. Chief complaint is pain in right chest and shortness of breath. On awakening in morning had chill, became feverish and dyspnœic, and developed pain in right chest on inspiration. On admission: signs of pleuropneumonia at right base. Temperature 100°–102°. Thought to have fluid, but puncture negative.

July 12, 1919: Puncture in posterior axillary line is negative.

July 14, 1919: Consolidation also of left base.

July 15, 1919: Pleuro-pericardial friction sounds on left.

July 24, 1919: Temperature continues 99°–103°.

July 25, 1919: Temperature declined by lysis, yesterday shot up again to 103°. Needle in ninth interspace in scapular line drew 350 c.c. pus. (Culture, pneumococci.) Transferred to surgical service (Doctor Ashhurst).

July 26, 1919: Right empyema encapsulated between lung and diaphragm. Operation (Doctor Ashhurst)—novocain, ¼ per cent. Excision of 5 cm. of tenth rib. Costal pleura normal but adhesions of lung to costal pleura above and in front of opening, and lung adherent to diaphragm. Could not be separated by fingers. Packed. Lung cut loose from diaphragm by scissors; 150 c.c. yellow, creamy pus. Tube and gauze wick. A few whiffs of ether toward end. Diaphragm felt normal for 5 cm. from ribs, then felt hard; this part was adherent lung.

August 3, 1919: Temperature has reached normal. Little discharge.

August 13, 1919: Tube removed. Has been up in chair several days and rapidly getting fat.

August 14, 1919: Temperature shot up to 103°. Tube replaced.

August 18, 1919: Last night and night before had chills; resident's attempts to get tube in far enough apparently ineffectual. Therefore, to-day, under gas, Doctor Ashhurst put finger into sinus, and found lung again adherent to diaphragm, and tore it loose, giving exit to bloody pus; and put tube again deep in wound, almost to dome of diaphragm.

August 25, 1919: Temperature has gradually reached normal. No discharge.

September 5, 1919: Tube removed. No discharge.

September 6, 1919: Temperature shot up to 103°. Tube replaced.

September 8, 1919: Temperature normal.

September 14, 1919: Tube removed.

September 15, 1919: Temperature shot up to 102°. Tube replaced.

September 17, 1919: Temperature normal. No discharge.

September 20, 1919: Out of bed.

September 27, 1919: Temperature stays normal, but sinus does not heal, though there is practically no discharge. Tube retained.

October 10, 1919: Tube shortened.

October 15, 1919: Tube removed and gauze wick inserted.

October 21, 1919: Bismuth paste injected to determine size of empyema cavity. X-ray shows sinus extends up to fifth rib anteriorly. (X-ray 1224 D.)

October 25, 1919: No discharge from wound since injection of bismuth.

October 30, 1919: Wound is firmly healed. Went home.

November 17, 1919: Returns on visit. Still healed. No symptoms.

February 29, 1920: Weight, one hundred and seventy pounds (one hundred and twenty-seven pounds on leaving hospital). Went to work the day after discharge from ward, and has been at work ever since. No disability. Lungs normal, except distant breath sounds at right base posteriorly. The rib has not yet reformed.

CASE XXXVII.—Empyema, right, massive. Recovered. Isador M., aged eleven years.

August 4, 1919: Admitted to the Episcopal Hospital, Doctor Robertson's service. Onset July 31st. On admission very ill, lobar pneumonia at right apex.

August 6, 1919: Puncture at angle of scapula gives 12 c.c. turbid fluid.

August 8, 1919: Puncture in axilla through fourth interspace and at angle of scapula in eighth interspace; 3 c.c. of slightly turbid pus obtained from each. Patient is better.

August 9, 1919: Puncture just lateral to angle of scapula gave 500 c.c. thick green pus. Much better after evacuation.

August 12, 1919: Puncture gives 350 c.c. of green pus. Temperature declining by lysis. Smear shows diplococci of pneumococcus type.

August 14, 1919: Temperature, 98°-102°.

August 16, 1919: Puncture gives 250 c.c. of pus, very thick and green; 20 c.c. of formalin in glycerine injected. Temperature fell from 103° to 99°.

August 18, 1919: No change. Examination by Doctor Ashhurst. Skodaic resonance over right apex anteriorly; interspaces on right side of chest obliterated. Dull in axilla and posterior to line of nipple, and posteriorly dull below the fourth interspace except close to vertebral column. Breath sounds distant. Post-pneumonic empyema. Duration, ten days. Transferred to surgical service (Doctor Ashhurst).

Operation (Doctor Ashhurst)—novocain, ¼ per cent. Resection of 4 cm. of tenth right rib posteriorly. One litre of pus (culture, pneumococci) evacuated on opening pleura. The cavity extended from diaphragm as high as finger could reach and also between diaphragm and lung (Fig. 22). Diaphragm was covered with thick gray slough, and the lower lobe of the lung stood out surrounded by pus on both phrenic and costal surfaces.

August 22, 1919: Free drainage. Doing very well.

September 1, 1919: Wound closing. Less discharge.

September 9, 1919: Tube removed.

September 13, 1919: Incision healed. Sent home.

March 21, 1920: Seven months after operation. Has gained fourteen pounds in weight since leaving hospital—present weight, eighty-three pounds. Lungs are normal, and rib appears to have reformed.

CASE XXXVIII.—Empyema, right. Recovered. Evelyn S., aged nineteen years.

November 16, 1919: Admitted to the Episcopal Hospital, Doctor Ashhurst's service. Sent from Philadelphia Hospital for Contagious Diseases, where she was taken October 31st for suspected diphtheria.

October 29, 1919: Onset with sore throat and headache.

October 31, 1919: Taken to Hospital for Contagious Diseases.

November 5, 1919: Pain in right side. Dulness.

November 13, 1919: Evidences of fluid in right chest. Puncture drew 20 c.c. yellowish purulent fluid (sterile). Throat has given nine negative cultures, never a positive culture.

.   On admission, chief complaint is pain in both arms and back. There is subpectoral abscess below right clavicle. Patient emaciated and very septic. Temperature, 103° F.

November 17, 1919: Seen by Doctor Fussell, who advised aspiration over right base, where signs were suggestive of fluid.

November 18, 1919: Dulness and distant breath sounds over lower posterior chest. Puncture draws pus. Diagnosis: right empyema.

Operation (Doctor Ashhurst)—novocain ¼ per cent. Resection of 3 cm. of ninth rib, below angle of scapula. Pleura thickened; 250 c.c. of greenish yellow, creamy, malodorous pus evacuated (same as by aspiration). Culture, no growth. Smear, organisms like streptococci but smaller. Cavity extends backward to spine and upward beyond reach of finger. Rubber tube sutured in wound. Right subpectoral abscess to be treated later. Diaphragm came just to level of rib resection, and felt flat across top to spine, whole cavity appears rigid, and may require secondary operation for closure. Still very ill (Fig. 23).

November 19, 1919: Had a chill.

November 20, 1919: Improving, free drainage of pus.

November 22, 1919: More drainage than usual from tube. Subpectoral abscess much smaller. Still very annoying cough.

November 25, 1919: Second operation. Large abscess from beneath left scapula drained under local anæsthesia. (Smear, diplococci and staphylococci.) First sign of this abscess developed seventy-two hours previously. Still very ill.

November 30. The subpectoral abscess has refilled.

Third Operation.—100 c.c. of pus from beneath right pectoralis major drained under local anæsthesia. (Smear, diplococcus and bacillus. Culture, no growth.)

December 1, 1919: Better. Still coughing. Incision in left back almost healed.

December 20, 1919: Out of bed in wheel chair.

January 9, 1920: Tonsils removed under local anæsthesia.

January 28, 1919: All incisions now firmly healed; the last to close was that of subpectoral abscess. Empyema incision has been healed for two weeks. Went home to-day.

March 21, 1920. Four months after operation. Incision has remained closed. Is round-shouldered, with slight scoliosis convex to the left. Gets tired easily.

CASE XXXIX.—Empyema, right. Recovered. Gertrude W., aged four years.

December 5, 1919: Admitted to the Episcopal Hospital, Doctor Ashhurst's service. Had whooping-cough and influenza in fall of 1919. Four weeks ago she began vomiting; physician made a diagnosis of congestion of lungs. Later he diagnosed pleurisy. On admission, anæmic, run-down child, with respiratory embarrassment. Respiratory movements almost absent on right. There is markedly diminished tactile and vocal fremitus of whole right chest, anteriorly and posteriorly. Percussion shows flatness over entire right chest. Puncture draws 75 c.c. of thick, greenish pus.

December 6, 1919: Operation (Doctor Moore, ward surgeon)—novocain, 1 per cent. Resection of 3 cm. of right ninth rib below angle of scapula 100 c.c. pus evacuated. (Smear, diplococci and staphylococci. Culture, mixed.)

December 24, 1919: Rise in temperature. Longer tube inserted.

December 27, 1919: Temperature down.

December 29, 1919: Tube removed.

January 7, 1920: Rise of temperature for past three days; 300 c.c. pus evacuated by forceps in sinus. Tube replaced.

January 13, 1919: Temperature normal since replacing tube. Tube removed to-day.

January 22, 1919: Out of bed for four days. Sent home, with incision healed.

April 11, 1920: Four months after operation; in good health; lungs normal. About four weeks after leaving hospital became feverish, and family physician picked a scab off the incision and evacuated a little pus; firmly healed again in three or four days.

CASE XL.—Empyema, left. Recovered. Thomas W., aged sixteen months.

December 31, 1919: Admitted to the Episcopal Hospital, Doctor Carson's service. Eleven days ago child developed fever and cough; physician called, who diagnosed pneumonia. After convalescence fever recurred, and physician suspected empyema. On admission, there is limited expansion of left chest, no fremitus on palpation, and dulness over entire chest continuous with heart dulness. Hyperresonance over right lung. Heart displaced 2 cm. to right. Very slight change in breath, sounds are clear and distinct. Has a cough.

Puncture of left pleura gives 100 c.c. turbid straw-colored fluid, no odor. (Smear and culture show diplococci.)

January 2, 1920: Not sleeping well; dyspnœic. Pulse not so good. Puncture gives 250 c.c. turbid odorless greenish straw-colored fluid; some relief of dyspnœa.

January 4, 1920: Slightly better. Fluid collecting again.

January 7, 1920: Puncture gives 150 c.c. greenish yellow, turbid fluid, no odor. Gradually improving.

January 8, 1920: Restless and dyspnœic. Very irritable. Seen by Doctor Ashhurst in consultation. Transferred to his surgical service.

January 9, 1920: Operation (Doctor Ashhurst)—novocain, ¼ per cent. Resection of 2 cm. of tenth left rib, midscapular line. Pleura 25 mm. thick. Thin serous pus evacuated. Cavity extends as far as finger can reach. Tube drainage.

January 12, 1920: Temperature normal since yesterday.

January 14, 1920: Tube removed. No pus has drained since operation.

January 29, 1920: Temperature rose to 104° yesterday, after being nearly normal since last note; 10 c.c. of pus evacuated from sinus by inserting forceps. Then temperature fell to normal. Tube replaced.

January 31, 1920: Transferred to Doctor Neilson's service.

February 19, 1920: Temperature has been normal four days after another flare up relieved by evacuating a little pus.

February 25 to March 9, 1920: Temperature, 100°–102° F.

March 9, 1920: Not doing well. Septic temperature. Nothing definite in chest findings, but X-ray examination indicates presence of pus. Under ether anæsthesia Doctor Hawfield (chief resident physician) ran finger into sinus, but found no pus. Tube left in sinus.

March 12, 1920: Free discharge of pus.

March 20, 1920: Temperature normal for past week.

March 26, 1920: Sent home, with tube still in sinus.

April 2, 1920: Tube out. Tiny sinus.

April 9, 1920: Wound healed.

CASE XLI.—Empyema, right. Recovered. Alice M., aged twenty-nine years.

February 6, 1920: Admitted to the Episcopal Hospital, Dr. J. B. Carson's service. Chief complaint: pleurisy pains. Eight days ago was taken suddenly with chill and feverishness. Some cough. Three days ago severe pain in right chest, constant since that time. On admission, consolidation, base right lung, with skodaic resonance above.

February 8, 1920: Puncture of right chest gives 250 c.c. serous fluid. (Smear shows a streptodiplococcus, probably pneumococcus. Culture is contaminated.)

February 10, 1920: Condition fair. Temperature falling by lysis.

February 18, 1920: Temperature since February 12th has been rising gradually, and since the 14th has been 100°–103°. Transferred to surgical service of Doctor Mutschler.

February 20, 1920: Operation (Doctor Ashhurst)—novocain, ¼ per cent. Patient prone. Resection of 4 cm. of eleventh right rib. Nearly 500 c.c. of creamy, yellow pus evacuated upon opening pleura, which was 2 or 3 mm. thick. (Culture, pure pneumococci.) Finger introduced palpates no lung as high as it can reach. Opening is at a level of diaphragm, which is flat, not domed, as normally. Large tube drainage.

March 5, 1920: Tube replaced by smaller one. Very little discharge. Up and about ward. Temperature has slowly fallen to normal.

March 19, 1920: Up and about ward. Very little discharge.

March 30, 1920: Tube removed.

April 14, 1920: Went home, wound healed in several days.

CASE XLII.—Empyema, right. Recovered. Theresa D., aged twenty-seven years.

February 7, 1920: Admitted to the Episcopal Hospital, Doctor J. B. Carson's service. Chief complaint: cough, backache and pain in the chest. Husband has pneumonia and three children have influenza. Patient has been sick in bed four days. Has a nursing baby.

Examination.—Limitation of expansion and impaired resonance over left chest.

February 11, 1920: Improved.

February 14, 1920: Not so well.

February 15, 1920: Consolidation at right base.

February 18, 1920: Signs of fluid at right base. Two punctures negative; third puncture found sero-pus. (Culture, pneumococci.) Transferred to surgical service of Doctor Mutschler.

February 20, 1920: Examination by Doctor Ashhurst. Entire right chest posteriorly is flat from spine of scapula down to base, and breath sounds are distant.

Operation (Doctor Ashhurst)—novocain, ¼ per cent. Patient prone. Resection of 4 cm. of tenth right rib near its angle. Pleura slightly thickened. Upon opening

ANALYSIS OF 43 OPERATIONS FOR EMPYEMA

No.	Name, age, date of operation	Side affected	Duration of illness before operation, including a preceding pneumonia	Nature of pus; and culture	Massive or encapsulated	Operation and Anesthetic	Result	Sinus healed	Remarks
1	John C., 5 years Sept. 22, 1906	R	6 weeks +	Metapneumonic, pus	Massive	Eighth rib. Ether. Pus, creamy, pale yellow, sour	Recovered	Under 10 months	
2	Joseph S., 5 July 26, 1907	L	3 weeks +	Metapneumonic.	Massive	Eighth rib. Ether. Pus, thick, inodorous	Died	....	Death in 1 week from enteritis.
3	Ed. W., 11½ July 25, 1908	L	2 weeks +	Metapneumonic diplococci and streptococci	Massive	Eighth rib. Ether. 100 c.c. thick, creamy pus	Died	....	Death in 2 weeks from pneumonia of other lung.
4	Kath. P., 6 July 24, 90	L	4 weeks +	Metapneumonic, pneumococci	Massive	Intercostal incision, 7th interspace; pus 500 c.c. Ether. Rib resected 1 month later	Died	....	Death in 2 months from sepsis.
5	Jos. T., 6 years July 24, 1909	L	5 weeks +	Metapneumonic. culture (?)	Massive	Eighth rib. Ether. Sad rib 90 c.c. and 1 mh l ter	Recovered	Over 9 months	
6	Elisa R., 3 yrs July 30, 1909	L	5 weeks +	Metapneumonic. culture (?)	Massive—"Necessitatis;" parietal	Sixth rib. Ether, 500 c.c. my ps	Recovered	?	Not traced.
7	Sam. S., 5 years July 30, 1909	L	11 days	Metapneumonic. mixed (colon)	Encapsulated, parietal	Eighth rib. Ether; Pus, thin ad fœld; do	Recovered	?	Not traced.
8	Wm. L., 50 years Sept. 14, 1912	R	2 months +	Metapneumonic	Encapsulated, interlobar, discharging through bronchus	Big hb ad 8h ribs. B sin 30.c.c. fœld pus	Died	....	Death in 2 days from sepsis.
9	Mic Y., 50 years Dec. 25, 1912	L	10 days	Metapneumonic, pus	Encapsulated, parietal	'Bth. rib. Gn. Semi-solid pus	Died	....	Death in 6 days from bed-sores, etc.
10	Mary OB., 5 years Jan. 22, 1913	L	2 weeks	Metapneumonic. pneumococcus	Massive	Ninth rib. Ether, 200 c.c. yellow, curdy pus	Recovered	8 weeks [1]	
11	Jno P., 7 years Feb. 14, 1913	L	3½ weeks	Metapneumonic. pus	Massive	Eleventh rib. Ether 500 c.c. yellow, creamy and curdy pus	Recovered	3½ months	
12	Walker H., 15 years Aug. 26, 1913	L	10 months	Tuberculous. Smear; micrococci Culture: no growth	Massive	Eleventh rib. Ether. Greenish pus	Recovered	4 weeks [1]	
13	Edna P., 7 yrs Ag. 27, 1913	L	6 weeks	Meta pne mo nic, diplococcus	Massive	Intercostal incision, 6th interspace. Eighth and ninth ribs resected 2 months later; bloody pus	Recovered	4 months after intercostal incision. 8 weeks after rib resection. [1]	
14	Margaret P., 12 years Nov. 1, 1914	L	12 days	Followed peritonitis (appendicitis?). streptococcus	Massive	Eighth rib. Gas. 150 c.c. pus. Later, drainage of intraperitoneal pelvic abscess	Recovered	10 weeks [1]	Streptococcus grown from blood. Also metastatic osteomyelitis of phalanx (staphylococci) and furunculosis

62

15	Hugh McI., 43 years, Nov. 8, 1914	R	4 weeks	Metapneumonic, pneumococcus	Encapsulated, parietal	Ninth rib. Eucain	Recovered	?	In good health one year later.
16	Joseph R., 19 years, Dec. 4, 1914	L	3 weeks	Metapneumonic, diplococci	Encapsulated, 2 parietal empyemata	Eighth rib. Eucain	Recovered	?	Tube fell into cavity after operation.
17	Gerald L., 28 mos., Dec. 11, 1914	L	3	Tuberculous for 7 years. Streptococcus	Massive, pulsating empyema necessitatis	Ninth rib. Eucain. Prune-juice pus smelling of hydrogen sulphide	Recovered	?	Not traced.
18	Tony V., 2 mos., Mr. 23, 1915	R	5 weeks +	Metapneumonic, streptococcus and staphylococcus	Encapsulated, inter-lobar	Seventh rib. Ether	Recovered	10 weeks¹	In good health 1 year later.
19	Joseph P., 9 years, Nov. 30, 1915	R	17 days	Metapneumonic, mixed (colon)	Massive	16th rib. Gas. 500 c.c. oloni smiling pus	Recovered	9 weeks	In good health 9 mos. later.
20	Francis P., 11 mos., Dec. 3, 1915	R	2½ weeks	Metapneumonic, streptococci, diplococci, staphylococci	Massive	Seventh rib. Ether. 90 c.c. pu. 7 wks later each rib. 150 c.c. tin fetid pus (streptococci oly)	Recovered	5 months (3 months after second operation)	In good health 1 year later.
21	Joseph B., 34 years, Dec. 10, 1915	L	3 weeks +	Metapneumonic, staphylococcus	Encapsulated, parietal, empyema necessitatis with independent pleural effusion	Eleh rib. del, 300 c.c. Red heal seventh thick yellow inod pus	Recovered	7 weeks	In good health 9 months later.
22	Edward S., 7 years, Dec. 11, 1915	R	3 weeks +	Metapneumonic, staphylococcus	Massive	Eighth rib. Gas	Died	1	Death 1½ days from noma of mouth.
23	James C., 3 years, Jan. 7, 1916	L	3 weeks +	Metapneumonic, pneumococcus	M ise	Tenth rib. Esther. 250 c.c. creamy pus	Recovered	9 weeks¹	Measles during convalescence. In good health 7 months later.
24	Philip G., 14 years, Jan. 14, 1916	L	4 weeks	Metapneumonic, tpus	lovi c, even ing ad be- diaphragm	Tenth rib. Novocain and gas. 500 c.c.	Recovered	7 months	Streptococcus from blood. In good health 4 years later.
25	Wm. B., 30 years, Jan. 14, 1916	R	9 weeks +	Metapneumonic, gus	B ted, in-stir	Ninth rib	Recovered	3 weeks¹	Not traced.
26	Kate D., 38 years, Aug. 5, 1916	L	6 weeks +	Metapneumonic, McC	E ter-lobar ted, in-gi- against	Se 8th ad 9th ribs. , dain	Died	1	Death 8 days, unrelieved. Pus not found at operation.
27	James McG., 30 years, Nov. 17, 1916	L	3 weeks	var ad culture, ito Mc	Encapsulated, between lung ad diaphragm	N ith and tenth ribs. ain	Recovered	5 weeks¹	In good health 3½ years later.
28	Wm. B., 20 years, Nov. 17, 1916	L	4 weeks	Mc gal	Encapsulated, inter-lobar ad	9th and fifth ribs. Eucain	Recovered	Over 4 months	In good health 3½ years later.
29	John L., 23 years, Dec. 20, 1916	L	3½ weeks	Metapneumonic, p	Encapsulated, two spto empyemata, both parietal	Ninth rib. Eucain	Recovered	7 weeks¹	In good health 3 years later.
30	Stanley K., 9 years, Jan. 10, 1917	R	3 weeks +	Metapneumonic, igja	M ise	Eleventh rib. Eucain. Reddish-brown pus	Died	1	

¹ Patients who continued under writer's supervision until death or healing of sinus.

ANALYSIS OF 43 OPERATIONS FOR EMPYEMA—Continued

No.	Name, age, date of operation	Side affected	Duration of illness before operation, including a preceding pneumonia	Metapneumonic or Tuberculous; and Culture	Massive or Encapsulated	Operation and Anæsthetic	Result	Sinus healed	Remarks
31	Robt. Smith, 7 ys Jan. 8, 1917	L	3 weeks+	Metapneumonic, negative	Massive	Eleventh rib. Eucain. Reddish-brown pus	Died		
32	Wm. L., 46 Jan. 24, 1917	R	3 weeks+	Metapneumonic, diplobacillus	Massive	Eleventh rib. Eucain. 250 c.c. creamy nauseous pus	Recovered	7 weeks¹	In good health 3 years later.
33	John B., 26 years Jan. 24, 1917	R	2 weeks+	Metapneumonic, pneumococcus	Massive	Eleventh rib. Eucain. 90 c.c. dly ylw pus	Recovered	Not traced	Desperately ill before operation (jaundiced).
34	Wm. D., 16 ys Jan. 26, 1917	R	3 weeks	Metapneumonic, pneumococcus	Massive	El with rib. Eucain. 90 c.c. creamy yellow pus	Recovered	6 weeks¹	Desperately ill before operation (bilateral pleuritis, endocarditis, and pericarditis). In good health 3 years later.
35	Edward H., 32 years April 8, 1917	R	10 weeks+	Tuberculous-metapneumonic diplococcus	Encapsulated, two distinct empyemata; (1) between lung and diaphragm; (2) parietal	Ninth rib. Eucain.	Recovered	7 weeks¹	No 1 years 1 r. (·ies in G. rado.)
36	Oliver C., 21 years July 26, 1919	R	3 weeks	Metapneumonic, pneumococcus	Encapsulated between lung and diaphragm	Tenth rib. Novocain. 150 c.c. creamy yellow pus	Recovered	12 weeks¹	In good health 8 the ter.
37	Isadore M. 11 years Aug. 18, 1919	R	19 days	Metapneumonic, pneumococcus	Massive—"Hour-glass empyema."	Tenth rib. Novocain. 1000 c.c. pus	Recovered	3½ weeks¹	In gd Wh 7 months tdr.
38	Evelyn S., 19 years Nov. 18, 1919	R	3 weeks	Metapneumonic, streptococci	Massive—"Hour-glass empyema necessitatis"	Ninth rib. Novocain. 250 c.c. yellow, creamy malodorous pus	Recovered	8 weeks¹	gy ill before. Nc ab- ss tr L. pus during convalescence. In fl ... Mo
39	Gertrude W., 4 years Dec. 6, 1919	R	4 weeks	Metapneumonic, diplococci and staphylococci	Massive	Ninth rib. Novocain. 100 c.c. pus	Recovered	6 weeks¹	In gd hlth 4 this tdr.
40	Thos. W., 16 months Jan. 9, 1920	L	3 weeks	Metapneumonic, pneumococci	Massive	Tenth rib. Novocain. Thin serous pus	Recovered	13 weeks	
41	Alice M., 29 years Feb. 20, 1920	R	3 weeks	Metapneumonic, pneumococci	Massive	Eleventh rib. Novocain. 500 c.c. creamy yellow pus	Recovered	7½ weeks¹	
42	Theresa D., 27 years Feb. 20, 1920	L	17 days	Metapneumonic, pneumococci	Massive	Tenth rib. Novocain. 900 c.c. thin turbid flaky pus	Recovered	7½ weeks¹	
43	James S., 34 years April 9, 1920	L	8 weeks	Metapneumonic, pneumococci	Massive—"Hour-glass empyema."	Tenth rib. Novocain. 1000 c.c. greenish-yellow creamy pus	Recovered		

¹Patients who continued under writer's supervision until death or healing of sinus.

it, thin turbid pus discharges, with some flakes of lymph, nearly 500 c.c. Finger introduced feels expanding lung, not bound down by adhesions. Large tube drain.

March 5, 1920: Tube replaced by smaller and shorter. Temperature normal ever since operation. .

March 19, 1920: Up and about ward. Very little discharge.

April 10, 1920: Tube removed.

April 14, 1920: Went home, wound healed.

CASE XLII.—Empyema, left. Recovered. James S., aged thirty-four years.

April 7, 1920: Admitted to the Episcopal Hospital, Doctor Hopkins's service. Onset February 6th, with influenza, followed by pneumonia with crisis in eight days. Did not get well. Thought by family physician to have tuberculosis. Two aspirations at home four weeks ago in posterior axillary line, left side, were negative.

April 8, 1920: Aspiration showed thick creamy pus. Aspirated in seventh interspace, posterior axillary line. Transferred to surgical service (Doctor Ashhurst).

April 9, 1920: Operation (Doctor Ashhurst)—novocain. Resection of 4 cm. of tenth rib in scapular line. Pleura thickened. Pus spurted 2 metres on opening pleura, creamy, greenish yellow pus. About 2 litres removed. Exudate surrounding lung on costal and diaphragmatic surface (Fig. 22). Tube inserted and anchored with silkworm-gut.

April 23, 1920: Tube shortened.

April 30, 1920: Smaller tube inserted.

May 12, 1920: Tube removed.

May 15, 1920: Went home; granulating wound. No discharge.

June 14, 1920: Wound healed.

OPERATION FOR EMPYEMA IN YOUNG ADULTS *

By Frank E. Bunts, M.D.
of Cleveland, Ohio

The great prevalence of pneumonia in many of the United States cantonments and the resulting incidence of empyema, reaching as high as 10 per cent. in the base hospital to which I was assigned, brought to the surgical service about 175 cases for operation. I am not able at present to give the exact data, but certain clinical facts connected with this series of cases seem to be of special interest.

All cases naturally occurred in young adults of army registration age, and while this may have no bearing upon the results, yet it must be granted that they should by the mere fact of their youth and of their having been admitted to service after elaborate physical examinations, be presumed to be better risks than the average case in civil practice, and to avoid the possibility of inherent differences in the varied cases found in civil practice, I have designated them in a group as young adults.

I. *Classification.*—In concurrence with the Chief of the Medical Service, patients with fluid in the chest were divided into three classes:

(a) Those with clear fluid and no microörganisms present.

(b) Those with slightly turbid fluid and various bacteria—staphylococcus, colon bacillus, or streptococcus hæmolyticus—present.

(c) Those with frank yellow pus and with bacteria present.

II. *Recognition, Diagnosis.*—Physical examination often failed to reveal the location of the accumulated fluid, though its presence was practically certain. The use of the aspirating needle was freely resorted to and a considerable number of punctures were frequently made without successfully locating the fluid. This was due, to a considerable extent, to the fact that many of the accumulations were encapsulated, and partienlarly to the frequency of interlobar collections of pus.

To obviate the frequent and not always innocuous punctures, early use of the X-ray examination was made in cases able to endure such examination. This greatly simplified and rendered comparatively easy the detection of the location of the empyema, and where stereoscopic plates could be made, immensely facilitated operative procedures.

III. *Treatment.*—Class (a). These were aspirated by the physician in charge, or upon request, by one of the surgical staff, but were not transferred to the surgical service.

Class (b). These were transferred to the surgical service, aspirated under primary ether anæsthesia, and injected with a small amount of glycerine and formalin (2 per cent. solution). They were watched carefully from day to day, and a failure to show improvement or an increase in the

---

* Read before the American Surgical Association, May 3, 1920.

severity of their symptoms was followed by immediate operation. In the neighborhood of 16 cases were treated in this manner, of which six or seven recovered without operation. Inasmuch as an occasional case under this classification recovered in which aspiration without the injection of formalin was carried out, it is impossible to say that the latter was a curative agent in the others. All that can be said is that a number got well under its use, and that it did not seem to do any harm in any instance.

Class (c). These were all operated upon within twelve hours after their detection, except, and this I believe to be of importance, *those cases where the high fever and physical signs showed the pneumonia to be still active or invading the opposite side.* In these the fluid was aspirated, sometimes repeatedly, until the pneumonic symptoms abated, and then aspiration was proceeded with. It was a self-evident fact in these cases that the empyema was not the determining factor in the critical condition in which these patients found themselves, and a radical operation, or indeed, any operation other than aspiration, would materially lessen thir chance of recovery. This we found to be true, from serious clinical experience.

Anæsthetic.—I have read and heard much discussion regarding the proper anæsthetic to be used in these cases, some saying that only local anæsthesia should be used, and almost all condemning the use of ether. In a few of the very worst cases when it seemed from the greatly debilitated condition of the patient that no general anæsthetic would be tolerated, I used local anæsthesia alone, but in all the others primary ether anæsthesia was used, and, I believe, without any ill effects whatever; the patient being wide awake at the end of the operation. I have not seen severe coughing or respiratory embarrassments result from the proper administration of ether, and the temporary and transient loss of consciousness, I believe, to be an act of mercy to the patient.

Method of Operating.—Local anæsthesia over area of rib to be resected, followed by light primary anæsthesia and rapid incision and excision of bone, insertion of a long ¾-inch rubber drainage tube which was sutured into the wound, tight suturing of the wound about it and a clamp to the tube to prevent escape of fluid.

Subsequent Treatment.—The patient was put in a semi-recumbent position or the head of the bed elevated by blocks, and the tube end inserted into a drainage bottle containing some antiseptic fluid and attached to the side of the bed. The clamp on the tube was opened up for a few moments every half hour, allowing a small amount of fluid to escape until the chest cavity was evacuated and danger of sudden respiratory or circulatory changes eliminated. The clamp was then removed entirely and drainage allowed to continue. At the end of a week or ten days, rarely earlier, the cavity was washed out twice daily with varying solutions, such as iodine, sterile water, normal saline, boracic acid, formalin and glycerine, and at two-hour intervals when the Carrel-Dakin method was used. The large number of cases operated upon gave excellent opportunity to try

67

out a series with each method. In from one to two weeks, when the discharge had greatly diminished, the large tube was removed and progressively smaller short tubes inserted.

Blowing into a bottle was insisted upon in every case, but not until the *unaffected side had been carefully strapped with adhesive plaster in a manner similar to that used in fractured ribs*, the object being to prevent emphysema of the well lung, if possible, and to hasten the expansion of the collapsed lung.

As soon as the patient was able to be up, light setting-up drills and breathing exercises were instituted. Beds were moved out of the wards on to the porches, foods were administered as frequently and in as great quantity as the patient could take them. Heroin, and occasionally morphine, were given during the first two or three days for pain or cough, threatened œdema of the lungs was combated with digitalis, atropine and oxygen, and in the later stages, iron, usually in the form of the syrup of the iodide, was given.

IV. *Results.*—There was a mortality of approximately 13 per cent. This included every case operated upon, regardless of post-mortem findings. No deaths occurred immediately after operation, two days to three weeks being the subsequent range of life when death followed operation, depending upon complications resulting.

New accumulations of pus, usually interlobar, were sought for and found by the use of the X-ray before using the needle in those cases which did not clear up under treatment, and secondary operations were sometimes necessary for their evacuation.

No case required extensive rib resection (Estlander operation), decortication, or other procedure, for obliterating the chest cavity. Two-thirds of all the recovery cases were either in France with their regiments or temporarily in a convalescent hospital with the wounds healed, and at the time of my detachment from the base hospital there were none who were in a condition which would not admit of their early discharge to duty or to a convalescent hospital without further operation upon the chest.

Complications.—Infective arthritis occurred in a small number of cases. Pneumonia on the opposite side and occasionally empyema on the opposite side made serious and, in one or two instances, fatal complications. Endocarditis and myocarditis were rare occurrences.

Autopsies.—Until countermanded, autopsies were held on all deaths following empyema. The results of these examinations were most illuminating and valuable. *In not one case could we ascribe the death to empyema.* It was invariably found that the drainage, so far as the part attacked was concerned, was satisfactory, but the cause of the death was a pyæmia rather than an empyema, broken-down and suppurating bronchial and mediastinal glands, pus in the pericardium, pultaceous areas in the spleen, abscesses in the liver, multiple abscess in the lungs, and free pus

68

in the peritoneal cavity, gave evidence of the general rather than the local character of the condition. I was informed by a Chief of Service in one of the cantonments, that these cases were not classified as death from empyema, but rather from pyæmia. If this be a proper disposition of them, then the mortality from simple cases of empyema was practically nil in the series of cases to which this paper refers.

Remarks upon Operations and Treatment.—The results of autopsy findings must be carefully considered before advocating any special line of treatment or operation. Following the great number of operations throughout the United States for empyema, a great array of opinions and operations was advocated and many claims for excellency presented which can scarcely be admitted in view of the fact that except under the most unfavorable circumstances and in the hands of the most inexperienced operators and of totally inadequate technic, deaths do not occur by reason of the method of operative procedure, but by reason of the inherent character of the pyæmia present, which precludes the possibility of efficient surgical intervention. This being the case, I do not present the method of operation outlined in this case as being superior to others, but in view of its low mortality, of the comfort of the patient, of its excellent permanent results, and of the cleanliness and absence of disagreeable odor in a ward full of these usually offensive smelling cases, I believe it to be worthy of consideration as a good method of operation.

THE ETIOLOGY OF CHRONIC EMPYEMA

By Walton Martin, M.D.
of New York, N. Y.

The impression that I have gathered, from studying my own cases of chronic empyema and from talking with other surgeons, is that chronic empyema is a very uncommon outcome of the acute infection of the pleura when the operation for drainage is performed and the after-care supervised by an experienced surgeon. I have talked over this question with men holding most divergent ideas regarding the treatment of acute empyema, and, if they are interested in the subject, they invariably tell me that with their method they never see chronic suppurative pleurisy develop.

This has suggested to me that in a large percentage of these cases the causative factor lies in the treatment of the acute condition. That is, in only a small percentage of cases are there present from the beginning conditions which will invariably lead to chronic empyema. The first thought, on seeing a large, unyielding cavity develop in the pleura following the drainage of an acute empyema, is that since the lung collapsed when the chest was opened it has remained collapsed because an open pneumothorax has been established; positive atmospheric pressure pressed the lung in, therefore, negative pressure must be established and maintained. Every recrudescence of the empyema question is regularly followed by a great many devices for so-called bloodless thoracostomy. Of course, the problem cannot be solved in this way alone. Statistics show, in fact, that more chronic empyemata result from continuous puncture aspiration drainage than from any other form of treatment except repeated aspiration.

I have thought, therefore, it might be of interest and profit to discuss other etiological factors, drawing my conclusions from a series of twenty-four cases on which I found it necessary either to do an extensive thoracoplasty or decortication.

The very definition of the condition is a debatable point. Is the persistence of pleural suppuration for two months, four months or six months indispensable? Is the ease with which it can be cured or the readiness with which the cavity can be disinfected the essential? One usually means, I think, by chronic empyema a persistent collection of pus in the pleural cavity with little or no tendency to heal; that is, an empyema in which, after the evacuation of the pus, the lung does not expand again and an infected cavity remains. These unfavorable anatomical conditions of the lung, pleura, and thoracic wall are reached much faster in some cases than in others, so that a definite time limit cannot be given, nor is there a definite pathological picture. There is obviously a gradual transition, with many intermediate forms, between the acute and chronic condition, but the essential feature is an infected cavity with rigid walls. If a collection of pus is not opened for several months or remains untreated until it bursts through the chest wall or lung, the pulmonary and visceral pleura, in response to the repeated bacterial irritation, become thickened and unyielding. The lung, compressed by the new-formed granulation tissue, is firmly held in a more or less collapsed condition. The pleura is converted into a thick layer of organized connective tissue. The deeper layers, those in contact with the lung, after a varying time become so well organized that they will not disappear even after the bacterial irritation ceases by giving free exit to the pus. This pleural response to irritation is probably dependent on the type and virulence of the bacteria and the special individual resistance of the pleura. However, there is a direct time relation between the duration of the infective process and these changes in the pulmonary and parietal plura, and, although there is a great variation in this time relation, yet it holds true that the ability of the lungs to expand has a direct relation with the interval between the onset of the empyema and the free evacuation of pus. If the pus be retained, for example, until it bursts through the chest wall a chronic empyema invariably results.

The thickening of the pleura in response to bacterial irritation and the binding- down of the compressed lung, so that when the chest is opened the lung no longer expands, is the pathological picture of chronic empyema. The inner surface of the suppurating pleural cavity is irregular and covered with pus and detritus. Its outer surface is made up of fibrillar connective tissue. It is not materially different from the walls of an abscess elsewhere in the body and obeys the same laws, so that the thickness and rigidity of the wall bears not only a definite relation to the duration of the infection, but to the amount of pressure or tension of the exudate set up by the bacterial irritation. Every time there is an increase in tissue tension about a nidus of pyogenic infection there is a local response manifested by an increase in the surrounding new-formed tissue walling it in. If the infected pleural cavity be opened and free passage be given to the exudate there will be found a direct relation between the adequacy of the drainage and the reaction and consequent thickening of the pleura. If intermittent or inadequate drainage be established the infection will not terminate, the pleura will continue to react to the bacterial irritation, and the granulation tissue forming the wall of the pleural cavity will become better and better organized. Now the conditions in the thorax are such that insufficient drainage is very liable to occur. Aside from the position of the original incision, whether a rib be resected or there be an intercostal incision, whether large drainage tubes be introduced or an attempt be made to make an air-tight joint about a tube, there is a marked tendency, as soon as wound healing begins, to close the drainage tract. The shifting planes of the thoracic wall and the crowding together of the ribs tend very quickly to break the continuity of the drainage path. The soft parts heal about the tube, and,

although it may be patent, it is often sufficiently compressed to interfere with the absolutely free exit of the pus which is essential to
lung expansion.

In Case XXI the patient presents an example of chronic empyema
resulting from inadequate drainage. One month after the first aspiration
a drainage tube was inserted. At the end of five months he still had a
small tube in the chest, the soft parts were contracted about the tube, the
rib had regenerated, forming a bone ring about the orifice in the soft
parts. Every few days he had a rise of temperature; he had lost his
appetite; he was anæmic; the muscles of his arm and side were atrophic;
his chest contracted. In short, he presented the usual picture of chronic
suppurative pleurisy. The retention of pus and the imperfect drainage
could readily be demonstrated by injections of a weak solution of methylene
blue. Notwithstanding coughing and straining, greenish pus was still pouring out of the wound three days later and the urine was stained for
several days, showing the absorption even through a thickened pleura. I
know of nothing more surprising than to see a patient four or five weeks
after an operation for empyema, with a small drainage tube still in the
chest, with the soft parts healed firmly about it, with abundant discharge
of pus, but with an afternoon temperature, a rapid pulse and no appetite,
change after reoperating and resecting a portion of a rib and establishing free drainage. The temperature becomes normal, the appetite returns, the lung often expands in a surprisingly short period. A similar
but slower result followed free drainage and sterilization of the cavity
in this patient.

There is yet another outcome of a focus of infection, uncommon to be
sure, but of great interest. The exudate does not break through the
surrounding wall nor is an external passage provided for it. The circumscribing wall becomes very greatly thickened, the virulence of the bacteria becomes more and more attenuated; finally, a static condition is
reached and the lesion is no longer active. It remains for months and
years latent. A most interesting problem is here presented regarding
the life-history and metabolism of non-spore bearing pyogenic bacteria
in one of these chronic abscesses. The examples of this condition that
we are familiar with are the chronic pyogenic bone abscesses. From
trauma or some obscure cause the delicate balance between the living
cells of the abscess wall and the microörganisms may be at any time
upset and the bacteria again begin to grow; tissue tension is again present, with its local and constitutional signs months and years, even, after
the original infection. There are records of circumscribed collections of
pus in the pleural cavity that have apparently been there for years and
that were discovered accidentally at autopsy. Brin reported the autopsy
of a woman, aged sixty-four years, operated on for stenosis of the common duct. The woman died on the fifth day. In the left pleural cavity
there was an abscess filled with thick yellowish pus and broken-down

material. It was situated between the diaphragm and the under surface of the lung. The surrounding pleura was 1½ cm. thick and the costal pleura calcareous. There was no communication with a bronchus. There was no record in the history of the patient of an illness other than that of the biliary colic.

A far commoner condition is the latent collection of pus following operation for acute empyema. A patient has an acute empyema; the pleural cavity is opened and drained. After a time the temperature is normal, the discharge diminishes or almost ceases, the drains are removed, and the external wound heals. The patient is discharged from a hospital service. He, however, after his return home never feels really well. His appetite is poor; from time to time he feels feverish; he has a slight cough. The physical signs over the affected side do not return to normal; the Röntgen ray may be indistinct and may only show great thickening of the pleura. One of my patients (Case XIX) with this condition was sent to Loomis Sanitarium for tuberculosis. He had had pneumonia and an operation for empyema six months previous at his own home. He remained at the sanitarium for four months, although no tubercle bacilli were found in the sputum. He then began to run a high temperature. An exploring needle was inserted into his chest near the old empyema scar and pus withdrawn. At operation there was a very large rigid-walled cavity involving the whole right pleura. In another (Case XI), a young Italian girl, there was an operation for empyema in December, 1913. After several months the sinus closed. She returned home, but never regained her health. She was readmitted two years later with a high temperature. An exploring needle inserted near the old scar withdrew pus. At operation there was a large empyema cavity, the lung was compressed against the vertebral column, the parietal and visceral pleura were enormously thickened.

Foreign bodies, usually drainage tubes, have been frequently found in the pleural cavity. It is usually taken for granted that they are responsible for the chronic suppurative pleurisy which always accompanies their presence. I have operated on two patients with this condition (Cases IV and VII). In one of them, a man, aged thirty-eight years, two tubes were removed. He had had a persistent sinus and chronic empyema for four years. The patient usually leaves a hospital with a draining sinus and a drainage tube in place. At one of his dressings no tube is found. From the fact that the sinus is narrow and that he has no realization of the cavern within, the doctor dressing the patient when the tube is lost assumes that the tube has fallen out, not in. He usually inserts a new tube. In other words, drainage tubes readily fall into chronic empyema cavities rather than cause them. Their presence there is an added factor, of course, in causing the persistence of the suppuration.

In nearly every series of chronic empyemata reported a certain number are caused by tuberculosis. A distinction should be made between tuberculosis of the pleura, secondary tuberculosis developing in a patient suffering from chronic suppurative pleurisy and suppurative pleurisy occurring in a patient suffering from tuberculosis. In my series there were three cases of tuberculous pleurisy. In two of these there was an associated pyogenic infection.

In 12 recurrences following acute empyema at the site of the primary operation, Stevens found the streptococcus hæmolyticus (the organism that caused the original infection) in 11; 1 was sterile. In 9 recurrences distant from the sinus, including undiscovered pus pockets from multi-locular empyema, 4 were due to the streptococcus, 3 were sterile, and 2 contained staphylococcus.

But the effort to base the prognosis and treatment on the type of infection made by Netter has not proved satisfactory. The infection is frequently mixed and there are extraordinary differences in virulence in different epidemics in both the pneumococcus and the streptococcus. The staphylococcus is rarely found unassociated with one or the other pyogenic microörganisms. Its presence in pure culture led Netter on two occasions to predict tuberculosis and in each instance his prediction proved true. The tendency of both the streptococcus and staphylococcus to persist in the tissue and the phenomena of reinfection and secondary infection with these organisms is significant. In making routine bacteriological examinations of granulating wounds one is struck with the ease with which reinfection takes place from some cause often difficult to discover: a piece of necrotic tissue, a minute foreign body or a small pocket with retained exudate. The wound surface which has been almost free from bacteria is suddenly swarming with them again. When the same type of bacteria start to grow luxuriantly we speak of reinfection; when a new organism is added we speak of secondary infection. We are all familiar with the effect of secondary infection in tuberculosis. Kiener reports two interesting observations of secondary infection following empyema: one, a staphylococcus infection, was grafted on a streptococcus; in another a staphylococcus was added to a tuberculous infection. In the subsequent persistent infection the staphylococcus was the prevailing organism.

In Cases II, VIII and XI, I have been able to follow, to a certain extent, the sequence of events in the development of the chronic empyema. In Case II, for example, at operation the lung was found compressed against the vertebral column; the cavity was very large, involving the whole chest. It was partially filled with foul-smelling pus; the pleura was greatly thickened. The patient was eighteen years old. He had been in good health before the onset of the acute empyema, three years before. The diagnosis of pus in the chest had been made early and an operation performed and the drainage tube inserted. After ten days this tube was replaced by another connected to a rubber suction bag and an effort had been made to make an air-tight joint between the thoracic wall and the drainage tube by iodoform packing, perforated rubber dam, and adhesive plaster. After several weeks the patient was allowed up and permitted to walk. The drainage tube was still in the chest and the suction bag still attached. He was operated on in May. In July he still had a tube in the chest. During this month the tube was removed and the external wound closed. He went home but continued in poor health. He returned to the hospital nine months later for cough and persistent temperature. The chest was opened, a piece of rib was resected, and a drainage tube inserted. The pus evacuated was brownish and very foul smelling. Again the suction bag was applied. There was the same sequence of events; he returned home, the wound again closed, but he never regained his health, although he was not actually sick. He had slight fever, persistent cough, and shortness of breath. In the patient referred to the exudate at the second operation was foul smelling. The original pyogenic infection had become secondarily infected by putrefactive organisms.

This question of secondary infection and reinfection and its relation to chronic empyema has been little studied. Of course, it presents unusual difficulties. Secondary surface contamination is almost certainly present in every granulation wound or cavity lined with granulations that communicates with the external air. This by no means necessarily denotes secondary infection. Forty years ago incision and drainage of the chest was unsatisfactory. It was soon generally recognized that the patients were reinfected after the operation. When both the operation and the after-treatment were carried out under antiseptic precautions there was an astonishing improvement in results. The study of the statistics between 1875 and 1895 is very instructive. I believe these cases I have referred to are examples of chronic empyema resulting from repeated reinfection of the pleura and intermittent drainage. A drainage tube is a foreign body. When a tube is retained in any wound until healing takes place it is soon compressed by contracting healing tissue. The pressure is finally sufficient to interfere with the nutrition of the granulations in contact with the tube; surface necrosis results. A condition of repair and interference with repair is established. The trauma is added to by the movement of the tube in the drainage tract; the greater the activity of the patient the more this displacement of the tube is likely to occur. By these repeated injuries of the granulations the protecting lining wall of round-cells is broken again and again. Surface organisms, usually the staphylococcus or streptococcus, penetrate the tissue and infection, not contamination, is established. If the tube be long the walls of the drainage tract are made up not only of thoracic wall, but the pleura. The exudate, made up of leucocytes and microörganisms, oozes between the tube and the granulating wall embracing the tube. Some of it trickles into the space still present in the pleura, is shut off by the granulations and imprisoned. There is a renewed intrapleural exudate sufficient to hinder expansion of the lung. When the tension of the exudate becomes sufficient it again escapes externally. One of the most admirable principles of the Carrel treatment is the scrupulous avoidance of secondary infection and damage to the granulations, and it seems to me, as soon as the healing wound has contracted so tightly about a drainage tube that it is inserted with difficulty, it is better to remove the tube or reoperate.

The influence of the anatomical arrangements of the adhesions between the pulmonary and parietal pleura at the time of the original infection has been suggested by Homan as an etiological factor of importance in determining the tendency of chemistry. If the lower margin of the lung be held down by adhesions to the diaphragm he believes that the prognosis is favorable; the lung will expand readily after drainage. If, on the other hand, the lung is collapsed and adherent and the lower margin is not in contact with the diaphragm, the prognosis is bad; chronic empyema is likely to occur. He shows a silhouette taken from a Röntgen-ray plate in one case of chronic empyema which represents one of the types seen in chronic suppurative pleurisy when there has been a large collection of pus in the chest. The lung is usually either compressed so that there is only a narrow band of lung tissue in contact with the vertebral column or, as in his illustration, drawn upward away from the diaphragm. The Röntgen-ray photographs in Cases VIII and XX are very like his diagram. Obviously a small sacculated empyema favorably situated for drainage offers a good prognosis. Also, obviously, a chronic empyema involving the entire pleural cavity, with lung completely collapsed, presents a more difficult problem than a circumscribed chronic empyema. His theory seems to me, however, to attribute a permanency to the original plastic adhesions, as if they were unmodified by the duration, character, and treatment of the infection, unaltered by protophytic ferment and proteolytic antiseptic solutions, uninfluenced by the mechanical factors of intra- and extrapulmonary pressure. A similar theory applied to the permanency of the original plastic adhesions about a focus of infection in the peritoneum would lead to conclusions at variance with common experience.

The shape of the empyema cavity has a significance in determining the readiness with which it can be drained and cured. If it is irregular, with secondary pockets or diverticuli, or presents a considerable cavity connected with the main cavity by a narrow channel, all the phenomena of intermittent drainage or incomplete drainage may be produced by the shutting off of a loculus or by the more or less complete blocking of a channel; drainage of the main pocket will evidently be inefficient. Multilocular empyemata and lung abscesses are frequent autopsy findings. In fact, the mortality in acute empyema seems to be largely due either to the fact that the empyema is only one of the localizations of a general infection which may lead to death with lesions in the lungs, pericardium, and meninges, or to undrained, circumscribed collections of pus. For example, in the necropsy findings reported in 16 fatal cases at Camp Sheridan, Ohio, 14 had one or more undrained collections of pus. In a fifteenth there was a miliary tuberculosis. In Case II, for example, an abscess was found in the left chest above the fourth rib containing 200 c.c. of pus. The pleural cavity below that point had been drained. There was a second pus pocket between the upper and lower lobe. If death does not occur and the pus from one of these secondary foci finds its way into the main cavity we have produced an irregular cavity imperfectly drained. In some of these cases a secondary opening occurs spontaneously through the lung, either a lung abscess breaking into the pleural or a loculated collection of pus finding its way through the lung and draining through a bronchus. Chronic empyema results when the microörganisms are attenuated and there is inadequate and intermittent drainage. Obviously, the virulence of the infection or the complete absence of drainage leads either to the death of the patient or the recognition and early treatment of the condition.

In Cases IV, V, VI, VII and IX the large empyema cavity was draining both through the chest and through the lung. In Case IX there was an abscess in the upper lobe that communicated with a bronchus and with the pleura, so that there was a dumbbell-shaped cavity draining at each end. In the case of Romain there was a similar condition, but the abscess was in the lower lobe. In these cases the large opening into a bronchus is an etiological factor in the persistence of the suppuration process. At times there is free drainage through the bronchus, at times it is blocked and the pus from the infected area in the lung backs up and empties into the pleural cavity. We have again produced the phenomena caused by intermittent collection, an exudate under tension about a focus of infection.

I believe, then, that the cause of the chronicity does not lie in any one factor, such as the variety of the organisms, the type of the exudate, the nature of the infection, or the anatomical arrangements of the original adhesions, but in the complex made up of all these causes, the underlying element being repeated infection and reinfection of the pleura, causing its thickening and rigidity and the binding down of the lung. We have abundant evidence from autopsy findings made within the first week of drainage in extensive infection of the pleura, from Röntgen-ray examination and from the physical signs that the lung will expand readily and quickly in favorable cases within the first week if there is a free passage made for the exudate, and this expansion occurs even under the ordinary aseptic or antiseptic dressing. From the figures of Cestan, in 1208 cases 1.8 per cent. were not completely cured after simple pleurotomy and drainage, whereas with aspiration drainage after incision the failures were 3 per cent., and after puncture drainage with aspiration the failures were 6 per cent. Stevens reported in 100 cases treated by simple incision that 56 healed satisfactorily, 34 healed after surface sterilization of the cavity with Dakin's solution; in 10 a thoracoplasty of moderate extent was indicated. In 23 cases treated by drainage and irrigation with Dakin's solution from the beginning there were 3 thoracoplasties for foci distant from the sinus. There were no recurrences at the site of the original operation.

Statistics, taking no account of the experience of the operator and the supervision of after-care of the patient or the original complications, may readily be misleading.

It was long ago pointed out by Schede that a closed pneumothorax, uninfected, rapidly disappeared. During the war Bastianelli found satisfactory restoration of lung expansion after an artificial pneumothorax which had been established and maintained for from twelve to fifteen days. Since we have made routine Röntgen-ray examinations I think many of us have been surprised when evidences of infection are no longer present, as shown by the mucoid nature of the wound secretion or by negative bacterial findings, to see that the lung expands satisfactorily if the outer wound is allowed to close, even in the presence of a considerable pneumothorax. When expansion has taken place and the infection has ceased, Röntgen-ray examination shows that the thickened pleura gradually returns to a layer so thin that it is no longer opaque to the Röntgen ray even when there has been long-continued infection and the pleura has been seen to be much thickened at operation (Case II).

I believe that chronic suppurative pleurisy, excepting when there are complicating conditions in the lung or an underlying tuberculous infection, should not occur. I feel sure that in the majority of cases there has been a failure to appreciate the fundamental principle involved in treating an infected cavity; that an absolutely free external passage for the exudate must be provided as long as infection is present; that scrupulous cleanliness must be observed in the after-care; that one must be always on the lookout for the possibility of secondary loculi and foci of infection and shut-off portions of the drainage tract; that in a widely drained cavity surface contamination does not lead necessarily to reinfection, but that in a poorly drained cavity reinfection and secondary infection are very liable to occur. I believe that surgeons with very different ways of operating and very diverging ideas regarding after-care get equally good results provided these essentials are borne in mind: That the entrance of air through the thoracic wound to any desirable degree can be assured by very simple means; that although the danger of early operation in streptococcus infection while pneumonia is still present has been recently generally recognized, this by no means implies the desirability of a long delay and treatment by aspiration after the pneumonic process is over and the exudate is purulent or seropurulent in character. I think no case should be allowed to leave a hospital with a drainage tube in the chest; that all patients with a closed, even if apparently sterile, pneumothorax should be kept under close observation until it disappears. I think that there should be a more general recognition that not only high temperature and obvious signs of infection indicate a pent-up collection of pus, but that a slight a ernoon temperature, a rapid pulse, loss of appetite, vague discomfort i the chest—in short, a failure to return to vigorous health—are very suggestive of a hibernating pleural abscess. Finally, that in the treatment of acute empyema will generally be found the etiological factors of the chronic condition.

In over one-half of the cases of chronic empyema in my series there was no complicating lesion, no infection with tubercle bacilli, no complexity of the original cavity.

OBSERVATIONS ON THE TREATMENT OF CHRONIC EMPYEMA

By George J. Heuer, M.D.

of Baltimore, Md.

In 1913 a patient who had been treated for pulmonary tuberculosis by artificial pneumothorax came to us with a tuberculous empyema. We resected a rib and drained an empyemic cavity containing over 1000 c.c. of thick greenish pus in which were myriads of tubercle bacilli. The lung, due to its long period of collapse, was incapable of expansion and the patient's condition did not permit a thoracoplastie operation. Under the circumstances, we tried repeated injections of Beck's bismuth paste, and were astonished at the result. The tubercle bacilli disappeared from the discharge, the discharge itself became a clear straw-colored sterile fluid, and the sinus tract spontaneously closed. The intrapleural cavity never became obliterated, yet the patient went about not at all inconvenienced by its presence (Fig. 1). So far as we can gather, this is the first case in which the complete sterilization of a chronic empyemic cavity followed the prolonged use of antiseptic substances. It demonstrated to us that it was possible to sterilize empyemic cavities and that sterile intrapleural cavities need not be surgically obliterated, but were quite compatible with good health.

Since that time we have been deeply interested in the treatment of chronic empyema. Our experience soon showed that we, at least, were not able within a reasonable time to sterilize all empyemic cavities by the injection into them of bismuth paste; and, guided largely by animal experimentation, we have therefore sought for other methods which would cure chronic empyema and still avoid the mortality and the mutilation of thoracoplastic procedures such as the Estlander and Schede operations. Our observations on the treatment of chronic empyema before and since the discovery of the Carrel-Dakin method of treating infected wounds, concern the description of and the results obtained by these methods.

1. *Bismuth Sterilization of Empyemic Cavities.*—In addition to the case described in our introductory remarks, we have attempted the sterilization of chronic cavities with bismuth paste in six cases. In five of them a preliminary rib resection to establish a satisfactory sinus was necessary. The method is now well known and we need not pause over it. We should, however, like to add our experience to that of others who have had favorable results. In one patient with a large tuberculous empyemic cavity similar to the one described, we failed to completely sterilize the cavity during the period (two months) he was under our care; yet there was marked improvement, as indicated by the fall in the temperature and the gain in weight. In the smaller empyemic cavities, however, and

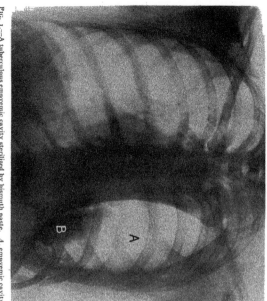

FIG. 1.—A tuberculous empyemic cavity sterilized by bismuth paste. *A*, empyemic cavity; *B*, a small mass of bismuth paste remaining in the cavity at the time of the closure of the sinus.

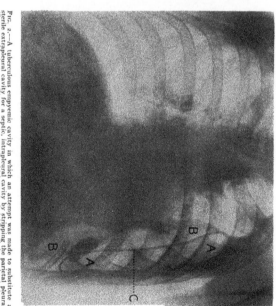

FIG. 2.—A tuberculous empyemic cavity in which an attempt was made to substitute a sterile extrapleural cavity for a septic intrapleural cavity by stripping the parietal pleura. (See text, Method 2.) The result, due to the thickness and rigidity of the parietal pleura, was a partial and not a total obliteration of the intrapleural cavity. *A*, extrapleural cavity; *B*, intrapleural cavity; *C*, the mobilized parietal pleura. (X-ray taken about ten days after operation.)

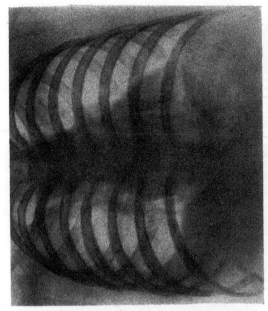

FIG. 3.—A chronic empyemic cavity treated by mobilization and excision of the parietal pleural followed by irrigations of the extrapleural cavity with Dakin's solution. (See text. Method 3.) The small dense shadow is the remains of the bismuth paste injected to determine the form and position of the cavity. (X-ray taken before operation.)

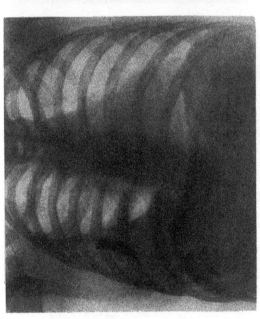

FIG. 4.—The end-result in the case shown in Fig. 3. (X-ray taken ten months after operation.) The cavity is obliterated. There is only a slight haziness to indicate what was found at operation to be a greatly thickened pleura.

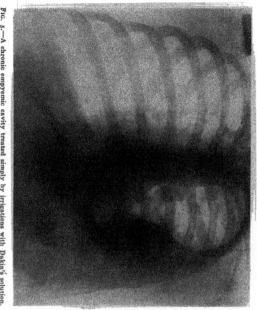

Fig. 5.—A chronic empyemic cavity treated simply by irrigations with Dakin's solution. (See text, Method 4.)

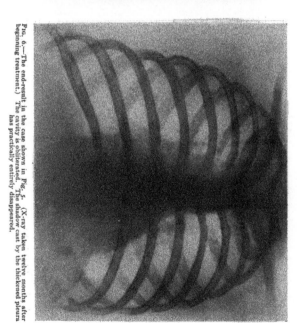

Fig. 6.—The end-result in the case shown in Fig. 5. (X-ray taken twelve months after beginning treatment.) The cavity is obliterated. The shadow cast by the thickened pleura has practically entirely disappeared.

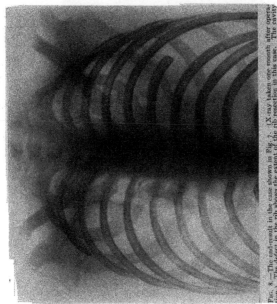

FIG. 8.—The end-result in the case shown in Fig. 7. (X-ray taken one month after operation). The defect in the rib shows the extent of the rib resection in this case. The cavity
is obliterated. The shadow cast by the thickened pleura has entirely disappeared.

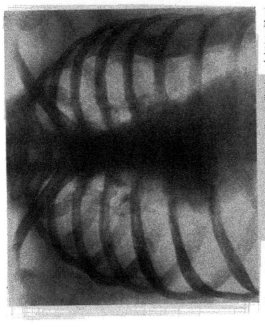

FIG. 7.—A chronic empyemic cavity treated by immediate sterilization and closure without
drainage. (See text, Method 5c)

especially in the long tubular intrapleural sinus tracts of tuberculous origin, we have been quite uniformly successful; and we have five cases at present which have been healed over long periods. Our total results, therefore, in seven cases are six successes and one failure. For the non-tuberculous cavities we have now, I believe, better methods of treatment; but if it is fair to judge from a small experience, the tuberculous cavities respond more quickly to bismuth paste than to Dakin's solution.

2. *Substitution of a Sterile Extrapleural Cavity for a Septic Intrapleural Cavity by Stripping the Parietal Pleura.*—It seemed possible from experiments on animals that an intrapleural cavity might be obliterated by stripping the parietal pleura according to the method of Tuffier and bringing it in contact with the visceral pleura. The contact of the two pleural surfaces might be maintained by suction upon the sinus or by the injection of air or nitrogen into the resulting sterile extrapleural cavity. A necessary requirement was that the sinus be at the lowermost point of the cavity. The operation was carried out away from the sinus tract and in a relatively aseptic field. After resection of 10 to 12 cm. of a single rib it was possible to strip the parietal pleura over a wide area. The procedure proved to be feasible if the parietal pleura were not too greatly thickened. In the presence of a rigid, board-like pleura, however, the result was that when mobilized the pleura stretched across the thoracic cavity as a cord subtends an arc, and could not be brought into contact with the visceral pleura. In two cases of this kind we were able to reduce the size of the cavities by one-half and three-fourths, but failed to completely obliterate them (Fig. 2). In one case the procedure was successful. In view of the probable failure of this method in many cases, it was abandoned. But our experience was not without value, for it taught us that the parietal pleura over chronic empyemic cavities may be stripped away from the thoracic wall, and that we had, therefore, a method of exposing the entire cavity through the resection of a single rib. It suggested also that the presence of the thickened parietal pleura probably largely prevented the expansion of the lung, and that the excision of this structure might, therefore, permit the expansion of the lung. It led to two of the following procedures (3 and 5).

3. *Excision of the Mobilized Parietal Pleura Over the Empyemic Cavity. Irrigation of the Extrapleural Cavity with Dakin's Solution. Secondary Closure.*—It appeared from our previous observations that the thickened pleura about an empyemic cavity probably prevented the obliteration of the cavity. By stripping the parietal pleura from the thoracic wall well beyond the limits of the empyemic cavity and excising it, it seemed to us that the cavity might more readily be obliterated. The result is an extrapleural cavity, presenting upon the mesial wall of which is an area of visceral pleura. The procedure, moreover, removes at least half of the infected pleural surface and allows the formation of granulation tissue from the thoracic wall. It is easier, I believe, than the Fowler or Delorme

operation. The Dakinization of the extrapleural cavity seemed necessary because of the presence of infection. In practice the operation has
been carried out as follows: After stereoscopic X-rays of bismuth injections of the cavity have been made to determine the size and position of
the cavity, the sinus tract is carbolized, encircled by an incision, and
dissected down to the pleura. Ten to 12 cm. of a single rib are excised and
the parietal pleura stripped away from the chest wall well beyond the
limits of the cavity. With as careful an observance of aseptic technic as
possible the parietal pleura is incised, the granulation tissue removed
from the cavity, and its entire inner surface carbolized. The parietal
pleura is then excised. The wound is closed except for an opening large
enough to permit the two tubes of our Dakin irrigating apparatus. This
procedure has been carried out in four cases; in two cases as a primary
procedure, and in two cases as a secondary operation following the failure of other methods. In all the cases the method was successful. The
cavities varied in size from 100 to 200 c.c. in volume, were elliptical rather
than spherical in shape, were of long standing (one to four years), and
were surrounded by a markedly thickened pleura. Sterilization of the
cavities and closure of the sinus tracts were effected in one case in
thirteen days, in one case in twenty-one days, in one case in forty days,
and in one case in sixty-seven days. We have examined personally or have
letters from all these cases. In none have the wounds reopened. The
patients have now been well for from six months to one and a half years.
We have a series of pre- and post-operative X-rays in three of the cases.
Although we cannot state accurately how soon after sterilization the
cavities were obliterated, we know that all were obliterated rather
promptly—almost surely within a month. In the later X-rays of these
cases the shadows indicating the thickened pleura have almost entirely
disappeared (Figs. 3 and 4).

4. *Preliminary Correction of the Sinus Tract and Cavity if Necessary.
Sterilization of the Cavity with Dakin's Solution. Secondary Suture or
Spontaneous Closure of the Sinus Tract.*—In the cases in which bismuth
X-rays showed a sinus leading directly into a single cavity, the tubes of
our irrigating apparatus were introduced into the cavity without preliminary operative procedures, and the sterilization of the cavity attempted. In the cases in which a long or tortuous tract led into the
cavity so that mechanical conditions for subsequent sterilization were
unsatisfactory, a preliminary operation with excision of the sinus tract
or the establishment of a new opening into the cavity at a point of election was performed. This method has been carried out in ten cases. In
one case no preliminary operation was necessary. In one case the cavity
was opened widely and the large open wound—the bottom of which was
formed by the cavity—subsequently closed by secondary suture. In eight
cases the sinus was excised and either enlarged or closed and a new
sinus established. In two of these eight cases rib resections (in one case

segments of two ribs; in one case of four ribs) were performed. In these two cases—in which the cavities were under the scapula—the rib resections may have hastened the obliteration of the cavities; but could not have influenced greatly the sterilization of the cavities. The results in the ten cases are as follows: One case insisted on going home three weeks after irrigations of the cavity were begun. At the time of his discharge the bacterial count was very low, but the cavity was neither sterile nor closed. This patient has not been heard from. One case, the only instance in this group of tuberculous empyema (secondarily infected with a hæmolytic streptococcus), was discharged two and a half months after beginning Dakin's solution irrigations. The bacterial count was rapidly reduced from infinity to one to two organisms per microscopic field; but for a month we were unable to do better than this and feared to close the sinus because of the presence of a hæmolytic streptococcus. A letter from this patient states that he is at present in a tuberculosis sanitorium and that the cavity is still draining. In one case the cavity was bacteriologically sterile and closed in one month after beginning Dakin irrigations, but reopened two weeks later. A secondary operation with stripping and excision of the parietal pleura cured this patient. In one case sterilization and closure were accomplished in three weeks. The wound, however, reopened and discharged, then closed spontaneously, and has remained closed for one and a half years. In the remaining six cases sterilization and closure were accomplished in fourteen days, twenty days, twenty-three days, thirty days, sixty days, and seventy days. By personal examinations or letters we know that in none of these cases has the wound reopened and that they have been well for from seven months to three years. Exclusive of the three cases in which sterilization was not accomplished, we know from X-ray studies that the cavities were not obliterated at the time of closure of the sinus tracts; in other words, that we closed or allowed to close a sinus over an intrapleural cavity. We know from subsequent X-ray examinations of four patients who have since returned for examination that the cavities—even though surrounded by a markedly thickened pleura—have spontaneously been obliterated and that the thickening of the pleura has largely disappeared (Figs. 5 and 6). Our total results, therefore, in these ten cases have been six complete successes and four failures. In one of the four failures the sinus, which reopened two weeks after its primary closure, closed spontaneously and has since remained closed. In another case included as a failure in this group, a subsequent operation resulted in the closure of the sinus and a complete cure. In only two cases, therefore, did we fail in the closure of the cavities before the patients left the hospital.

5. *Immediate Sterilization of Chronic Empyemic Cavities with Pure Carbolic Acid. Closure without Drainage.*—Our experience with the progressive sterilization of empyemic cavities led us to attempt the immediate sterilization and complete closure of chronic empyemic cavities at

the time of operation. This procedure has been attempted only in small (up to 200 c.c. in volume) and favorably situated cavities. The operation has been carried out as follows: The sinus tract is carbolized, surrounded by an incision, tied off, and recarbolized. With a new set of instruments the sinus tract is followed down to the pleura, care being exercised not to open it. Ten to 12 cm. of a single rib are resected and the parietal pleura stripped from the thoracic wall beyond the limits of the cavity. With the wound held widely open with a rib spreader and with the greatest care not to contaminate the field, the parietal pleura is incised from one end of the cavity to the other (at the same time excising the sinus tract), and the cavity—previously cleansed by Dakin irrigations—opened widely. Holding up the edges of the incised parietal pleura the granulation tissue lining the cavity is wiped out and then the cavity is carbolized throughout with pure carbolic acid. The excess of acid is wiped out with alcohol or salt sponges. The parietal pleura has been treated in various ways; it has been allowed to simply fall into the cavity; it has been sutured to the visceral pleura, so as to bring the two layers of the pleura accurately into apposition; or it has been excised. The extra-pleural cavity is wiped dry. The wound is closed without drainage. This procedure has been carried out in five cases, but in two cases operated upon before I went abroad, and successfully so far as immediate results are concerned, our records have not yet been found. In two of the three cases in which we have complete records the wound healed by primary intention and remained healed. In one case the wound healed per primum, but on the fifth day after operation an area of induration appeared in the subcutaneous tissues along the healed incision. Before the incision was opened cultures from the fluid in the cavity showed that the cavity was sterile. With the opening of the incision the cavity became secondarily infected, but was sterilized with Dakin's solution and later closed by secondary suture. By personal examination we know the end-results in these three cases. In the two cases in which the wounds healed by primary intention, the wounds have remained healed and the patients are well three and a half years and four years after operation. In the case which developed a secondary infection the wound has remained healed since the secondary closure of the cavity (Figs. 7 and 8). We know the fate of the cavities in these three cases. In one the cavity after operation became filled with blood, as proved by aspiration, but later was completely obliterated; in one, if we properly interpret the clear space in the X-rays, the cavity did not fill with fluid, but remained an air space until its obliteration (Figs. 9 and 10); in one the cavity remained filled with a blood-tinged serous fluid until its obliteration.

To summarize our observations, we may say that twenty-four patients with long-standing chronic empyema have been treated by one or another—in a few instances by two—of the methods described. There has been no operative mortality. Through the efforts of Miss Spicer, my

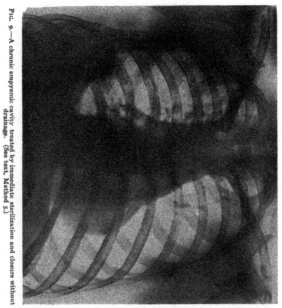

FIG. 9.—A chronic empyæmic cavity treated by immediate sterilization and closure without drainage. (See text, Method 5.)

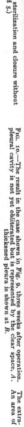

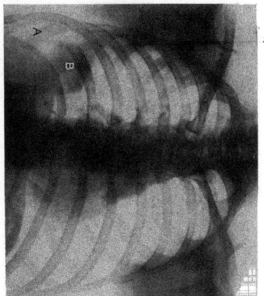

FIG. 10.—The result in the case shown in Fig. 9, three weeks after operation. The extrapleural cavity is not yet obliterated but is represented by the clear space, A. An area of thickened pleura is shown at B.

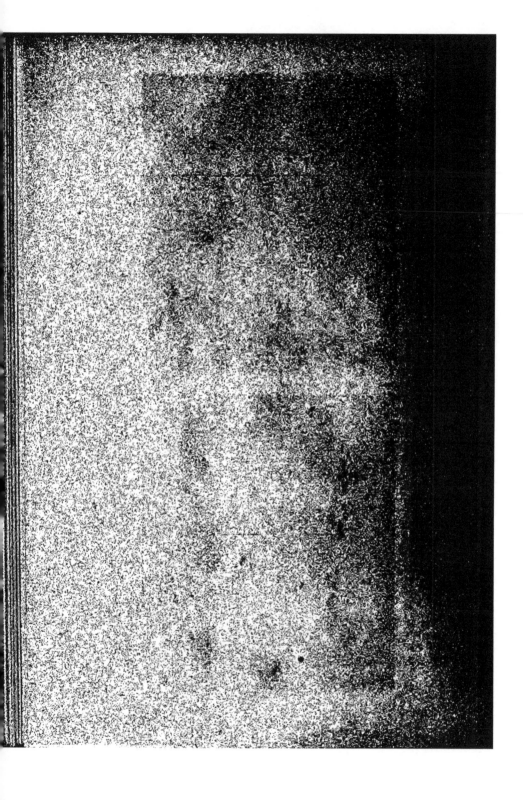

secretary, and Miss McEvoy, my social service aide, I have with one exception either examined personally or have received letters from all these patients. Twenty patients were discharged from the hospital with their wounds healed. In nineteen of these patients the wounds have remained healed, and eighteen patients are well from seven months to four years after their discharge from the hospital. One patient died of pulmonary tuberculosis two years after his discharge from the hospital; in one patient the sterile cavity became reinfected by the rupture into it of a tuberculous focus, and death occurred following an extensive thoracoplastic operation, three years after the sterilization of the cavity. Four patients were discharged from the hospital with their cavities infected and draining. Two of these patients are in tuberculosis sanitoria with their cavities still draining; one patient has since died of pulmonary tuberculosis. One patient discharged against our wishes three weeks after his admission has not yet been heard from. With the exception of this last patient, whom undoubtedly we could have cured had he remained in the hospital, our only failures occurred in patients with active pulmonary tuberculosis in whom a tuberculous empyema followed prolonged artificial pneumothorax treatment.

Not less interesting than the facts that empyema cavities of long standing can be sterilized and that subsequent to sterilization and closure of the sinus tracts they are spontaneously obliterated—and by expansion of the lung rather than by retraction of the thorax—is the fact that eventually there is almost a complete restoration to the normal. The late X-rays in our series show that the markedly thickened pleura certified at operation practically entirely disappears. In four cases we have indeed aided in this restoration to the normal by excising the thickened parietal pleura; but in cases in which such excision has not been done the thickened pleura has nevertheless disappeared (Figs. 3 to 9, inclusive).

In conclusion, we may add some observations on the complications following the irrigation of empyemic cavities with Dakin's solution. *Hemorrhage* from the cavity has occurred in three cases in the above series. It was not excessive nor alarming and spontaneously ceased so soon as the irrigations were discontinued. It invariably occurred late in the process of sterilization—at a time when the organism count was five per microscopic field or lower. It has not yet in our experience been a serious factor in the treatment of empyemic cavities by Dakin irrigations. In two cases the irrigations were discontinued for from twenty-four to forty-eight hours, then recommenced and without a repetition of the bleeding. In one case recurring, slight hemorrhages caused us to discontinue the irrigations and a single injection of bismuth paste was followed by closure of the sinus. *Bronchial fistulæ* have developed in the course of the irrigations with Dakin's solution in two cases. In one case there was a history of a previous bronchial fistula which had apparently been closed for three months. In the other case there was no history to

85

indicate that a bronchial fistula had previously been present. This complication has, in our experience, prevented for a time, at least, the continuation of the irrigations because of paroxysms of coughing, the taste of the solution, and the fear of strangulation. In the two cases in which bronchial fistulæ have occurred, injections of bismuth paste have been substituted for the irrigations.

EMPYEMA *

A SYLLABUS OF OPERATIVE TREATMENT

By Howard Lilienthal, M.D.
of New York, N.Y.

THIS is an attempt to standardize the selection of operative methods in the surgery of empyema of the thorax. It is presented here for discussion and criticism. It consists of: (1) A classification of the conditions demanding operation. (2) A list of procedures with a brief description of each. (3) A synoptic table showing the types of the disease paired with their appropriate operations.

In such a presentation as this there can be given no complete plan for carrying any save the simplest cases to their conclusions; but complications, such, for example, as the discovery of an unsuspected sacculation, may put the case in another class which can be treated according to the table. It is also recognized that there can be no absolute rule for the treatment of any given case because the conditions are never twice exactly alike; but this does not forbid our attempt to construct a model. Bacteriology is not considered because it has nothing to do with our subject. It is of prognostic value only. Every case is assumed to have been röntgenologically studied except in acute intrathoracic tension, when therapeutic aspiration is urgent even without the X-ray. Anæsthesia in minor operations should be local, even with rib resection. Intrapharyngeal differential pressure by ether vapor or nitrous oxide and oxygen is preferable for the more serious procedures. The Carrel-Dakin method is recommended as a most valuable post-operative aid but it should not be employed when the instillation of even small quantities of the fluid with a wide opening for its escape from the thorax is followed by severe coughing. Also in children and in a few susceptible adults the long-continued application of this treatment seems to cause a general deterioration. Such patients improve on discontinuing this remedy. Empyema can best be treated in a hospital.

CLASSIFICATION OF CONDITIONS DEMANDING OPERATION

(Tuberculosis, syphilis, actinomycosis, etc., are not included.)

Acute empyema	A. Seropurulent effusion / B. Frankly purulent effusion	a. General or large.
		b. Sacculated, single or multiple.
		c. With purulent expectoration (hidden lung abscess or empyema emptying through a bronchus).
		d. With lung abscess (intrinsic).
		e. With lung abscess (bronchiectatic).
		f. From extrapleural sources other than lung, by direct extension.
		g. With tension pneumothorax.
		h. Traumatic.

---

* Read before American Surgical Association, May 3, 1920.

87

HOWARD LILIENTHAL

Chronic empyema ....
- I. With closed thorax.
- II. With pleurobronchial fistula and closed thorax.
- III. With open thorax (fistula).
- IV. With pleurobronchial fistula and open thorax.
- V. With fibrosis and permanent contraction of lung.

A List of Procedures with a Brief Description of Each

PROCEDURE No. 1.—Diagnostic Aspiration. Only a few c.c. to be removed. Syringe to be detached and needle to be withdrawn while 2% lysol is slowly injected through it into the puncture tract to prevent infection and phlegmon of the chest wall (5 to 15 c.c. may be injected).

PROCEDURE No. 2.¹—Therapeutic Aspiration. Use fine trocar and canula with rubber tube attached so as to empty the chest by patient's expulsive efforts and by gravity. No forcible suction to be employed. Air permitted to replace the fluid removed or if desired the air may be expelled from the chest by the patient's straining with closed glottis or even by his normal respirations, the tube being pinched during *inspiration* until no more bubbles appear on straining or on *expiration* from end of tube held under water. The canula is then quickly withdrawn. (X-ray will demonstrate the efficacy of this method of getting air out of the thorax.)

PROCEDURE No. 3.—Minor intercostal thoracotomy and tube drainage (with or without airtight closure).

PROCEDURE No. 4.¹—Resection of rib with its periosteum. Tube drainage.

PROCEDURE No. 5.¹—Major intercostal thoracotomy with rib retraction (rib spreader) and full exploration of chest cavity with mobilization of lung if desirable.

PROCEDURE No. 6.⁴—Noncollapsing major thoracoplasty, with costotomy but no resection of ribs. Mobilization of lung.

PROCEDURE No. 7.—Various forms of collapsing thoracoplasty. (Schede, Estlander, Wilms, etc.)

Synoptic Table

(Showing the Types of the Disease Paired with Their Appropriate Operations.)

Condition	Operation
Acute Seropurulent Effusion.	
a. General or large	Procedure No. 2. Repeat if necessary until frank pus is present or no more fluid accumulates.
b. Sacculated, single or multiple	Procedure No. 2 applied to larger cavities. Repeat if necessary until pus is present or no more fluid accumulates.
c. With purulent expectoration (hidden lung abscess or empyema emptying through a bronchus)	Procedure No. 2. Repeat until pus is present (or no more fluid accumulates), then Procedure No. 5.
d. With lung abscess (intrinsic)	Procedure No. 4. This is preliminary as a rule, but it may prove curative.

88

OPERATIVE TREATMENT OF EMPYEMA

Condition	Operation
e. With lung abscess (bronchiectatic)	Procedure No. 5 with a view to dealing later on or at the same time with pulmonary condition (lobectomy).
f. From extrapleural sources other than lung by direct extension...	Procedure No. 4. Generous resection and dealing at once with the cause (e.g., subphrenic abscess).
g. With tension pneumothorax......	Procedure No. 2 followed by Procedure No. 3.
h. Traumatic	Procedure No. 2 followed by Procedure No. 3 or 5 according to extent of trauma.

Acute Frankly Purulent Exudate.

a. General or large	Procedure No. 3 followed if course is unsatisfactory by Procedure No. 5. (Fluoroscopic study important.)
b. Sacculated, single or multiple	If single, Procedure No. 4. If multiple, Procdure No. 5.
c. With purulent expectoration (hidden lung abscess or empyema emptying through a bronchus)...	Procedure No. 4
d. With lung abscess (intrinsic)	Procedure No. 4. Generous resection with simultaneous or deferred drainage of abscess.
e. With lung abscess (bronchiectatic)	Procedure No. 5. Possibly as first stage of lobectomy.
f. From extrapleural sources other than the lung by direct extension.	Procedure No. 4 with immediate attention to cause.
g. With tension pneumothorax......	Procedure No. 2, later No. 3 or No. 5, according to X-ray.
h. Traumatic	Procedure No. 4. (Revision probably necessary.)

CHRONIC EMPYEMA

I. With closed thorax (simple)........	Procedure No. 5.
II. With pleurobronchial fistula and closed thorax. (X-ray diagnosis pyopneumothorax.)	Procedure No. 3, later No. 5.

Condition	Operation
III With open thorax (fistula)	Procedure No. 6.
IV. With pleurobronchial fistula and open thorax (thoracic fistula)	Procedure No. 6.
V. With fibrosis and permanent contraction of lung. (Demonstrated at operation by impossibility of inflating lung with intrapharyngeal pressure after "decortication"; and after weeks of further effort by blowing and coughing exercises)	Procedure No. 7.

POSTSCRIPT.—The use of Beck's paste or of 5 to 10 per cent. iodoform in vaseline is recommended in certain narrow cavities which have previously been rendered bacteria free or nearly so. This form of treatment is often successful even when there is an open bronchus at the end of the tract.

BIBLIOGRAPHY

[1] Lilienthal, Brickner and Kellogg: Thoracic Injuries. Report of Cases Treated by Surgical Team 39, etc. *Jour. of the Am. Med. Asso.*, March 22, 1919, vol. lxxii.
[2] Lilienthal, Howard: Thoracic Fistula and Chronic Empyema. ANN. SURG., July, 1919.
[3] Lilienthal, Howard: Empyema. ANN. SURG., Sept., 1915.
[4] Lilienthal, Howard: Thoracic Fistula and Chronic Empyema. ANN. SURG., July, 1919.

FATAL POST-OPERATIVE PULMONARY THROMBOSIS *

By Albert J. Ochsner, M.D.

of Chicago, Ill.

SURGEON-IN-CHIEF OF AUGUSTANA HOSPITAL AND ST. MARY'S HOSPITAL; PROFESSOR OF CLINICAL SURGERY
MEDICAL DEPARTMENT, UNIVERSITY OF ILLINOIS

AND

Chester C. Schneider, M.D.

of Milwaukee, Wis.

It has seemed worth while to consider our experience with post-operative pulmonary thrombosis in connection with a review of the most important papers which have been written upon this subject with a view to bring out any points of value in the direction of prophylaxis, as none of the methods of treatment of the condition, once it has been established, seem to have proved successful.

It seems clear from all of the many careful observations that are recorded in the literature, as well as from our own experience, that the condition does not depend upon any one cause, although most observers seem to agree upon several causes which are more important than others. In order that these views may be brought out clearly, we have stated each together with the name of its author in as concise a form as possible before stating our own observations and conclusions.

Causation.—The causes of pulmonary thrombosis in their order of importance are: (1) Local infection; (2) anæmia; (3) slowing of blood stream; (4) subnormal general physical condition; (5) cachexia; (6) micro-organisms in the blood; (7) excess of white blood-cells; (88 inefficient hæmostasis; (9) traumatization of tissues with retractors, etc.; (10) injury to veins of extremities due to badly arranged operating table; (11) injury to intima of veins; (12) excess of calcium salts in the blood.

History.—The condition has been recognized and discussed for generations. Van Swieten [8] in 1705 recognized that clots occur in the vessels during the puerperium and wrote gravely on their prognosis.

In 1784 Dr. Charles White, a distinguished London physician, did not associate pulmonary embolism with phlegmasia alba dolens.

Virchow in Berlin and Meigs in Philadelphia wrote on the subject of blood clots stopping the stream of the circulation; Virchow advocating that the obstructing clot must always travel to the heart and the pulmonary arteries; Meigs advocating that it may be formed *in situ* in the heart or pulmonary artery as well. Virchow upheld the embolus theory, Meigs the thrombosis theory.

Virchow [29] first showed the relation between thrombi and emboli, pointing out that emboli not infrequently have their origin in the soft-

* Read before the American Surgical Association, May 4, 1920.

ening, breaking down, and detachment of venous thrombi. He stated that in embolism the plug consists, not of blood clots, but of so-called vegetation or concretion of fibrin which has been washed off from the valves of the heart or from the endocardium and carried forward by the arterial current until the vessels become too small in calibre to allow it to advance any further.

Anatomy.—Cohnheim and Litten [9] experimentally demonstrated the fact that the arterial ramifications of the pulmonary artery do not anastomose. They are end-arteries.

The bronchial arteries supply the parenchyma of the lung with not insignificant quantities of blood. Virchow called them the nutrient arteries of the lung. They showed that pulmonary infarcts do not result in the death of the lung, when death of the animal itself does not result, but prevent the functioning of the infarcted area for purposes of oxidation. They conclude that despite the absence of parenchymatous changes in infarcted lungs, where the quantity of infarcted lung is sufficient, death must result from disturbance of respiratory function. The bigger the obstructed artery or the larger the number of smaller obstructed arteries, the greater is the effect upon respiration, and so it happens that where multiple emboli occur successively, even without parenchymatous changes in the lungs, death must eventually ensue from respiratory insufficiency.

Anningson [1] claimed that in the pulmonary artery the clots are most commonly found at the point where it breaks up into its branches.

Mann [10] states that deaths due to pulmonary embolism should be divided into three groups: (1) Immediate death occurring when only a small portion of the pulmonary circulation is obstructed. (2) Death caused within a few minutes and due to complete or almost complete blocking of the pulmonary circulation. (3) Delayed death, the result of an increase, by thrombosis, of an initial blockage by an embolism of a portion of the pulmonary circulation.

Experimentally, it was impossible to produce death or seriously imperil the life of the animal by emboli until the pulmonary circulation was greatly obstructed.

There is a wide difference of opinion regarding the frequency with which pulmonary thrombosis occurs primarily or is due to an embolus.

Virchow [20] divided obstruction of the pulmonary artery into four groups:

1. Following compression of a branch of pulmonary artery, coagulation of the blood may occur.

2. The introduction of a deleterious substance sets up an inflammation and this causes coagulation of the blood.

3. Spontaneous coagulation of blood from causes within the blood itself.

4. Obstruction occurs through a more or less compact mass which is carried into the pulmonary vessels and becomes lodged in them.

The majority of plugs in the trunk or main divisions of the pulmonary artery found in cases of sudden death, present the anatomical characters of emboli, associated perhaps with secondary thrombi, but there remain a certain number of cases of sudden or gradual death from primary thrombosis of the pulmonary artery or from thrombosis extending into a main division from an embolus in a smaller branch.

Welch [21] showed that bland embolism in medium-sized and small branches of the pulmonary artery in normal lungs and without serious impairment of the pulmonary circulation usually causes no symptoms and no changes in the parenchyma of the lungs.

Virchow [20] pointed out that emboli fill the pulmonary arteries without adhering to the walls when they are young, while the vessel walls show no changes, but when the emboli are old they cling to the wall which shows inflammatory changes.

Emboli usually stop at the bifurcation of a large artery, usually the vessels of the second and third order (Paget). Before and behind these fresh blood coagulation may occur.

Welch [21] shows that an embolus is the starting-point of a secondary thrombosis, which usually, although not always, completes the closure of the vessel, if this was not affected by the embolus itself, and extends on each side to the nearest branch.

Humphrey [1] said thrombosis occurred most commonly at the junction of the profunda and saphena veins with the femoral. The presence of valves at the meeting-point of two veins helps to bring about the condition.

Anningson [1] thinks that inflammation might follow the clotting, but was not the cause of it.

Clots may be absorbed, leaving the veins as normal as before.

Glynn [14] believes that emboli in the pulmonary artery may be distinguished from primary thrombi by the fact that the former are coiled or fractured or riding astride of a bifurcating vessel.

Fowler and Godley hold that embolism is commoner than thrombosis (pulmonary), but spontaneous thrombus does occur. West considers spontaneous thrombosis exceedingly rare.

Welch [21] believes in the usually accepted opinion that the majority of plugs found in the pulmonary artery and its main divisions in cases of sudden death are emboli.

Recently, Mery [14] in France and Newton Pitt in this country have maintained that spontaneous thrombosis is not infrequent, that in fact it may be commoner than embolism.

Box,[5] after making careful autopsies of several cases of so-called pulmonary embolism, came to the conclusion that these cases are a combination of thrombosis with embolism. He considers that a clot first forms in the pulmonary artery or in the right side of the heart and some sudden movement causes detachment of this clot which enters and completely plugs one or both pulmonary arteries.

He explains that a clot forming in the pulmonary artery or right ventricle very soon after the operation may become absorbed without producing symptoms, but it may increase in size, become detached and then plug the pulmonary artery.

Wilson [22] thinks it is probable that obstruction of the pulmonary artery sometimes occurs without proving fatal.

According to Foulkrod,[22] embolism of the pulmonary artery is invariably fatal. When involving the small blood-vessels in the lungs it may produce atelectasis, infarct, abscess or gangrene and the patient may recover.

Welch [23] states that asphyxia, cerebral anæmia, or interference with the coronary circulation are the factors concerned, but the exact apportionment to each of its due share in the result is not easy, nor very important.

Dr. Wm. Zahn [25] made a very extensive study of the formation of thrombi. His work will always stand out as a classic upon this subject and should be studied in detail in considering this subject.

Incidence.—In McLean's [25] experience emboli and embolic abscesses follow 2.2 per cent. of all laparotomies.

Ritzman [24] reported fifty-five cases in 6000 autopsies. All patients were over thirty years of age, and most were between fifty and seventy. There were as many females as males.

Bang[1] reported eighty-eight cases of embolism, one-half of which occurred in persons between twenty and thirty years of age.

In Lichtenberg's[23] collection of 23,680 operations, including 16,000 laparotomies, there were 2 per cent. of pulmonary complications and among the laparotomies 5.5 per cent.

Among 1000 operations on the vermiform appendix, Muhsom[25] reported thirty-one cases, five of which were fatal.

Mauclair[22] has collected fifty cases after the radical cure of inguinal hernia, twelve out of twenty-five fully reported being fatal.

The prognosis of post-operative pulmonary embolism is extremely grave; in 233 cases collected by Lenormant, death occurred in 106 or 45.5 per cent.

The order of frequency in which emboli are found in the different arteries may be given as follows: pulmonary, renal, splenic, cerebral, iliac and lower extremities, axillary and upper extremities, coeliac axis with its hepatic and gastric branches, central artery of the retina, superior mesenterics, inferior mesenterics, abdominal aorta, coronary, and the heart.

Lotheisen[18] collected sixty-six cases of pulmonary embolism, of which fifty-five were fatal:

1. Following fractures, thirty-six cases; thirty fatal.
2. Contusion, six cases; five fatal.
3. Tendon and muscle lacerations, four cases; four fatal.
4. Following operations, twenty cases; sixteen fatal.

Of Lotheisen's sixty-six cases, only six were under thirty, the majority being over forty. Of his sixty-six cases, forty-one were males, twenty-two females, and three unspecified.

Bang[1] found ten cases of embolus in 600 autopsies—1.66 per cent.

According to Wilson,[38] in operations on blood-vessels, alimentary canal, and genito-urinary organs, from 1 to 2 per cent. of all cases give more or less distinct evidence of emboli, about 7 per cent. of which are in the lungs.

About 10 per cent. of post-operative emboli which give clinical symptoms cause death.

Foulkrod[13] found thirty-seven cases of proved or suspected pulmonary embolism. According to his observations, thrombosis and embolism (not confined to pulmonary) occur in from 1 to 3 per cent. of cases, including both post-operative and obstetric. Obstruction of the pulmonary circulation alone occurs in a very much smaller percentage of cases.

Beckman, quoted by Van Sweringen,[36] reports six cases of pulmonary embolism occurring at Rochester in the first eight months of 1910 out of 4530 consecutive cases operated upon.

Kelly and Cullen report four deaths from pulmonary embolism out of 901 hysterectomies.

Howard showed that venous thrombosis occurred thirty-four times in 3774 patients with appendicitis and that a little less than one-eighth of these were cases of pulmonary embolism.

Albanus found that pulmonary embolism followed in 2 per cent. of abdominal operations.

Burkhard gives in 236 operations for uterine fibroids twelve cases of embolism (Keen's Surgery).

In Bidwell's[2] practice pulmonary embolism or thrombosis has occurred in .5 per cent. of abdominal operations.

The risk of pulmonary thrombosis after an appendectomy in the quiet stage is not merely a nominal one, since three such cases occurred in Bidwell's practice and represent a mortality of nearly 1 per cent. after operation, the death rate from other causes being only .4 per cent.

POST-OPERATIVE PULMONARY THROMBOSIS

Out of 700 obstetrical cases, Church[1] saw only one case of pulmonary embolism. These cases are evenly divided between primiparæ and multiparæ.

Playfair[25] states that as far as present statistics go, thrombosis and embolism seem more common in primiparæ than multiparæ.

Lotheisen[18] states that emboli occur, as a rule, in adults. Only one case of a child with pulmonary embolism could be found in the literature—a year-and-a-half-old boy with diphtheria and pneumonia.

Bidwell[5] thinks that pulmonary embolism after abdominal operations may be more frequent than is generally supposed and that its apparent rarity may be due to the surgeon's natural dislike to attract attention to his fatal cases.

McLean's[20] studies and observations have convinced him that a far greater percentage of post-operative ailments than we are accustomed to attribute to embolism really owe their origin to that cause.

Etiology of Thrombosis.—Welch[33] states that slowing and other irregularities of circulation in combination with lesions of cardiac or vascular wall or with the presence of microörganisms or other changes in the blood are important predisposing causes of thrombosis and frequently determine the localization of the thrombus.

2. Changes which impair or destroy the smooth surface of the normal inner lining of the vessel play an important part in the etiology of thrombosis (inflammation, atheroma, calcification, necrosis, other degenerations, tumors, compression and injury).

3. Infective thrombi (thrombophlebitis) develops during the progress of pneumonia, typhus, acute rheumatism, erysipelas, cholera, scarlatina, variola, tuberculosis, syphilis, nearly all acute and chronic infections. Likewise in chlorosis, gout, leukæmia, senile debility and chronic wasting, and cachectic diseases, particularly cancer, thrombosis is a recognized complication.

4. Chemical changes in the blood-ferment thrombi. Alterations in the formed elements of the blood caused directly or indirectly by toxic substances are of great significance in the etiology of pulmonary thrombosis.

a. Increase of blood platelets—there is a parallelism between the disposition to thrombosis and the number of platelets in certain diseases.

b. Calcium content is an important factor in coagulation of blood.

As factors in the causation of thrombosis, Lotheisen[18] considers:

1. A change in the blood constituents.

(*a*) Anæmia (puerperal hemorrhage or uterine hemorrhage due to myoma uteri).

(*b*) Gestation (physiological changes in blood and leucocytosis).

(*c*) Chlorosis.

(*d*) Prolonged fevers, malaria, cholera.

(*e*) Elephantiasis (Fayrer, three cases).

(*f*) Cachexia-malignant tumors.

2. Slowing of blood stream.

(*a*) Weak heart.

(*b*) Fatty degeneration—pregnancy.

(*c*) Pregnancy—gravid uterus pressing on veins.

3. Change in the vessel wall.

(*a*) Phlebitis.

(*b*) Trauma.

(*c*) Atheroma.

Wilson[35] states that the most important factors concerned in extensive post-operative thrombosis are:

(*a*) Injury of vascular walls.

(*b*) Slowing and stagnation of blood-stream.

(*c*) Disintegration of the corpuscles of the blood from toxic substances.

(*d*) Bacteræmia.

Foulkrod[13] enumerates as pathological conditions influencing coagulation the fol-

95

lowing: Preëxisting thrombosis, toxæmia or infections—under this heading he includes infections of the endometrium and broad ligament veins and particularly bronchial infections, profound mental depression, placenta prævia or other conditions producing excessive hemorrhage, mechanical pressure from the weight of the uterus, and slowing of the heart action.

Playfair [23] believes further thromboses of heart and pulmonary artery are sometimes due to dysentery; typhus and typhoid fever may also cause death by thrombosis of pulmonary artery.

According to Ritzman's [24] observations, the causes were various: vitium cordis, myodegeneration, arteriosclerosis, anæmia and cachexia, conditions causing phlebitis, injuries and operations. Nearly all the affections were related to vascular disease of some sort.

Church [6] claims that thrombosis is induced in puerperal state, rheumatism, fevers and other blood dyscrasiæ, such as erysipelas, diphtheria, pneumonia—increase of fibrin in the blood one third.

Bidwell [4] says pulmonary embolism is unpreventable since the active cause as well as the means of prevention are not known.

It is the opinion of Bidwell that thrombosis occurs only in consequence of changes in the blood-vessels, the blood, or both. A thrombus, of course, is formed by the development of fibrin; but fibrin does not exist in healthy blood, but is produced by the action of fibrin ferment on fibrinogen. Fibrin ferment does not exist in the blood, but is the result of a combination of calcium salts with nucleo-proteid. Calcium salts are normal constituents of the blood, but nucleo-proteid is not, and it is probably produced by degeneration of leucocytes and of blood platelets. In normal circumstances a considerable quantity of nucleo-proteid can be disposed of in the circulation, probably by the action of the endothelial lining of the blood-vessels; this power is, however, diminished by injury, by inflammation, and by retarding of the blood-stream.

Therefore, thrombosis forms when the walls of the blood-vessels have been injured; also in cases of sepsis, by increase of CO_2 in the blood, by general conditions, such as chlorosis and anæmia, and lastly by specific fevers, more especially typhoid.

Bland Sutton,[5] in his Hunterian lecture, is convinced that the formation of thrombi in the great veins after pelvic operations is due in all cases to sepsis.

Faure [11] describes two fatal cases occurring within a few days operated between February 12 to 24, 1919, during the influenza epidemic after the clinic had been free from such fatalities for many months, thus attributing these cases to influenza infection. At the same time, there were three additional cases of phlebitis and numerous cases of wound infection during this period, while the clinic had been free from all of these complications for months.

McLean [20] has shown how, except in the presence of an infection, it was impossible to produce experimentally a thrombus and a resulting embolus, and for this reason claims that a perfectly aseptic operation is rarely followed by an embolic process.

He insists that endothelial damage, on which so much stress is generally laid, is not, *per se*, a cause of thrombosis. Infection and necrosis (or the toxins derived from an infection and necrotic process) are probably the most important factors in thrombus production. A slowing of the blood-stream is a contributory cause, but of itself will not cause a thrombus to form.

Fromme [13] introduced a silk thread into the jugular vein of rabbits. A sterile thread produced a thrombosis only in anæmic animals or in those in bad physical condition, while the thread impregnated with any form of bacteria regularly produced thrombi.

Talke [25] said he had placed culture of staphylococci near thirteen arteries and thirty-one veins in thirteen animals, and he removed these after nine to twelve hours. Twenty-two veins and eleven arteries were thrombosed. The vessel wall and the surrounding tissues showed typical inflammation, but the thrombosis occurred before the microörganisms had entered the lumen of the vessel, hence seemed to be caused by the toxins.

Bidwell[*] quotes some surgeons who assert that all cases of thrombosis are really septic in origin, but states that it is difficult to agree with this statement, since it occurs in aseptic cases and in such a case as a gastric ulcer.

Libanoff[*] explained the formation of thrombokinase in large hæmatomata leading to the danger of local or distant thrombosis and pointed out the necessity of evacuating these to avoid their absorption. Commenting on this, Murphy asks: " Why has one clinic so many cases of thrombosis and embolism and the other clinic so few? " May it not be due to imperfect hæmostasis by one operator and the perfect capillary hæmostasis of the other? In the first instance, large hæmatomata form, and the latter give up the thrombokinase and thrombosis follows; while in the other no hæmatomata form and consequently no thrombokinase is given out, and therefore no activity of thrombogen occurs with the calcium salts to form a thrombus.

Volker[*] said he was surprised to find in necropsies on animals dead of embolism that there was invariably some brownish liquid blood in small quantities at the bottom of the wound, and it occurred to him that there might be some relation between the debris of these small hæmatomata and fatal embolism. He believed the debris from the hæmatomata should be looked upon as the cause of embolism.

Dr. Joseph Price, quoted by Volker,[*] called attention to the dangers of these small "blood pools" in the pelvis following operations as early as 1893 and placed great stress upon the danger from them and the importance of leaving the field of operation perfectly dry.

After delivery the blood dyscrasia is increased by, the absorption of effete matter in the process of uterine involution. Severe hemorrhage and syncope with slowing of the blood-stream increase the tendency to coagulation. Plugs normally found in natural labor in the open orifices of the uterine sinuses after separation of the placenta may find their way into the systemic circulation.

Zurheile[*] claims that retardation of blood-stream is the main factor in the production of a thrombosis, so that the blood plates pile up mechanically in the more sluggish blood. His experiments show the uselessness of striving to prevent thrombosis by reducing the coagulating property of the blood; as we are unable to act on the blood plates, all we can do is to prevent the blood-stream from becoming sluggish.

Aschoff[*] suggests that it may be possible to prevent thrombosis by changing the physical condition in the circulation, combating any tendency to slower pulse rate. He does not think that thrombosis is always of infectious origin, but a superimposed infection transforms a primary insignificant thrombosis into a dangerous thrombophlebitis. He supports the theory advanced by Virchow that the slowing up of the stream is the principal factor in the development of thrombi.

All cases observed by Glynn[*] of pulmonary thrombosis had been bed-ridden, and passive congestion of the lungs may have been a predisposing cause of thrombosis. It is also a fact that nine cases had been anæsthetized.

Bardeleben[*] showed that streptococci introduced into the blood-stream produce a thrombosis only if the stream is slowed down, otherwise non-virulent varieties are destroyed, while virulent varieties produce severe bacterææmia if highly virulent streptococci become lodged upon the vessel wall.

Bidwell[*] points out the fact that when thrombosis attacks a femoral vein, the left is most usually affected, and this is explained by the course of the left iliac vein being less direct than that of the right and also by the fact that the flow of blood through it is likely to be retarded by the pressure of a loaded sigmoid.

Playfair[*] believes that central thrombosis (cardiac and pulmonary) should be looked upon as a complication which is liable to attend the performance of surgical operations in general, but more especially those done on cachectic subjects or those involving much shock or hemorrhage.

He also states that both thrombosis and embolism are much more common in patients who are anæmic and weak either from hemorrhage or other cause.

Duncan[1] argues that it is due to anæmia, which so frequently affects women suffering from uterine fibroids, and supports his views by quoting a case of a woman with fibroids dying from pulmonary embolism while in the hospital awaiting operation.

Clark, quoted by Van Sweringen,[21] believes that thrombosis in non-septic epigastric veins is due to propagating thrombus of the deep epigastric veins originally produced by the traumatism resulting from operative manipulations and especially the use of heavy retractors.

Others maintain that post-operative thrombosis is caused by the pressure of retractors on the edges of the abdominal wound causing injury to the deep epigastric veins; the thrombus forms first at the seat of injury and afterwards spreads down to or around to the femoral vein.

It is generally supposed that patients suffering from uterine fibroids are peculiarly liable to thrombosis and embolism; this is explained (1) by the increase of calcium salts in the blood, as shown by the tendency to calcareous degeneration of the fibromata, and (2) by some degeneration and weakening of the cardiac muscle fibre which is commonly associated with the condition and, according to several authors, to the fact that the stump left after the removal of the uterus has not been carefully covered with peritoneum after accomplishing perfect hæmostasis, thus favoring infection.

Anningson[1] thought it possible that the tendency to coagulation during the puerperal state and in pneumonia, erysipelas, etc., was due to excess of white corpuscles in these conditions.

Virchow[20] believed that the fibrin clots or pulmonary emboli were secondary to thrombosis elsewhere. This thrombosis occurs in the veins or right heart, and is carried to the pulmonary arteries by the blood-stream.

To substantiate this he reports that out of seventy-six sections performed in August in the Morgue of the Berlin Charities he encountered eighteen venous thromboses and six lung or pulmonary thromboses.

Obstruction may or may not cause change in the parenchyma.

When the blood in one vein clots, the coagulum extends beyond the mouth of the next vein, so that, as the blood from this vein passes by, small pieces of coagulum can easily be detached. Virchow has been able to match the edges of pulmonary emboli with those of venous thrombosis from which they originated.

Wilson[21] states 80 per cent. of emboli have their source in venous thrombosis, 10 per cent. are cardiac and 10 per cent. scattered and undeterminable. Long, loosely formed thrombi from medium-sized veins are those chiefly concerned in embolism. When large, loose thrombi in resting patients, any unusual exertion or change of position may cause a dislocation of large masses which become dangerous emboli.

Church,[4] quoting Playfair in his "Science and Practice of Midwifery," says, "I have shown from a careful analysis of twenty-five cases of sudden death after delivery, in which accurate post-mortem examination has been made, that the cases of spontaneous thrombosis and embolism depend upon the period after delivery at which the fatal result occurs. In seven of these cases there was distinct evidence of embolism, and in them death occurred at a remote period after delivery, in none before the nineteenth day. This contrasts remarkably with the cases in which post-mortem examinations afforded no evidence of embolism. These amounted to fifteen out of twenty-five; in all of them, with one exception, death occurred before the fourteenth day, often on the second or third. The reason for this seems to be that in the former, time is required to admit of degenerative changes taking place in the deposited fibrin, leading to separation of an embolus; while in the latter, the thrombosis corresponds in time and to a great extent no doubt also in cause to the original thrombosis from which in the former the embolus was derived. Many cases I have since collected illustrate the same rule in a very curious and instructive way."

Playfair [*] expresses the following opinion:

Obstruction of the pulmonary artery after delivery may depend upon either embolism or spontaneous thrombosis.

The former usually occurs at a much later period after delivery than the latter, and spontaneous thrombosis probably corresponds with and is due to some cause similar in its nature to that which produces the obstruction of the peripheral veins in true cases of embolism.

Church [*] states thrombosis may occur simultaneously at the periphery (veins) and centre (heart and lungs) of blood-stream. Dr. W. J. Playfair cites cases of pulmonary obstruction that have not proved fatal immediately and in which shortly afterwards phlegmosia dolens commenced, showing thereby that coagulum was first formed in the centre and then at the periphery.

Thrombosis rarely occurs till one week after an operation; from the tenth to the fourteenth day is the usual time, but sometimes it is as late as one month. Recovery is generally complete in from two to three weeks. As a rule, these cases do not suffer from pulmonary complications, and in those rare cases in which sudden death does occur after a femoral thrombosis, it is probable that a thrombosis coexisted in the pulmonary artery.

Etiology of Embolism.—Lotheisen [*] makes the following observations: Most emboli originate from the veins of the lower extremity. In his sixty-six cases, forty originated there.

Following parturition or gynæcologic operations, emboli have originated from thrombosis of veins about the uterus.

The hemorrhoidal plexus has also been indicted several times.

Bumm describes two cases following operation on the rectovaginal septum.

Embolism usually occurs after a previous period of rest in bed followed by sitting up, straining at stool, or muscular effort, manipulation or massage of the leg, rubbing in ointment or even the application of a bandage or zinc gelatine boot (Velpeau).

Wyder [*] saw pulmonary embolism following colpoperineal plastic.

Symptomatology of Thrombosis.—Pain, swelling, masses in superficial veins (or deep veins).

Thrombosis—sudden pulse rise with normal temperature, later temperature rise with embolism. After this temperature may descend while the pulse remains elevated (Mahler[34]).

Welch [*] gives one of the clearest descriptions of symptoms. Death may be instantaneous from syncope. More frequently the patient cries out, is seized with extreme precordial distress and violent suffocation, and dies in a few seconds or minutes. Or when there is still some passage for the blood, the symptoms may be prolonged for several hours or even days before the fatal termination. The symptoms of large pulmonary embolism are the sudden appearance of a painful sense of oppression in the

99

chest, rapid respiration, intense dyspnœa, pallor followed by cyanosis, turgidity of the cervical veins, exophthalmos, dilatation of the pupils, tumultuous or weak and irregular heart action, small empty radial pulse, great restlessness, cold sweat, chills, syncope, opisthotonous and convulsions. The intelligence may be preserved or there may be delirium, coma, and other cerebral symptoms. Particularly striking is the contrast between the violence of the dyspnœa and the freedom with which the air enters the lungs, and the absence of pulmonary physical signs, unless in the more prolonged cases, it be the sign of œdema of the lungs.

Wyder[14] enumerates the symptoms of pulmonary embolism as follows: (1) dyspnœa (cardiac apnœa); (2) anxiety; (3) cyanosis; (4) dilated pupils; (5) powerful and irregular heaving of heart; (6) pulse imperceptible; (7) death following syncope.

Auscultation during pulmonary embolism reveals often a blowing murmur during systole or systole and diastole at the base. Henning heard this in 4 cases out of 33.

In Lotheisen's 66 cases it was reported 3 times. Pain in the region of the scapula or in the right or left hypochondrium. Consciousness is usually retained to the last. Rarely delirium, syncope, or convulsions occur. Sense of coldness complained of; they frequently shiver.

Regarding the diagnosis, Meyer[20a] considers next to the clearly demonstrable enlargement of the right heart, the accentuation of the second pulmonary sound of importance.

Differential Diagnosis.—Wyder[14] states that atheroma of coronary arteries gives a similar picture. These patients usually give a history of previous similar attacks.

Schumacher[30] calls attention to the fact that the diagnosis of pulmonary embolism may be difficult because a suddenly occurring internal hemorrhage, also myodegeneration of the heart, can produce like symptoms.

Prophylactic Treatment.—Many suggestions have been made in the direction of prophylactic treatment, of which the following are the most important.

Wyder[14] lays down the following rules:

(a) In chlorosis give iron.

(b) In cases of pregnancy avoid operation in the neighborhood of the uterus, anus, and vulva if possible. Such operations may cause miscarriage, which aids in liberation of emboli.

(c) In cases of operation avoid hæmatomata, because thrombosis is readily set up in adjoining veins.

(d) In cases of venous stasis in the lower extremities elastic bandages and massage are recommended to avoid thrombosis. If thrombosis is suspected, however, these should not be employed (v. Jurgensen). The author condemns massage in all cases for fear of liberating emboli.

(e) For the same reason, Puternan goes so far as to avoid massage in all cases of fracture until three weeks after injury.

(f) In cases of thrombosis all movements should be avoided. Patients should not sit up in bed. Straining at stool should be avoided by the use of proper cathartics.

(g) Elevation of the leg has no value.

(h) Cold compresses changed every hour or two and laid on the anterior surface of the leg, so as not to make necessary the elevation of the leg, are advised.

Rest in bed is mandatory as long as symptoms of thrombosis or capillary thrombi are present. Even after the swelling has disappeared the patient should remain in bed for several days.

Tally recommends as a prophylactic measure that good contraction of the uterus should be sought after labor.

In endocarditis undue muscular effort, including straining at stool and severe coughing should be avoided.

Thane [27] suggests the undesirability of prolonged use of Trendelenburg position, as it may predispose to pulmonary embolism.

Ward [11] speaks of the abandonment of extensive exposure of the levator ani muscle during perineoplasty to prevent bruising of the numerous small veins exposed.

The length of time that a limb should be kept immobilized should be gauged by the disappearance of swelling, tenderness and fever which often takes one or two months. The return to normal activity should be by easy stages.

Grober [16] advises where possible the excision of the original site of thrombosis.

When thrombo-embolism occurs, keep patient absolutely at rest in bed and give morphia for distress.

Welch [12] advises the following points in the treatment of thrombosis:

(a) Prophylactic measures should be directed toward maintaining good nutrition, strengthening the heart's action and warding off secondary infection.

(b) He mentions the use of citrated milk; 20 to 40 grains of citrate to the pint in diseases conducive to thrombosis.

(c) Absolute rest, suitable position, and immobilization of the thrombosed extremity, and nourishing diet to ward off embolism.

Caution patient against moving the leg; palpation of affected limb should be of the gentlest sort and is better omitted altogether. The patient should not be allowed to walk in less than forty days. After the danger of embolism is passed, massage and bandaging may be employed to advantage.

Wilson [30] enumerates the following precautionary measures:

(a) Reduction of vascular traumatism to minimum at operation.

(b) The encouragement of very early free movement on the part of the patient.

(c) The post-operative administration of drugs to increase the coagulability of the blood is of questionable value as far as thrombosis and embolism are concerned.

(d) Measures leading toward the reduction of bacteræmia. Eliminate foci of infection, treat with vaccine, etc.

Bidwell [8] insists that methods of prevention are of more importance than methods of treatment, and these include the treatment of anæmia before operation, giving excess of fluids, the use of citrates, and getting the patient up as soon as possible after operation. At the same time lime salts, magnesium carbonate and milk should be avoided.

He states that the tendency to coagulation is decreased by oxygen, by improving the force of the circulation, by alcohol, by excess fluids and reduction of solids, by citric acid, rhubarb, acid fruits and wines and by tobacco.

Wyder [34] considers the most important prophylactic measures to recognize the presence of thrombosis and avoid everything which may loosen emboli.

Thorough blood study in cases of anæmia he advises to postpone operation until this is relieved. Administer iron in these cases.

To prevent femoral thrombosis after an operation Bidwell [8] believes that we should avoid the risk of injury to the edges of the wound by placing gauze pads beneath our retractors, and by using them as gently as possible; we should avoid an exclusive milk diet; we should keep the lower bowel unloaded, so as to minimize the interference with the blood-stream through the common iliac vein by pressure from the sigmoid; we should give excess of fluids, especially by rectum, and we should avoid calcium salts and carbonate of magnesia. The patient should have plenty of fresh air and should be given citrates, if milk is allowed.

Th. Kocher agreed with Volker [29] and went still further, saying that he sought for locations where there may have been old thrombi, e.g., in the varices of the leg. He thinks it clearly indicated to cure such varices before subjecting the patients to major operations during which they may succumb to embolism. For this purpose he makes use of ligatures of the large saphenous by Trendelenburg's method by multiple intermediate ligations of the varices.

Playfair[22] agrees that the main element in the treatment of such cases is the most rigid rest and a nourishing supporting regimen.

Paul Zweifel[11] reports eighteen pulmonary thrombosis deaths in 1832 cases operated upon a table interfering with the veins of the lower extremities and only three in 860 cases operated upon a table which did not have this feature. In the former series, the deaths from this cause amounted to one in 100; in the latter series, one in 286.

He advises the following precaution which, according to his enormous clinical experience, will greatly reduce the occurrence of pulmonary thrombosis. Avoid all pressure upon the veins of the lower extremities, such as occur from permitting the legs to hang over the lower end of the table in operations in the Trendelenburg position with the use of the tables which drop the lower end.

He gives further statistics, according to which he lost five cases from thrombosis in 450 abdominal sections; three in operations for uterine fibroids, one for carcinoma of the uterus, and one for extirpation of a cyst in a patient seventy-five years of age. Following this high mortality, notwithstanding the fact that the extremities were not traumatized during the operation, a change in the technic was followed by only five deaths from thrombosis in 2060 laparotomies and only one in 484 operations for uterine fibroids, and this in a patient who had suffered eight weeks previously from a cerebral embolus. All the five deaths mentioned occurred in decrepit, anæmic, or cachectic patients.

The change in technic consisted in the absolute control of oozing of blood and in applying a purse-string suture covering absolutely all raw surfaces in the pelvis.

R. Olshausen[24] attributed the frequent occurrence of pulmonary thrombosis to the use of an operation table which caused the knees to be flexed in placing patients in the Trendelenburg position, causing a compression of the veins of the lower extremities; 2443 with 14 pulmonary thromboses; of these there were 571 uterine fibroids, with seven thromboses. Following these cases he reported fibroids with no thromboses in cases operated on a table without compression of the veins of the legs.

Therapeutic Treatment.—According to Wyder,[24] upon the occurrence of pulmonary embolism rapid therapeutic measures are necessary.

1. Subcutaneous injections of ether and camphor in oil. Von Kenézy gave ether injections hourly for two days and claims that the patient felt definite alleviation after each. Oeder gave .2 gram camphor every five minutes or 2.4 grams in one hour, and claims a recovery with this. Caffein and digitalis may be used intravenously.

2. Morphia .02 gram, used by most clinicians, counteracts shock, and if death supervenes, makes this less painful.

After infarction combat dyspnœa and distress with opiates.

Lead acetate may be administered. He does not hold artificial respiration useful, because death does not occur from respiratory obstruction but rather lack of oxygen in the blood.

Bidwell[8] states with regard to treatment, while he recognizes that little can be done when the whole of the right pulmonary artery is blocked; oxygen, strychnine, and saline injections are always given, and in one case life was prolonged fifteen hours.

Church[9] urges the use of oxygen gas inhalation for these patients on the basis of its demonstrated value in the treatment of pneumonia.

Meyer[20a] describes the removal of pulmonary emboli by Trendelenburg's operation in detail. Trendelenburg performed twelve operations of this kind on man without a permanent recovery.

He states that the coagulation of blood and recurrence of embolic accident can be avoided by injection of hirudin.

He distinguishes three classes of pulmonary embolism:

1. The one causing immediate exitus which evidently is due to shock, as not infrequently only a partial thrombosis of the artery may be found at autopsy.

2. The one causing death within a few minutes. Here thrombosis is perfect, separating pulmonary and greater circulation. The right heart becomes quickly overdistended.

3. The one of protracted course which is more frequently observed. Here one of the main branches of the artery and subdivisions become suddenly clogged, only gradually total obstruction sets in.

As a matter of fact, only the third category will furnish cases with indication for operation and the task of establishing this indication is rendered difficult on account of the experience that some of these patients get better under conservative treatment. He considers operation imperative if medical treatment fails to bring improvement.

Four times this operation was performed at the Zurich Clinic, but the patients could not be saved.

TABLE OF CASES OF DEATH DUE TO PULMONARY THROMBOSIS DURING THE FIVE YEARS 1915 TO 1919 IN THE AUGUSTANA HOSPITAL

	Date	No.	Sex	Age	Diagnosis	Operation	Operator	Post-operative days	Predisposing cause of embolism
1	7/15/15	43793	M	42	Osteochondroma of left ileum	Excision of osteochondroma	A. J. O.	4	Phlebitis.
2	9/ 4/15	44273	M	46	Gastric ulcer; cholecystitis, chronic appendicitis	Posterior gastroenterostomy cholecystectomy; appendectomy	N. M. P.	6	Perforated ulcer with preoperative loss of weight.
3	4/13/16	46790	F	33	Cholecystitis, retroversion, rectocele	Cholecystectomy perineorrhaphy	N. M. P.	2	
4	7/ 7/16	47388	F	44	Carcinoma of rectum	Colostomy	A. J. O.	3	
5	5/21/17	50718	M	65	Hypertrophied prostate	Suprapubic prostatectomy	N. M. P.	15	Cachexia; phlebitis left leg.
6	6/12/17	50802	F	33	Gestation; 3rd degree laceration perineum	Parturition perineorrhaphy	R. H.	14	Perineal sepsis.
7	4/28/18	54315	F	51	Cholelithiasis; carcinoma of rectum	Cholecystostomy panhysterectomy	A. J. O.	7	Anæmia; cachexia.
8	12/16/18	56932	F	43	Floating kidney; cholecystitis; appendicitis	Nephropexy; cholecystotomy; appendectomy	A. J. O.	12	Preoperative loss of weight, 35 pounds.

Year	Operations	Obstetrical deliveries	Laparotomies	Hysterectomies
1915............	3,665	153	1204	94
1916............	3,510	187	1218	88
1917............	3,303	211	927	133
1918............	3,303	278	871	107
1919............	2,915	270	1055	106
	16,696	1099	5275	528

Seven deaths in 16,696 operations = 1 case in 2385 = 0.042 per cent.
One death in 1099 obstetrical cases = 1 case in 1099 ± 0.1 per cent.
Five deaths in 5275 laparotomies = 1 case in 1055 = 0.1 per cent.
One death in 528 hysterectomies = 1 case in 528 = 0.5 per cent.

We have reviewed the histories of all cases of death due to pulmonary thrombosis which occurred during the past five years in the Augustana Hospital following surgical operations, including the years 1915 to 1919, eight cases. These are represented in the accompanying table. Of these, four cases occurred in my own service, three in the service of my colleague, Dr. N. M. Percy, and one in the obstetrical service in a patient in which a very extensive perineal laceration had to be repaired immediately following delivery. It is likely that the thrombosis had no relation to the operation, because deaths from this cause have occurred many times after delivery of cases in whom no surgical repair was made, but in order to make our statistics complete the case had to be included.

During these years 16,696 operations were performed in all in the Augustana Hospital with 5275 laparotomies, and of these 528 were hysterectomies which in all other statistics we have encountered showed the largest percentage of deaths from pulmonary thrombosis.

During the same period 76 cases of so-called pernicious anæmia were operated for splenectomy, cholecystectomy and appendectomy in patients who, according to all statistics, should have resulted in a considerable number of deaths from pulmonary thrombosis. Among these cases, most of which were operated by my colleague, Dr. N. M. Percy, there occurred no deaths from this cause.

In every case, however, the operation had been preceded by one or more transfusions of whole blood without the addition of citrate of soda.

Recognizing the etiological importance of the twelve conditions mentioned at the beginning of this paper, whose validity seems to have been established by many authorities noted for their keenness of observation, it would seem worth while to investigate whether death from pulmonary thrombosis could have been avoided in any or all of these cases had every possible precaution been taken to eliminate each one of these etiologic factors to the greatest possible extent.

1. *Local Infection.*—It seems certain that even the slightest amount of local infection may cause a thrombosis in a neighboring vein which may be loosened and serve as the cause of a fatal pulmonary thrombosis when it becomes lodged in the pulmonary vein. Although there is no evidence in any one of our cases that this has actually occurred, yet it seems important to still further perfect aseptic methods of operation. Of course, hæmostasis must be accomplished as a result of a normal thrombosis of the ends of the cut vessels, but it does not seem likely that such a thrombus will ever become loosened, so that it can cause death due to pulmonary thrombosis.

2. *Anæmia.*—Most of the patients, especially Cases II, V and VII, showed some degree of anæmia. It seems likely that it might have been possible to correct this by more careful preliminary treatment or by transfusion of whole blood.

3. *Slowing of Blood Stream.*—It has been claimed that keeping patients for a long continued operation in the Trendelenburg position would interfere with the blood stream in the extremities to such an extent that this serves as a predisposing cause. In none of our cases, except

104

Case II, could this have been the cause, as none of the other operations were of long duration.

4. *Subnormal General Physical Condition.*—This obtained in Cases II, VII and VIII, but aside from the possible improvement which could have been secured by the preliminary transfusion of whole blood, it is doubtful whether this cause could have been eliminated to a marked extent.

5. *Cachexia.*—The only treatment which could be of any benefit would again be the transfusion of whole blood. Two of our own cases belonged to this group, and were similar cases to come under our care in the future, we should make use of prophylactic transfusion of whole blood.

6. *Microörganisms in the Blood.*—None of our cases belong to this group, but we believe that in several cases of this class we have obtained great benefit by the transfusion of whole blood, although it is, of course, impossible to state that thrombosis has been prevented in any given case, although it failed to appear in any of these following transfusions.

7. *Excess of White Blood-cells.*—This cause did not exist in any of our cases.

8. *Inefficient Hæmostasis.*—Until very recently we had not fully appreciated the importance of this etiologic factor, and it is quite possible that some of our deaths may have been due to an error in this direction, although fortunately our method of closing the stump in hysterectomy for many years has corresponded to that upon which Zweifel[37] lays so much stress, and it is possible that we may have escaped many deaths from pulmonary thrombosis in this class of cases without being entitled to any credit for this.

9. *Traumatization of Tissues with Retractors, Etc.*—It seems likely that we have not exercised proper care in this direction, because until recently we have made use of heavy retractors for holding open the abdominal wound. These have now been discarded, and although we cannot trace any case directly to this cause, it seems likely that our technic has been bad in this direction.

10. *Injury to Veins of Extremities Due to Badly Arranged Operating Table.*—Zweifel and others have traced a number of their cases directly to the use of a table in which the knees are bent, so that the veins are compressed during the operation. They found a marked reduction of fatal cases upon abandoning this particular table. We have never used this type of table, but it seems proper to again direct attention to this apparent cause.

11. *Injury to Intima of Veins.*—Rough handling of tissue in the vicinity of the wound undoubtedly often causes an injury to the intima of veins, and it seems worth while to train one's self and one's assistants to avoid this as well as all other forms of unnecessary traumatization of tissues.

12. *Excess of Calcium Salts in the Blood.*—So many authors mention this as an etiologic factor that it may be important to consider it. So far we have paid no attention to this element.

It seems likely from our observations that in the future we will be justified in systematically adding the transfusion of 600 c.c. of whole blood to our preliminary treatment in a considerable proportion of cases belonging to a class which has in the past made up our list of deaths from pulmonary thrombosis and that the other precautions will be carried out with greater care.

It is likely that this will result in a considerable reduction in the death rate from post-operative pulmonary thromboses.

A short analysis regarding the etiology of the thrombophlebitis as shown in our eight tabulated cases is as follows:

CASE I.—A man, forty-three years of age, who had an enchondrosteoma 21 by 11 by 7 cm. removed from the lateral surface of the left ileum. The wound was aseptic and there is nothing in the history which could serve as a predisposing factor, except the fact that ten years previously the patient had suffered from thrombophlebitis of the veins in both legs and that the venous circulation had been impaired ever since this occurrence. The wound was aseptic, but his thrombophlebitis must have lighted up again. Had this patient received careful preliminary treatment for several weeks, it is quite likely that the thrombophlebitis might have been prevented.

CASE II.—A man forty-five years of age, giving a history of gastric ulcer complicated with cholecystitis and chronic appendicitis, had lost considerable in weight and was anæmic as a result of loss of blood from his gastric ulcer. The gall-bladder was thick, universally adherent, sacculated and filled with black viscid bile. The mucosa was granular. This gall-bladder was removed. The appendix was sacculated and universally adherent. In this case, the patient died six days after the operation from pulmonary thrombosis. This patient had anæmia and mild cachexia, also a great amount of disturbance because of the extensive operation and extensive adhesions. The operation lasted one hour and a half, consequently several factors were present which would account for the pulmonary thrombosis. A preliminary transfusion of whole blood and performing the operation in two stages, a gastro-enterostomy at the first stage and a cholecystectomy and appendectomy after the patient had fully recovered from the first operation, would probably have prevented the unfavorable result.

CASE III.—A woman, thirty-three years of age, showed nothing in her history which would predispose to the development of thrombophlebitis. She had a normal cholecystectomy for the relief of gall-stone disease and perineorrhaphy performed with an anterior suspension of the uterus. She died from pulmonary thrombosis two days following the operation. It seems likely that some of the veins in the vicinity of the broad ligaments or rectum must have been injured during the operation. The case emphasizes the importance of protecting the veins.

106

CASE IV.—A woman, forty-four years of age, with carcinoma of the rectum. This patient showed but very slight cachexia and was otherwise in fair condition. A simple colostomy was performed. The patient was under the influence of the anæsthetic less than half an hour, and there was nothing that one would reasonably expect to cause a thrombosis except that the mesentery of the sigmoid was transfixed and a strand of gauze and glass tube were passed through to keep the intestines from slipping back into the abdominal cavity. Evidently, a thrombus was loosened from one of these veins. Whether preliminary transfusion of whole blood might have prevented this, it is difficult to say.

CASE V.—A patient sixty-five years of age had a simple suprapubic prostatectomy from which he made a very satisfactory recovery for fifteen days, when he died suddenly from pulmonary thrombosis. On the afternoon of the fourteenth day a phlebitis developed in the femoral vein, which undoubtedly accounts for the embolus which gave rise to pulmonary thrombosis.

CASE VI.—A patient, thirty-three years of age, who suffered from a severe laceration of the perineum during delivery which was repaired immediately, died fourteen days later from pulmonary thrombosis. In this case there was severe suppuration of the perineal wound. Whether the infection from this source was responsible for the pulmonary thrombosis or whether the latter condition resulted from a loosened thrombus from the uterus, we have been unable to determine.

CASE VII.—A patient, fifty-one years of age, suffering from gallstones and cancer of the rectum with marked anæmia and cachexia, died of pulmonary thrombosis seven days after the operation, which consisted of a cholecystectomy and panhysterectomy. In this patient the anæmia should have been corrected by transfusion of whole blood and panhysterectomy should have been performed at the first operation and cholecystectomy after the patient had regained strength.

CASE VIII.—A patient forty-three years of age, suffering from a floating kidney which could be moved over the greater portion of the abdominal cavity, from cholelithiasis and appendicitis. She had lost 35 pounds in weight previous to the operation. The operation performed consisted of cholecystostomy, appendectomy, and suturing the kidney in place. The gall-bladder contained a large number of stones. In this case, good judgment would have undoubtedly prevented the pulmonary thrombosis, because with the patient in this condition, the appendix and gall-stones should have been removed first and the floating kidney operated at a second operation.

BIBLIOGRAPHY

[1] Anningson: Lancet, London, 1881, i, 16.
[2] Aschoff, L.: Med. Klin., Nov. 7, 1909, Beitrage zur Thrombosenfr., 1912.
[3] Bang: Afhandl. fur Doktorgraden Kjobreharn, 1880.
[4] Bardeleben: Arch. f. Gyne., 1907, lxxxiii, p. 36.
[5] Bidwell: London Pract., 1909, lxxxii, 214-223.

OCHSNER AND SCHNEIDER

[6] Bland-Sutton: Lancet, Jan. 16, 1909.
[7] Bumm: Centralblatt fur Gyne., 1894.
[8] Church: Tr. Edin. Obst. Soc., 1891, 2, xvii, 210–221.
[9] Cohnheim and Litten: Arch. f. Anat., etc., Berlin, 1875, lxv, 99–115.
[10] Cohnheim: Untersuchung uber die Embolishen Processe, Berlin, 1872.
[11] Faure, J.: Paris Medical, July 24, 1919.
[12] Fromme: Physiol. A. Path. d. Woch., Berlin, 1910, 168.
[13] Foulkrod: Am. J. of Obst., New York, 1911, lxxix, 855–857.
[14] Glynn: Liverpool Med. Chir. Jour., xxvii, 204–218.
[15] Grober: Deutsch Med. Wchnschr., Feb. 19, 1914.
[16] Ledill: Am. J. Med. Sciences, Phila., 1872, lxiv, 325–365.
[17] Libanoff: Jour. de Chir., Jan., 1914.
[18] Lotheisen: Beitrag. z. klin. Chir. Tubing., 1901–2, xxxii, 655–686.
[19] Mann, J.: Ex. Med., 1917, xxvi, 387.
[20] McLean: Lancet Clinic, 1916, cxvi, 221.
[20a] Meyer: Tr. Am. Surg. Assoc., xxxi, 1913, 233–248.
[21] Murphy: Surg., Gyn. and Obst., Jan. 8, 1915; Pract. Medicine Series Surgery, 1915, p. 92.
[22] Olshausen: Venhandl d. Gese. f. Chir., 1908, xxxiv, 15.
[23] Playfair: Tr. Path. Soc., Lond., 1867, xviii, 68–75; Lancet, July 27, 1867, 94; Lancet, Aug. 10, 1867, 153.
[24] Ritzman: Berl. Klin. Wchsch., July, 1911.
[25] Talke: Beitr. z. Klin. Chir., 1902, xxxvi, 339.
[26] Tally: Musser and Kelly, 1917, iv, 551.
[27] Thane: Anst. Med. Gazette, 1912, 126.
[28] VanSweringen: J. Ind. State Med. Ass., Fort Wayne, 1912, v. 157–160.
[29] Virchow: Neue Notizen Gibiet d. Natur u. Heilkunde, 1846; Beitr. z. Exp. Path. u. Phys., Berlin, 1846, 1–90.
[30] Volker: Semaine Medicale, April 29, 1914.
[31] Ward: Am. Jour. Obst., 1913, lxvii, 561.
[32] Welch: Thrombosis and Embolism; Allbotts System of Med., 1909, vi, 691–821.
[33] Wilson: ANNALS OF SURGERY, Dec., 1912, lvi, 809–817.
[34] Wyder: Volkmann's Sammlung Klin. Vortrage n. f., 146–1896.
[35] Zahn: Virchow's Arch., 1875, lxii, 81.
[36] Zurheile: Med. Klin., Nov. 7, 1909.
[37] Zweifel: Arch. f. Gyne., lxiii, 151; Arch. f. Gyne., cxi, 391.

THE CALLOUSED ULCER OF THE POSTERIOR WALL OF THE STOMACH *

BY WILLIAM J. MAYO, M.D.

OF ROCHESTER, MINN.

FROM July 1, 1914, to July 1, 1919, 647 operations were performed in the clinic on 638 patients with gastric ulcers, with an average operative mortality of 4.7 per cent. All patients who died in the hospital following operation are statistically classified as having died from operation, without regard to the cause of death or length of time after operation. During this same five-year period 2734 operations were performed on 2720 patients with duodenal ulcers, with an operative mortality of 1.2 per cent.

In twenty-eight of the series of 638 gastric ulcers the ulcers were mul-

108^{a}

CORRIGENDA

MAYO ON THE CALLOUSED ULCER OF THE POSTERIOR WALL OF THE STOMACH.

In the Annals of Surgery for July, 1920, page 109, 3d line from the top, 3.2 per cent. instead of 4.7 per cent. as the average mortality in the Mayo clinic of operations for gastric ulcer.

3 pounds. Fourteen patients had marked secondary anæmia, and anæmia was present in all, often accompanied by a cachexia. The maximum hæmoglobin was 66, the minimum 26. The pain was in the epigastrium in fifty-six patients, in the back in twenty-four; it radiated to the right in fifteen cases, to the left in eight, and downward in eight; in eleven it was given indefinitely as in the stomach and mid-abdomen. Food gave relief in fifty cases. The obstruction was not extreme in any case, although distinct lagging of food or obstruction varying from slight to moderate was demonstrated in 35 per cent. of the series.

Hour-glass stomachs were excluded from the series. Acids averaged about normal for the age, and there was little difference between the acid

---

* Read before the American Surgical Association, May 3, 1920.

(five points above) of the patients who had hemorrhages and those who did not. Nineteen patients (20 per cent.) had gross hemorrhages; seventeen vomited blood, and twelve, whether or not they vomited blood, had blood in the stools. The clinical diagnosis was correct in seventy-one cases. Cancer was diagnosed in six cases, pyloric obstruction in two, gall-stones or gastric ulcer in four, and duodenal ulcer in two. The X-ray diagnosis was correct in seventy-one cases; duodenal ulcer in two, and "negative stomach" in ten. No X-ray was made in two cases. The ten cases in which the diagnosis was negative represent a type which is now better understood. Within the last three years the X-ray technic has improved and diagnosis by this means is established in above 90 per cent. of lesions of the stomach.

To epitomize: The main characteristics of ulcer of the posterior wall of the stomach are: Chronicity, lesions usually large, more or less continuous distress, occasional exacerbations from localized peritonitis, and anæmia often accompanied by marked cachexia.

Even at operations it is sometimes difficult to determine whether the condition is ulcer or cancer until the lesion is actually exposed and a specimen secured for immediate microscopic examination. In our early experience in some cases clinically diagnosed as ulcer in which gastro-enterostomy only was done, the patients died later from carcinoma of the stomach, but at a time remote from the operation. It must be admitted that this is an impressionistic view because there was no specimen removed for evidence that the growths in question were not cancerous at the time the operations were performed. But since the ulcers were not removed, why did the patients live so long before the cancers became manifest? The opposite mistake certainly was made, because in some cases (7) that were clinically diagnosed cancer and in which gastro-enterostomy was done, the patients lived too long after the operation for the original diagnosis to have been correct. And here is just the difficulty in trying to settle the question of the frequency with which chronic ulcers of the stomach undergo malignant degeneration. Clinical diagnosis is notoriously defective, post-mortem evidence cannot prove the original disease, and operations that do not permit the actual excision of the lesion or the removal of a specimen for microscopic examination are open to objection. No matter how we view the question *a priori*, however, the experience of Robson, Moynihan, Fouchet, Deaver, and others, and the experience in our clinic is too large for the data to be controverted by the opinion of clinicians who have not had specimens removed and accurately examined during the life of the patient. Aschoff very properly points out that if the lesion is cancer originally the base of the ulcer will prove to be cancer. Wilson and MacCarty have shown in our cases of cancer on ulcer that cancer existed in the overhanging margin of the ulcer and not in the base.

An interesting side-light is thrown on the problem of peptic ulcers by

110

Balfour's investigation of the frequency of hemorrhage following operation for ulcer of the duodenum and stomach. He found, in cases of duodenal ulcer in which nothing but gastro-enterostomy was done and in which there had been hemorrhage before operation, that 1 in 8 had hemorrhage afterward, although all the other signs and symptoms were abated. In cases of gastric ulcer, however, hemorrhage occurred in only 1 in 12 following operation. Balfour explains this discrepancy as due to the fact that gastric ulcer, because of its carcinoma liability, was subjected to radical removal, while duodenal ulcer, having little or no cancer liability, was not usually excised. Balfour found that if duodenal ulcers were excised the liability to secondary hemorrhage disappeared and the mortality of cautery excision with gastro-enterostomy was not greater than gastro-enterostomy without excision. That all varieties of gastric ulcer are more serious than duodenal ulcers has been shown by data compiled from our cases by Hunter, Actuary of the New York Life Insurance Company; the death rate from duodenal ulcer in the first four years after operation was practically the same as the normal, as a matter of fact, better, while for gastric ulcer the average death rate in the four years was three times normal. A study of these tables cannot fail to leave a well founded suspicion that at least a minority of the patients died from cancer of the stomach.

Summary of Results in 85 Cases of Calloused Ulcer on the Posterior Wall of the Stomach in Which Operation was Done from July 1, 1914, to July 1, 1919.

		Per cent.
Cases	85	
Operations	87	
Deaths in hospital	4	4.7
Deaths after leaving hospital	10	11.7
Living patients reporting their condition	43	50.5
Improved	14	32.5
Unimproved	3	6.9
Cured	26	60.4
Patients not located	28	32.9

A. *Cautery or Knife Excision.*—Cautery alone or knife excision alone has a limited field of usefulness in cases of small ulcers in all situations. It has given good results when care is exercised not to disturb the nerve supply and the muscular efficiency. Opening the stomach and applying the cautery to the base of the adherent ulcer is not a sound procedure.

B. *Gastro-enterostomy.*—At times the general or local condition of the patient may indicate posterior gastro-enterostomy, or the extent of the posterior lesion may warrant anterior gastro-enterostomy.

C. *Resection.*—Resection of the pyloric half of the stomach by the methods of Billroth or the Polya-Balfour gives good results in suitable cases, and is the operation of choice when the pyloric region is involved. But when the ulcers lie high on the body of the stomach the operation removes a large part of the uninvolved organ that is capable of good

111

WILLIAM J. MAYO

function. Resection in continuity (sleeve resection) of the ulcer-bearing
area of the stomach, if the ulcer is in the middle third, is an excellent
method, as has been shown by our experience and corroborated by
Stewart. A circular piece of the stomach, including the ulcer, is removed
and the proximal and distal parts of the stomach are united end-to-end
with catgut.

D. Excision and Gastro-enterostomy.—After a good specimen has been
secured for microscopic diagnosis the ulcer is excised with the cautery,
the defect is closed with catgut sutures, and a posterior gastro-
enterostomy performed. Excision of the ulcer and gastro-enterostomy
would seem the logical procedure in the average case, but experience has
shown that the method may fail to give complete relief if the ulcers are on
the posterior wall of the stomach, because the reformation of crippling
adhesions that immoblize the posterior wall sometimes follow.

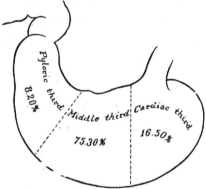

FIG. 1.—Diagram of location of ulcers found on the posterior
wall of the stomach, at operation, from July 1, 1914, to July
1, 1919.

OPERATIVE TECHNIC

The procedure herewith described combines excision of the ulcer and gastro-enterostomy and is satisfactory at least in that it usually prevents subsequent posterior fixation of the stomach. The approach to the posterior
wall of the stomach can be made either from above or below. I have
tried both, and perhaps because I have had a larger experience with the
upper approach I prefer it.

The gastrohepatic omentum is divided (Fig. 2), if necessary the
gastric artery is tied, and the adhesions high on the lesser curvature are
separated to secure adequate operating space. After all the adhesions are
cleared away I insinuate my finger around the adherent ulcer. This

112

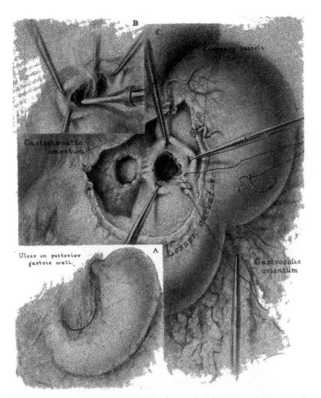

FIG. 2.—A. Lines marking proposed incisions in gastrohepatic omentum for exposure of ulcer which is removed for microscopic examination, and in gastrocolic omentum to draw the left-hand portion of the omentum proper into the lesser peritoneal cavity. B. Excising the ulcer with cautery. C. Crater of the ulcer on the posterior wall of the stomach separated from the pancreas for three-quarters of its extent, thereby exposing ulcer cavity in the pancreatic surface.

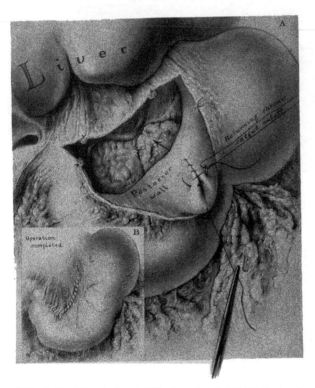

Fig. 3.—A. Ulcer being sutured transversely and omentum drawn behind the stomach covering the pancreatic incision and operative field. B. Operation completed.

hooks the involved stomach and pancreas in such manner that they can be drawn up into the wound and exposed. The stomach and its posterior attachments are held up by the finger, or by a gauze tape, and the ulcer is shaved off from the pancreas deep enough to include all the base. Sometimes in the huge ulcers the pancreas cannot be sufficiently exposed for the safe excision of the entire base of the ulcer. In such cases the pancreatic defect is carefully seared with the cautery. I have never seen fat necrosis or any harmful evidence of pancreatic leakage follow these manœuvres. The margin of the ulcer is caught with forceps in order to further its exposure. If the stomach contains a considerable quantity of fluid which has not been removed by the preliminary use of the stomach tube, the fluid should be removed by suction. Frozen sections of the base of the ulcer, of the involved pancreas, and of the margin of the ulcer area in the stomach are subjected to microscopic examination, and after this the ulcer is excised with the cautery. The posterior wall of the stomach above the ulcer will be found dilated and pouched, and the gap in the stomach is easily closed with through-and-through catgut sutures, bringing the cauterized margins of the stomach directly into contact. A second row of catgut sutures turns this line in. The direction of the suturing which prevents narrowing naturally suggests itself (Fig. 3). An opening is then made below the greater curvature through the gastrocolic omentum, and the tip of the omentum is drawn upward behind the stomach and fastened in a manner to cover the whole of the operative field. This insures speedy union and permanently separates the posterior wall of the stomach from the pancreas and liver. A posterior gastro-enterostomy completes the operation. Even if the field of operation is considerably soiled I make a proper toilet and do not use drainage; I have had no occasion to regret the omission.

BIBLIOGRAPHY

Aschoff, L.: Ueber die mechanischen Momente in der Pathogenese des runden Magengeschwürs und über sine Beziehungen zum Krebs. Deutsch. med. Wchnschr., 1912, i, 494–496.

Balfour, D. C.: Surgical Treatment in the Bleeding Type of Gastric and Duodenal Ulcer. Jour. Am. Med. Assn., 1919, lxxiii, 571–575.

Deaver, J. B.: Early Recognition of Carcinoma of the Stomach. New York Med. Jour., 1919, cix, 749–751.

Hunter, A.: Gastric and Duodenal Ulcers: Mortality after Operation. Association of Life Insurance Medical Directors, 1919.

Moynihan, B.: Disappointments after Gastro-enterostomy. Brit. Med. Jour., 1919, ii, 33–36.

Pauchet, V.: Traitement de l'ulcère chronique de l'estomac (gastroctomie suivie de gastro-jéjunostomie termino-latérale). Presse med., 1916, xxiv, 445–450.

Robson, A. W.: The Operative Treatment of Ulcer of the Stomach and Its Chief Complications. Brit. Med. Jour., 1906, ii, 1345–1350.

Stewart, G. D., and Barber, W. H.: Segmental Resection for Gastric Ulcer. ANNALS OF SURGERY, 1916, lxiv, 527–536.

Wilson, L. B., and MacCarty, W. C.: Pathologic Relationships of Gastric Ulcer and Gastric Carcinoma. Am. Jour. Med. Sc., 1909, cxxviii, 846–852.

8   113

FAILURE OF PRIMARY ROTATION OF THE INTESTINE (LEFT-SIDED COLON) IN RELATION TO INTESTINAL OBSTRUCTION *

BY EMMET RIXFORD, M.D.

OF SAN FRANCISCO, CAL.

PROFESSOR OF SURGERY IN THE STANFORD UNIVERSITY MEDICAL SCHOOL

WHATEVER be the cause of the inhibition of the primary rotation of the mid-gut it is perfectly obvious that when this condition is accompanied, as is usually the case, by failure of fixation of the mesentery, the conditions are ideal for the production of volvulus of large portions of the intestine. In this condition, which for brevity's sake is often called "left-sided colon," the mesentery on the right side ordinarily does not adhere to the posterior peritoneum. Why, we do not know, unless it is because we have to do with the mesentery of the small intestine.

In the normal condition of rotation of the intestine when the hepatic flexure of the colon grows over to the right or is pushed over by growth of that portion of the transverse colon which lies to the right of the duodenum, the superior mesenteric artery through its large branch which becomes the middle colic artery furnishing a relatively fixed point, the large intestine itself generally adheres on the right side, though not so uniformly as the descending colon adheres on the left side, and it is not unlikely that adhesion of the intestine occurs before that of the mesentery. At least the irregularity of the mesenteric adhesion leaving, as it often does, crypts and fossæ which are sometimes of surgical importance in relation to internal hernia, suggests that the intestine adheres first. The mechanism of this adhesion is also unknown. It is hardly competent to say that it is congenital. The fine cicatricial bands which are commonly observed about the ascending and descending colon suggest that the cause of the adhesions is some pre-natal inflammatory process, pre-natal peritonitis, if you will. Possibly the large bowel is less actively mobile and more penetrable by irritating substances. Certainly there is much material absorbed by the colon in pre-natal life desiccating the fluid contents of the small bowel into the stiff paste of meconium which is retained for a long time in the colon. If a pre-natal inflammation of the outer wall of the large bowel is presupposed it would readily enough account for these adhesions and other congenital bands which are frequently found. Such explanation has been offered for the production of this most interesting congenital anomaly, the failure of rotation of the mid-gut. An example of an adventitious band occurred in the second case here reported, where there was found a cord-like mass of tissue leading from the posterior wall of the abdomen to the posterior surface of the cæcum which lay in the right iliac fossa notwithstanding the fact that the small intestine lay completely to the right of the colon. The band was

* Read before the American Surgical Association, May 3, 1920.

manifestly the result of adhesion of the cæcum. Such a band of adhesion would furnish perfect conditions of obstruction by herniation of loops of bowel through the opening between it and the mesentery, but also if it were accompanied by " left-sided colon " with failure of attachment of the mesentery it would furnish a fixed point about which the entire intestine might be twisted, making a double volvulus—right and left.

Under normal conditions that part of the intestine between the lower part of the duodenum and that portion of the transverse colon which is

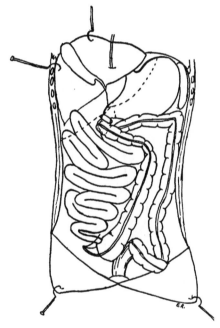

FIG. 1.

supplied by the mesocolic artery rotates to the left, *i.e.*, so as to form a left-handed spiral at the point of crossing of the large and small intestines, throwing the duodenum to the left beneath the superior mesenteric artery, so that afterwards the artery is found to pass down directly over its anterior surface. The angle of this left-handed rotation is said to be 180 degrees, but, as a matter of fact, it is 270 degrees or more, for in early embryonic life when the intestine is attached to the umbilicus by the vitelline duct the mesentery lies in the sagittal plane. As the gut grows and the loop of the small bowel and cæcum become drawn out and rotation takes place, as it were, about the vitelline duct or Meckel's diverticulum as an axis, what was originally the left side of the mesentery becomes not merely the right side (rotating 180 degrees, which would place the large bowel simply in front), but by further rotation of 90 degrees becomes the posterior layer, *i.e.*, it adheres to the posterior layer of the peritoneum and lies in the coronal plane or beyond.

It is said that bands of adhesions are sometimes the effective cause of the inhibition of rotation, but of the three cases of "left-sided colon" here reported such were not made out in the first case, although a most

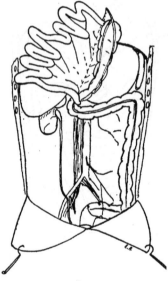

Fig. 2

careful autopsy was made. In the second case observation is simply lacking, since in the hurry of a desperate operation there was neither time nor justification on other grounds for extended search after interesting phenomena. In the third case, however, there were very definite bands, one on each side, nearly an inch wide, consisting of simple fibrous tissue which if of inflammatory origin must have been very old, even pre-natal, for they presented no evidence of inflammatory reaction, no thickening, no cicatricial contraction, no adventitious blood-vessels. Had they been the result of bacterial inflammation secondary to the volvulus they would almost certainly have contracted sufficiently to have caused strangulation of the intestine or fatal obstruction. But admitting that these bands were

116

the cause of the failure of rotation of the intestine there is still a question as to their origin.

In the three cases here reported, all that I happen to have seen of "left-sided colon," the condition was found at operation for intestinal obstruction. In the first case the obstruction was not the result of the congenital anomaly, but was due to carcinoma of the transverse colon. In the other two the failure of rotation of the gut and fixation of the mesentery was the predisposing if not the direct cause of the obstruction.

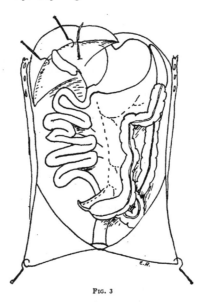

FIG. 3

CASE I.—A man of sixty-two years, merchant of Seward, Alaska, who had always enjoyed rugged health, came to operation for obstruction of the transverse colon which had been progressive for a year. The distention was greatest on the right side and in the upper abdomen. Incision for a proposed right inguinal colostomy showed the right flank filled with distended hypertrophied coils of small intestine, the cæcum not to be found, a large, hard, fixed tumor in the region of the transverse colon, liver filled with metastases, an immense elastic coil of distended colon on the far side of the small bowel, evidently the ascending colon. The hepatic flexure was successfully brought to the lateral abdominal wall in front of the small bowel, sutured into the incision and opened some hours later. The patient escaped peritonitis but succumbed on the fourth day to broncho-pneumonia. Autopsy showed "left-sided colon," no cicatri-

117

cial or other bands about the duodenum or jejunum, carcinoma of transverse colon involving the mesentery and invading the portal · vein with shower of metastases in the liver.

In brief, the " left-sided " colon in this case in no wise interfered with a long and active life, but the unusual and not to be anticipated · location of the colon with reference to the distended loops of small intestine added much to the difficulties of the operation for relief of the obstruction.

CASE II.—A woman of forty-one years, mother of one child, had always been strong and well till depleted by hemorrhage from a large myoma. Hysteromyomectomy rendered difficult by extensive adhesions from an old pelvic inflammation entailed considerable traumatism to the lower peritoneum. Because of the weakened condition of the patient time was not taken for exploration of the upper abdomen nor removal of the appendix. Patient made an excellent primary recovery, but on the fifth day developed a temperature of 102° and on the sixth 105°, pulse 124, leucocytosis, vomiting, evidence of infection of the uterine stump, abdominal distension more marked on the right side. Enemas, hot compresses, withdrawal of food gave much relief. The distention which remained was thought to be due to inflammatory ileus or to obstruction from adhesions about the cæcum. Patient so far recovered as to be able to take food for about a week, but the symptoms of obstruction became more marked and secondary septic symptoms coming on the abdomen was opened on the nineteenth day. The distention was entirely in the cæcum and small bowel. The cæcum was adherent to the anterior abdominal wall where it had perforated. The appendix which was 6 inches long was inflamed and adherent by its tip to the uterine stump. It was first removed to get it out of the way and then it was found that the obstruction of the colon was due to volvulus, a right-handed twist. The twisting was difficult to explain because the relations of the terminal ileum and cæcum were normal and the mesentery of the cæcum was attached to the posterior abdominal wall by a cord nearly an inch in diameter and 6 inches or more long. The rotation in the volvulus, therefore, could only have occurred by the gut (cæcum and portions of the small intestine) passing around itself as an axis, the mesenteric cord being a sort of pivot, at a time anterior to the attachment of the appendix to the uterine stump. The most likely explanation is that in withdrawing gauze pads which were used to hold the intestines back in the first operation, they rubbed or pulled on the bowel sufficiently to give it the right-handed twist. When the volvulus was untwisted the large bowel was found to be necrotic in spots and had to be resected. There were embarrassments in making the necessary lateral anastomosis, for the ascending colon was in the pelvis and adherent and led upward toward the splenic flexure on the left side of the small intestine. Anastomosis was accomplished and patient made a normal recovery. She was well when last seen, some six years later.

CASE III.—A boy of five years, whose history from birth was that of a delicate child who suffered from early infancy from recurring attacks of colicky pain and vomiting. His nutrition was always the greatest concern of his parents, but he managed to grow somewhat in spite of his starvation. He was bright mentally and had learned to refrain from eating whenever he felt one of these attacks coming on, and that was pretty frequently, for when the stomach was empty the attacks sooner subsided. He had never known what it was to have a full meal. When he came under our care he was just recovering from his severest attack of obstruction. He was far below normal in weight, had almost no fat; his face was pinched and purplish, and his extremities blue and cold. He was too weak to be up more than a short time each day. Loth to move, he was quite content to lie in bed and watch other children play. The abdomen was distended above, but was concave below, the abdominal wall tense as in the atrophy of starvation, but not spastic. No tumor could be made out. No icterus.

From the history and the findings it was evident that the child was suffering from some form of chronic obstruction high up in the intestine, not complete, but probably due to some congenital anomaly. We thought possibly congenital stricture of the duodenum or hypertrophic pyloric stenosis. After administering fluids by rectum we opened the abdomen and found the explanation of the obstruction in a volvulus of the intestine at a point just below the biliary papilla. Included in the volvulus was the entire small intestine, the ascending and part of the transverse colon. Only the stomach, pylorus, and upper duodenum were distended; the remainder of the intestine was collapsed.

The entire mass of the intestine, having no other attachment than at the point of the twist, which consisted of a cord hardly more than an inch in diameter, was lifted bodily out of the abdomen. The posterior peritoneum was continuous from the descending colon across to the right side of the abdominal wall, and because of the absence of fat was transparent, so that the right kidney and ureter, the aorta and the vena cava and their branches were clearly visible in their normal relations as in an anatomical drawing. The left kidney was not visible, being covered by the descending colon and its mesentery. When lifted out of the body the intestinal mass could be twisted about at will freely in any direction. The mesentery seemed to be disposed somewhat in the form of a trough with V-shaped cross-section ending at the ileocæcal valve with the superior mesenteric artery running along the apex of the angle and in the coronal plane, making nearly a straight line for the meso-appendix in which it found its termination.

Untwisting the bowel to the left through a complete circle (360°) two bands of fibrous tissue came into view, one on each side, binding the duodenum to the transverse colon so that they were in contact. The bands were cut, care being taken not to injure the mesenteric artery and vein, and this permitted the loops of intestine to be separated an inch or more. The intestinal mass was then laid

EMMET RIXFORD

in the abdomen in the normal relation of rotation, the ascending
colon to the right, the small bowel to the left, the superior mesenteric
artery passing in front of the duodenum. The tissues assumed this
so-called normal position quite readily. The boy reacted normally;
in fact, began almost at once to make up for his five years of starvation. He grew like the blossom stalk of an aloe, and is now a
strapping, normal boy of thirteen.

MESENTERIC THROMBOSIS *
WITH A REPORT OF 6 CASES

BY GEORGE G. ROSS, M.D.
OF PHILADELPHIA, PA.

THROMBOSIS of the mesenteric vessels is a condition of interest to the surgeon, not only because of its comparative rarity, but also because of its gravity, the difficulty of diagnosis, and the corresponding lack of success in its treatment.

Two cases of mesenteric thrombosis are noted in the records of the Lankenau Hospital in a period of ten years (1909 to 1919), during which time there were about 30,000 surgical admissions.

The anatomic points in this connection are well known and need be only hastily reviewed. The superior mesenteric artery alone supplies the small intestine and practically all of the large bowel with the exception of the descending colon, sigmoid, and rectum. The duodenum has a double blood supply. The superior mesenteric artery is stated to be an end artery, the inferior mesenteric is said not to be.

The superior mesenteric artery, then, is not only much more frequently the seat of the thrombosis, but the condition in this vessel or its branches should be correspondingly more serious than when it occurs in the inferior mesenteric area. The latter statement would be difficult of proof, because in either location the condition is of such gravity that recovery is extremely rare.

There seems to be no doubt that arterial blocking in the mesentery is far more common than obstruction of the venous circulation. Statistics have been given to show that it is twice as frequent (other authors state the ratio to be five to one).

In the reported cases there has often been no effort to differentiate between thrombosis of the mesenteric vessels and embolism. Indeed, this must often be impossible. The symptomatology is the same in either case and even at operation or autopsy it is difficult to determine whether in a given case we are dealing with a primary thrombotic or embolic condition. Venous conditions are, of course, thrombotic.

Arterial obstruction occurs either by embolic plugging of the vessel or thrombotic obliteration or by thrombosis developing at the site of lodgment of an embolus (Smith, *Wisconsin M. J.*)

Venous obstruction is said to be either of the ascending or descending variety. Whatever the nature of the beginning of the process, its course, prognosis, and treatment are the same.

There have been described also certain forms of vascular stoppage

* Read before the American Surgical Association, May 3, 1920.

more chronic in character, but all of those with which the surgeon has to deal are acute in their course.

Perhaps of more interest as a classification is the division of these cases into those in which the process is the primary one surgically; *i.e.*, the one for whose diagnosis and treatment the surgeon is called, *vide* Cases I, II, III, IV, and V, or those in which the condition follows directly after some surgical condition (Case VI), already dealt with as a complication or secondary involvement.

A great deal of attention has been given to a consideration of symptoms and diagnostic points in connection with mesenteric thrombosis. Elaborate classifications and tabulations of histories and groups of cases have failed to bring out a symptom complex upon which even a probable diagnosis can safely be made in a fair percentage of the cases seen. It is true that in some of the instances, especially those that are post-operative, slow in onset and of the venous form of thrombosis, there are no symptoms which would even lead us to suspect the true condition interfering with the patient's recovery.

A consideration of the sequence of events in thrombotic conditions will at once point out the chief fact in symptomatology and diagnosis and one practically always overlooked.

When a thrombosis occurs, the blood supply of a certain segment of intestine is stopped or diminished to a great degree. With the diminution in blood supply of such a segment there comes the natural lessening of function, manifested as lessened peristalsis. If the segment of bowel affected be other than a very minute one, peristalsis ceasing in it soon causes stoppage, due to local paralytic ileus, and we find that the case develops the signs of intestinal obstruction. Of the further changes, gangrene, perforation, etc., little need be said. They are terminal stages only.

To repeat—the symptoms of mesenteric thrombosis, in so far as they may be grouped, are the symptoms of an acute intestinal obstruction.

We have not even arrived at a point of diagnostic skill that enables us to differentiate with certainty the variety of intestinal obstruction when such an obstruction is known to exist. How much more difficult it must always be to recognize definitely the occurrence of such a rare cause of diminished or absent intestinal action as mesenteric thrombosis. But we should always be able to recognize the fact that there has taken place a grave occurrence within the abdomen demanding immediately *definitely* planned and executed *surgical* attention.

In the five cases which I have to report pain is a prominent symptom as it is in every acute intestinal obstruction.

In Case I (Germantown Hospital, January, 1919) the patient was taken sick ten days before admission with a severe attack of abdominal pain in the region of the umbilicus, and then becoming general throughout the abdomen. Similar (?) attacks have been noted for fourteen years prior to admission.

In Case II (Germantown Hospital, February, 1919) the attack began suddenly, with abdominal pain, nausea, and vomiting.

In Case III (Lankenau Hospital, 1915) the chief complaint is given as pain over whole abdomen. It is described in detail in the history as beginning seven days before admission as an epigastric pain of gradual onset, becoming worse three days after the beginning of the pain.

In Case IV the illness is described as beginning two days before admission with pain in the right lower abdomen, soon followed by vomiting. In this case the pain remained localized in the right lower abdomen.

In Case V (University of Pennsylvania Hospital, service of Doctor Deaver) the patient was seized with a severe pain in the epigastrium.

It is evident, then, that we have in all five cases a very definite history of pain as an early symptom, in only one of the instances described as of gradual onset.

A brief consideration of the case histories themselves will make plain the fact that these are cases of obstruction not often diagnosed.

CASE I.—Operated upon by my assistant, Dr. Wm. B. Swartley, at the Germantown Hospital. About ten days before admission the patient began with a severe attack of abdominal pain in the region of the umbilicus, radiation and becoming general, although worse near the midline and about the umbilicus. There was much tenderness and rigidity. The patient had not been constipated. Shortly after admission to hospital there was a peculiar looking tarry stool.

The patient states that for the last years she has had frequent attacks of severe abdominal pain, coming on suddenly, causing her to go to bed, and to be away from her duties seven to ten days. At these times the pain was located in the central part of the abdomen and in the right lower quadrant, the abdomen was sore and rigid, the bowels often constipated. She had anorexia and at times vomiting during these attacks. Such attacks occurred three to four times a year. The history otherwise is unimportant; no menstrual disturbances; one child, living and well.

Physical examination shows a fairly well-nourished woman of forty. The patient is extremely anæmic, but not jaundiced. The tongue is coated. The patient has pyorrhœa of a marked degree. Chest shows slight dullness over the apex of the right lung. No râles. The heart shows slight enlargement to left and a soft systolic endocardial murmur which is not transmitted. The abdomen is distended and tympanitic. Much general tenderness and rigidity on deep pressure and an area of dullness in the right flank suggesting fluid. No peristalsis is heard. No palpable masses or liver enlargement were found. The pain on pressure is slightly more severe to the right of the umbilicus. Vaginal examination negative. The leucocyte count on January 5, 1919, was 15,000; on January 6, 1919,

123

was 9000; hæmoglobin, 26; red blood count, 2,690,000. Occult blood test on fecal matter was negative on January 6, 1919, but a note on January 13th states that there were definite signs of intestinal hemorrhage. The urine showed a faint trace of albumin.

A right rectus incision was made and an appendix showing chronic obliterative appendicitis was removed. One foot of the lower portion of the ileum was found to be black and almost gangrenous, due to a thrombosis of the branch of the mesenteric artery supplying the portion of the bowel. There was a V-shaped infarcted area in the mesentery. The patient's condition did not permit of resection and the wound was closed and paitent put to bed. Under intravenous saline and stimulation the patient lived about four hours.

The appendix removed was 30 and 5 mm. The canal was obliterated. The coats white fibrous and thickened, and the appendix somewhat hooked, due to a shortening of the meso-appendix. This case shows several features of great interest. The history shows first a pyorrhœa, a possible original focus of infection. The condition of the removed appendix and the history suggest previous attacks of acute or subacute appendicitis. The heart murmur suggests a possible endocarditis and the original to be an embolus instead of a simple thrombosis of the mesenteric vessel.

The findings on admission show clearly the picture of a late stage of obstruction. The bloody stools and anæmia secondary to intestinal hemorrhage are said by some authors to suggest thrombosis. Such a marked anæmia, however, would be more likely to be taken, other things being equal, as pointing to possible malignant disease. Most striking, however, is the ten-day interval between onset and operation, rendering cure out of reasonable expectation.

CASE II.—Miss C. J., aged sixty years. The patient was admitted to the Germantown Hospital February 21, 1919, having first been seen on that day by Doctor Moxey, who at once realized the gravity of her condition. The patient was sent in with a diagnosis of acute obstruction—this being entirely correct. The patient when first seen by her physician had been ill about two days. The onset had been sudden, with severe abdominal pain, nausea, and vomiting. The patient had been constipated and had without avail used both purgatives and enemata.

Physical examination showed a heavily built woman evidently very ill, in fact, in extremis. She was dyspnœic and cyanotic. The abdomen was distended and tympanitic, but not rigid. No peristalsis, the patient complained of nausea, but there was no retching or vomiting. A fatty endocarditis may have been a factor in causing the respiratory embarrassment.

Operation was undertaken as a forlorn hope. The patient died before anything could be done to relieve her condition. The small intestine, for approximately 10 feet, was found to be gangrenous, swollen, but not markedly distended. The mesenteric arteries were thickened, rigid, hard, and thrombosed, and there was no demonstrable attempt at the formation of a collateral circulation. The cæcum and ascending colon were thickened and distended and the hepatic flexure moderately bound down by adheisons but not obstructed.

This case shows the involvement of a far greater extent of gut than Case I, a complete shutting off of the blood stream and a fulminating course. Had this patient consulted a physician at once some hope could have been entertained for her, since her condition would have been evident at any time after the onset of the disease and early operation with resection might have been possible.

CASE III (Lankenau Hospital, operated on by Dr. John B. Deaver). —B. B., aged forty-six years, admitted February 13, 1917. Two days before admission the illness began with pain in the right lower abdomen. The pain continuing, after a few hours the patient began to vomit. He was given purgatives, but the patient's bowels did not move and the pain continued more or less constantly up to the time of admission. The patient complained of no fever or chill, but showed marked anorexia. His previous medical history notes: "Two previous attacks—one a month ago, and six months ago."

On admission the patient is seen to be fairly well nourished. The abdomen was somewhat distended with a tumor-like fullness in the right iliac fossa. There was rather marked tenderness and rigidity in the lower right abdomen where a mass was vaguely palpable. Peristalsis was present in the upper and left portions of the abdomen. Rectal examination revealed distinct tenderness to the right and very slight tenderness to the left side.

Operation—*four days* after admission—February 17, 1917. Under ether anæsthesia. A McBurney incision was made and enlarged upward; at a point a hand's breadth above the cæcum in the ascending colon, partial necrosis was evident, and on slight manipulation the bowel wall gave way and fecal material poured out into the field of operation. A glass drainage tube was placed in the pelvis and purulent fluid evacuated. A large rubber tube was placed in the rent in the ascending colon and the bowel closed about the tube and then sewed to the parietal peritoneum. Gauze was packed about the tube.

Peritonitis steadily became more marked after the operation and the patient succumbed.

Post-mortem inspection through the wound showed thrombosis of the mesenteric veins leading to the ascending colon.

The salient points of the history here cited are few but important. They are: (1) The simulation of an attack of acute appendicitis. The history is not typical but was sufficiently deceptive to have caused the postponement of operation for four days and the employment of a McBurney incision. (2) The early localization of symptoms correctly indicating the position of the abdominal lesion itself.

The operative procedure—drainage alone—was the correct one, the outlook hopeless at the time of operation.

CASE IV.—G. A., aged fifty-two years (Lankenau Hospital, case of Dr. John B. Deaver). Admitted October 22, 1915; died October 23, 1915. The patient's illness began seven days before admission with pain in the epigastrium, gradual in onset. Purgatives were given and the patient's bowels moved freely. Three days after the onset of the illness the patient seemed to get worse and the whole abdomen became painful. The patient began to vomit dark material and vomited everything taken by mouth thereafter. No one spot could be given as the seat of the most intense pain. There was no jaundice or chill.

The previous history mentions frequent attacks of indigestion and the use of alcohol.

Physical Examination.—The patient is a very large man, evidently in great pain. Complexion sallow; tongue heavily coated. The abdomen is greatly distended and generally tender, this tenderness being more marked in the epigastrium and left lower quadrant. Peristalsis absent. Blood-pressure, 125–80.

The patient died twenty hours after admission, not being operated on. Autopsy showed mesenteric thrombosis with gangrene of the proximal four to six feet of ileum.

A rather concise history here shows an obstruction with a typical symptom at the onset unrecognized. Three days after the onset the severe obstructive and peritonitic manifestations render it evident that operative intervention could have accomplished nothing.

CASE V.—D. H. G., aged fifty-one years (University Hospital, operated on by Dr. John B. Deaver). Admitted September 25, 1918. The day before admission the patient was seized with a severe pain in the epigastrium. In the course of an hour or so this pain became generalized, affecting both the upper and lower right quadrant. The pain was paroxysmal in character, leaving the patient with a dull ache between the paroxysms. One such paroxysm of pain lasted an hour. The patient has vomited several times, once following a dose of magnesium sulphate and again following a dose of mustard water. No fecal vomiting. Bowels have not moved since beginning of illness.

Past medical history is unimportant as bearing on the present illness. Physical examination: The abdomen is tender and rigid in the epigastrium and the right iliac regions, the point of maximum tenderness being in the left upper quadrant. Little, if any, abdominal distention was present, but the upper abdomen was tympanitic on percussion. Auscultation shows peristalsis of an exaggerated and gurgling type. Blood examination: White blood count, 13,280; 76 per cent. polymorphonuclears.

After admission an enema was given with but slight result and no relief of symptoms. Lavage disclosed gastric contents having a decidedly fecal odor and appearance. A diagnosis of intestinal obstruction was made and immediate operation performed.

Operation by Dr. John B. Deaver. Ether anæsthesia. A right rectus incision was made. No mechanical obstruction was found, but there was a thrombosis of a branch of superior mesenteric artery supplying a segment of the ileum. There was considerable hemorrhage into the mesentery and a small amount of free blood in the abdominal cavity. The segment of bowel affected was in fair condition, apparently being taken care of by the collateral circulation. Doctor Deaver expressed the opinion that no further surgical procedure would benefit the patient, and the operation was terminated. During the operation the patient received 750 c.c. of salt solution intravenously.

The first two days after operation were somewhat stormy for the patient, but after this he rallied and made an uneventful recovery.

He was discharged on the fourteenth day after operation, in very good condition. When last heard of through the family physician, he had had no return of symptoms.

This, the only case operated upon that recovered, is of note in several ways: (1) The correct diagnosis of intestinal obstruction, was made early and operation was performed at once. At operation good judgment based upon experience saved the patient from an extensive and uncalled-for procedure. The case proves, upon the living patient, a fact noted at autopsy; namely, that the collateral circulation, perhaps more often than would be supposed, has overcome the effects of mesenteric thrombosis.

CASE VI.—Mrs. C., aged thirty-seven years (Germantown Hospital). This patient had been operated upon for a pelvic condition. Intra-abdominally a cyst of the left ovary was excised, the appendix removed and the round ligaments shortened by the Gilliam method. There was also done a trachelorrhaphy and colporrhaphy, and perineorrhaphy. For six or seven days her convalescence progressed favorably. She had been catheterized regularly. Upon one occasion the nurse, after having by mistake introduced the catheter into the vagina, made the error of introducing it into the urethra without resterilizing it. The following day the patient had a well-developed septic cystitis; with a rise of temperature, chill and frequency of urination, with severe burning pain. Forty-eight hours later she had another chill with phlebitis of the left saphenous vein. The phlebitis continued an upward course into the iliac veins with involvement of the inferior mesenteric veins—through the middle hemorrhoidal vein which is the avenue of communication between the systemic and portal circulation. Her abdomen became distended and tympanitic and extremely tender. There was intense pain, nausea, and vomiting. The bowels were moved by enema and at no time did she show signs of intestinal obstruction.

Blood culture showed a colon bacillæmia. The diagnosis of thrombosis of the inferior mesenteric veins seems justified by the symptomatology and the sequence of events, although positive corroboration must be lacking because of the patient's recovery without a second operation.

A careful consideration of the foregoing case reports and of the numerous similar cases on record would lead us to a number of definite conclusions. They may be summarized as follows:

1. Arterial mesenteric thrombosis is a lesion causing a form of acute

GEORGE G. ROSS

intestinal obstruction, rare, but occurring with sufficient frequency to
make it imperative to remember its possible occurrence.

2. Its symptom complex is that of an acute intestinal obstruction,
slower in onset than the purely mechanical forms of acute obstructive
ileus (adhesion, volvulus, etc.).

3. Venous mesenteric thrombosis is a condition of vaguer symptomatology and slower course than that formed in arterial obstruction. It
tends more to spontaneous cure, and is more likely to be a secondary
or post-operative condition. When, however, its remedy by the establishment of collateral circulation does not occur, it gives the same final
symptoms as does the arterial form of obstruction.

4. The treatment of mesenteric thrombosis is the treatment of any form
of acute intestinal obstruction—early operation. The procedure employed must vary with the condition found at operation.

(a) If the vitality of a segment of gut has been gravely affected,
resection is indicated.

(b) If the patient's condition contra-indicates resection, the gut
should be drawn out of the abdomen, fastened to the edges of the wound
and a Paul's tube introduced, resection to be performed later.

(c) In the one case of this series that recovered nothing was done to
the intestine and spontaneous cure resulted. While it is true that this
may at times occur, and the judgment of the operator may indicate such a
course, such isolated instances do not refute the general rule of early,
radical procedure.

To Contributors and Subscribers:

All contributions for Publication, Books for Review, and Exchanges should be
sent to the Editorial Office, 145 Gates Ave., Brooklyn, N. Y.

Remittances for Subscriptions and Advertising and all business communications
should be addressed to the

ANNALS of SURGERY
227-231 S. 6th Street
Philadelphia, Penna.

GOITRE *

A CLINICAL STUDY OF ONE HUNDRED AND THIRTY-NINE CASES

By Miles F. Porter, M.D.

of Fort Wayne, Ind.

The group of cases forming the basis of this study is made up of those cases only the records of which are on file in my office in the card system which I have been using since November, 1912. This group was chosen because it was believed that it would be thoroughly representative, and especially because of the availability of the records for the purpose of study. No case is considered which presented itself after August 18, 1919. Total number of cases 139—females 121, males 18. This makes the proportion of males to females 1 to 6.7. The preponderance of females, it will be noted, is slightly less than that given by Dock,[1] which is 6 or 8 females to 1 male. It is pretty generally believed, especially since our experience with the draft, that the preponderance of females over males is not so great as it was formerly thought to be. Of the 139 patients, 74 of them presented themselves because of symptoms developing in a heretofore symptomless goitre or because a quiescent goitre had begun enlarging. In 47 of the 81 operative cases in which the history covers this point, the symptoms calling for operation developed on old symptomless goitres. In seventeen cases no mention is made in the histories bearing upon this point.

The youngest patient was 16, the oldest 70, both females. The average age of all patients was 35.5 years, average age of males 33.7 years, average of females 35.8 years. Of the 121 females 82 were married, 39 were single. In other words, 67.7 per cent. of the female goitre patients of this group were married. The statistics show that in Indiana about 65 per cent. of the females between 15 and 50 are, or have been, married. These figures seem to indicate that the marriage state itself is not particularly conducive to the development of goitre. Fifty-nine (72 per cent.) of the married females in this group were parous and eight (9.8 per cent.) sterile. Norris[2] says that one marriage in seven or eight is sterile and that from 50 to 75 per cent. of this sterility is due to the woman. Calculating from the figures given by Norris we find that 90.63 per cent. of married women are fruitful. In this

---

* Read before the American Surgical Association, May 4, 1920.
[1] Modern Medicine, p. 837, vol. iv.
[2] Surgery, Gynecology and Obstetrics, 1912, vol. xv, p. 706.

group of cases the percentage of fruitful marriages is 18.63 per cent. less than this, *viz.*, 72 per cent., indicating that goitre may be a causative factor in childless marriages.

Of the 139 cases 99 were treated surgically: Thyroidectomy was done in 81, injections of boiling water in 18 and in 3 cases both forms of treatment were used. In 2 of these the thyroidectomy followed the injection of boiling water and in 1 boiling.water was injected into the right lobe at the time the left was removed. In one patient the right lobe was removed some months after the removal of the left by another operator. Of the cases which came to operation there were 10.8 females to 1 male—a somewhat greater preponderance of females than occurs in the same group when operative and non-operative cases are considered together. A very large proportion of the specimens removed by operation were submitted to microscopic examination—perhaps 90 per cent. or more, though I cannot speak with exactitude. No case of so-called metastatic colloid goitre was encountered and I will add that I never have seen one. Five cases were pronounced malignant. All of these patients were females, all were married—four were multipara. One woman had been pregnant once and had aborted herself. Three of the patients presented toxic symptoms—two of them also had exophthalmus and two patients presented no toxic symptoms but came for operation because of pressure symptoms plus the disfigurement. In four of the patients the symptoms which caused them to consult a surgeon developed in a goitre of long standing. In two of these cases only the suspicion of malignancy was entertained prior to the operation either because of the rapidity of growth or the nodular feel of the tumor or both. The average age in these five malignant cases was forty years. The first of these operations was done in July, 1913, and the last in April, 1917. On one I am unable to get any report and the remaining four are living and well, although one of them reports that at times " it seems as though her neck is enlarged," but I have not had the opportunity to examine her. The other three show no signs, local or otherwise, of a return of the trouble and one has passed through a normal delivery since her operation. Balfour[3] gives the cancer incidence in a group of goitre patients from the Mayo Clinic as 1.19 per cent. Ochsner and Thompson[4] say that it is less than 1 per cent. In this group of cases it is 3.64 per cent. Considering the large incidence of malignancy in this group together with the percentage (100) of cures, one is led to question the diagnosis in some, at least, of these cases. It is well to note here, however, that while all of these patients have passed the three-year period, only one has passed the five-year period, while two are within a few months of the end of the five-year period. Microscopic sections on which the diagnosis of malignancy.was based are herewith presented, together with the pathologist's diagnoses. (See Figs. 1, 2, 3, 4 and 5 with accompanying legends.) Having presented the evidence I prefer, without further argument, to leave

[3] Collected Papers of the Mayo Clinic, vol. x, 1918, p. 393.
[4] Thyroid and Parathyroid Glands, p. 33.

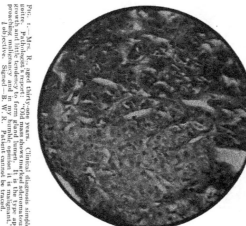

FIG. 1.—Mrs. R., aged thirty-one years. Clinical diagnosis simple goitre. Pathologist's report: "Old mass shows marked adenomatous growth and little tendency to form gland lumen. It is the type approaching malignancy and in my humble opinion it is malignant." ⅓ objective. Signed—B. W. R. Patient cannot be traced.

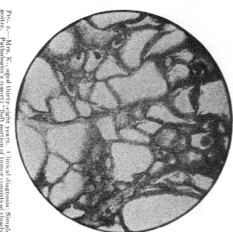

FIG. 2.—Mrs. K., aged thirty-eight years. Clinical diagnosis: Simple goitre. Pathologist's report: "Soft portion of tumor consists of closely packed adenomatous structure with very small lumen and free cellular growth in intercellular tissue. I consider this malignant."— B. W. R. ⅓ objective. Patient's report: "Some pain in throat. Somewhat enlarged." Four years after operation.

130⁵

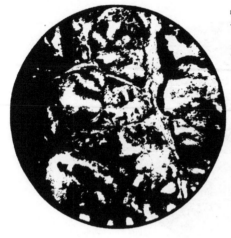

Fig. 4.—Mrs. S., aged twenty-seven years. Clinical diagnosis: Exophthalmic toxic goitre. Pathologist's report: "Adenocarcinoma—papillomatous outgrowths," ⅔ objective. Signed—B. W. R.

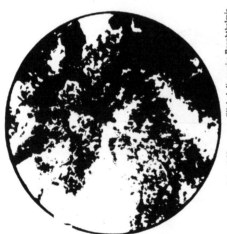

Fig. 3.—Mrs. S., aged fifty years. Clinical diagnosis: Exophthalmic toxic goitre. Malignancy suspicioned because of rapidity of growth and nodulation of tumor. Pathologist's report: "Malignant adenoma —badly broken down. Section from less degenerated portion—⅔ objective." Signed—B. W. R.

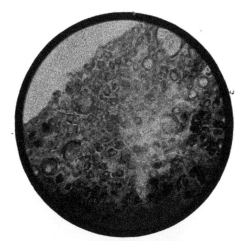

FIG. 5.—Mrs. N., aged fifty-nine years. Clinical diagnosis: Hyperthyroidism with suspicion of malignancy because of recent rapid
increase in size of goitre of thirty years standing and the nodular
character of the tumor. Pathologist's report: Irregular diffuse growth
of epithelial cells which are definitely malignant. These seem to
originate from the cells lining the gland acini and are arranged in a
rather alveolar form. There is relatively little colloid. The fibrous
stroma is abundant in parts and Very scant in others. Diagnosis:
Carcinoma of thyroid. Signed—B. M. E.

the judgment in the case in the hands of fellows who have had a larger experience than I. Simply adding that the microscopic diagnoses in four of the five cases were made by Dr. B. W. Rhamy, of Fort Wayne, who is a pathologist of large experience, and in the remaining case by Dr. B. M. Edlavitch, also of Fort Wayne, and who has had considerable experience.

One patient only of the operative cases presented symptoms of parathyroid trouble after operation. They were very mild and subsided in a couple of days. In two of the thyroidectomies there were symptoms of injury to the recurrent laryngeal nerve. One seems to be permanent, at least she is seldom able to speak above a whisper now more than three years after the operation; in the other case there was partial aphonia, which lasted but a few days. In both the posterior capsule was left at operation and in neither did I have any suspicion that the nerve had been injured until the aphonia was noted. It is important to add that the patient with the permanent aphonia had experienced attacks of loss of voice on several occasions prior to the time she came for operation. I have not been able to trace all of the operative cases and therefore cannot speak with accuracy as to the results, but inasmuch as I asked all of the patients to keep me informed of their progress, and especially to inform me if they did not get as well as they thought they. should, and do know positively of the results in the majority, I feel warranted in saying that the operative treatment has been very satisfactory. One patient is still suffering, after thyroidectomy, with toxic symptoms with quite a considerable enlargement of that portion of the right lobe which was left at the time of the operation. One patient who presented a typical picture of the so-called neurotic type was, after extensive study by my confreres and myself, subjected to thyroidectomy for a small goitre which was present. Three months later he reported as having gained $11\frac{1}{2}$ pounds in weight but as being no better so far as nervousness and weakness was concerned. In none of the cases with marked exophthalmus was this symptom entirely cured, but most of these patients declare that their eyes have always been prominent and are satisfied with the degree of retrogrssion that followed the treatment. There were no operative deaths attributable to the boiling water injections. Two patients whose goitres had been injected died some time after the last injection was given. One with pronounced cardiorenal involvement which had existed for some months prior to her first visit to me. In this case no post-mortem was made. The other patient who died following the boiling water injections had received in all three injections. She presented the usual picture of pronounced thyrotoxicosis including exophthalmus. The patient presented no symptoms of reaction after either of the injecetions and went to her home town and died four days after the last treatment. Post-mortem examination was made by her attending physician, from whose report the following abstract is made: "Universal enlargement of the mesenteric lymph-nodes. Right kidney much mottled, pyramids very dark, capsule easily stripped, left kidney very hard, not so large and not so much mottled. Spleen enlarged with numerous light spots hard to the touch, left adrenal large, right not so much enlarged. Heart enlarged, muscular tissue normal. Remains of old lung and pleural lesions. The thymus gland, especially the right lobe, much enlarged—as long as the index finger. Thyroid enlarged, very firm, cuts with difficulty. Colloid material absent. Tissue has the appearance of boiled veal or pork." Urinalysis made in this case, twenty-four days before death occurred, revealed a normal urine. The findings in this case indicate that the cause of the patient's death lay in the pathology found in the thymus and adrenals and raises the question as to the possibility of procuring relief through a thymectomy. At no time when I saw her did I regard her as a safe risk for even so slight an operation as ligation.

One of the patients treated with boiling water injections was in extremis when I saw him, with very aggravated symptoms of thyrotoxicosis, including anorexia, emaciation, diarrhœa and mental aberration partaking of the nature of active maniacal type. After the third injection this patient went to his home town, continued to improve until he was considered a reasonably safe surgical risk, when he had a thyroidectomy at the hands of his home surgeon with results reported to me several weeks later as entirely satisfactory. Several patients who received boiling water injections were advised to have thyroidectomies done later. Five followed this advice, the rest were satisfied with the improvement following the boiling water injections and refused further surgical interference notwithstanding the fact that in several patients the goitre was large enough to be quite unsightly. There were three deaths following thyroidectomy—one death occurring during the operation, one 30 minutes after and one two hours after operation. The anæsthetic used in two of these fatal cases was ether and in one novocain. Post-mortem was not permitted in either case. I know now that operation should not have been attempted in either of these cases. One of the patients had been cured a year before her visit to me by boiling water injections given by her family physician and was very insistent that a radical operation be done if possible, and I allowed myself to be persuaded to remove her goitre under local anæsthesia after twenty days' rest and treatment in the hospital. Of the other two fatal cases neither improved under rest, etc., and I was persuaded to undertake a radical operation when I should have done either a ligation or boiling water injection. There were no fatalities after June, 1916.

In patients who are good risks and who stand thyroidectomy well there is, in my opinion, no objection to doing other operations which are necessary at the same time. I have done hernioplasty, salpingectomy and hemorrhoidectomy immediately following thyroidectomy several times and have had no cause to regret my action. In this group of cases 65 were toxic, 26 exophthalmic, 37 simple, and the remaining 11 were unclassified. The boiling water treatment was given only in toxic and exophthalmic cases. Seventeen thyroidectomies were done for simple goitre. A study of this group of cases throws no light on the question as to the relationship between goitre and local infections. Indeed, it is pertinent to say here that my whole goitre experience has left me undecided as to whether or not there is any causal relationship between local infections and goitre except infections of the thyroid itself and infections of the generative organs. There are patients in this group wherein a cure of frequent attacks of tonsillitis followed thyroidectomy and other patients in which removal of the tonsils was followed by a subsidence of the thyroid symptoms and still others in which the thyroid symptoms were not benefited by the removal of the local infection and again others in which the removal of the thyroid had no influence on the local infection present.

In the thyroidectomies local anæsthesia was employed in seven cases, both local and general in two, and in the remaining sixty-seven cases ether was used. Routine blood examinations were not made, for the reason that after quite a number of these examinations had been made the conclusion was reached that nothing of prognostic or diagnostic significance was to be gained thereby. In no case did a reaction of consequence occur and in no case was there alarming hemorrhage at the time of operation. In two patients, both young females, troublesome hemorrhage occurred a few hours after the operation. In one the hemorrhage was brisk and required a tampon, which was removed after forty-eight hours, after which the case progressed normally. In the other case the hemorrhage partook more of the nature of an oozing which kept up for forty-eight hours and in spite of what seemed an ample drain of rolled rubber dam a hæmatoma was formed and was followed by a low grade infection which prolonged the recovery several days. Stimulating treatment following operation was seldom used, perhaps in five or six cases all told.

ADENOMA WITH HYPERTHYROIDISM *

By CHARLES H. MAYO, M.D.

OF ROCHESTER, MINN.

THE report from the Surgeon General's Office of the physical condition of the first million draft recruits made us appreciate the fact that we have actual goitre regions in America. Goitre is most prevalent in the northwest states and next in the Great Lakes region; in some of the southern states and in the New England states the disease is rare.

I first operated for goitre in 1888 and I wish to express my appreciation here of the teaching of that great master surgeon, the late Theodor Kocher, who called special attention to the avoidable complications in surgery of the thyroid. Before Kocher's death approximately 5000 operations had been performed for goitre at his clinic.[16] Reports show that there are variations in the changes in the thyroid in different countries; thus cancer and simple goitre were proportionately much more common in Kocher's reports than in those of this country. It was only after 1900 that Kocher strongly advocated surgical treatment of exophthalmic goitre.[14] The condition shown by Plummer to be adenoma with hyperthyroidism had been described in foreign clinics as atypical exophthalmic goitre and was classified by various authorities into more or less ill-defined groups, designated as secondary morbus basedow (Gauthier and Buschau), formes frustes, or incomplete (Marie[20]) goitre heart (Kraus, Gittermann, and Stern), sympathicotonic and vagotonic (Eppinger and Hess), goitre basedowifié (Marie[21]), and basedowized (Kocher[13]). These groups include psychoneurosis, early exophthalmic goitre, and hyperthyroidism from adenoma. Gittermann more nearly than the others describes the symptoms, but he attributes the condition to a cardiac cause and recommends cardiac therapy in contradistinction to the preëxisting theory that the cause of exophthalmic goitre is to be found in the central nervous system. Adenomas with hyperthyroidism had not been definitely enough described to be commonly recognized since they were considered an atypical type. No pathologic findings other than those noted in adenoma without hyperthyroidism have been found to characterize adenoma with hyperthyroidism; the latter contains areas of varying degrees of degeneration and sometimes scattered areas of hypertrophy, but similar areas are also found in the non-toxic adenomas.

Plummer has had an opportunity to observe in the clinic not only the majority of cases of adenoma with hyperthyroidism and of exophthalmic goitre, but also several thousand cases of adolescent goitre and simple goitre in which operation was not advised. As a result of his clinical observation the present standardization of goitre has largely come about.

* Read before the American Surgical Association, May 4, 1920.

In 1906 Plummer noted that from 17 to 20 per cent. of the patients whose condition was clinically diagnosed at that time exophthalmic goitre had atypical symptoms; goitre, loss of weight, tachycardia, nervousness, and tremor were present without exophthalmos. These cases of adenoma with hyperthyroidism were discussed by Plummer at the meetings of the American Medical Association in 1911 and in 1912.[24]

About a century and a half ago exophthalmic goitre was described as a clinical entity by Parry, long afterwards by Graves, and later by Basedow. Möbius, in 1887, suggested that in exophthalmic goitre the gland is probably over-active in secretion, and Greenfield, in 1893, observed that diffuse parenchymatous hypertrophy and hyperplasia are present and that the gland contains little colloid. Wilson, in 1908, confirmed and elaborated Möbius' theory by the publication of a report on the first large series (294 cases) studied; he also showed that in a certain percentage of cases clinically called exophthalmic goitre the glands did not show diffuse parenchymatous hypertrophy and hyperplasia on microscopic examination. MacCallum, in 1905, was content to place such cases in the hyperplastic class if a small amount of hyperplasia was found. Kocher did the same in 1912.[18] It should be stated that there is a small percentage of cases, an intermediate group, between exophthalmic goitre and thyrotoxic adenoma which leans to one or the other condition, hyperplasia with adenoma or small adenomas with areas of hyperplasia.

Up to January, 1920, the surgeons of our clinic performed 9613 operations for simple goitre, including adenoma with hyperthyroidism; 10,135 operations have been performed for exophthalmic goitre during the same period. Previous to 1912 adenomas with hyperthyroidism were included with exophthalmic goitre. Many of the patients with exophthalmic goitre had more than one operation, such as ligation, before resection.

The services of Kendall, a trained biochemist, were secured and a laboratory was opened in the clinic for the study of the chemical nature of the gland. In December, 1914, the active principle of the thyroid gland, thyroxin, was first isolated by the use of barium salts, and three years later a small amount of thyroxin was synthesized. The synthesis was repeated and the structural formula confirmed in April, 1919.

Plummer, in 1916, presented his theory that the thyroid secretion is active in metabolism and that it vitally concerns the available energy of the cell,[28] and during this year he started a metabolism laboratory with Doctor Boothby and Miss Sandiford, of Boston, in charge. All varieties of goitres, including those with related complicating diseases, were studied. The basal metabolic rates in the patients with myxœdema were especially helpful; by giving definite amounts of thyroxin intravenously or by mouth it was possible to bring their basal metabolic rates to normal within given periods, and by continuing the tests the rapidity with which the thyroxin is exhausted was shown. The amount burned daily, the amount in the gland, and the amount in the body of the normal person

135

were soon determined. Previous observers, Magnus-Levy and others, have pointed out the excessive oxidation shown by metabolism in cases of hyperthyroidism, but no one had been able to state the degree. Plummer was enabled to determine the degree in exophthalmic goitre above the basal metabolism and to standardize the disease in appearance, severity, and activity, thus standardizing also the degree of thyroid deficiency in myxœdema.

Plummer in his various communications since 1909 has shown that the condition of hyperthyroidism may occur in adenoma without diffuse parenchymatous hypertrophy and hyperplasia;[25] this was supported by Goetsch in 1916, who called attention to the marked increase over normal in mitochondria in the thyroid gland in cases of exophthalmic goitre and of toxic adenoma. Bensley has shown the granules to be numerous in the thyroid cells, and others have shown that they are increased in number in the active or growing cells in general, whether representing work activity or proliferative activity is not determined.

The essential points in the clinical differentiation of exophthalmic goitre and adenoma with hyperthyroidism presented by Plummer in 1913 are[26] (1) The difference in the average ages of the patients when the goitres were first noticed. Enlargement of the thyroid was noted from five to ten years earlier in life by the patients with non-hyperplastic goitre than by the patients with hyperplastic (exophthalmic) goitre; (2) the time elapsing between the appearance of the goitre and the onset of hyperthyroid symptoms; in cases of exophthalmic goitre the symptoms of hyperthyroidism followed the appearance of the goitre within an average of nine-tenths of a year, while in cases of non-hyperplastic adenoma with hyperthyroidism an average of fourteen and one-half years elapsed before the symptoms of hyperthyroidism appeared; and (3) the relative frequency of exophthalmos in exophthalmic goitre contrasted with its almost absence in non-hyperplastic adenomas with hyperthyroidism.

Exophthalmos occurs within three months of the appearance of hyperthyroidism in an average of 50 per cent. of the cases of exophthalmic goitre and within two years in 87 per cent. Exophthalmos, even of questionable degree, was rarely noted in cases of non-hyperplastic adenoma with hyperthyroidism. In 1915 Plummer published a brief résumé of an immense mass of evidence to show the differences in the average blood-pressures in these two syndromes and the definite tendency to hypertension in adenoma with hyperthyroidism, which is not found in exophthalmic goitre.[27] The marked differences in the clinical pictures of exophthalmic goitre and of non-hyperplastic adenoma with hyperthyroidism led Plummer, in 1916, to point out, in an extremely valuable article, the probability of the different etiology in the two diseases; he had previously given the working hypothesis: "The active agent of the thyroid gland is a catalyst which accelerates the rate of formation of a quantum of potential energy in the cells of the organism." In May, 1916, Plummer

TABLE I.

Average Metabolic Rate and Blood Pressure in Adenoma and Exophthalmic Goitre Before and After Treatment [1]

	Adenoma — Without hyperthyroidism: Before treatment	Adenoma — With hyperthyroidism: Before treatment	Adenoma — With hyperthyroidism: Two weeks after thyroidectomy	Exophthalmic goitre — Two ligations, 2 months' rest and thyroidectomy: Before treatment	Ten days after second ligation	After 2 months' rest	Two weeks after thyroidectomy	Before treatment	After second ligation and 2 months' rest	Two weeks after thyroidectomy	One ligation and thyroidectomy: Before treatment	Ten days after 1 ligation	Two weeks after thyroidectomy	Thyroidectomy: Before treatment	Two weeks after thyroidectomy
Number of cases averaged in each group	18	201	75	36				55			52	22		52	
Age, years	43.8	47.7	47.4	35.0				36.7			38			33	
Duration of goitre, years	16.9	17.9	19.7	2.8 (1.6)²				3.0 (1.0)			3.5 (1.1)			3.2 (1.4)	
Age at onset of goitre, years	26.9	29.8	27.7	32.2 (33.4)				33.7 (35.7)			34.5 (36.9)			29.8 (31.6)	
Duration of symptoms, years		2.0	2.2	1.6 (1.3)				1.4 (1.0)			1.7 (1.3)			1.3 (1.0)	
Age at onset of symptoms, years		45.7	45.2	33.4 (33.7)				35.3 (35.7)			36.3 (36.7)			31.7 (32.0)	
Systolic B. P.	143	156	160	147		148		148			140	138		133	
Diastolic B. P.	85	86	86	73		73		75			67	72		72	
Pulse pressure	58	70	74	74		75		73			72	66		61	
Pulse rate	91	102	113	126		126		124			121	116		109	
Haemoglobin	75	73	74	70		71		74			74			74	
B. M. R.	+2	+28	+7	+66	+50	+42	+19	+66	+42	+16	+52	+41	+16	+36	+8
Systolic B. P.	127	143	146	133			75	134		129	124	124	120	122	
Diastolic B. P.	77	80	81	61			51	71		76	75	64	73	73	
Pulse pressure	50	63	65			59	93	63	109	53	49	60	47	49	
Pulse rate	78	97	102	115				109		90	90	109	92	88	
Weight	78		80	51.7 (48.1)	55.8			49.2	53.9		113			109	

¹ This table is extracted from a paper presented by Dr. W. M. Boothby at the Harvard Medical Society, February 17, 1920, Boston.

² The cases in this group of more than five years' duration are omitted from the averages given in the brackets because the duration of the goitre is confused by a pre-existing adenoma.

137

presented a paper before the Association of American Physicians in which he stated that the thyroid plays an important part in metabolism; that the evidence of high metabolism dominates the clinical syndrome of hyperthyroidism; that the rate of metabolism is dependent on the thyroid hormone, and that this function is not specific for certain tissues, but is common, to all the cells of the organism. DuBois in June, 1916, published the report of the results of his studies of the basal metabolism. The condition of adenoma with hyperthyroidism as described by Plummer is as follows: "Thyroid adenoma with hyperthyroidism is a disease associated with adenoma, characterized by an increased metabolic rate and excited by an excess of the normal thyroid hormone in the tissues. It is clinically evidenced by nervousness, tremor, tachycardia, loss of strength and weight, and a tendency to hypertension; in the later stages myocardial disintegration appears."[3] It is a disease of middle life. The underlying cause or stimulus activating adenomatous growth and over-secretion is not known. Pathologically the thyroid contains single or multiple adenomas in various stages of development or degeneration. The tissue outside the adenomas may be normal or colloid thyroid or contain areas of scattered hyperplasia. The histologic classification and the cellular content are still under investigation.

In the patients with adenoma with hyperthyroidism there was a gradual and appreciable change in symptoms two or three years previous to examination, the patients became nervous and excitable, and in the early stages they were ambitious to work, although unable to maintain physical or mental effort for a long period. These patients have good appetites and think they should be gaining in weight, but find that they are actually losing weight. The skin is warm with a tendency to perspiration. The heart beats faster and harder than normally, especially on slight exertion; it later palpitates, even when the patient is at rest. The blood-pressure often shows hypertension. The symptoms appear gradually and insidiously, usually becoming definitely worse about one year before the patients appear at the clinic; later there are an increase in nervousness and mental instability, moderate tremor, loss of strength, and dyspnœa on exertion; the heart beats rapidly and hard but the beat is not so accentuated as in exophthalmic goitre. In the long standing and more severe cases there is evidence of cardiac insufficiency with more or less œdema of the legs and ankles, often accompanied by myocardial disintegration, shown by irregular rhythm due to the premature contractions or auricular fibrillations.[31] Exophthalmos and gastro-intestinal crises, noted in exophthalmic goitre, are absent. As the duration of hyperthyroidism is prolonged, and the metabolic rate gradually increases, the increased functional demand is supplemented by actual myocardial changes (Willius[32]), resulting from the presence of an excess of the thyroid hormone.

The average age of the patients with adenoma with hyperthyroidism at the time of the examination in two groups of 201 cases and 75 cases, was forty-seven and seven-tenths and forty-seven and four-tenths years, respectively; 77 per cent. were more than forty.

The average age of patients with adenomas without hyperthyroidism in whom the adenomas were of sufficient size to justify operation, or for whom the operation was advised as a protection against future hyperthyroidism was slightly less, forty-three and eight-tenths years in a group of 167 cases; this is higher, however, than the average age of all patients with adenomas without hyperthyroidism who come to the clinic.

Exophthalmic goitre brings the patient for examination ten years earlier in life than does thyrotoxic adenoma. Four groups of exophthalmic goitre patients averaged between thiry-three and thirty-six years of age. In thyrotoxic adenomas a goitre is present eighteen· to nineteen years before the patient appears for operation; the symptoms of hyperthyroidism have been present about three and one-half years, or twice as long as even the enlarged gland has been noticed in the patients with exophthalmic goitre.

The average metabolic rate following operation and partial thyroidectomy, or removal of the adenomatous mass, falls from $+35$ per cent. to $+7$ per cent., usually within two weeks. This rapid drop in metabolism is in contrast with the result obtained from thyroidectomy in cases of exophthalmic goitre with an average basal rate of $+36$ before operation; the rate is within normal limits within two weeks in only 45 per cent., although it is below $+14$ per cent. in 76 per cent. The basal metabolic rate in a series of cases is shown in Table I.

BIBLIOGRAPHY

[1] Basedow: Exophthalmus durch Hypertrophie des Zellgewebes in der Augenhöhle. Wchnschr. f. d. ges. Heilk., 1840, vi, 197-220. -

[2] Bensley, R. R.: The Thyroid Gland of the Opossum. Anat. Rec., 1914, xiii, 431-440.

[3] Boothby, W. M.: A Study of the Metabolic Rates in Adenoma of the Thyroid with Hyperthyroidism. Presented before the Harvard Medical Society, Boston, February, 1920.

[4] Buschau, G.: Ueber Diagnose und Theorie der Morbus Basedowii. Deutsch. med. Wchnschr., 1895, xxi, 336-338.

[5] DuBois, E. F.: Metabolism in Exophthalmic Goiter. Arch. Int. Med., 1916, xxvii, 915-964.

[6] Eppinger, H., and Hess, L.: Vagotonia, a Clinical Study in Vegetative Neurology. Translation by W. M. Kraus and S. E. Jelliffe. Jour. Nerv. and Ment. Dis., 1915, xlii, 47-50.

[7] Gauthier, G.: Des goitres exophthalmiques secondaires ou symptomatiques. Lyon méd., 1893, lxxii, 41-48; 87-89; 120-127.

[8] Gittermann, W.: Struma und Herzkrankheiten. Berl. klin. Wchnschr., 1907, xliv, 1487-1490.

[9] Goetsch, E.: Functional Significance of Mitochondria in Toxic Thyroidadenomata. Johns Hopkins Hosp. Bull., 1916, xxvii, 129-133.

[10] Graves, R. J.: Lectures. Med. and Surg. Jour., 1835, vii, Lecture xii.

[11] Greenfield, W. S.: Some Diseases of the Thyroid Gland. Lancet, 1893, ii, 1493-1497, 1553-1555.

[12] Kendall, E. C.: Isolation of the Iodine Compound Which Occurs in the Thyroid. Jour. Biol. Chem., 1919, xxxix, 125-146.

139

[12] Kocher: The Pathology of the Thyroid Gland. Brit. Med. Jour., 1906, i, 1261-1266.

[13] Kocher, A.: Ueber Morbus Basedowii. Mitt. a. d. Grenzgebiet. d. Med. u. Chir., 1902, ix, 1-304

[14] Kocher, A.: Die histologische und chemische Veränderung der Schilddrüse bei Morbus Basedowii und ihre Beziehung zur Funktion der Drüse. Virchow's Arch. f. path. Anat., 1912, ccviii, 86-296.

[15] Kocher, T.: Ueber Kropf und Kropfbehandlung. Deut. med. Wchnschr., 1912, xxxviii, 1312-1316.

[16] Kraus: Ueber Kropfherz. Berl. klin. Wchnschr., 1906, xliii, 1413.

[17] MacCallum, W. G.: The Pathological Anatomy of Exophthalmic Goitre. Johns Hopkins Hosp. Bull., 1905, xvi, 287-288.

[18] Magnus-Levy: Über den respiratorischen Gaswechsel unter dem Einfluss der Thyroidea sowie unter verschiedenen pathologischen Zuständen. Berl. klin. Wchnschr., 1895, xxxii, 650.

[19] Marie, P.: Contribution à l'étude et au diagnostic des formes frustes de la maladie de Basedow. Thèse de Paris, 1883.

[20] Marie, P.: Maladie de Basedow et gôitre basedowifié. Rev. neurol., 1897, vi, 91.

[21] Möbius: Über das Wesen der Basedow-Krankheit. Centralbl. f. Nervenheilk., 1887, x, 228.

[22] Parry, C. H.: Enlargement of the Thyroid Gland in Connection with Enlargement or Palpitation of the Heart. Collections from the unpublished medical writings. London, 1825, ii, 111.

[23] Plummer, H. S.: Discussion following paper by Marine: The Anatomic and Physiologic Effects of Iodin on the Thyroid Gland of Exophthalmic Goitre. Jour. Am. Med. Assn., 1912, lix, 325-327.

[24] Plummer, H. S.: The Clinical and Pathologic Relationship of Simple and Exophthalmic Goitre. Am. Jour. Med. Sc., 1913, cxlvi, 790-796.

[25] Plummer, H. S.: The Clinical and Pathologic Relationship of Hyperplastic and Nonhyperplastic Goitre. Jour. Am. Med. Assn., 1913, lxi, 650-651.

[26] Plummer, H. S.: Studies in Blood-pressure. I, Blood-pressure and Thyrotoxicosis. Tr. Assn. of Am. Phys., 1915, xxx, 450-457.

[27] Plummer, H. S.: The Function of the Thyroid, Normal and Abnormal. Tr. Assn. of Am. Phys., 1916, xxxi, 128-133.

[28] Stern, R.: Differentialdiagnose und Verlauf des Morbus Basedowii und seiner unvollkommenen Formen. Jahrb. f. Psychiat., 1909, xxix, 179-273.

[29] U. S. War Department, Office of Surgeon General: Bulletin 11: Physical Examination of the First Million Draft Recruits: Methods and Results. Washington, Government Printing Office, 1919.

[30] Willius, F. A.: Auricular Fibrillation and Life Expectancy. Minn. Med., 1920. (In press.)

[31] Willius, F. A.: Observations on Changes in Form of the Initial Ventricular Complex in Isolated Derivations of the Electrocardiogram. Arch. Int. Med., 1920, xxv, 550-564.

[32] Wilson, L. B.: The Pathological Changes in the Thyroid Gland as Related to the Varying Symptoms in Graves' Disease; Based on the Pathological Findings in 294 Cases. Am. Jour. Med. Sc., 1908, cxxxvi, 851-861.

SPECIAL CONSIDERATION OF TOXIC ADENOMA IN RELATION TO EXOPHTHALMIC GOITRE *

By George W. Crile, M.D.

of Cleveland, Ohio

For a long time it has been noted that following the removal of simple goitres, especially those of large size, some patients have reported an improvement in general health beyond what one would anticipate from the mere removal of the enlarged gland. In some cases the improvement has semed to pertain principally to the nervous system; in some cases to the heart. At first it appeared that this improvement must be in part psychic, *i.e.*, relief from the disfiguring growths; and in part mechanical relief from pressure, relief from interference with the circulation through the large venous trunks, relief from interference with the respiratory exchange.

But with increasing experience it was realized that there was like improvement in cases in which there was no psychic stress; no interference with the circulation in the venous trunks; no interference with the respiratory exchange. It appeared, therefore, that the improvement must be due to the loss of thyroid activity. A comparative study showed also that the changes referred to above more frequently followed the removal of adenomata than the removal of colloid goitres; and that they were most marked after the removal of hyperplastic glands.

The only proved function of the thyroid gland is the fabrication of iodine into an iodine-containing compound which is adapted to the needs of the organism. In hyperplastic goitres this function is most active; but that adenomata also perform the characteristic thyroid function has been shown by the researches of Marine and Allen Graham.

Marine has found that adenomata contatin iodine, not as much as is found in colloid goitres, but enough to suggest that they are functionally active; and Graham found that adenomatous tissue affects differentiation in tadpoles as it is affected by normal thyroid tissue. Clinical evidence of the functional activity of adenomata is found in the frequent development of symptoms identical with those which are characteristic of exophthalmic goitre, and in the disappearance of these symptoms after the removal of the adenoma.

In hyperthyroidism due to hyperactive adenomata either iodine or thyroid extract may cause an aggravation of the symptoms.

In view of these facts, the following questions arise: Are these clinical symptoms of so-called toxic adenomata due to a degeneration of the adenoma—such as may occur as a result of the degeneration of fibroid

* Read before the American Surgical Association, May 3, 1920.

tumors? Are they due to such changes as are produced by a chronic toxæmia from infection of the gall-bladder, of the teeth, tonsils, bones, etc., or by intestinal toxæmia? Or are they due to the thyreo-iodine which is fabricated by the adenoma?

That the last of these queries suggests the true interpretation appears to be indicated not only by the identity of symptoms referred to above, but also by the fact that the well-developed " toxicity " from the toxic goitre produces a sensitization of the organism to adrenalin identical with that present in cases of hyperplastic goitre which are associated with exophthalmos and the other characteristic symptoms. In fact, with the exception of exophthalmos, all the characteristic symptoms of true exophthalmic goitre may be present in cases of " toxic adenoma "—increased basal metabolism, tachycardia, increased respiration, nervousness, tendency to fever, low thresholds, emaciation, increased appetite.

On the other hand, in the toxæmias from the toxins of degeneration and in chronic infections, the appetite is not increased, and, as a rule, the basal metabolism is not increased. In certain cases of high blood-pressure, cases of myocarditis, or of neurasthenia, in which the only evidence of the thyroid involvement was the presence of a small goitre, I have excised the gland with good results.

Moreover, if in a case of true exophthalmic goitre, the gland is not hyperplastic, but there is an adenoma, the removal of the adenoma relieves the patient in exactly the same way and to the same degree as the removal of the hyperplastic gland.

The removal of the adenoma gives relief also in those cases of adenomata in which the basal metabolism is not increased, the appetite is not increased, and there is no increased sensitization to adrenalin, but in which there is present myocarditis, or a high blood-pressure or neurasthenia. It would seem as if adenoma caused by every grade of toxæmia progressively from myocarditis, increased blood-pressure, nervousness, and increased metabolism to true exophthalmic goitre. These progressive stages of the disease are analogous to the degrees of infection which vary from mild oral sepsis to empyema of the gall-bladder, acute peritonitis or acute osteomyelitis. It would seem, therefore, that the various types of goitre should logically be regarded as varying degrees of the same or of similar processes.

In view of these facts it would appear that, certainly as far as treatment is concerned, no differentiation should be made between exophthalmic goitre with hyperplasia or thyrotoxicosis from adenomata; that the same regimen of management which has proven effective in the treatment of exophthalmic goitre will produce like results in the treatment of toxic adenoma.

The general management of exophthalmic goitre and the principles upon which it is based have been presented in other papers; but the line of treatment is summarized here to emphasize the importance of its inclusive application.

Special Points in Treatment.—(a) In advanced cases of toxic goitre, whether of the so-called adenomatous or exophthalmic type, the internal respiration is abnormally sensitive, as is indicated by the adrenalin test (Goetsch), and by the baneful effects of diminished exchange of air as a result of emotion or of injury. Therefore, the operative procedure should be graded according to the severity of the disease.

(b) The anæsthetic should be nitrous oxide which, as a rule, should be administered to the patient in bed, the transference to the operating room being made after anæsthesia is established.

(c) In moderate cases the entire operation may be completed at one séance.

(d) In more severe cases, the thyroid activity is diminished by a preliminary ligation in bed, under nitrous oxide analgesia and local anæsthesia.

(e) In extremely grave cases it may be necessary to diminish the thyroid activity by multiple steps; ligation of one vessel; ligation of the second vessel; partial lobectomy; complete lobectomy; when necessary allowing intervals of a month or more between any two of these stages. If, during operation, the pulse runs up beyond the safety point, the operation is stopped and the wound dressed with flavine, the operation being completed after a day or two, when conditions are safe. In some cases, though the thyroid is resected, it is advisable to dress the unsutured wound with flavine and make a delayed closure in bed the following day under analgesia.

(f) In multiple stage operations the length of interval is determined by the degree of physiologic adjustment.

(g) In certain cases lobectomy is performed in bed.

(h) Psychic control is required throughout to diminish the intense drive by establishing confidence and hope. An *anociated* regimen should be prescribed for the pre-operative, inter-operative, and post-operative periods.

(i) If after operation there is inaugurated an excessively high temperature, with greatly increased pulse and respiration, then on the principle that heat increases chemical activity and electric conductivity, and that these in turn increase heat, such patients are literally packed in ice—packed early. This procedure has been found to exercise a remarkable control over the destroying metabolism.

This post-operative phase of exophthalmic goitre is closely analogous to heat-stroke in symptoms and in control; and both heat-stroke and the so-called post-operative hyperthyroidism are the antithesis of surgical shock in which by contrast the heat centre is functionally impaired. In the latter, heat is as useful as cold is in the former.

The principles outlined above and the development of the treatment are based on the study of my personal series of 2477 thyroidectomies, including 1306 for exophthalmic goitre. The last series since the foregoing completed plan has been routinely used, during the period beginning February 21, 1919, and continuing through April 23, 1920, consists of 562 thyroidectomies with 5 deaths, including 300 for exophthalmic goitre with 3 deaths. Throughout this final series no case has been refused for operation—the operability has been 100 per cent.; the mortality rate of the total series has been 0.88 per cent.; of the cases of exophthalmic goitre, 1 per cent.

RESULTS OF OPERATIONS FOR ADENOMA WITH HYPER-
THYROIDISM AND EXOPHTHALMIC GOITRE *

By Edward Starr Judd, M.D.
of Rochester, Minn.

Before drawing conclusions with regard to the results of the treatment of goitres producing symptoms of hyperthyroidism it might be well to define the conditions as they are generally understood at the Mayo Clinic. Changes in the thyroid which apparently produce two definite clinical syndromes that are usually attributed to alerations in the secretory activity of the gland are: (1) Hyperthyroidism of exophthalmic goitre in which the symptoms are characteristic; the changes in the thyroid are always the same and result in a general diffuse hypertrophy and hyperplasia of the gland and (2) adenoma of the thyroid with hyperthyroidism,[5] first described as a clinical entity by Plummer[6, 7] (1911–1912) ; in many respects adenoma with hyperthyroidism resembles exophthalmic goitre,[8] but on careful examination can be readily recognized as a distinct disease. The activity of the thyroid gland in this condition is confined to the new growths or adenomas in which the hypertrophy occurs, instead of in the normally functionating part of the thyroid.

There is a third syndrome which is often mistaken for hyperthyroidism due to thyroid changes. The patients in this group present nervous manifestations, although the nervousness is of the kind seen in the psychoneurotic person, with tremor and tachycardia, although of a different kind from that met with in hyperthyroidism. The differential diagnosis is at times difficult because the thyroid gland is generally enlarged, due to an increase in colloid; the basal metabolic rate, however, is always normal. The importance of considering this third type apart from the goitres with hyperthyroidism is evident from the fact that this latter group responds to general medical treatment, and surgery is contraindicated.

The symptoms in cases of adenoma with hyperthyroidism apparently result from an increased production of a normal or nearly normal thyroid hormone. While organs such as the other ductless glands and certain parts of the central nervous system may show some changes, the gross changes in the thyroid are constant and permanent and establish a basis for surgical treatment.

The presence and degree of hyperthyroidism in exophthalmic goitre may be determined by several means. The clinical features offer an accurate estimate of the amount of disturbance produced by such changes in the gland. In considering the hyperthyroid cases, the natural course of the disease must be taken into consideration first. Hyperthyroidism occurs in exacerbations. The toxic symptoms develop gradually and after a

---

* Read before the American Surgical Association, May 4, 1920.

certain time, usually a few months, they reach their climax. If the patient survives the attack, the toxic features gradually subside after a short period, although there is almost never a return to normal, and definite evidence of the hyperthyroidism persists until the beginning of the next attack. Occasionally a spontaneous cure with the disappearance of all evidence of the disturbance occurs.

Loss of weight and strength and increased pulse-rate often reveal the degree to which the toxæmia has progressed. The loss of body weight is particularly important, and by carefully noting this symptom an estimate can be made not only of the degree of toxicity, but also of the relative length of the particular attack. This finding also influences the line of treatment to be followed. It is a well recognized fact that the surgical mortality is unduly high if patients with exophthalmic goitre are operated on while the toxæmia is progressive, or at the peak of a hyperthyroid wave.

Loss of strength indicated by weakness of the extensor muscles and the patient's inability to raise his body up a step, or his inability to walk a short distance, is also an important test of the degree of toxicity. The pulse-rate, nervousness, and tremor are influenced by so many other factors that they do not have the value that loss of weight and loss of strength have in determining the degree of hyperthyroidism.

In a consideration of the cases of adenoma with hyperthyroidism, a different problem is presented, namely, the clinical course of the disease. The thyrotoxic cases are usually those in which an innocent enlargement of the thyroid has existed for a long time. In our series patients with this type of goitre had had an enlargement on an average of almost twenty years before it was associated with symptoms of hyperthyroidism. In the cases of exophthalmic goitre this interval was usually less than one year. Acute crises of hyperthyroidism are not so apt to occur in cases of toxic adenoma as in cases of exophthalmic goitre; the toxic features develop more slowly and are progressively noticeable. Frequently the cardiac symptoms predominate and not infrequently those cases are regarded as "heart disease." There is also a tendency for these cases to be hypertensive.[9] The basal metabolic rate is always increased, but does not average so high as in exophthalmic goitre.

Within recent years much attention has been given to the changes in the basal metabolic rate[5] in both groups of hyperthyroidism,[1, 5, 8, 10] and it is contended by those who have had the most experience in this work that the basal metabolic rate is an absolutely accurate method of determining the presence and the degree of thyroid disturbance. Plummer and Boothby have carried out this study extensively and they believe that in general the thyroid is the main controlling factor in basal metabolism, although other conditions may influence the rate to a certain degree, and that any hypertrophy in the gland will be evident by an increase in the activity, and any reduced thyroid function will be evident by a lower metabolic rate than normal. The degree of hyperthyroidism estimated from the clinical features, and the degree of hyperthyroidism determined from the changes in the basal metabolic rate practically always correspond. The adrenalin test is apparently at variance with both the clinical picture and the metabolism studies. In our experience the test when used to determine the presence of toxæmia resulting from thyroid changes has responded almost the same in patients with known hypothyroidism, in normal persons, and in patients with hyperthyroidism. The psychoneurotics have seemed to give the best response to the test. It does not as yet seem advisable to employ the test to determine the presence of toxæmia with a view to operative procedures, for the psychoneurotics, so far. as we can determine, do not have thyroid toxæmia. Studies on this subject have recently been reported from our clinic by Boothby and Sandiford,[4] and by Sandiford.

This study of the operative results in exophthalmic goitre and adenoma with hyperthyroidism is based on two selected groups of 100 cases each: One hundred consecutive cases were selected from the list of exophthalmic goitres in which operation was done in 1914, and 100 consecutive cases of adenoma with hyperthyroidism in which operation was done in 1917 and 1918. The list was chosen from 1914 for the exophthalmic group because it seemed that six years is sufficient time to demonstrate the success or failure of operative procedures. The cases in the group of adenoma with hyperthyroidism were chosen from the years 1917 and 1918 because a study of the metabolic rate had been made in all cases; the average time elapsed since operation is two years.

The cases were studied first on the basis of the clinical history and the pathologic findings, and only the cases in which these two findings agreed were selected. Diffuse parenchymatous hypertrophy was definite in all of the thyroids removed in cases diagnosed exophthalmic goitre by the clinician. All the cases of adenoma with hyperthyroidism showed on pathologic examination adenomatous tissue of various types and sometimes scattered areas of parenchymatous hypertrophy; diffuse parenchymatous hypertrophy, such as is typical of exophthalmic goitre, however, was not present.

Letters of inquiry were sent to the patients in each group. Replies were received from all the patients with adenoma with hyperthyroidism and from eighty-eight of the patients with exophthalmic goitre. In the latter group twelve letters were returned unclaimed.

Eighty-eight of the patients with adenoma with hyperthyroidism were females whose average age was forty-eight and eight-tenths years. The twelve males averaged forty-eight and four-tenths years. Eighty-three of the patients with exophthalmic goitre were females averaging thirty-four and three-tenths years, and seventeen were males, averaging thirty-six and six-tenths years.

In adenoma with hyperthyroidism, as Plummer has pointed out, the adenoma usually becomes evident early in life, but the symptoms of hyper-

147

thyroidism do not develop until middle age. In this series of cases of adenoma with hyperthyroidism the goitre was first noticed at an average age of twenty-nine and eight-tenths years, and the patients came for treatment nineteen years and four months later, after noticing symptoms for two years and five months. In the cases of exophthalmic goitre the enlargement was noted at an average age of thirty-one and two-tenths years; and the patients came for treatment three years and eight months later, after noticing symptoms for one year and nine months.

In the majority of cases clinical examination revealed an enlargement of both the right and left lobe of the thyroid (Table I):

TABLE I

	Cases of exophthalmic goitre	Cases of adenoma with hyperthyroidism
Right and left lobes	79	49
Right lobe, isthmus, and left lobe	11	14
Right lobe	4	17
Left lobe	3	10
Isthmus	1	5
Right lobe and isthmus		4
Left lobe and isthmus		
Not stated	2	

Consistent metabolic readings were not taken in exophthalmic cases in 1914, but records of ninety-eight pre-operative and forty-four post-operative cases of adenoma with hyperthyroidism were obtained. In some cases several readings were taken and in others only one, so that the figures given represent an average of those taken in each case. The average pre-operative rate was + 32.7, and the average post-operative rate was + 9.2. Some of the post-operative rates were obtained within three weeks after operation, and others within a year or two, but the average number of days post-operatively was twenty-two. These figures agree very well with those obtained by Boothby in a careful analysis of the basal metabolic rates in adenoma and in exophthalmic goitre and with those published by Sandiford.

The choice of operation depends on several important factors, and no fixed rule can be made for any group of cases. The type of operation not only varies for each group, but also for each patient and the stage of the disease. Whereas in the group of cases of adenoma with hyperthyroidism thyroidectomy was done with small risk, in the group of 100 cases of exophthalmic goitre primary or secondary ligation was deemed advisable in sixty-four. Primary thyroidectomy was performed in only thirty-six of this group. This is a higher percentage of ligations than we ordinarily consider necessary, and indicates that this particular group of cases largely represents the severe type. While primary thyroidectomy is the operation of choice and may be done with a comparatively low mortality in the early cases of exophthalmic goitre, in our series only about one in

148

three patients presented himself at a time in the course of the disease to warrant dispensing with the preliminary ligation.

In most cases the best operative results are obtained by subtotal thyroidectomy, which is accomplished by removing all except the posterior part of each lobe. The immediate benefit derived from the operation is greater and the recurrences fewer than if lobectomy is done.

Questions in the letters of inquiry were :
1. Do you consider yourself cured as a result of operation?
2. Do you consider yourself improved?
3. Do you consider your condition unchanged?
4. Do you consider yourself worse?

Besides these questions, the patients were given a list of symptoms to report on, such as palpitation, rapid heart, and prominence of the eyes. Various factors which might have influenced their replies were considered; for instance, if the patient reported himself cured and his pulse record and symptomatic condition indicated otherwise, he was not placed among the patients cured.

In Table II are tabulated the interesting facts revealed from a study of the clinical histories with a view to ascertaining which of the most noticeable pre-operative symptoms persisted after operation and which disappeared.

TABLE II

	Symptoms in exophthalmic goitres		Symptoms in adenoma with hyperthyroidism	
	Pre-operative	Post-operative	Pre-operative	Post-operative
Nervousness	98	39	88	45
Tremor	93	21	83	6
Dyspnœa	84	29	76	28
Palpitation	89	26	80	29
Tachycardia	79	24	72	23
Loss of strength	89	13	79	17
Loss of weight	89		92	
Vomiting	34		8	
Prominence of eyes	70		6	
Change of voice	25	12	6	11
Heart moderately enlarged	38		14	
Heart markedly enlarged	19		9	
Murmurs	33		28	
Œdema	20		34	
Exophthalmos	67	25	3	
Thrill	48		4	
Bruit	72		10	
Average normal weight, pounds	137.3	Average gain 27.3 in 61 cases	151.1	Average gain 31.6 in 82 cases
Average weight at operation, pounds	121.8	Average loss 10.5 in 5 cases	131.7	Average loss 11.5 in 3 cases
Average pulse rate	122.6		111	
Average systolic blood pressure	145.2		157.2	
Average diastolic blood pressure	75.6		82.4	

149

EDWARD STARR JUDD

The most common symptoms persisting in each group are nervousness, tremor, dyspnœa, palpitation, tachycardia, loss of strength, and loss of weight. It was difficult to estimate the amount of nervousness that persisted after the operation, and whether the nervousness that many of the patients spoke of was due to any remnant of the disease, because the patients who were apparently otherwise entirely well often complained of some nervousness. Practically the same may be said regarding dyspnœa, palpitation, and tachycardia. All patients who mentioned having any of these symptoms after operation are included regardless of the fact that most of them stated that they were entirely well.

TABLE III

Exophthalmic Goitre

Patients cured .... 58 (65.8 per cent.)
Patients markedly improved .... 12 (13.6 per cent.)
Patients slightly improved .... 5 (5.6 per cent.)
Patients died from all causes during the six years.. 15 (15 . per cent.)

More than 65 per cent. of the patients suffering from exophthalmic goitre were free from all evidences of the disease six years after operation. Besides these, 13.6 per cent. are markedly improved; some of them feel entirely well; 5.6 per cent. are slightly improved, although they still have considerable evidence of hyperthyroidism; many of the group have only occasional acute exacerbations. Undoubtedly most of these patients would be benefited by the removal of more of the gland. Fifteen patients have died since the operation, two in the hospital, the others since going home. Some of these deaths were probably due to hyperthyroidism, but deaths from all causes have been included.

TABLE IV

Adenoma with Hyperthyroidism

Patients cured .... 83 (83 per cent.)
Patients markedly improved .... 5 (5 per cent.)
Patients slightly improved .... 1 (1 per cent.)
Patients not benefited .... 2 (2 per cent.)
Patients died from all causes during the two years .. 9 (9 per cent.)

CONCLUSIONS

1. Thyroidectomy will cure more than 65 per cent. of patients with the more severe types of thyroidism. If the patients could be treated earlier and with a better understanding of the plan of treatment, in all probability this percentage would be increased considerably.

2. More than 80 per cent. of patients with adenoma with hyperthyroidism can be relieved of their toxic symptoms and a cure obtained by thyroidectomy. A higher percentage of cures would undoubtedly be obtained if the patients were all operated on before there is any evidence of œdema or terminal degeneration.

150

OPERATIONS FOR EXOPHTHALMIC GOITRE

BIBLIOGRAPHY

[1] Boothby, W. M.: The Clincal Value of Metabolic Studies of Thyroid Cases. Boston Med. and Surg. Jour., 1916, clxxv, 564–566.

[2] Boothby, W. M.: The Value of the Basal Metabolic Rate in the Treatment of Diseases of the Thyroid. Med. Clin. North America, 1919, iii, 603–618.

[3] Boothby, W. M.: A Study of the Metabolic Rates in Adenoma of the Thyroid with Hyperthyroidism. Presented before the Harvard Medical Society, Boston, February, 1920.

[4] Boothby, W. M., and Sandiford, Irene: The Effect of Subcutaneous Injection of Adrenalin Chlorid on the Heat Production, Blood-pressure, and Pulse Rate in Man. Proceedings of the American Physiological Society. Am. Jour. Physiol., 1920, li, 200–201.

[5] Boothby, W. M., and Sandiford, Irene: The Laboratory Manual for the Determination of the Basal Metabolic Rate. Philadelphia, Saunders, 1920 (In press).

[6] Plummer, H. S.: Discussion Following Paper by Marine, D.: The Anatomic and Physiologic Effects of Iodin on the Thyroid Gland of Exophthalmic Goitre. Jour. Am. Med. Assn., 1912, lix, 325–327.

[7] Plummer, H. S.: The Clinical and Pathologic Relationship of Simple and Exophthalmic Goitre. Am. Jour. Med. Sc., 1913, cxlvi, 790–796.

[8] Plummer, H. S.: The Clinical and Pathologic Relationship of Hyperplastic and Non-hyperplastic Goitre. Jour. Am. Med. Assn., 1913, lxi, 650–651.

Plummer, H. S.: Studies in Blood-pressure. I. Blood-pressure and Thyrotoxicosis. Tr. Assn. Am. Phys., 1915, xxx, 450–457.

[10] Plummer, H. S.: The Function of the Thyroid, Normal and Abnormal. Tr. Assn. Am. Phys., 1916, xxxi, 128–133.

[11] Sandiford, Irene: The Basal Metabolic Rate in Exophthalmic Goitre, with a Brief Description of the Technic Used at the Mayo Clinic. Endocrinology, 1920, iv, 71–87.

[12] Sandiford, Irene: The Effect of the Subcutaneous Injection of Adrenalin Chlorid on the Heat Production, Blood-pressure, and Pulse Rate in Man. Am. Jour. Physiol., 1920, li, 407–422.

TOXIC GOITRE*

By WALLACE I. TERRY, M.D.
OF SAN FRANCISCO, CALIF.

IT is now fairly well recognized that two distinct types of goitre may give rise to toxic symptoms, *viz.*, the hyperplastic thyroid and adenomata. It is further recognized that the symptom-complex may be almost identical with either type of goitre, except that exophthalmos is not present in cases of adenoma of the thyroid, unless there is also hyperplasia of the thyroid tissue itself. It is seldom that the adenomata will produce extreme degrees of toxicity. We owe to Plummer the recognition of the rôle of the adenomata in the production of toxic symptoms, and we are also indebted to Goetsch for his further researches along these lines.

There are, however, many practitioners who do not appreciate the difference between the hyperplastic goitre and the adenomata from the standpoint of treatment. They consider them entirely innocent and advise that they be let alone or may prolong the medical treatment of them until a goitre heart has developed and a cure for the patient is no longer possible. I have thus emphasized the toxic adenomata, because, to my mind, they are not curable by medical means, including the X-ray. Until we have some new measure of real value at our command, it seems to me that the treatment of toxic adenomata should be surgical from the outset. In those occasional combinations of adenomata with hyperplasia, thyroid activity can be lessened by rest and suitable irradiation, but the adenomata will pursue their course despite the treatment.

We all know of apparently spontaneous cures of true exophthalmic goitre, but probably many of these relapse after some years of good health; it has been my experience to operate in two cases where the free interval was nineteen years. It has been stated that exophthalmic goitre is a self-limiting disease and that spontaneous cures result after five or six years in from 60 to 70 per cent. of the cases. Such a statement I think must be founded on a rather limited experience or else the term cure does not mean all it should. Too often do we see patients with unstable nervous systems, irritable and weakened hearts, slight exophthalmos and about normal-sized thyroids, who are supposedly cured, and yet under some toxic stimulus these patients will rapidly go down hill. We see the same thing after surgical treatment, due to insufficient removal of thyroid tissue in some cases, but more often to the fact that the bad nervous systems and the bad hearts were there before the operation. .To employ a Hibernianism, the treatment of toxic goitre should begin before it becomes toxic.

* Read before the American Surgical Association, May 4, 1920.

152

The surgical treatment of mildly toxic goitre is usually most gratifying, but the very severe cases require time, patience, and a recourse to all sorts of expedients to tide them along to a point where it is safe to operate. This safe point is often most difficult to judge, despite the pulse record, the improved weight, and lowered basal metabolic rate, the reaction to epinephrin, and the apparently strong heart. We have no accurate means of determining the resistance of an enfeebled nervous system to psychic or physical trauma, and our estimate of the resisting power of the myocardium is often inaccurate.

To consider personal statistics, up to March 31, 1920, I have done 748 operations for goitre, and of these 527 were for toxic goitres on 504 patients. There were 22 deaths among the toxic cases—a mortality rate of 4.3 per cent., whereas there was but one death among the 216 patients with simple goitre—a mortality rate of less than ½ per cent. The difference is, of course, striking, but what we should expect, unless one refuses to accept bad risks along with the good ones. The good risks may come in groups, as, for instance, during the period from January 22, 1917, to April 15, 1918, I did 108 operations on 103 patients with toxic goitre without a single fatality, whereas in the next succeeding series of 103 patients there were 8 deaths.

Since 1904, when I did my first operation for goitre, I have classified the toxic cases under four degrees of severity, viz., mild, moderate, marked, and extreme. The classification may be open to question, but it was based on personal judgment, using such factors as pulse-rate, blood-count, tremors, vaso-motor changes, excitability, exophthalmos and more recently basal metabolism. In accordance with this classification, it is found that 155 patients were designated mildly toxic, 86 moderately, 212 markedly, and 51 presented a picture of extreme degrees of toxicity. There were 13 deaths among these 51 extremely toxic cases, 1 of them following the ligation of both superior thyroid arteries and 3 following the injection of boiling water. Some of the remaining 9 deaths might have been prevented by doing less severe operations than resections or lobectomies— they are evidence of the fallibility of my judgment.

Of the 504 cases of toxic goitre, I have accurate pathological reports in 376. The reports show typical hyperplasia in 158 cases, to which should be added 31 cases in which the thyroid was in a resting state, approaching the normal in its microscopical picture. This resting state had been brought about either by the administration of iodine, as shown by Marine a number of years ago, or other medical measures, particularly rest, by irradiation, or by minor surgical procedures. There were 172 cases of toxic adenomata and 13 cases of adenomata with varying degrees of hyperplasia, which latter may be designated "mixed" types.

As a result of the investigation of the prevalence of goitre among army recruits, we know that it is more common in certain parts of the United States than we had anticipated. It was found, for instance, by

Kerr and Addis that 20.4 per cent. of over 22,000 recruits examined had goitres—these were from eleven northwestern and Pacific states. Only a small number of these had toxic symptoms. If such a proportion obtains in young men, it is reasonable to suppose that they are still more common in young women. It will be the work of the hygienist to solve this problem and when it is done there will be fewer goitres which demand surgical attention.

THE MANAGEMENT OF TOXIC GOITRE FROM THE SURGICAL POINT OF VIEW*

By Charles H. Frazier, M.D.
of Philadelphia, Pa.

In a recent contribution to a current periodical the relative merits of X-ray and surgical treatment are presented from a series of cases, the mortality of which was about 15 per cent. A mortality so high, either after X-rays or operation, seems prohibitive, and the conclusions therefore negligible. So much thought and labor has been given in recent years to safeguarding the patient in the management of toxic goitre that we have a right to expect a better showing. As a matter of fact, surgery to-day is not only the safest but the most effective way of saving life and restoring health. In my own clinic during the past five years, the mortality after resection for toxic goitre was only 1 per cent. and a fraction. My experience with the pathological lesion of the thyroid includes a series of 339 cases which form the basis of these remarks.

The absorbing interest of the thyroid gland has aroused inquiry in the minds of many. From the laboratories, the internists and the surgeons there is a continuous output of contributions, of greater or less moment, in mass indicating the widespread interest in the many-sided aspects of thyroid disease. As most entertaining, though chiefly of historical value, is the " Operative Story of Goitre," by Halstead. Here is recorded Gross' point of view as to the propriety of removing a goitre. About half a century ago he wrote, " Every step he takes will be environed with difficulty, every stroke of his knife will be followed by a torrent of blood, and lucky will it be for him if his victim live long enough to enable him to finish his horrible butchery. Thus, whether we view this operation in relation to the difficulties which must necessarily attend its resection, or with reference to the severity of the subsequent inflammation, it is equally deserving of rebuke and condemnation. No honest and sensible surgeon, it seems to me, would ever engage in it."

What a transformation there has been from this picture of butchery to the refined technic of the modern thyroidectomy!

The interrelationship between the thyroid and the adrenals has long been recognized. In differentiating between the sympathetic and vagus hypertonic types of hyperthyroidism, Kostling (Grenzgebiete 21, 1910) a number of years ago considered an adrenalinæmia as the most important sign of the former and called attention to the dilatation of the iris on the installation of adrenalin. More recently Goetsch has recommended the test as a point in diagnosis in the border-line cases, cases resembling in some respects true

---

* Read at the Conjoint Meeting of the New York Surgical Society and the Philadelphia Academy of Surgery, February 2, 1920.

hyperthyroidism, but without definite recognizable signs. Did this test prove infallible, we would have a valuable guide in the selection of cases for operation in this borderline group. I welcomed it as such, for in a certain number of instances, with but trifling enlargement of the gland, but without a clear picture of hyperthyroidism, I have been in a quandary as to the propriety of operating. I have applied the test routinely during the past few months, but have found it yet of little aid, and my skepticism has been aroused by negative reactions even in a typical exophthalmic syndrome.

To me one of the most practical problems of the surgery of toxic goitre is the determination of the degree of toxicity. This has a practical bearing upon the choice of operation. Kocher (*British Medical Journal*, Oct. 1, 1910) told us ten years ago that in the blood picture we had a very important aid as to prognosis and laid emphasis especially upon the relative increase in the lymphocytosis, he looked upon the degree of lymphocytosis as an evidence of the degree of toxicity. While it is quite true that, as a rule, the degree of the lymphocytosis bears a relationship to the gravity of the case, I have not found it by any means a constant guide as to the operative risks or as to the tolerance of the patient to surgical therapy.

What may prove to be a more dependable objective test is the determination of the basal metabolism, and the new Benedict apparatus, which we have installed as part of our equipment, has simplified this method of determination to a considerable degree. The estimation of the basal metabolism is, however, of more importance as a means of differential diagnosis in cases of obscure clinical picture with thyroid enlargement. In one of my series there was a great deal of doubt as to the relationship between the enlarged gland and a train of symptoms that were by no means typical. In this case the metabolism was not above but subnormal, so that an operation not only would have given no relief but would have been distinctly harmful. Metabolic studies serve the useful purpose, therefore, of enabling one to make a fairly accurate differential diagnosis between true hyperthyroidism and, for example, simple neurasthenia.

Means and Aub (*Arch. Int. Med.*, Dec., 1919) make the significant statement that for the most part patients with goitres, but without clinical signs of thyrotoxicosis, not only have a normal metabolism but that such cases do not subsequently become toxic.

Studies of the basal metabolism, I believe, should be made routinely in all cases of hyperthyroidism or for that matter of hypothyroidism, with just the same regularity as one should take the white-cell count in appendicitis or examine the urine in diabetes. This is true not only because of its value in differential diagnosis but because of the parallelism between the other signs of toxicity and the basal metabolism. For example, in the cases which clinically I would regard as severe, I find the basal metabolism runs something like this: plus 66, 78, 74, 68, 80, 73, 81, 93, etc., while of those cases of moderate severity it varies from plus 45 to plus 65 and the mild cases run below 45. To this statement it should be remembered, however, there are noted exceptions and for this reason particularly one must still hold some-what in abeyance the evaluation we are to place upon these metabolic studies in the management of new cases. For example, two patients with precisely the same metabolic rate may not be equally good surgical risks. Occasion-ally one sees a patient with a high metabolic rate with an unusually good tolerance to operation and vice versa. Again, a patient with a given metabolic rate may at different times be a good or a bad surgical risk. I have not been able to demonstrate that the metabolic rate always increases *pari passu* with exacerbations or crises. For these and other reasons the composite picture must be our guide as to what shall be our plan of action. Careful observation of each patient for at least a week, and two weeks, preferably, with attention to the cardiovascular symptoms, the vasomotor disturbances, the nervous and mental instability, in association with the blood picture and metabolic studies, will give us often much more satisfying and dependable data than any single objective test.

For practical purposes elaborate classifications of the toxic cases is unessential. The toxic adenomata may present operative problems quite as grave as those of hyperplastic type. Some of the most serious cases with which I have had to deal have been of the adenomatous group, with high metabolic rates and profound disturbances of the myocardium, cardiac rhythm and function, and while the technical difficulties of resection are not as great as with the toxic hyperplasias, the patients require just as much atten-tion in the preliminary treatment and after-care.

Every available agency must be called into play in the nursing of these patients back to health. Rest, of course, is helpful in the preparation of patients for operation, but of itself will reduce the basal metabolism from only 10 to 15 per cent. Even this slight improvement should be taken advan-tage of. With hydrobromate of quinine I have had no demonstrable results and I was interested in the observation (Means and Aub) that the effect of rest plus hydrobromate of quinine had no more influence on the basal metabolism than rest alone.

In the extremely toxic cases I always prescribe X-ray treatments, but the results have not been altogether satisfactory. It is in those cases in which there is the slightest suspicion of an enlarged thymus that irradiation should be employed. There is not the least doubt that an enlarged thymus is responsible for many of the sudden deaths following operation and irradiation should be prescribed and practised in all such cases preliminary to operation.

With regard to the X-rays therapeutics in general, all the reports which I have seen deal in generalities and do not give in detail the end results. The writers of these reports would lead us to believe that the results are almost uniformly good and one would infer better than the results of surgery. The insinuation is made also that X-ray therapy is without danger in itself. To this, however, I take exception; in the first place, Holmes and Merrill (*Journal A. M. A.*, 73, 1963, 1919) tell us that the gland may be destroyed and a state of hyperthyroidism produced if the treatment is pushed too fast.

The changes go on in the gland some time after treatment is discontinued. Secondly, the toxæmia may be increased to a dangerous degree by the first treatment and cases have been recorded (Secher) where the reaction following Röntgen therapy has been fatal. Thirdly, the increase in connective tissue makes subsequent operation more difficult.

The problem uppermost in our minds to-night is the surgical treatment. There can be no doubt as to the propriety of operation; the results are too striking to place the surgeon in a defensive attitude. It is a question only under what circumstances and by what method one shall proceed. That surgical procedure shall not be brought into disrepute, we should avoid certain pitfalls, and among these I would mention first of all the neurasthenias with enlarged glands between which there is no relationship of cause and effect. Fortunately the differentiation can now be demonstrated by objective tests. In the second class I would place the mildly toxic cases of adolescence, for here we have a physiological enlargement and the need of the economy is not less thyroid tissue in most instances but more iodine.

The third group among the undesirable include the thymic cases, and I have already referred to the necessity of preliminary X-ray treatment; in the fourth group I would place the wreckage, the cases in the terminal stage of the disease, the utterly hopeless cases; and in the fifth group the cases of hypothyroidism. I will not elaborate upon these several groups. Their recognition implies often careful, intensive study, but if our records of surgical achievement are to be above criticism, those groups should not be included among our operable cases.

In recommending operation shall we discriminate between the mild, moderate and severe cases? In the very mild cases, operation is not urgent; by change of occupation and other simple remedies (the care of teeth infection, the removal of infected tonsils and the like) there may be some improvement. But even without improvement, if the condition remains stationary and does not handicap the patient, operation remains one of choice rather than of necessity. But in the moderate cases I have always urged operation, because these are on the threshold of a condition that must always be considered potentially grave. There is no doubt at all that a certain percentage of cases recover spontaneously; nor is there any doubt that a certain percentage are improved or recover by what is called medical treatment, essentially rest; but it is equally true that these are subject to recurrences or relapses; and, whether the patient has been under medical treatment or not treated at all, every crisis of hyperthyroidism through which the patient passes leaves that patient a poorer surgical risk. This point must always be borne in mind by those who advise a "course of medical treatment." The degenerative changes, which take place in the vital organs during the period of procrastination, are permanent and preclude the ultimate and complete recovery of the patient. For these reasons, therefore, I take a firm stand as to the propriety of early operation.

Whether to begin the operative treatment with a resection or with a preliminary ligation, I think admits of no discussion. It has been my practice to resort to preliminary ligation when there is the least doubt as to the propriety of a resection, and as time goes on I find the number of preliminary ligations is increasing rather than decreasing and single ligation I prefer to double ligation at one or two weeks' intervals. As a rule, with a metabolic rate over 60, I always practice preliminary ligation, and in cases of lower metabolic rate when the other signs of great toxicity are evident in the rapid pulse, much loss of weight, restlessness, sleeplessness, and particularly marked vasomotor disturbances. The operation is performed in the patient's room, and according to our " anoci " technic the patient does not know that she has had more than an unusually severe " inhalation " treatment. I believe there are sound anatomical reasons for selecting the superior pole and I always surround the pole with two ligatures and divide all the tissues between, which includes thyroid tissue, cervical sympathetic fibres, lymphatic vessels, in addition to the arteries, that is the main trunk and its posterior branch.

. There is but one objection, and only one, to preliminary ligation, and that is the additional scars. But the greater safety far outweighs any consideration of cosmetics. To make the scars less conspicuous, I place them always in a crease in the neck. Almost invariably one of two creases will be found near enough to the level of the pole to answer our purpose, and if the incision follows the crease accurately the scar will be quite inconspicuous.

I need not dwell upon the improvement after ligation, as you know in most cases it is striking as to pulse-rate, weight, basal metabolism and other indices of improvement. There is but one point that should be emphasized in this connection. The resection should follow at an interval of not more than two or three months. The maximum improvement is noted about that time and there may, and in most cases will be, relapses as the compensatory circulation increases in volume. In a few cases the patient may feel so much better that she or he will not return. This is a risk one takes in the practice of ligation. In some the improvement will not be so apparent, but as the vascularity of the gland has been appreciably diminished, the final operation will be attended with less bleeding. The difference in degree of improvement is difficult to account for, except perhaps on an anatomical basis, since the four arteries are subject to considerable and frequent variation. The superior arteries may both be very small, the inferior correspondingly large or vice versa. Whatever the explanation, I find great variations in the results. In the exceptional case the condition may be temporarily aggravated as in a recent observation where the metabolism rose from 49 to 66 after a single ligation.

But even though the preliminary ligation may not have been followed by as much improvement as had been anticipated, this step in the management of goitre serves a useful purpose. The reaction of the patient to the minor procedure is a very good index of the degree of reaction that may be anticipated after the final thyroidectomy. In some instances the thyroidectomy,

CHARLES H. FRAZIER

if the reaction is slight, may be performed two weeks rather than two months after the ligation.

The ultimate and total result of surgical interference follows the resection of the gland. In the preparation of the patient our " anoci " technic following the principles of Crile is strictly observed without variation. It matters not by what seductive method the gland is " stolen," the advantages of the principles involved cannot be overestimated, and with a trained staff of assistants and nurses the patient need not know the gland has been removed until she returns home. The measure of success in the surgical treatment of hyperthyroidism is in direct proportion to the amount of tissue removed. The incomplete or partial relief of symptoms, the relapses or recurrences must be charged to the failure to remove enough tissue. The resection should be bilateral even though the pathology seems confined to one lobe. I have never removed too much and more than once in earlier days too little. At least symptomatically there have been no instances of myxœdema, although in one instance the basal metabolism was minus. It is difficult to express in figures what proportion of tissue should be removed; some say four-fifths, some five-sixths. This, I believe, is too much if based on the size of the lobes with their pathological accession. If one leaves a thin layer of thyroid tissue, lining that portion of the capsule which remains after resection, there will be quite enough for the body economy. All operations are performed under nitrous oxide anæsthesia. According to our technic and to our conception of the advantages of the control of psychic influences local anæsthesia is distinctly contra-indicated.

In the final analysis the value of the surgical treatment of the toxic goitre must be estimated in terms of end results. The mortality now is far below that of any other method of treatment and each year the mortality is lowered. As for the end results, I have not been able to review my entire series, but in the analysis made before the war 80 per cent. of the patients heard from were recorded as recovered, either altogether or sufficiently to enable them to resume their occupations. The degree of recovery, be it remembered, must depend upon whether at the time of operation the ravages of the disease had damaged beyond repair the vital organs.

A "TOURNIQUET OPERATION" IN TOXIC AND OTHER GOITRES *

By Leonard Freeman, M.D.
of Denver, Colo.

When operating upon a toxic goitre it usually is better to remove a part of each lobe than the whole of one lobe, not only for cosmetic reasons, but because diseased glandular tissue is less liable to be left behind. Also, secretion is diminished in the remnants of the gland from the division of blood-vessels and from cicatricial contraction.

Hence, partial, bilateral thyroidectomy is the operation of choice, and it becomes a matter of importance to develop a rapid and safe technic adapted to the limitations of the average surgeon. With this object in view, I desire to call attention to a method which I have employed for a number of years, accumulating experience having convinced me of its value. I have used it one hundred and eighty-two times and have found it applicable to all kinds of goitres—large, small, soft, vascular, and hard—with the exception of those which are calcified. In this series of cases I have never injured the recurrent laryngeal nerve or, to my knowledge, the parathyroids, and I believe such danger to be practically negligible, even with comparatively inexperienced operators.

Operative Technic.—The preliminary steps are those employed in most goitre work—collar incision, exposure of the gland and dislocation of its lobes. It seldom is necessary to divide any muscles, as is done often in other procedures.

From this point on, the technic differs. It has for its object the placing of a tourniquet around the base of each lobe, before partial excision, so as to control hemorrhage by compression of *all* the vessels without injury to the nerves or parathyroids. This is done by means of two wires, one on either side of the base of the lobe, held in place by elastic bands passing through the glandular substance.

The necessary equipment (Fig. 1) consists of a number of ordinary strong rubber bands, two or three inches long and somewhat thicker than the lead in a pencil; two pieces of wire of a similar diameter and three or four inches in length, with the ends turned over into small loops to prevent injury to gloves or tissues (large hairpins will suffice); and a pair of small alligator forceps.

The consecutive steps are as follows: (1) Elevate one of the thoroughly dislocated lobes with the fingers or with appropriate forceps. (2) Plunge the alligator forceps directly through the base of the lobe near

* Read before the American Surgical Association, May 4, 1920.

11   161

its centre and close to the trachea, grasp a rubber band and pull it through, so that an end projects from either side. Repeat the manœuvre near each extremity of the lobe, so that its base remains transfixed by three loops (Fig. 2). (3) The wires, which must be long enough to project well beyond the lobe at either end, are now passed through the three loops on each side (Fig. 2). (4) With the lobe well elevated, and an assistant holding the ends of the wires together, the central band is pulled taut and clamped close to the wire with hæmostatic forceps, thus binding the wires firmly together (Fig. 3). The two remaining bands are manipulated differently. After pulling on them until they are tense, each strand is wrapped in an opposite direction about the projecting ends of the wires before clamping, so as to insure the constriction of the vessels at either pole (Fig. 3). (5) The portion of the gland beyond the tourniquet is then excised with scalpel and scissors, leaving only a sufficient cuff on either side for the insertion of a hæmostatic suture (Fig. 4). One can take one's time in doing this, the bleeding being perfectly under control. An important point is that the elastic contraction of the rubber bands maintains the hæmostatic pressure of the wires even though much tissue is removed from between them.[1] (6) With a long catgut suture the raw area is whipped over, utilizing the lateral " cuffs " in the procedure (Fig. 4). It may be desirable to go back over the first suture-line, so as thoroughly to control the bleeding, but it seldom is necessary to tie any vessels separately, not even the thyroidal trunks. (7) After unclasping the forceps which hold the rubber bands, the wires and bands are removed. There usually is no bleeding of consequence from the punctures through the gland substance, but if any should occur it can be checked by pressure or a suture. (8) The wound is then closed and drained. (9) An enlarged isthmus may require separate handling, or it may be removed along with a lateral lobe, by including it within the grasp of the tourniquet, as I have often done. I do not consider it necessary to divide the isthmus in any but exceptional cases.

The advantages of this method of operating are several: (a) Bleeding from all the vessels is completely controlled. (b) No hæmostatic forceps are required after applying the tourniquet, thus avoiding an embarrassing profusion of instruments, not to mention the danger of injuring a nerve in their application. (c) The wires cannot slip when the gland is cut away, because they are held in position by the elastic bands passing through the stump. (d) The safety of the recurrent laryngeal nerve and parathyroids is assured by the wedge-shaped excision, and even if they should be caught in the grasp of the wires the pressure is not great enough to damage them permanently.

This constriction without crushing is important, and is one of the reasons why the wire tourniquet is superior to the use of large forceps

[1] The elastic bands are superior to fishing-line, which I used exclusively until recently (Colorado Medicine, Jan., 1916).

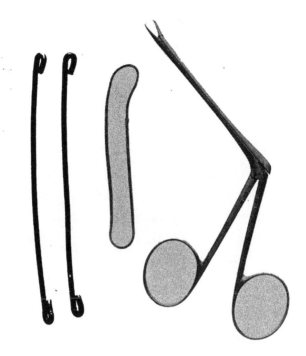

FIG. 1.—Showing wires, rubber bands and alligator forceps.

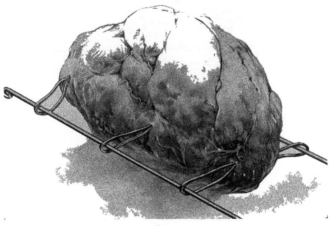

FIG. 2.—Rubber bands drawn through base of lobe and wires inserted through the projecting loops on either side.

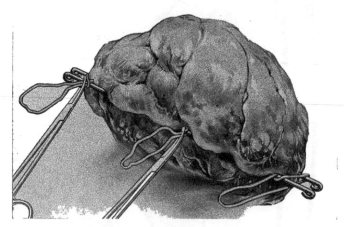

FIG. 3.—Rubber bands drawn taut and held by forceps, the end bands having been wrapped around the extremities of the wires.

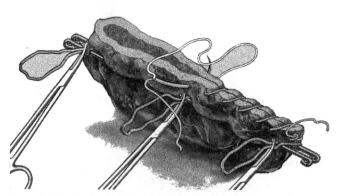

FIG. 4.—Showing wedge-shaped excision and method of inserting hemostatic suture. (For the sake of clearness the "cuff" is pictured unnecessarily wide and thick.)

which are sometimes similarly employed; for if the forceps are closed tightly enough to prevent slipping they will crush, which is undesirable in toxic goitre, and may injure the nerves and parathyroids. In addition, forceps occupy more room than wires and often are difficult to apply, because of the thickness of the lobe and because they cannot be bent to conform to varying conditions.

Anyone who sees fit to try this method of operating will find it easy, safe, comparatively bloodless, and rapid. Its merits will be especially appreciated in the soft and vascular goitres of toxic type.

THE RELATIONSHIP BETWEEN RANULA AND BRANCHIO-GENETIC CYSTS *

By JAMES E. THOMPSON, F.R.C.S. (ENG.)

OF GALVESTON, TEXAS

THE name " Ranula " is usually applied to a cyst with mucous contents which is found underneath the mucous membrane covering the floor of the mouth on one side of the frenum of the tongue. The wall of the cyst is thin and is loosely attached to the surrounding tissues. It consists of fibrous tissue of a loose variety. The inner surface is often covered by a single layer of tesselated epithelium. The contents are of mucus of the consistence of white of egg. These cysts vary in size. They rarely cross the midline. When large they extend outwards and downwards. Wharton's duct and the sublingual gland can usually be seen superficial to the cyst but apparently not structurally connected with it. The cyst usually lies entirely within the buccal cavity on the upper surface of the mylohyoid muscle (Fig. 1, A). Not infrequently a prolongation of the cyst extends around the posterior border of the mylohyoid, producing a swelling in the submaxillary region (Fig. 1, B) which may reach the size of a small mandarin orange. Occasionally the submaxillary swelling may consist of two separate cysts, one of which alone communicates with the intrabuccal cyst (Fig. 1, C).

Various theories have been advanced from time to time to account for the presence of ranula. Up to the present time none has been satisfactory. It has always appeared to me that a cyst which presents such consistent anatomical and pathological features must have one and only one origin; and, therefore, I have never believed that a ranula could at one time be derived from Wharton's duct, at another from the sublingual gland, at another from one of the mucous glands, and at still another from an adventitious bursa (Fleischmann's). I have satisfied myself in every case of ranula that has come under my observation that neither Wharton's duct nor the sublingual gland are responsible, by finding that these structures were healthy and normally placed. To refuse to believe that some cysts may not have their origin in the mucous glands of this region would be unwise. One meets with examples of mucous cysts of considerable size arising in the mucous membrane of the mouth. These cysts, however, are very superficial, very closely connected with the mucous membrane and do not separate it from the subjacent tissues. In other words, they do not show the frank burrowing qualities of true ranula. As to Fleischmann's bursa I may say frankly that I have never seen it, and further, that many anatomists in a life's experience have failed to satisfy themselves as to its real existence.

---

* Read before the American Surgical Association, May 5, 1920.

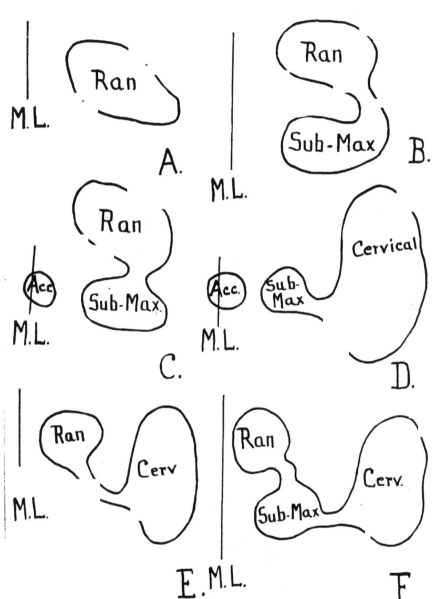

FIG. 1.—(Original V. K.) A diagrammatic representation of the anatomical distribution of the cysts met with in the deep cervical, submaxillary and sublingual regions. *A*, represents a simple ranula. *B*, a ranula and submaxillary cyst communicating with one another by a neck. *C*, a ranula and submaxillary cyst communicating with each other; also a small isolated cyst in the submental region. *D*, shows a deep cervical cyst communicating with a submaxillary cyst; also an isolated submental cyst. *E*, shows a deep cervical cyst communicating with a ranula by a long narrow neck which traverses the submaxillary region. *F*, shows a deep cervical cyst communicating with a submaxillary cyst which in turn opens into a ranula. The letters *M L* mean "middle line of the neck." For purposes of comparison all the cysts have been drawn on the left side of the body.

With the hope of throwing some light on the origin of ranula I venture to present a careful analysis of a group of cases which I believe will prove that a direct relationship exists between cysts of undoubted branchiogenetic origin and cysts in the submaxillary region and the floor of the mouth. In 1906[1] I reported two cases of cysts of the upper region of the neck that were identical with each other in their anatomical and pathological features. In each case the cyst was deeply placed in the upper portion of the neck under cover of the parotid gland and the ramus of the jaw. In one case the cyst communicated with a ranula under the tongue by a narrow communicating track which passed across the submaxillary region (Fig. 1, E). In the other case there was no ranula, but the cyst opened in front by a short passage into a large cyst occupying the submaxillary region (Fig. 1, D). In front of this a small accessory cyst was found in the middle line underneath the symphysis of the jaw (Fig. 1, D). Since that time a number of cases of cervical cyst have come under my observation identical in every particular as to structure and location. Each cyst had associated with it either a submaxillary cyst or a ranula, or both, with which it communicated freely. In Fig. 1, D, E and F, drawings of the different types of cyst are shown which picture in a striking manner their close relationships with one another. Two of these types, D and E, were described in my original paper and I have verified the accuracy of my original description by cases seen subsequently. Type F has been added since, and inasmuch as it embodies all the most typical features of these compound cysts it will be used as the basis of a common clinical and pathological description.

The history and anatomical findings are as follows: Mrs. L. F., aged thirty-one years, white, came under my care suffering from a ranula under the left side of tongue, which was the size of a walnut. The submaxillary region of the same side was also occupied by a cystic swelling which increased in size when pressure was made on the ranula. The two cysts evidently communicated freely. In addition there was a swelling between the angle of the jaw and the mastoid process, which obliterated the natural hollow in front of the lobule of the ear. The ranula had been noticed a few years previously and several attempts had been made to cure it by tapping and snipping out parts of the walls of the cyst. The swellings in the submaxillary and parotid regions were of recent onset. Recognizing the nature of the case I suggested operation. The neck was opened by a semicircular incision such as is employed for ligature of the lingual artery. The ranula and submaxillary cyst were dissected out in one piece. It was found necessary to remove the submaxillary salivary gland to facilitate the dissection. The posterior part of the submaxillary cyst led into a narrow neck, which penetrated the deep compartment of cervical fascia separating the submaxillary gland from the deep cervical fascial space to open finally into a large cavity which lay in the upper part of the neck under cover of the parotid gland and the inferior maxilla. This contained

---

[1] Texas State Journal of Medicine, December 7, 1906.

thin mucus and its walls were smooth and firmly attached to the surrounding tissues. The boundaries of the cavity were as follows: *Above*, one could feel the base of the skull represented by the under surface of the petrous portion of the temporal bone. All the bony irregularities were clearly distinguishable. *Below*, the cyst wall turned on itself about the level of the greater cornu of the hyoid bone. *Externally*, one could feel distinctly the inner surface of the ramus of the inferior maxilla covered by the internal pterygoid muscle, the projection of the spine of Spix and the deep surface of the parotid gland. *Posteriorly*, the anterior surface of the mastoid and styloid processes were clearly palpable. *Internally*, the cyst extended for a short distance in front of the transverse processes of the upper cervical vertebræ. The internal carotid artery could be felt very close to the posterior wall of the cyst. A small portion of the cyst wall was removed and stained for epithelium. No epithelial lining could be demonstrated. Complete removal being clearly an impossibility, the mucus contents were evacuated and the interior of the cavity thoroughly scrubbed with gauze soaked in tincture of iodine. A drainage tube was inserted. This was retained two days and then removed. After considerable reaction the wound healed up by first intention and the patient left hospital at the end of three weeks apparently cured. I heard from the patient about a year afterwards and found that the cervical part of the cyst had refilled and that she was contemplating another operation.

All the cysts seen so far have been so characteristically alike that the above description is accurate in its main essentials for every one of them as regards the cervical compartment. Considerable variation has been present in the submaxillary and lingual regions. Fig. 1, *D; E* and F represent the types observed so far. It is almost certain that further experience will reveal others.

Microscopic examination of the lining membrane of the cyst wall has been rather unsatisfactory. In most cases we were unable to find epithelium. When present it was of the tesselated variety. The fibrous tissue was fairly dense and the fibrous bundles were separated by large lymph-spaces containing very few cellular elements.

I have made a somewhat exhaustive search of reported cases, but so far I have been unable to find cases that correspond anatomically to those reported above. The anatomical boundaries of the cervical portions of these cysts are so unusual, definite and consistent as to negative mere coincidence as to structure and origin and to make it reasonably certain that they result from a definite cause and therefore are likely to be met with true to type in the practice of every surgeon. It is more than probable that they are not rarities but that they have escaped accurate description. A study of *A, B, C, D, E* and F in Fig. 1, leads one to the inevitable inference that each picture is a complement of all the rest, like fragments of a picture puzzle, and that the different cysts have a common origin. They give us the impression of being daughter cysts which have been segregated from a mother cyst and carried by some agency into regions remote from their original home, during which process obliteration of one or more of the daughter cysts or even of the mother cyst has occurred, producing a final picture corresponding more or less closely with one of those in the figures. The potentialities of such a mother cyst are present in the neck of the human embryo of four weeks at a period when the external gill cleft depressions are existent and the cervical sinus is in process of formation The persistence of the cervical sinus in whole or in part is probably responsible for all branchial cysts and fistulæ, and, inasmuch as the stages in its development are inseparably connected with those of the branchial arches and clefts, it will be necessary to add a description of the life history of the latter to enable us to handle the subject intelligently.

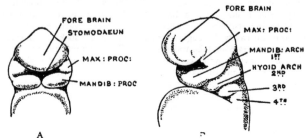

FIG. 2.—(From Keith's Human Embryology.) The branchial arches and stomodæum of a human embryo of the third week. Front and side Views.

In the third week of fœtal life the branchial arches make their appearance (Fig. 2). The pharyngeal region of the embryo resembles that of an adult fish, but whereas in fishes the arches are separated by clefts, here they are separated by depressions. These depressions, generally spoken of as internal and external cleft depressions, are visible on the outer aspect of the neck and the inner aspect of the pharynx. They are separated by a membrane which is lined on its outer side by epiblast and on its inner side by hypoblast (Fig. 3). In the normal course of development the membrane never disappears, so that it is incorrect to speak of gill clefts in the human embryo in the same sense that we use the term in referring to fishes. In the rare instances in which the membrane is perforated a complete cleft is formed which may persist in the adult and may be the forerunner of a branchial fistula. The growth of the neck is so rapid that by the end of the sixth week all external evidence of the branchial arches and cleft depressions has disappeared.

BRANCHIAL ARCHES

Six arches are usually described, of which four can be distinguished on the surface of the neck (Fig. 2). The posterior ends of the two anterior are connected with the bony skeleton, but those of the posterior four lie free in the tissues. Each arch contains: (1) a basis of cartilage; (2) a vascular arch; (3) nerves; (4) muscle elements (Fig. 3). *The first arch* is the mandibular. Its basis (Meckel's cartilage) forms the foundation of the lower jaw, although the greater part disappears. The posterior end persists as the malleus and the anterior end as the part of the lower jaw which carries the incisor teeth. The nerve of the arch is the third division of the fifth. The artery of the arch disappears but the origin of the external maxillary (facial) marks the place where it arose from the ventral aorta (external carotid). The *second arch* is the hyoid. Its posterior end persists as the stapes, the middle portion as the styloid process and stylohyoid ligament, and the anterior end as the lesser cornu of the hyoid bone. The nerve of this arch is represented by the facial and auditory (7th and 8th). The artery of the arch disappears, but the lingual artery marks the place where it arose from the ventral aorta. The *third arch* is represented in the adult by the great cornu and body of the hyoid bone. Its nerve is the glosso-

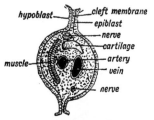

FIG. 3.—(From Keith's Human Embryology.)
Schematic section of a Visceral arch.

pharyngeal (ninth). The artery of the arch persists as the first part of the internal carotid. The superior thyroid arises from its place of origin from the ventral aorta. The *fourth arch* is represented in the adult by the upper part of the thyroid cartilage. Its nerve is the superior laryngeal branch of the vagus. The vascular arch is represented on the right side by the first part of the subclavian artery, and on the left side by that part of the arch of the aorta between the origin of the left carotid and the point of entrance of the ductus arteriosus. The *fifth arch* is represented in the adult by the lower portion of the thyroid cartilage. Its nerve is the inferior laryngeal branch of the vagus. The *sixth arch* is represented in the adult by the cricoid and arytenoid cartilages and the cartilaginous rings of the trachea and bronchi. Its nerve is the inferior laryngeal branch of the vagus. The vascular arches of the fifth arch probably disappear early. Those of the sixth persist. On the left side it forms part of the right pulmonary artery and the ductus arteriosus; on the right it shares in the formation of the right pulmonary artery.

The *muscles of the arches* deserve special consideration. At first they are limited to the area of their respective arches, but with the increase in

169

length of the neck of the embryo and the differentiation of different structures such as the tongue, palate and larynx, many of the muscles are carried into regions remote from their origin. As they always carry their nerves with them, we can distinguish the embryonic origins of all the muscles of the neck by their nerve supply. From the first arch (mandibular, fifth nerve) are derived the muscles of mastication, the myohyoid and the anterior belly of the digastric, the tensor palati and tensor tympani. From the *second arch* (hyoid—seventh nerve) are derived the stapedius, the stylohyoid, the posterior belly of the digastric, all the muscles of facial expression and the platysma. From the *third arch* (ninth nerve) are derived the stylopharyngeus and some of the muscles of the soft palate. From the *fourth arch* (superior laryngeal

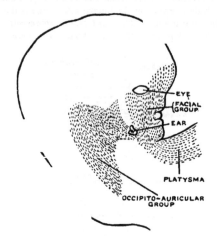

FIG. 4.—(From Keith's Human Embryology.) The expansion and migration of the platysma sheet in a human embryo of six weeks.

nerve) are derived some of the muscles of the soft palate, the constrictors of the pharynx and the cricothyroid. From the *fifth arch* (inferior laryngeal nerve) are derived the intrinsic muscles of the larynx.

Great irregularity is shown in the movement or migration of these muscles, and this is strikingly exemplified in the soft palate where one of the muscles (tensor palati, fifth nerve) is derived from the first arch, while the rest are derived from the third and fourth arches (ninth and tenth nerves). The most extensive migration is seen in the muscles derived from the second arch (hyoid) (Fig. 4). A remarkable muscular bud makes its appearance which grows upwards into the face and scalp over the surface of the first arch and downwards into the neck over the surfaces of the posterior arches. From it the occipitofrontalis, all the muscles of expression and the

170

platysma are derived. The branches of the seventh nerve carried with these muscles identify their origin.

To these disturbing agents in the orderly arrangement of parts is added another muscular migration which arises in the seventh, eighth and ninth body segments which are situated behind those supplied by the tenth and

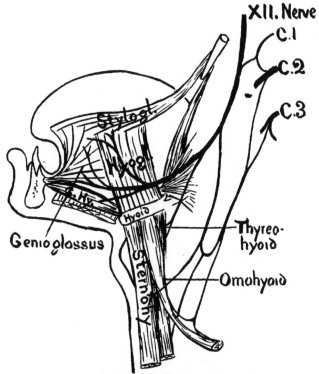

Fig. 5.—(Original V. K.) Modified from Cunningham. Showing the muscles supplied by the hypoglossal nerve (XII) to illustrate the migration of the muscles derived from the seventh, eighth and ninth body segments. It must be noted that the infrahyoid muscles are probably derived from the cervical segments behind the hypoglossus group.

eleventh nerves (Fig. 5). These segments are supplied by the twelfth nerve (hypoglossal). The path and extent of this migration is clearly indicated by the course of the hypoglossal nerve and the situation of the muscles supplied by it. It may be divided into two parts: an upper (lingual) from which the geniohyoid, the geniohyoglossus, hyoglossus and all the intrinsic muscles of the tongue are derived; and a lower (infrahyoid) which forms

171

JAMES E. THOMPSON

the depressors of the hyoid bone. One of these muscles, the omohyoid, extends downwards as far as the scapula. The actual path of migration of the upper (lingual) division is charted accurately by the course of the main trunk of the hypoglossal nerve. The descendens hypoglossi is a similar guide to that of the lower division. The upper muscular division penetrates into a bud of hypoblast which is situated on the posterior surface of the fused anterior ends of the first, second, and third arches. This bud, called the lingual bud, is developed from two separate parts (Fig. 6), an anterior (buccal) which arises from the anterior ends of the first visceral arch (tuberculum impar), and a posterior (pharyngeal) which arises from the anterior ends of the second and third arches. The epithelium covering these buds retains its original nerve supply. That to the anterior which forms the anterior two-thirds of the tongue comes from the nerve to the first arch (fifth lingual), while that to the posterior which forms the posterior third

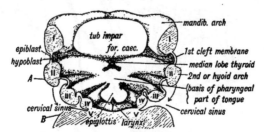

FIG. 6.—(From Keith.) The floor of the pharynx in a human embryo of the fourth week. Five branchial arches are shown separated by cleft depressions. The early stages of the development of the cervical sinus are shown; also the separate hypoblastic eminences that form the anterior and posterior parts of the tongue.

of the organ is derived from the nerves of the second and third arches and is represented by the chorda tympani (seventh) and the glossopharyngeal (ninth). The resulting organ offers an interesting picture of a muscular mass innervated by the twelfth nerve and covered by mucous membrane supplied by the fifth, seventh and ninth nerves.

The muscular migrations have been described in some detail because our final argument is based on the hypothesis that they are responsible for carrying cysts from one region of the neck to the other.

BRANCHIAL CLEFTS

Four cleft depressions can be recognized in the embryo. The *first cleft* (hyomandibular) persists. Its external depression is represented by the external auditory meatus. In connection with the internal depression the Eustachian tube and the tympanum are developed. The membrana tympani is supposed to represent the cleft membrane. The second, third and fourth clefts disappear and usually leave no trace of their existence. In a very

172

young embryo (fourth week) the second arch (hyoid) grows downwards and covers the third and fourth and comes into contact and fuses with the body wall behind the fifth. By this growth, which is analogous to that forming the gill covers of fishes, the orifices of the second, third and fourth cleft depressions are covered up and a space is shut off into which they open. This is called the "*cervical sinus*." A knowledge of the ultimate fate of the cervical sinus is of fundamental importance in explaining the characteristics of branchiogenetic cysts. Under normal conditions it disappears. If it persists a cyst or a fistula may result. The sinus may open externally on

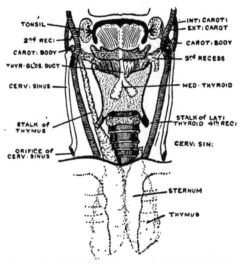

FIG. 7.—(From Keith's Human Embryology.) A diagrammatic representation of the structures developed in connection with the inner cleft recesses. Note on the right side of the figure a branchial fistula due to perforation of the second branchial cleft and persistence of the cervical sinus. This figure should be studied in connection with Figs. 8 and 9.

to the neck or internally into the pharynx. The external opening is invariably along the line of the anterior border of the sternomastoid muscle. It may be placed anywhere between the angle of the jaw and the sternal notch, but it is usually about the middle of the neck. When an internal opening is present it is usually due to perforation of the second cleft membrane, and the pharyngeal orifice is situated in the tonsillar crypt (Fig. 7). Internal openings due to perforation of the third and fourth cleft membranes are infrequently seen. The pharyngeal orifices of these openings are situated lower down in the sinus pyriformis. The tracks leading from the cervical sinus into the pharynx through the membranes of the second, third and fourth clefts would in the adult neck course in widely diverse directions. That pass-

173

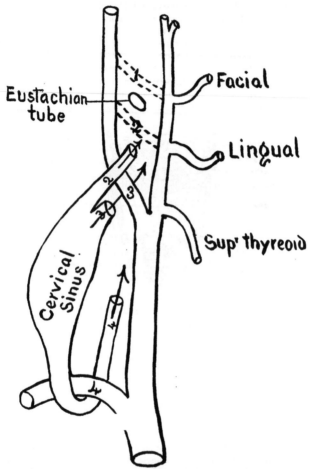

FIG. 8.—(Original W. K.) A diagrammatic representation of the cervical sinus to show the anatomical paths which would be taken by fistulous passages passing through persistent second, third and fourth clefts. This figure shows the relationships of these fistulæ to the Vascular arches of the neck. The large figures are on the Vascular arches; 2 is on an obliterated trunk; 3 is on the commencement of internal carotid; 4 is on the right subclavian. The smaller figures near the arrows are on the fistulous tracks. Note that track 3 passes below the fork of the carotids and track 4 passes below the subclavian artery (right side).

ing through the second cleft always courses upwards between the arch of the carotid arteries and penetrates the pharyngeal muscles above the glossopharyngeal nerve; that passing through the third cleft courses upwards below the in-

ternal carotid, above the superior laryngeal nerve and below the glossopharyngeal nerve; that passing through the fourth cleft must pass downwards, hook
around the subclavian artery on the right side and the aorta on the left and
course upwards alongside the inferior laryngeal nerve. When both internal and
external openings are present a fistulous track passes from the surface of
the neck to the pharynx. When there are neither internal nor external
openings present, but th.. sinus persists either in whole or in part, a cyst
results. In Figs. 8 and 9 an attempt has been made to show in a diagrammatic

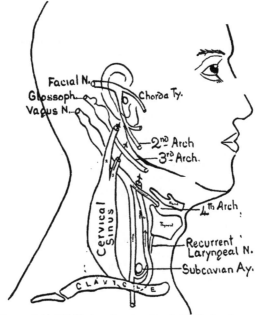

Fig. 9.—(Original W. K.) A complementary picture to Fig. 8 to show the anatomical relationships of persistent branchial fistulæ to the nerves of the neck.
Arrows are placed in the fistulous tracks leading from the cervical sinus. Note
that track 3 passes beneath the glossopharyngeal nerve and above the superior
laryngeal branch of the vagus; also that track 4 passes downward below the
subclavian artery (right side).

manner the relationships of the fistulous tracks of branchial origin with the
nerves and arteries of the branchial arches. A careful study of these
plates will convince us that the description of the fistulæ in question has
hitherto been very loose and inaccurate. This is particularly the case with
those due to the persistence of the third and fourth clefts. The statement
that a fistula due to the persistence of the cervical sinus always passes
upwards between the fork formed by the external and internal carotids,

175

JAMES E. THOMPSON

can only be true on strict embryological grounds when the second branchial cleft persists. That almost all fistulous tracks take this direction is absolute proof of the persistence of this cleft in the great majority of cases. Too few careful records of dissection are available to enable us to speak authoritatively as to the frequency with which the third cleft persists; while I am not acquainted with any observation showing a fistulous track passing around the subclavian artery or the aorta, the only possible route when the fourth cleft persists.

There is abundant evidence to justify us in attributing lateral cysts and fistulæ situated in the middle of the neck, to the persistence of the cervical sinus and the branchial clefts. But it is more difficult to explain how cysts situated close to the base of the skull and those in the submaxillary and lingual regions can be derived from the same source. It will be conceded that the cysts under consideration conform to the type of branchio-genetic cysts in anatomical structure and contents. Therefore, the difficulty in accepting them as truly branchio-genetic will disappear if a satisfactory explanation can be offered as to the manner in which they are carried from their original location, and disintegrated into two or three separate fragments. It appears to me, if we admit the possibility of these cysts being carried from a lower level to a higher by muscular agency in the rearrangement of the muscular planes of the neck, that the problem is easily solved. After due deliberation I have adopted the theory that ranula, submaxillary cyst and deep cervical cyst of the type described, are derived from the cervical sinus which has been carried from its original position by the muscles of the branchial arches and those of the hypoglossal segments during the process of their migration. On this theory the deep cervical cyst which has such characteristic anatomical boundaries would be carried upwards by the palate muscles, all of which except the tensor palati (first arch) are derived from the third and fourth arches, whereas the cysts found in the submaxillary and lingual regions would be carried upwards by the muscles of the tongue derived from the hypoglossal group which belongs to the seventh, eighth, and ninth body segments.

LATE RESULTS AFTER THE RADICAL OPERATION FOR CANCER OF THE BREAST *

By Willy Meyer, M.D.

of New York, N. Y.

Last fall, when preparing the data for a clinic I intended to hold during the Congress of American Surgeons in this city (October, 1919) on late results of operation for the radical cure of cancer of the breast, I tried to reach all my former ward patients, but soon was obliged to give up the efforts in this direction. It proved absolutely impossible—with the ever-shifting population of a large city like New York—to trace the patients operated upon in the wards.

This experience again impressed me with the great desirability, nay, necessity, of the "Follow-up System" so auspiciously inaugurated by a number of large hospitals in our country.

Under the circumstances I was obliged to content myself with the data available from my private patients, whom I had personally followed up for the last twenty-six years.

Two radical operations have been before the profession since the fall of 1894. Their principal point of difference is the direction in which the surgeon proceeds. The one method starts from the chest and works toward the axilla, leaving the clavicular portion of the pectoralis major behind; it requires entering the space between pectoralis major and minor muscles; the latter usually is divided and then sutured. As a matter of necessity this method involves quite some loss of blood.

The other method, which I have practised since September 12, 1894, starts from the axilla and works toward the sternum. The tendons of pectoralis major and minor are divided in the early stage of the operation, necessitating complete excision of both muscles. Blood- and lymph-vessels are primarily divided within the axilla. The lymph-nodes and axillary fat are lifted out in connection with the tumor, before the cancerous breast itself is handled. The entire mass is removed without entering what I call the "infected area." Hemorrhage is reduced to a minimum.

The final results of the operation from the sternum toward the shoulder, as reported, have been good. Still small cancerous glands have repeatedly been found between pectoralis major and minor muscle, and where cancerous lymphatic glands have developed there must be present suspicious lymphatic vessels. I feel that it must be better for

* Remarks made at the Joint Meeting of the New York Surgical Society and Philadelphia Academy of Surgery, February 3, 1920, and before the Surgical Section of the New York Academy of Medicine, April 2, 1920.

the patient if the space between the two muscles is not entered and the entire diseased area is excised in its normal anatomical relation.

Previous to 1894 excision of the breast for carcinoma was at last done in two stages, but at the same sitting, first, the removal of the breast with axillary contents; then the excision of the pectoralis major muscle. This arrangement forced the surgeon to widely enter " the infected area " and caused an unnecessarily great loss of blood. Personally, I did not see a single lasting cure after this mode of advance. The radical operation changed the results with one stroke. Most forcibly was this brought home to me by comparison of my personal statistics before and after September, 1894. The first two cases subjected to the modern radical operation were completely cured, and Case IV of this series had enjoyed freedom from cancerous recurrence for many years when she died of old age.

The following personal cases are alive and well to-day, from twelve to twenty-five and one-half years after operation:

CASE I.—Operated upon September 12, 1894, when thirty-eight years of age (now a lady sixty-four years old). It is the first case operated upon by the method outlined above. She is alive and well to-day, twenty-five and one-half years after operation (Fig. 1).

CASE II.—Operation done in 1895, at the age of forty-eight years (now a lady seventy-three and one-half years old). The patient is alive and well to-day, twenty-five years after operation (Fig. 2).

CASE III.—Operation in July, 1902, when thirty-three years old (now a lady of fifty-one years). Patient alive and well to-day, eighteen years after operation (Fig. 3).

CASE IV.—Operation in December, 1903, at the age of thirty-six years (now a lady of fifty-three), perfectly healthy and free from recurrence to-day, seventeen years after operation (Fig. 4).

CASE V.—Operation in July, 1908, at the age of thirty-five years (now a lady of forty-seven years of age), perfectly healthy to-day, twelve years after operation (Fig. 5).

All patients have the full use of their arm, and are able to assume the posture of the " Statue of Liberty."

CASE VI (Fig. 6).—Operated upon in September, 1917; is added merely to show the present line of incision with Handley's addition down to a point midway between umbilicus and xiphoid process, for the excision of the fascia covering the upper portion of the recti muscles, in conjunction with the other mass. I consider this addition decidedly recommendable, because it makes the operation more radical and usually enables us to close the wound without grafting.

Five other cases have remained free from recurrence for four, six, eight (2), and sixteen years, respectively, and then died of other diseases.

Another patient, a pronounced diabetic at the time of operation, was well for six years after the same when she succumbed to the diabetes, without having developed any signs of a recurrence of cancer.

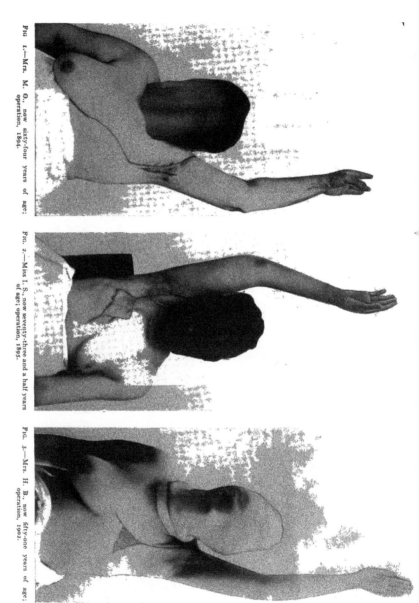

Fig. 1.—Mrs. M. O., now sixty-four years of age; operation, 1894.

Fig. 2.—Miss I. S., now seventy-three and a half years of age; operation, 1895.

Fig. 3.—Mrs. H. B., now fifty-one years of age; operation, 1902.

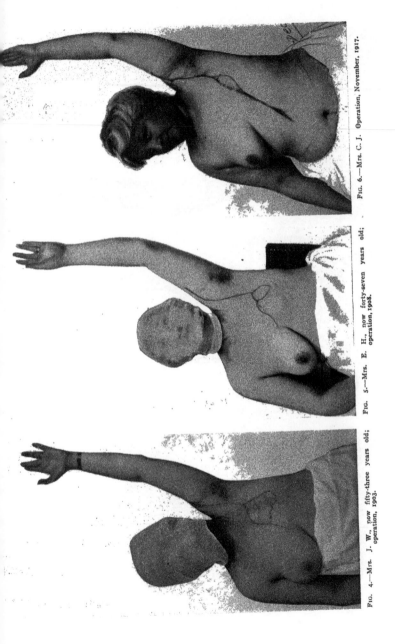

FIG. 4.—Mrs. J. W., now fifty-three years old; operation, 1903.

FIG. 5.—Mrs. E. H., now forty-seven years old; operation, 1908.

FIG. 6.—Mrs. C. J. Operation, November, 1917.

. Still another patient, operated upon for cancer of the right breast in March, 1899, returned to me in December, 1900, with a carcinoma of the left breast, which I then also extirpated. She was well and free from recurrence when last heard from, in the spring of 1907, six and one-quarter years after the second operation.

A few days ago, I met a lady, now almost eighty years old, in perfect health, who had been operated upon by me for a scirrhus of the breast at the age of seventy-three years (seven years ago).

These results, to my mind, prove the efficiency of the method; they prove that the *radical operation for cancer of the breast can cure* patients thus afflicted. If not all cases are saved, this is due:

1. To the stage of the disease in which the patients reach the surgeon;
2. To the virulence of the agent that produces carcinoma.

Paget's Disease (Epithelioma of the Nipple).—In this connection I will not fail to say a few words regarding Paget's disease, this most malignant of all cancers of the breast known to us. If ever early and radical operation is imperative, it is in these cases, as will be seen from the following three observations which I made in the last two years.

CASE I.—Female, aged thirty years, mother of five children, had been in the hands of a quack and had been treated by caustics. When I saw her in January, 1918, the disease in the breast and axilla had far advanced. After the radical operation, the other breast soon became affected and, one year later, also was excised. Then, not long after, the disease became disseminated and she died from cancer en cuirasse.

CASE II.—Female, aged thirty-eight years, had been in the hands of one of our best X-ray specialists in the city. One and a half years after the cure of the nipple by radium treatment there was a local recurrence and a very extensive cancer of the breast with infected glands in the axilla and along the subclavian vein. Radical operation, done by me December, 1918, followed by renewed X-ray and radium treatment. She now has developed intrathoracic metastases.

CASE III.—Male, aged forty-five years. He had been in the hands of an experienced surgeon who had extirpated the breast only, without axillary glands, evidently because none could be found at that time. One and three-quarter years later the patient presented a far-advanced carcinoma. The radical operation then performed could not save him; he died from general metastases eight months later.

In operating upon mammary carcinoma, I make it a point to circumcise the skin widely at the base of the breast. I prepare two ample flaps and enfold them extensively, then divide the fasciæ at the base of the two flaps and extirpate them together with the mass.

I do not think that involvement of the supraclavicular glands presents a contra-indication to operation; on the contrary, I consider it the surgeon's duty to operate when these glands are infected. Halsted, as well as the late Rodman, also Perthes abroad, have observed cases that remained well for a number of years after the extirpation of these glands.

In none of the cases who have remained well from twelve to twenty-five and one-half years after operation, were the supraclavicular glands found infected at the time of the operation, and, hence, they were not removed.

Personally, I have not operated upon a single case in which there were no infiltrated axillary glands.

As I have stated in a previous paper, to my mind statistics regarding the results of the radical operation for cancer of the breast are worthless. They do not prove anything. What *does* determine the fate of the patients is the so-called virulence of the disease. One and the same surgeon may do an equally radical operation in two seemingly early or apparently equally far-advanced cases; and one may remain well and free from recurrence for, say, twenty-five years, while the other may develop a regional recurrence and metastases within a few months.

All we can say is that cancer, being a local disease in the beginning, may be cured by radical operation if done at an early stage.

THE REQUIREMENTS OF TECHNIC IN OPERATIONS FOR CANCER OF THE BREAST.*

By Jabez N. Jackson, M.D.
of Kansas City, Mo.

THE primary object of any operation for cancer should be the permanent cure if possible, of that cancer. This purpose should never be lost sight of.

ESSENTIAL PRINCIPLES

In the accomplishment of this purpose, two primary principles present themselves.

First: The operation must be sufficiently thorough to insure the complete removal of all probably infected tissues within the limits of reasonable surgical access.

Second: Dissemination of the infection during the operation must be guarded against; likewise contamination of the wound with liberated cancer cells which may be left to regraft the disease.

In the evolution of a surgery which will fulfil these demands in cancer of the breast, the pioneer work of American surgeons, such as our fellows Professor Halstead and Willy Meyer, has largely blazed the way. Their work, based on accurate knowledge of the pathology of cancer and its routes of extension, supplemented by the later studies of the English surgeon, Handley, has pretty well standardized the extent of resection required.

EXTENT OF OPERATION.—The standard excision of to-day, therefore, involves the following:

1. *Skin.*—A wide area of skin covering the breast. In this respect American surgeons are inclined to go rather farther than the English. Many insist on a complete removal of the entire skin over the mammary gland. The English surgeons, as a rule, demand less skin removal, but insist on an extensive deeper resection. At least a wide area surrounding the underlying focus of infection must be removed. With present methods, complete ablation can be followed with equally satisfactory subsequent management.

2. *Mammary Gland.*—The entire mammary gland must, of course, be removed. It is well to remember that there are often outlying lobes, and these must not be overlooked.

3. *Pectoral Muscles.*—It has been pretty fully demonstrated that lymph vessels containing cancer cells may be found running through the pectoralis major muscle and between the two pectorals. These muscles should, therefore, be included in the ablation. The clavicle portion of the pectoralis major is probably free from suspicion, and, for good reason, is by many not sacrificed. Its retention particularly saves a very trouble-

* Read before the American Surgical Association, May 5, 1920.

181

some vacant space just below the clavicle, which is hard to obliterate, and causes tedious convalescence. Some divide the pectoralis minor for axillary dissection and then resuture. We are unable to note any disadvantage to the patient in its absence, and its removal makes clean axillary dissection much better.

4. *Axillary Glands, Fat and Fascia.*—All lymph-bearing structures from the axillary fossa requires clean and complete dissection. After the pectoral muscles have been divided and retracted, an incision to the outer side and parallel to the axillary vessels and nerves divides the loose fascia down to the line of cleavage of these structures. Then dissection on this plane inward clears them completely of all fat, fascia and glands. This clearing is carried high up beneath the clavicle towards the subclavian vessels and supraclavicular space. Branches from the axillary vessels are clamped close to their origin and divided, thus enabling one to make a complete dissection. This tissue clearing is continued down the under side of the scapula until the subscapular muscle stands out clearly and below and posteriorly the latissimus dorsi. Likewise the thoracic wall is cleared of all loose tissue, including the pectoral muscle above, leaving the ribs and intercostal muscles bare. This muscle and fascia clearing runs quite to the median line.

5. *Supraclavicular Space.*—Some surgeons, as routine, make a similar clearing of the subclavian triangle above the clavicle. We believe this adds little to safety, and perhaps much to embarrassment. We prefer the post-operative raying of these areas.

6. *Abdominal Fascia.*—Handley claims that metastatic spread is largely along fascial planes, and that by this route the abdomen is reached. Hence he advises further the removal of the fascia of the rectus on the side involved, down to the umbilicus, and in part the corresponding fascia of the external oblique. We have done this in certain cases, but do not believe the practice has become general with American surgeons as yet.

DISSEMINATION AND CONTAMINATION.—In operating we must further remember that *dissemination* may take place during the operation through uncut lymphatics, or *contamination* of the wound may occur with cancer cells escaping from cut lymphatics.

Dissemination may occur by milking the lymphatics in the manipulation of the infected breast during operation. Manipulation or squeezing of the breast should, therefore, be carefully avoided. More important, however, in preventing this complication is the suggestion, original, we believe, with Willy Meyer, to begin work in the axilla, dividing the lymph vessels at their highest point before the breast is handled at all. Thus the routes of dissemination are cut off. We go further and completely circumscribe the breast in our primary dissection, early dividing as well the pectoralis major at its sternal attachment, so as to cut off the route of dissemination through the chest wall into the thorax. The breast itself is therefore not handled at all until its peripheral zone has been completely shut off from its lymphatic connections.

Contamination.—We are also of the opinion that perhaps many of the cases of local recurrence are due to cancer cells escaping from the cut lymphatic vessels during the operation. These implanted in the wound after its closure serve as grafts, which in their home soil readily develop into new growths. While this idea is not demonstrable, it is at least thoroughly plausible. To prevent such contamination we are wont to utilize two resources. *First:* Incision at the outset is made complete as planned, and the flaps on all sides which remain are dissected up to the extent required. They are at once covered with hot gauze pads to protect their surface from contact of escaping cells. As the dissection proceeds, we extend the process of gauze protection, covering both the area of the wound to remain, and as well the cut surfaces of the ablated breast to prevent the escape into the wound of the cells from divided lymphatics. *Second:* Fearing that despite these precautions there may yet occur contamination, we thoroughly irrigate the wound before suturing, with a stream of water of some force, accompanied by light mopping with gauze. In our experience, local external recurrences are rare, and we feel that perhaps these precautions have aided in the results.

SECONDARY CONSIDERATIONS

Admitting the fulfillment of the above essentials in the details of operative technic, looking to the primary object of the cure of cancer, an ideal surgical procedure yet involves other considerations. We know that of all factors of success, an early operation is the best possible promise of a permanent cure. Surgery must, therefore, win women to the idea of an early operation. In considering this purpose we must recognize the psychological and utilitarian aspects of surgery. Surgery must be made as attractive as possible, or perhaps better expressed, less repulsive. We have seen many results in the past in which this aspect of the case was not impressive. An arm disabled, with contracting and binding scars (which rendered it almost useless) ; long and tedious wound healing, with prolonged hospital stay and mounting hospital expenses—sapping the ofttimes limited financial resources; repulsive scars from excessive skin grafting, with ribs showing through and the heart beats almost visible; is it remarkable that with these pictures shown in their friends, women should shrink from surgery in their own needs? Our results in cancer are not brilliant at best, but they are the best that science offers up to date. As surgical results we can probably only improve them through universal resort to early operation. We must, therefore, bend our efforts to make the primary results of surgery at least as attractive as possible.

Of these utilitarian and psychological factors, that of first importance is the preservation of a good function of the arm.

Preservation of Function.—Painless, free, unrestricted movements of

the arm constitute good function. Excess of scar tissue or improper
placement are the chief factors producing disability. To prevent these
troubles, several points should be observed.

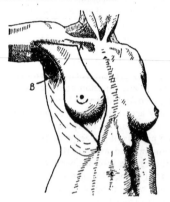

No. 1.

FIG. 7.—Incision of new method, meeting
demands in certain cases.

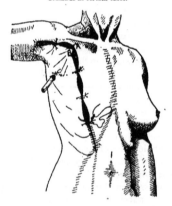

No. 2.

FIG. 8.—Illustrating method of closure.

First.—The line of scar should not run transversely from arm to chest.
If it does, the inevitable contraction of scar tissue is inclined to draw the
arm towards the chest and prevent full elevation, abduction, and external
rotation. A line of suture running in the long axis of the arm up to the

184

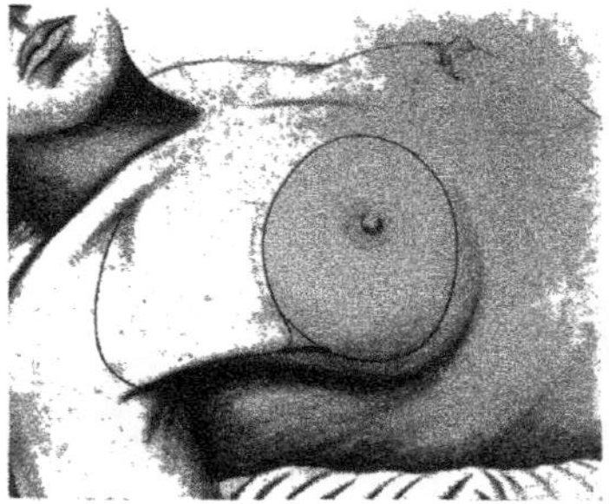

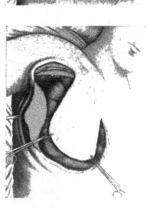

Fig. 1.—Outline of incision, marked with a scratch stroke of the knife, in author's original operation.

Fig. 2.—Quadrilateral flap of the skin and superficial fascia stretched out by tenaculum forceps and transferred inward to cover defect created by removal of skin and breast.

Fig. 3.—Method of insertion of figure-of-eight coaptation sutures.

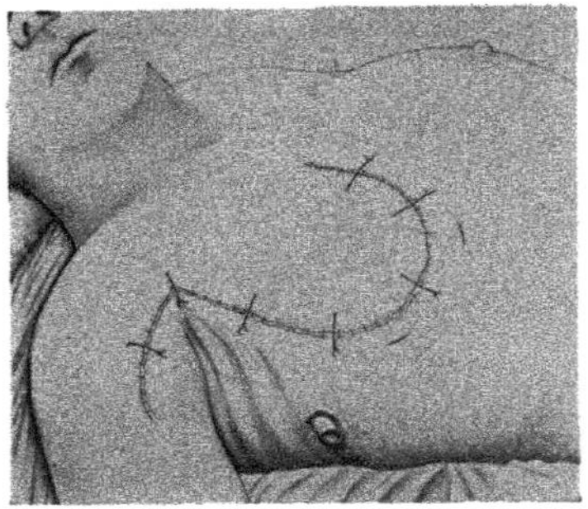

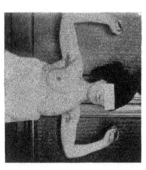

Fig. 4.—Flap sutured in place, with drainage-tube inserted.

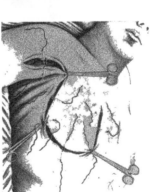

Fig. 5.—Photograph illustrating exact method of mapping out flap in author's original method.

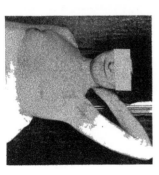

Fig. 6.—Demonstrating unrestricted use of arm and relation of scar to the arm when thus used.

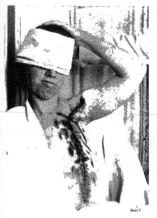

Fig. 9.—New method immediately after closure with position of placement of arm. Photograph likewise shows stab wounds to insure drainage of venous engorgement of flap.

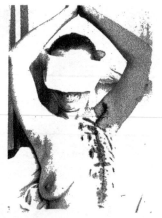

Fig. 10.—Showing complete elevation of arm one week after operation.

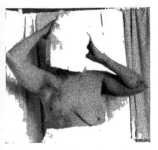

Fig. 11.—Position of arms two weeks after operation. At this time mobility was complete and voluntary, as illustrated. Author's new method.

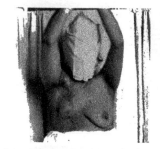

Fig. 12.—Position of arms two weeks after operation. At this time mobility was complete and Voluntary, as illustrated. Author's new method.

level of the shoulder-joint and then on to the chest, would appear ideal.

Second.—The proper obliteration of the emptied axillary fossa presents a problem. Unless satisfactorily accomplished, the large cavity must be finally obliterated by organization of new tissue with scar formation, which further restricts mobility. What may be even more troublesome to the patient is the compression by such scar tissue of the brachial plexus, with much ensuing pain, or the compression of axillary vessels with impairment of circulation. A paper by our lamented Murphy, presented before the Western Surgical Society in 1904, emphasized these particular points. As a corrective, he advised leaving a flap from the lower border and outer end of the pectoralis major muscle, which was carried closely around the axillary structures and sutured to protect these from scar contractures. To us it seemed that this expedient was subject to criticism in that it left the portion of this muscle likely to be infected. Endeavoring to meet the obvious demands in a better manner led to our original work on this subject, which evolved the technic which we presented to the Western Surgical Society in December, 1905, and published in the *Journal of the American Medical Association,* March 3, 1906.

The complete obliteration of the axilla fossa, by bringing the skin from the under side of the pectoralis major, or the floor of the axilla, up to a longitudinal incision in the line of the arm, covered these vessels snugly and we consider it the chief value of that technic. When this was done in this way, we found the skin covering the front of the pectoral fold lax, and rather accidentally we slid it over to cover the area of the breast excision, and thus the flap evolved. While the flap proved an aid in covering the area of denudation, and this contributed to the value of the operation, the chief virtue sought and developed was in placing the scar line properly and in readily obliterating the axillary fossa.

Third.—In the rapid restoration of function we have found another expedient valuable. If the case is dressed after the operation with the arm down to the side, we find it hard to get a timid patient to raise, abduct or externally rotate the arm. They are thus very slow in being educated to get the arm upward or backward, and hence are unable to dress their hair or otherwise wait upon themselves. To remedy this we have from the outset kept the arm up at right angles to the trunk. They are put to bed with the arm in this position; then early passive motion is begun, while between times the arm is kept up. With our method there is no tension even with the arm in this extreme abduction, and rapid improvement in arm function is pronounced.

Short Convalescence.—Methods which insure prompt wound healing, and correspondingly shorten convalescence, save time and hospital expense— both matters ofttimes of much concern. These indications are best met by methods which permit *primary closure* of the wound without undue tension and primary union. It is remarkable how much can be done to facilitate suture by proper under cutting in dissecting up the flaps in *any* operation. With a wide skin removal, however, this can in some cases not be accomplished except by some *plastic method*. To these plastic methods some have objected, saying: "When one seeks to close a wound at the end of his operation, he will probably not be radical enough in the operation." If this were true, there would be nothing to say. But on the contrary, it is much more probable that a surgeon will do a radical operation *always* if he is possessed of resources which still permit closure without tension and primary union in most cases.

In either plastic flaps or undermined flaps we will sometimes have inadequate terminal vessel supply for every inch of skin margin, and hence there may be some small area of consequent necrosis. These areas when present are small. In many instances they result from venous engagement with secondary capillary compression and obstructions. *Multiple small stabs* scattered over the flap will permit drainage of venous engagement and obviate these areas of gangrene quite decidedly. It is a small point, but worth noting.

Cosmetics.—Finally, of the minor factors is that of cosmetics. Women are naturally quite sensitive of their person. A disfiguring scar produces repulsion and horror both in the individual as well as in other women who see it. A wound covered by a skin graft is certainly not a thing of beauty at best, and may be a determining factor in keeping others from needed surgical attention. We believe that in the present day, with methods available, skin grafting should almost never be necessary.

AUTHOR'S OPERATIONS.—*First Method.*—In meeting all these requirements of an ideal operation in cancer of the breast, after nearly fifteen years' experience with it, we yet believe the method we first published in 1906 comes more nearly serving than any we know. In detail of technic there have been several changes noted in the preceding lines, and we will not enter into any further description than may be obvious from the pictures herewith presented, supplementing the former article. Theoretically it has been perhaps criticised, as are all plastics, that in seeking closure infected tissues are left behind. On the contrary, we do a more radical operation than any we have witnessed in other clinics, and do so because we know we can yet secure easy closure. Perhaps it might be thought that the flap itself might be the site for local recurrences. In answer we might note that the skin which forms the flap is not removed in any described technic to our knowledge. We admit to having seen cases done elsewhere in which the flap had been apparently taken too far inward and came from the mammary region. But correct observance of our method discloses that the outer incision runs quite out to the deltoid and its inner parallel should be entirely outside of the mammary gland. In experience we have seen only two recurrences in the flap, and excision of the small nodules in both these cases showed that they had origin in the fascia of the chest and not in the tissues of the flap. Both of these experiences were in early cases, and we believe were due to con-

186

tamination. Since employing the methods suggested we believe these recurrences will be rare at least. In fact, it has been rather noteworthy in our experience how rare have been external or so-called skin recurrences, and that in these instances, how immune the flap area had been. In fact, we believe the method readily applicable to all cases except in those of most extensive skin involvement, or in those rare cases in which the extension may be out on the skin over the anterior axillary fold itself.

Second Method.—In just such a case as this we were obliged to forego the flap entirely in a case about a year ago. We have remarked before that, after all, the flap is the least valuable feature of our operation. We found in this instance we were still able to preserve the more characteristic advantages of our original operation, and this method we wish briefly to present. The diagrams presented reveal the nature of the incision better than can be expressed in words. By this method all of the skin over the pectoral area as well as that of the mammary region is removed—a more radical skin removal than any heretofore presented. In closure of the wound, however, it is observed that the axillary fossa is obliterated exactly as in our first method. Likewise the scar in the long axis of the arm to above the shoulder and thence to the chest presents the same advantages of scar location to favor functional utility of arm. With the usual rather extensive undermining, we have found that even this large wound closes rather readily without practically any tension, and we have secured primary union in all cases. As a matter of fact, to prove it out we have employed this method in most of our cases in the past year, whether specially indicated or not. We find quite as good functional results. It does not present quite so attractive a cosmetic appearance.

TRAUMATIC FAT NECROSIS OF THE FEMALE BREAST AND ITS DIFFERENTIATION FROM CARCINOMA *

By Burton J. Lee, M.D.

AND

Frank Adair, M.D.

of New York, N. Y.

The object of this report is briefly to set forth the clinical, operative, and pathological findings of two cases of traumatic fat necrosis of the breast, recently encountered at the Memorial Hospital. Although much has been written concerning the differentiation between the benign lesions and mammary carcinomata, a careful search of surgical and pathological literature has failed to reveal any reference to this subject, for it has apparently hitherto been unrecognized.

We have the hope that the data presented and the discussion stimulated by the study of these two cases may result in a better understanding of the clinical and pathological aspects of this subject and lead to its more accurate diagnosis in the future.

Clinically the simulation to carcinoma is very startling, and we desire to place special emphasis upon this point. In one of the cases, a radical amputation of the breast, muscles and axillary contents was performed, the operator believing that the tumor was malignant. In the other patient only local removal of the mass was practised, at first, but gross examination of the cross-section, in the operating room, led one of the writers to a diagnosis of carcinoma, which was confirmed by another surgeon, but not concurred in by a third. The breast was removed, but the muscles were not sacrificed. A more careful analysis of the gross and microscopic appearances made the real character of the lesion apparent.

CASE I.—E. B. The woman was a white, native-born American, aged fifty-two years, and was a widow. She was admitted to the Memorial Hospital August 29, 1919.

Chief Complaint.—A growing mass of considerable size in the right breast.

Family History.—Negative for carcinoma.

Past History.—Previous illnesses: She was operated upon at the Memorial Hospital, six years previously, for an abscess of the right side of the neck. She had had several miscarriages. Her past history was otherwise negative.

Breast History.—She had had no lactations and there had never been any ailment with either breast.

Present Illness.—In May, 1919 (three months before her admission

---

* Read before the American Surgical Association, May 5, 1920.

188

to the hospital), she received a definite trauma to the right breast. This occurred while she was sitting in a street car. A woman carrying a child fell heavily against the patient, delivering a severe blow with her elbow against the right breast. This incident was not followed by tenderness or pain. Three months later (three days before her admission to the hospital) the patient noticed a lump, about the size of a lime, at the site of the former injury, in the upper outer quadrant of the right breast. This mass has been unassociated with pain.

Physical Examination.—The patient was a well-developed, well-nourished white woman, weighing about 190 pounds. Her general physical examination was negative, with the exception of the lungs, which showed on percussion slightly increased dulness between the scapulæ, together with a few scattered sibilant râles. Röntgen-ray examination of the chest showed no evidence of tuberculosis or metastasis. The Wassermann was twice reported negative.

Breasts: The mammary glands were of large type. A tumor was present in the upper outer quadrant of the right breast, measuring about 5 by 4 cm. There was no retraction of the nipple, nor was there any discharge from it. The mass showed moderate fixation to the skin, with some slight surface dimpling. There was some attachment to deeper structures. No axillary or supraclavicular nodes were palpable. The left breast was normal.

Provisional Diagnosis.—Primary carcinoma of the right breast.

Operation.—On September 23, 1919, the right breast, muscles, and axillary contents were removed by Doctor Bolling.

Pathological Examination. Gross Examination.—Three centimetres above and outside of the nipple situated in the breast was a tumor mass 2 cm. in diameter, irregular, circumscribed, but not encapsulated. It merged along one border with the fat tissue and elsewhere with the breast tissue. The tumor was opaque, brownish yellow, as in a xanthoma, and there was irregular hyperæmia along the upper edge. The growth lacked definite cicatricial character and chalky streaks.

The whole breast was uniformly fibrosed and contained no cysts. The axillary nodes were slightly enlarged and apparently not cancerous.

Microscopic Examination.—Sections showed broad areas of fat necrosis, surrounded by a broad zone of new cellular connective tissue, in which large vessels showed active obliterating endarteritis. Along certain segments of necrotic areas there was granulation tissue containing several large giant-cells. A search for spirochæte in the tissues was negative.

The patient was discharged from the hospital October 1, 1919, eight days after operation, having had an uneventful convalescence.

Subsequent Notes.—The patient was readmitted on November 10, 1919, because of persistent hemorrhage from the vagina. Examination revealed a small bleeding-point on an otherwise normal cervix. On either side of the vaginal vault were fungoid epithelial growths and half way down the posterior wall was another small tumor.

Sections taken from the vaginal growths were reported to be basal-celled carcinoma.

The patient was treated with radium by Doctor Bailey, and is still under his observation.

March 31, 1920, no evidence of disease in the vagina and cervix was apparent. The final outcome of the vaginal tumor will have to be subsequently reported.

Doctor Ewing has stated that the vaginal growth bears no relation of any sort to the traumatic fat necrosis of the breast, but these data are included as a part of the follow-up history of the case.

CASE II.—R. R.   The woman was a Roumanian, aged thirty-six years and was married.   She was admitted to the Memorial Hospital January 15, 1920.

Chief Complaint.—A lump in the right breast, which was steadily increasing in size.

Family History.—Negative for carcinoma and tuberculosis.

Past History.—Occupation: housework.   Habits: abstemious. Weight: her usual weight was 211 pounds, and this was approximately her weight at admission.

Previous Illnesses.—She had always been well, with the exception of two extra-uterine gestations, both of which necessitated operative procedure.

She had never had any miscarriages.

Her past history was otherwise negative.

Breast History.—There had been three lactations: the first one fifteen years ago, the last one four years later, the duration of each having been about a year.

The nipples had always protruded.

There had never been any unusual breast incident during her nursing period.

Present Illness.—June 22, 1919 (about seven months before her admission to the hospital), her last operation for ectopic pregnancy was performed. Pleurisy and pneumonia developed and she became dangerously ill. She was given a hypodermoclysis under the right breast, three quarts of saline being introduced. No unusual pain was associated with this administration. One month later (six months before admission) she first accidentally noticed a small lump, the size of a walnut, in the upper and inner part of the right breast at the site of the previous injection. This mass had caused no pain whatever, but had been steadily increasing in size.

Physical Examination.—The patient was a robust, middle-aged woman, of unusually large build. Her appearance indicated perfect health. The general physical examination was negative. The lungs were clear throughout and fluoroscopy of the chest was negative.

Breasts: Large and pendulous.   The left breast was normal.

The right breast showed no retraction of the nipple, nor was there any elevation of it. About 3 cm. to the inner side of the right nipple was a mass, 3 by 2 cm. in diameter, making it approximately the size of a small hen's egg. The tumor was roughly cylindrical, fairly sharply circumscribed, and had a distinct firm edge. The mass was hard in consistency. It lay just beneath the skin on the

190

upper inner aspect of the breast, near its posterior surface. The tumor showed slight skin adherence, but was, however, movable in the breast and not attached to deeper structures. There was one small soft lymph-node in the right axilla.

Provisional Diagnosis.—The provisional diagnosis was carcinoma of the breast, although the circumscribed character of the mass suggested the possibility of a benign adenoma.

Pre-operative Treatment.—The patient received the usual pre-operative Röntgen-ray cycle for the chest, breast, axillary and supraclavicular regions, the cycle being completed on January 21st. Operation was performed nine days later.

Operation.—Under ether anæsthesia a local excision of the tumor was made through the anterior aspect of the breast, going well wide of the involved area. This local excision was done because the mass was so sharply defined that it seemed possible that malignancy might not be encountered. The tumor was immediately sectioned after its removal, and was found to consist of two sharply outlined solid areas, while between them lay a small cavity containing thick, oily fluid. As the knife passed through the solid tumor tissue one had the same impression of cutting a hard, granular substance that one experiences in sectioning a carcinoma. Although none of the minute yellow points so frequently seen in carcinoma could be distinguished, its extreme hardness made me feel fairly certain that the case was one of cancer of the breast. Another surgeon present concurred in this gross diagnosis. However, Doctor Stone did not believe the tumor was carcinomatous.

An amputation of the breast was then performed down to and including the fascia covering the pectoralis major muscle. The muscles themselves and the axilla were not disturbed. Further operative procedure was to depend upon the report of the pathologist.

Post-operative Diagnosis (by the Operator).—Carcinoma of the breast: Following the operation the operator was considerably concerned about the outcome of the case, having a fairly definite conviction that a more radical operation should have been performed. He was therefore very anxious to learn the result of the gross examination, anticipating criticism of the incompleteness of the operation. He was greatly surprised, however, to be told that the breast itself should not have been removed, that local excision of the tumor was all that had been indicated and that the lesion had no malignant features.

Pathological Examination. Gross Examination.—There was an indurated area, 2 by 1 by 4 cm., slightly cicatricial, not quite hard enough for carcinoma; well circumscribed, almost entirely encapsulated, apparently a fat lobule, which suggested a tumor process. On cross-section the texture was opaque, xanthematous and light yellow in color, not translucent, without definite chalky or silvery points. Adjoining was a smaller fat lobule, with a few similar slightly opaque points. Adjoining also was a cyst, 1 cm. wide, containing creamy contents, having a smooth blood-stained wall.

191

Gross Diagnosis.—Chronic inflammation in fat tissue. The remainder of the breast was normal.

Microscopic Examination.—The structure of the lesion showed chronic productive inflammation in fat tissue. There were no evidences of carcinoma. The fat-cells were proliferating, replacing fat, and many small giant-cells were present. There was much diffuse new fibrous tissue, which accounted for the opacity. In places there were collections of lymphocytes and occasionally a few cysts. The large cyst was lined by large epithelial cells of the sweat-gland type. A few accompanying breast alveoli showed round-cell infiltration.

There was no unusual incident in the patient's convalescence.

Incidence.—At the Memorial Hospital the ratio of traumatic fat necrosis of the breast to mammary carcinoma is as 2 to 330, or 0.6 per cent.

Pathology.—In our study of the pathology presented in these two cases we are greatly indebted to Dr. James Ewing, pathologist at Memorial Hospital, and he has outlined the following points in the gross examination of traumatic fat necrosis of the breast.

Gross Appearances.—The differential diagnosis of the gross lesions in these two cases presented an interesting problem. A careful study of the details of the naked-eye appearance led to the conclusion that in neither case was the lesion carcinomatous.

In the case of E. B. the presence of a rather large area of opaque discolored fat tissue, nearly diffluent in the centre, was satisfactory evidence that the chief material was necrotic fat. This area along one side was sharply demarcated from normal fat tissue, as is infiltrating mammary cancer; but this zone failed to show the positive signs of carcinoma, such as cicatricial contraction, grayish lustre, and fatty and chalky points and streaks. Likewise the rather broad zone 2 to 3 cm. of cellular granulation tissue did not present the form, outline, or texture of carcinoma. Accordingly, a gross diagnosis against a neoplastic process was rendered.

In the case of R. R. the gross diagnosis was more exacting, but was accomplished by careful adherence to the criteria of gross anatomical diagnosis of mammary cancer. Here there was one separate area, 2 by 2 cm., of necrotic fat, which was readily recognized. A second area presented greater difficulties. This was an oval area of 2 by 1 cm., firm and cicatricial in appearance, with exanthematous texture and considerably resembling carcinoma. However, it was observed that this area was fairly well encapsulated; that in size and form it was exactly similar to the adjoining fat lobules; and that it did not present the smooth opaque texture of carcinoma nor the chalky points or streaks. On these data the diagnosis of chronic inflammation of fat tissue was given. Paraffin sections revealed a productive inflammatory process with multiplication of many cuboidal fat-cells lying in alveoli, which would have been difficult to distinguish from alveolar carcinoma in a frozen section.

Microscopical Appearances.—Areas of necrosis in fat tissues were to be

192

seen with new connective-tissue cells, growing in and about these areas of necrosis. This growth of new tissue was very abundant, and with the giant-cells which one saw scattered throughout the tissue a luetic granuloma might superficially be suggested. Many of the giant-cells were markedly flattened, the syncytial tissue being closely applied along the borders of huge vacuoles, which corresponded to large tissue spaces containing diffluent fat. These giant-cells were, therefore, of the so-called foreign-body type. Certain portions of the sections show proliferation of the nuclei of fat-cells, these same cells showing also an opaque zone close to the periphery of the cell, probably representing certain changes in fat saponification.

The blood-vessels show an obliterating endarteritis which was apparently of recent origin and a perivascular infiltration with lymphocytes.

Diagnosis.—Trauma appears to be an essential and distinctive etiological factor in connection with fat necrosis of the breast. A history of the appearance of a mammary tumor with no preceding definite trauma would practically eliminate fat necrosis as a possible diagnosis. Although trauma is not infrequently encountered in the history of a mammary cancer, it is often indefinite and frequently absent. A recent exception to this rule was met in a young woman, aged twenty-six years, who received a terrific blow upon the breast by a hard-hit baseball. Six months later she developed, at the exact site of the injury, an encapsulated papillary cystadenocarcinoma of the breast. It is well known that this particular type of cancer is one of the less malignant varieties. In general, however, the surgeon should weigh carefully the evidence of distinct trauma to the breast and remember the possibility of a fat necrosis and the secondary chronic inflammatory changes attending it.

Clinically, traumatic fat necrosis of the breast very closely simulates mammary carcinoma and the differentiation may be very difficult. The symptoms of fat necrosis which strongly suggest malignancy may be enumerated as follows:

1. *Rapid Increase in Size.*—The mass of traumatized fat increases rapidly because of the proliferation of new connective tissue associated with the chronic inflammatory process. A period of several weeks or months may elapse from the time of the receipt of the injury to the appearance of the tumor; and from that time on the increase in size strongly suggests the possibility of malignancy.

2. *Skin Adhesions.*—Both the patients under report exhibited the same skin adherence which one sees in many cases of malignant disease of the breast. The tumor mass seemed held to the skin by several lines of adhesion and gave the impression of a solid tumor with superficial surface closely adherent to overlying skin. This feature so often regarded as pathognomonic for malignancy was striking in both instances.

3. *Consistency.*—The consistency of the tumor in each instance was as hard as in the average case of malignancy. Although some of the benign

13   193

fibro-adenomata are very hard, the two characteristics above mentioned are lacking in this type of growth. Upon the other hand, one must bear in mind the exceedingly soft, brain-like encapsulated carcinomata which are the most malignant of all types of mammary cancer. In general, hardness in a breast tumor suggests malignant possibilities, and traumatic fat necrosis with the reaction attending it produces a distinctly hard mass.

4. *Lack of Pain.*—No pain was experienced in the cases of fat necrosis. This gave an exact parallel to malignancy, because tumors of the latter type in their early stages exhibit an entire absence of pain. Only in the later, more advanced periods does a cancer of the breast cause pain.

5. *Adhesion to Deeper Structures.*—One of the patients showed definite fixity of the tumor to the underlying muscles. This symptom is almost invariably regarded as a sign of malignancy, and its presence, therefore, strongly influenced the surgeon in reaching a diagnosis of malignancy.

The points of differentiation from malignant disease may be outlined as follows:

1. The history of trauma is more exact and definite than with the average carcinoma.

2. The tumor in fat necrosis is fairly well circumscribed, while the mass in carcinoma is usually more diffuse.

3. The tumor is rather more movable in the breast than is usual with carcinoma.

4. Axillary nodes, if present, have not the hard consistency of those associated with cancer. This differential point would, of course, be of no value in a very early mammary cancer without metastasis in the nodes.

5. The characteristic gross appearances of fat necrosis upon cross-section of the tumor have already been outlined under the paragraph on pathology.

DISCUSSION.—Several points worthy of discussion may briefly be referred to:

In connecting the appearance of a tumor with a history of trauma one should bear in mind the four medicolegal points usually required:

1. The history of trauma must be sufficiently definite and of a severity adequate to produce the tissue damage.

2. The site of the trauma and the location of the lesion must be identical.

3. A proper time relationship must exist from the receipt of the trauma to the appearance of the tissue changes.

4. Proof should be at hand that the tissue was normal before the receipt of the trauma.

All of these requirements, save the fourth, are met in the cases of fat necrosis, and it is obviously impossible to fulfill the fourth requirement.

When the wide distribution of subcutaneous fat is considered, one may well ask the question, Does fat necrosis from traumatism ever occur in the tissue? Our colleague, Doctor Farr, of the New York Hospital, has completed a paper, about to be published, in which several cases of traumatic fat necrosis in subcutaneous tissues are reported. Boxers and wrestlers must be subject to a tremendous number of traumatisms to the superficial fat. It seems probable that some defensive mechanism must exist to prevent the development of necrosis in fat tissue following trauma. In the cases in this report it seems fair to assume that some peculiar conditions may have been present, permitting the trauma to bring about the lesions described.

In the first case lues might be thought of as a possible etiological factor, on account of the miscarriages, the granulomatous appearance of the tissue and the obliteration of endarteritis. However, two Wassermanns in expert hands were negative, and a careful search for spirochætes failed to reveal any organism.

The second patient showed nothing in the tissues quite comparable to the extensive granulomatous changes found in the first patient, and here syphilis could be dismissed at once.

We feel, therefore, that a leutic element in these cases may be positively dismissed as having no bearing upon the pathology of this disease.

CONCLUSIONS

1. Traumatic fat necrosis of the female breast is a definite clinical entity.

2. It must always be included with the benign lesions of the breast.

3. Clinically, it more closely resembles carcinoma of the breast than any other tumor, and must be differentiated from it.

4. A distinct history of trauma to the breast and a well-circumscribed, firm mass, showing rapid increase in size, unassociated with pain and without axillary nodes that are firm, suggest the possibility of fat necrosis.

5. Local removal of such a mass is justifiable if a proper gross diagnosis can be made in the operating room. Should the gross examination reveal carcinoma, complete amputation may then be performed.

6. The diagnosis of traumatic fat necrosis of the breast by gross examination is possible. The gross features of this lesion should, therefore, be clearly understood by every surgeon.

7. Further lines of research, along chemical as well as along morphological lines, may throw additional light upon the real nature of this process.

HYPERPLASTIC TUBERCULOSIS OF THE SMALL INTESTINE *

By Joseph Ransohoff, M.D., F.R.C.S. (Eng.)

OF CINCINNATI, OHIO

THE protean manifestations of tuberculosis, which elsewhere demand surgical intervention, are not often staged in the alimentary canal. The terminal ulcerations without any trace of reparative effort found in nearly 40 per cent. of cases of fatal pulmonary tuberculosis are practically never surgical.

In the tuberculous peritonitides which call for operation, the causative intestinal lesion has either undergone repair or cannot be found. There remain, then, two conditions which are distinctly surgical. First, the strictures from healed tuberculous ulcers, almost always found in the small intestine either singly or in numbers, and second, the more or less localized processes, which because of their chronicity permit of excessive efforts at repair, and therefore assume the guise of neoplasms. It is to this class of cases that the term "hyperplastic tuberculosis" has been given.

Practically all of the cases reported since Hartman and Pillet [1] first called attention to and named this condition have been found in the cæcum and the terminal coil of the ileum. Just why this segment of the intestine should be the chosen seat for tuberculosis, typhoid, and actinomycotic lesions probably is difficult to answer. Less resistant, perhaps, because of its fixed position, the first stasis in the thereunto fast-moving intestinal current, favoring germ growth, and last, but perhaps not least, the trouble-brewing appendix, may separately and together be invoked in explanation of this striking fact.

Cæcal tuberculosis in contrast with the widely disseminated terminal type in pulmonary cases is nearly always primary, and appears in otherwise fairly healthy individuals of between twenty and forty years. A few cases have been recorded between ten and twenty. Guinon and Pater saw one in a child four years old (Hartman).

Since Hartman [2] was enabled to analyze two hundred and twenty-nine operations for cæcal tuberculosis before the London Medical Society, and very many more cases have been reported since, there would be no justification in adding one or more of this region. Of tuberculosis of hyperplastic type and limited to the small intestine, I have been enabled to find only one other case, that of Soubeyran. [3] The patient was a female, aged twenty-five years. The lesion involved 9 centimetres of the ileum. Resection was followed by death nineteen days after the operation.

The case which I beg to present involves the small intestine only, and that at a part far removed from the cæcum.

* Read before the American Surgical Association, May 3, 1920.

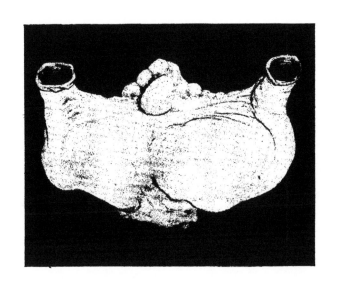

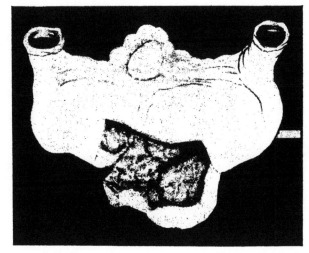

196ª

HYPERPLASTIC TUBERCULOSIS OF THE SMALL INTESTINE

B. S., aged nine years, was admitted to the General Hospital, Pediatric Service, October 13, 1919. The chief complaint was pain in the stomach. Family history negative. Had whooping cough three years ago. Last winter patient had scarlet fever, followed by enlargement of the cervical glands. After continuing for five months the gland was removed, and was shown to be tuberculous. Cardio-respiratory functions normal. X-ray of chest shows no enlargement of the lymph-nodes.

Digestive System.—Patient eats fairly well, but does not drink milk. The bowels move three or four times a day, usually with loose stools. For past two or three years patient has been troubled with cramps in the stomach, coming on four or five times a day, and having no relation to bowel movement, but coming on soon after food intake and irrespective of the kind of food. Pain is often very severe, causing him to double up. It usually lasts about an hour, and is finally relieved by the application of hot-water bottle. Pain sometimes comes on suddenly during sleep. It seems to be localized in a small area immediately to the left and slightly below the umbilicus. Patient does not vomit at any time. Renal and vesical functions normal.

Present Condition.—Patient is a white male child, apparently about five years of age, but in reality about nine. Expression rather listless, greenish-yellow cast to skin. On the left side of the neck there is an oblique scar, marking the site of previous operation. One small gland palpable in the anterior triangle in the left side of neck.

Chest.—Bony framework very prominent, owing to lack of nutrition, development poor. Scapulæ winged, shoulders markedly "rounded," right more so than left, showing tendency to retraction at the apices of lungs. Veins plainly visible. Spine exhibits marked hyposcoliosis, right shoulder droops more than left. Expansion fair, lagging over left apex. Percussion elicits impaired resonance posteriorly to left of spinal column in interscapular space. Auscultation, puerile breath sounds heard throughout chest, no râles heard.

Abdomen.—Pot-belly in type, rigidity interferes with palpation, no special tenderness at any point and muscular tension about equal on the two sides. On the left side there is a mass about the size of an apple, can be felt to the left of the midline, below the umbilicus. The mass appears fixed.

Blood Examination.—Hæmoglobin, 65 per cent.; red cells, 3,100,000; white cells, 7250; polymorphonuclears, 74 per cent.; large lymphs, 7 per cent.; small lymphs, 15 per cent.; eosinophiles, 4 per cent.

Temperature slightly elevated and irregular, ranging to 100° in the evening. Pulse accelerated most of the time, in the neighborhood of 100. Stool is well formed, devoid of parasites. Test of blood negative. Wassermann negative. Von Pirquet positive.

X-ray examination October 21, 1919, of the intestinal tract, following injection of opaque enema and the giving of barium shows the tract to be normal in position and size, and presents no evidence of filling defect. Barium meal passes normally through small intestine.

November 5, 1919, transferred to Surgical Service for exploratory operation. Tentative diagnosis: Retroperitoneal tuberculous glands. Ether anæsthesia. When complete relaxation of the abdominal muscles was achieved, it was found that the tumor mass, irregularly nodulated, was distinctly movable. Through a median incision the mass was easily delivered and was found what appeared to be a discrete growth of the small intestine, situated in the lower part of the jejunum. It involved about seven inches of the gut, and with the exception of a broad omental adhesion at one part, it was not attached. The lymph-nodes in the mesentery were enlarged in lessening degree from the intestinal attachment toward the root. About ten inches of the intestine were resected, together with the mesentery and an end-to-end anastomosis, with sutures, made in the usual way. A thorough exploration of the abdominal cavity failed to reveal any other pathological lesion, nor were any lymph-nodes discernible. The recovery of the patient was uneventful. His condition six months after the operation is satisfactory. He attends school regularly, is free from pain, and presents no evidence of recurrence.

Pathological Report.—The specimen removed is a segment of the small intestine, about ten inches in length. It presents the gross appearance of an irregular tumor mass. On section the tumor mass is found to consist entirely of the enormously thickened intestinal wall. This is very rigid and is cut with some difficulty. In thickness this wall varies from 1-3 of a centimetre to 1 centimetre. At the central part there is an attached tag of omentum, 3 centimetres wide. Directly underneath this there is an indurated ulcer. There is a loss of substance in the mucosa, measuring 1 centimetre by 1½ centimetres. The mesenteric glands on section are of uniform consistency and present no evidence of caseation or other necrotic changes. The rest of the mucosa, to the naked eye, appears unbroken. The surface has a glazed and uniform appearance; the valvular folds normal to this part have quite disappeared. Here and there are minute polypoid elevations.

Microscopic Report—In the sections of the tissue fixed with formalin and stained with hæmatoxylin and erythrosin, the much thickened wall of the gut is seen to be composed entirely of small round-cells and polymorphous epithelioid cells (Fig. 3). Only very rarely a multinucleated giant-cell can be found (Fig. 4). This sarcoma-like tissue extends from the muscular coat to and into the villi of the mucosa, replacing, for the most part, the tissue of the intestine. In only one section are villi able to be seen, and here the submucosa is filled with epithelioid cells, numerous lymphocytes and a few polymorphonuclear leucocytes. The sections show only a slight amount of connective tissue, but many blood-vessels are present. In a few areas there is a transition from cells that resemble spindle-cells (from the outer surface of the wall of the intestine) to uniformly round-cells (in the more central portion of the tumor mass). In other areas the tissue is degenerated, the cells being indistinct, and their nuclei staining very poorly. There is no definite structure or arrangement of the cellular elements, but only a diffuse cellular proliferation.

Bacteriological Report.—Attempts were made to stain acid fats and other bacteria with negative results. It must be said that failure may have been due to the method of fixation used.

Remarks.—The above case presents several points of interest. The outstanding clinical sign, which should have led us to a correct pre-

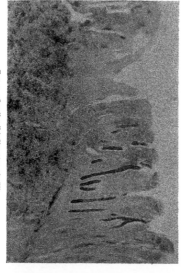

Fig. 3.—Small-cell infiltration of villi.

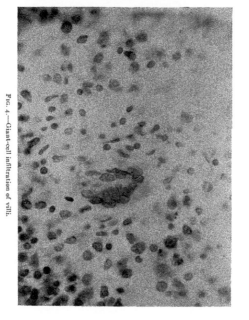

Fig. 4.—Giant-cell infiltration of villi.

198a

operative diagnosis, was the severity and frequency of the intestinal cramps, which were present for a year or more. The growth appearing fixed until complete abdominal muscular relaxation was obtained, under anæsthesia, and the previous existence of enlarged glands in the neck, led us to believe the mass to be probably of retroperitoneal type. This case well represents, therefore, the clinical value of abdominal examination under anæsthesia. "Prof. Wherry."

In contradistinction to the value of X-ray examinations in diseases of the stomach and of the large intestine, it is found in this instance, as is generally the case, that neither fluoroscopic nor the taking of radiograms is of much service in lesions of the small intestine.

I have termed this a case of hyperplastic tuberculosis. Of its originally being tuberculous in character, there can be no question. A study of microscopic sections, however, makes one feel that in many ways the cells resemble those of an ordinary type of lymphosarcoma. A differentiation from microscopic appearances alone seems impossible, and it is a question in my mind whether it is not possible that we are dealing with the development of a sarcomatous condition in what was primarily purely tuberculous. Of the tuberculosis, one must be certain, because of the clinical history and the ulcer, and perhaps the policeman-like characteristic work of the omentum, as shown in the illustrations. Unfortunately, because of faulty preparation of the specimen when removed, the bacillus could not be demonstrated.

The absence of metastasis at the time of the operation, and the continued well-being of the patient, lead me to hope that the suspicions of malignancy are not well founded. Nevertheless, there have been a few cases reported, particularly of the intestine, in which tuberculosis was associated with sarcoma, and particularly lymphosarcoma.

According to Mikulicz,[4] a combination of tuberculosis and sarcoma, especially of lymphosarcoma, is not unusual. Nothnagel in one case found a lymphosarcoma developed in the base of a healed tuberculous ulcer. A further difficulty is that sarcoma of the small intestine appears in a diffuse form over quite extensive segments of the gut.

The question of the relation of tuberculosis to malignant disease is not a new one. Since the days of Rokitansky, and after him Virchow, there has been a general belief that tuberculosis and malignant growths do not develop in the same soil. As a rule, this is unquestionably true, but by numerous cases it has been shown that they are not incompatible. The most recent publication upon this subject, although it relates more to carcinoma than to sarcoma, in relation to tuberculosis, comes from the Mayo Clinic, in an article by Broders.[5] He reports on twenty cases of tuberculosis and malignant disease occurring in the same organ or tissue eight times, or 40 per cent.; in seven cases, or 35 per cent., the two conditions were actually associated in the same microscopic field.

199

JOSEPH RANSOHOFF

BIBLIOGRAPHY

artman and Pillet: Bull. de la Soc. Anat., 1891, p. 471.
artman: British Medical Jour., 1907, vol. l, p. 849.
ubeyran: Monpel. Medicine, vol. xiv, p. 470.
ikulicz: Handbuch der Praktischen Chir., vol. iii, p. 373.
roders: Mayo Clinic, 1919.

ACUTE INTESTINAL OBSTRUCTION. THE CAUSE OF THE CONTINUED HIGH MORTALITY; HOW THIS MAY BE REDUCED *

By John E. Summers, M.D.
of Omaha, Neb. ·

Almost the last written words of the late Dr. John B. Murphy were upon subjects included in the title of this paper, and I want to make a short quotation from what he wrote: " From most reliable statistics we find 40 per cent. mortality in acute intestinal obstruction. One may well ask will this appalling mortality ever cease? Why does it exist?· Because the diagnosis is not made in time for a life-saving operation. The technic in this line of operation is superlatively good, but the clinical recognition is extremely tardy." Personally, I believe that both the operative technic in certain instances, and the post-operative treatment can be greatly improved, thus contributing towards lessening the mortality.

In a paper published in the ANNALS OF SURGERY, February, 1915, entitled " The Mortality Statistics of Two Hundred and Seventy-six Cases of Acute Intestinal Obstruction," Doctor Deaver shows that of these 276 cases there were 118 deaths—a mortality of 42 per cent. All of these patients were admitted into the German Hospital under his care, during a period of ten years. There were 156 cases of strangulated hernia and 120 of the different types of internal strangulation. In 241 cases there were adequate records of the average time from the onset of the condition to the time of operation. In the cases that recovered it was sixty-one and seven-tenth hours, or over two and one-half days, and in the cases that died ninety-seven hours, or four days and one hour. Doctor Deaver remarks, " Under such conditions it is to be wondered at that so many cases had a fortunate outcome." In a letter of recent date, Doctor Deaver writes me and says: " In my hospital and private practice I have not noticed any decrease in the mortality of acute intestinal obstruction since 1915; nor have I noticed any difference in acute appendicitis; both conditions are either not recognized early or have been badly treated by purgation; as you and I both know. The younger men who have graduated in the last two or three years I am sure will be the ones to reduce this mortality. I quite agree with you, much has to be gone over before the essential is grasped."

Sir Berkley Moynihan says that " To operate early in a case of intestinal obstruction is an experience that few surgeons often enjoy." He says that, " There are few surgeons who can show a mortality lower than 50 per cent."

In every country where medical education is acknowledgedly in keep-

* Read before the American Surgical Association, May 3, 1920.

ing with the age, the same story is told—patients with intestinal obstruction come to operation too late—hence the chief reason for the high
mortality. One report from St. Bartholomew's Hospital, London, gives
a recovery of only 15 cases out of a total of 60. In France and Italy the
same kind of reports are to be found.

Before this audience it would be a supererogation upon my part to
attempt to add anything in the differentiation of acute intestinal obstruction from other pathology as generally recognized, but I would strongly
recommend the teachings of the late Dr. J. B. Murphy as published in his
Clinics, as the best expositions of the diagnosis of acute intestinal obstruction. I would also like to recommend particularly the writings of
our fellow member, Dr. John B. Deaver.

When the diagnosis is made within the first twenty-four hours, the
operation done promptly, the obstruction relieved and the gut viable, the
patient usually recovers. The small mortality results from the same
causes as when the operation is done later, only there is added in the
latter the condition of enormously distended intestines filled with poisonous gases and fluids. In no circumstances should the bowel ever be
left in this condition. It should be largely evacuated through one or
several small incisions which are later closed with perhaps a drain in
one, fastened in with purse-string sutures. I do not like the employment
of an enterotomy tube, as recommended by Moynihan, for the immediate
drainage of the distended bowel. If the same patient has been copi-
ously vomiting foul, fecal-smelling fluids, my judgment is that through
a high left rectus incision a 20-22 (French) catheter should be introduced
into the jejunum as near the origin as recognizable, and fastened in as
indicated above. Nature points out the route; the drainage direction has
become retrograde; the intestinal current is reversed—its drainage will
remove the source of the fatal auto-intoxication which is killing the
patient; the absorption, too, from the upper small intestine, considered
so fatal, is greatly reduced. *The vomiting ceases.* This is a positive proof
of the efficacy of the procedure. It is remarkable the large amount of foul
fluid that will drain out of a catheter so placed; very much more and in a
much shorter time than will take place through a drain introduced in the
lower part of the distended gut. When we consider that Nature is trying her best to rid the bowel of its poisonous contents and relieve the
pressure against the obstruction by reversing the current and expelling
the fluids and gases by vomiting, not to assist her by opening the jejunum
would appear unfair. I am convinced, also, that in advanced cases the
introduction of a catheter drain into the jejunum will not infrequently
save life, provided no attempt is made to open the abdomen for exploration or other surgical effort. The cause of the obstruction can be taken
care of later. Of course, there is always the risk of a fatality from peritonitis secondary to gangrene. Post-operative peritonitis with paralytic
obstruction and foul vomiting should be given the hopeful help of a

jejunostomy. It can be used as a prophylactic measure when post-operative peritonitis may be anticipated. My attention was first called to this jejunostomy procedure by a paper of Victor Bonney's in the *British Medical Journal*, April 22, 1916, entitled "Fecal and Intestinal Vomiting and Jejunostomy." He had advocated and practiced the procedure and published it in the Middlesex Hospital Reports in 1910. He reported six successful cases. Bonney's technic was the establishment of drainage through a jejunal fistula, which later required a second operation to close.

McKinnon, of Lincoln, Nebr., who has saved a number of lives by the technic I have outlined, says that the catheter comes away after two or three days, and that the opening in the jejunum closes shortly afterwards. My experience is the same. We know that the opening closes likewise when the catheter is properly placed in the bowel lower down. Bonney divides the obstructed intestine into three segments: the lower, middle, and upper; the lower more or less collapsed, the middle containing gas, the upper containing fluid. My experience is that the lower and middle segments contain gas chiefly; the upper segment most of the fluids.

"The character of the vomited matter indicates the condition of the upper part of the intestinal tract, for where the vomiting is fecal or intestinal the stomach forms the highest part of the fluid-containing segment. This upper segment does not necessarily reach as high in every case of intestinal obstruction when it first comes under clinical observation, nor need it at first include any part of the small intestine; for if the primary obstruction is situated low down in the large intestine, the total area of distention may not at first extend above the ileocæcal valve. In such the 'segment of toxicity' will comprise the cæcum and descending colon. In this phase the vomit is neither fecal nor intestinal, but simply the stomach contents. In all cases of obstruction, however, the stomach and jejunum will eventually be included in the fluid-containing segment, and so soon as this occurs the fact is made patent by the change in the character of the vomit, which at first becomes intestinal and finally fecal.

"This upward extension of the limits of the fluid-containing segment is due to a rapid upwardly extending infection of the canal by organisms of the lower intestine."

As Bonney says, "The drainage opening must tap the fluid-containing segment."

When the obstruction is in the sigmoid a drain should be put into the cæcum. My time is too limited to more than suggest the intra-abdominal technic indicated by conditions presented. When the mechanical cause of the obstruction has produced gangrene of the annular or napkin-ring area type, resection should not be done, but the gangrenous area should be invaginated as an intussusceptum and the gut properly sutured so as to form an intussusception. The gangrenous part sloughs off and the integrity and continuity of the canal is restored. I introduced this technic, reporting cases, in a paper published in the *Journal of the American Medical Association,* 1907. It is a reliable procedure and its principles can be broadened. I have recently shown in the December, 1919, number of the *Nebraska State Medical Journal* how the principle can be applied when resection is deemed advisable. Girdin, of Rio de Janeiro, adopted my suggested method of resection without opening the gut, and Pauchet recently reported in the *Bulletins et Mémoires de la Société de Chirurgie de Paris* three cases of megalocolon resected after this manner. The making of an anastomosis, thus side-tracking an obstruction, is a wise thing to do if the releasing of the obstruction threatens to injure the bowel so that a resection might be necessary. The saving of time is one of the most important elements in the carrying out of a successful operation.

I am a great believer in the scientific principles upon which Crile bases his operative and post-operative treatment in general surgery, and more particularly so in its application in grave cases of abdominal surgery. The profession, except, perhaps, in goitre surgery, has not grasped the importance of Crile's work.

Crile says that, " By employing water, hot-packs, and morphine in post-operative treatment—this latter to reduce the respiration 10–14 per minute—the surgeon can play the patient almost at will. The control of the drive, as marked by the changes in the respiratory rate in particular, is dramatic. Morphine lowers the respiratory rate, decreases the peristalsis of the intestines, reduces pain, and secures physiological rest and sleep, the prime means of recuperation."

This same kind of post-operative management is the one I have been using for some time and gives me great confidence in handling dangerous cases. As far as the employment of morphine is concerned, it has always been *my* practice to employ it as Crile indicates. Alonzo Clark was my teacher and I have always followed his teachings in the treatment of peritonitis. I have never been guilty of giving salines in the treatment of peritonitis, which was for some years in vogue as the result of the recommendations of several surgeons and physicians then in high authority. I am convinced that by early operation and the doing of only the essential, doing it rapidly and well, the establishment of proper drainage, and the employment of the " anociated " treatment, the mortality of acute intestinal obstruction can be reduced 25 per cent., perhaps 50 per cent. In reply to a recent personal note to Doctor Crile, he writes me: " In our clinic the high mortality attending the critical situation presented by acute intestinal obstruction did not begin to fall until we became cognizant of the damage resulting from auto-intoxication *per se.* With the recognition that this danger by so much lessened the patient's chance for recovery, we employed the shortest possible operation, avoided lipoid solvent anæsthetics, employed hot packs, and the Alonzo Clark opium treatment after the operation, with sodium bicarbonate and glucose per rectum. A study of over 219 operations for intestinal obstruction shows a falling mortality rate beginning with the adoption of the methods outlined above."

Among a number of cases of intestinal obstruction seen during the past year I want to briefly report, as illustrative of types, six operated cases.

CASE I.—Acute obstruction in a case of carcinoma of the sigmoid. A large, heavy man, aged fifty-four years. Late operation (Clarkson Hospital) third day of obstruction; exploration disclosed a carcinoma of the sigmoid adherent to the abdomino-pelvic wall; small bowel and colon much distended and dark in color. Cæcostomy; three weeks later resection of the sigmoid; deep cauterization with soldering irons of the area where the carcinoma was adherent to and infiltrating the abdomino-pelvic wall. Later closure of the cæcostomy. Man now in perfect health. Operation done one year ago.

CASE II.—Woman, aged fifty-five years, in poor general health; acute obstruction from carcinoma of splenic flexure of the colon. Exploratory incision (Clarkson Hospital); colon much distended; cæcostomy; two weeks later resection of the colon; death in a few days from exhaustion.

CASE III.—Woman, aged forty years, marked abdominal distention; foul vomiting. Late operation (University Hospital). Median incision—small bowel very dark and enormously distended. Nearly two basinfuls of contents evacuated through three small incisions; openings sutured; anastomosis by suture around a loop of small gut adherent to the left abdominal wall—so tightly adherent as to cause obstruction, and in a condition so threatening perforation that I feared to attempt its release. Patient left the table in a collapsed condition, but recovered.

CASE IV.—Young man entered the Clarkson Hospital; he was very sick, having been ill for ten days with appendicitis; there was a large abscess bulging in the lower middle abdomen; incision and drainage of the abscess was done; a fecal fistula developed, evidently in the lower ileum. The bowels moved naturally and through the fistula; later only through the fistula. Operation—anastomosis by suture around the fistula; death some days later from exhaustion. Post-mortem disclosed the anastomosis perfect, fistula in ileum only a few inches from the ileocæcal valve.

CASE V.—Woman, aged thirty-eight years, operated in a neighboring city (Fremont). Acute obstruction for forty-eight hours; foul vomiting; considerable distention. Incision disclosed that the obstruction was due to a band, probably from a pelvic operation done four years previously; the band was divided. Although the intestines were distended and dark, I did not drain them, and I believe I took an unwarranted chance in not doing so. The woman recovered.

CASE VI.—A man sixty-five years of age came to the Clarkson Hospital with an appendiceal abscess which was opened and drained. Before the wound closed he developed an acute intestinal obstruction. A jejunostomy as described was done at night, under local anæsthesia, the patient being in bed. Relief was prompt; the obstruction was overcome and the jejunostomy incision closed satisfactorily.

CONCLUSIONS

1· Teachers of medicine and surgery should impress by personal acts the philosophy of early diagnosis and prompt surgical treatment.

2. A safe two- or three-stage operation is preferable to any radical procedure which would add much risk as a completed operation.

3. When vomiting has reached the stage of being foul, fecal smelling, always drain the small bowel as high up in the jejunum as it is recognizable. Nature points out this route.

4. Anæsthesia should be local—plus gas oxygen if necessary.

5. Post-operative. Opium should be administered after the Alonzo Clark formula. Large quantities of normal salt solution should be given by hypodermoclysis. Sodium bicarbonate and glucose in 5 per cent. solutions should be administered by the Murphy drip method. Under this treatment the skin will be active if kept warm, and reaction from shock and toxæmia favored.

CAUSES OF DEATH BY ACUTE APPENDICITIS AFTER OPERATION *

STUDY OF TWO HUNDRED AND FIFTY-FIVE Cases

BY ARCHIBALD MacLAREN, M.D.

OF ST. PAUL, MINN.

THE best pathologists tell us that there are five varieties of peritonitic inflammation caused by pyogenic germs, and that it is not always possible to distinguish between them and that all five types may exist in the same case at the same time.

A. B. Johnson's surgical diagnosis gives the following varieties: (1) Localized abscess. (2) Diffuse spreading acute peritonitis with fibrino purulent exudate. (3) Acute peritonitis with cloudy serous exudate. (4) Fibrinous type, alone, fibrin existing in thick masses. (5) Accumulations of slightly cloudy sterile serum.

Johnson says that one of the most frequent causes of peritonitis is the rupture of a gangrenous appendix. Some of the worst cases of peritonitis that we have had to deal with were caused by the rupture of an appendix which was not gangrenous but which contained from one-half drachm to one teaspoonful of pus. Such appendices may lie dormant for months following a preceding acute attack, but ulceration eventually occurs with the sudden discharge of the contained pus directly into the free peritoneal cavity. The first pain, under such circumstances, meaning the commencement of a septic peritonitis.

When we include in the study of acute appendicitis cases which do not show pus at operation, we are deceiving ourselves, and confusing the subject by including cases in which there is almost no mortality, with cases that are extremely dangerous. In our clinical experience it has often been impossible to determine whether in certain border-line cases we were dealing with appendiceal abscess or some other form of appendiceal peritonitis.

In this list we have eliminated all cases of relapsing appendicitis, even when operated upon, during an acute attack. We have limited this study to septic peritonitis due to perforated appendices, and to appendiceal abscesses, including no case in which pus was not present.

We have not been able to lay down any definite rule which we should always follow in treating the individual appendiceal case. Each one must be decided on its own merits. We have occasionally postponed operation when we felt sure that the attack was subsiding. But if the case was growing worse (and from a short study), was progressing toward a fatal termination, we have not hesitated to operate at any time during

---

* Read before the American Surgical Association, May 3, 1920.

the attack. In this list of 255 cases no case has been denied operation. Every one has been given a surgical chance. In studying the thirteen cases in this series which have died, we will not be sure but that two of these patients might have had a better chance of escape if they had been delayed according to Ochsner. But, on the other hand, we cannot forget some four cases which died in the hospital under our care years ago, when we were trying out " the waiting for the eighth day policy."

Incision.—When it has been decided that an operation should be performed for acute appendicitis we advise making a simple straight incision over the appendix just to the outside of the right rectus muscle. Do not use a cross muscle incision for this class of cases. We have had two deaths due to the cellulitic, or gas bacillus, infection with excessive sloughing of the loosened-up muscular and fascial planes in the McBurney incision. In one case reported later in this paper the cellulitis ran around into the tissues of the back, and the patient died on the eighteenth day with a clean peritoneal cavity. We would also advise against sewing these wounds up tightly. We feel sure that we have saved some of these worst septic peritonitis cases by not putting in any stitches at all, simply relying upon adhesive strapping to keep the intestines in the peritoneal cavity. The strapping does not interfere with drainage, and the ultimate wound results are amazingly good. In treating these cases we should remember that we are trying to save the patient's life, not to avoid hernia. The operative hernia can be repaired at some future date. The patient has only one chance of escape.

In treating these bad septic peritonitis cases we should remember that animal experimentation has tended to prove that peritonitis in itself is not necessarily fatal, only when the animal has a raw surface under his liver, following cholecystectomy in the presence of septic peritonitis, was the case sure to die, and usually in the first twenty-four hours (experiments P. P. McNeen, Ricketts Laboratory), which proves what we have known clinically for many years, " that the peritoneum protects the system against bacteræmia." A great measure of success in the treatment of septic peritonitis cases depends upon the wise handling of the complications of the disease. After thorough drainage the peritonitis usually quickly subsides. But occasionally an undrained accumulation of pus will form in either kidney pouch, above or below the liver, but usually in the pelvis. When we have recognized these accumulations early and drained them, the case usually has recovered. When we have not found them early enough, the case has died even after drainage. We have always found at post-mortem an unrecognized abscess which, if we had discovered early enough and drained, the case perhaps might have recovered. Intraperitoneal drainage uphill will work well for from twenty-four to possibly forty-eight hours, but after that time the intestinal coils become so firmly adherent to each other around the drain that all intraperitoneal pressure is destroyed and we are then trying to drain an iron pot through a drain put in at the top. We have frequently seen an old ten to fifteen day appendiceal abscess case discharging profusely through an upper drainage opening, while the pelvis was filled with a large abscess bulging against the anterior rectal wall (Figs. 1 and 2).

More than one-half of our deaths have been late deaths, the patient dying, not from acute peritonitis, but rather from exhaustion due to prolonged intraperitoneal suppuration. A few die from intestinal obstruction due to bands, but more frequently these obstruction cases are septic ileus. Our cases have died chronologically after operation: One on the eighth day; one on the tenth day; one on the twelfth day; one on the eighteenth day; two on the twenty-first day; one on the thirty-third day.

As regards time of operation after perforation we have operated during the first forty-eight hours 69 times with 5 deaths, or, a mortality of 7.1 per cent. Third day, 29 times; fourth day, 11 times; fifth day, 14 times; sixth day, 8 times; seventh day, 7 times; total, 69 operations during the dangerous period of Ochsner with the same mortality, 7.1 per cent. One case that died of opium poisoning the same night which she was operated upon, has been excluded from this classification. Of the remaining 117 cases all have been operated upon on and after the eighth day with two deaths, or a mortality of less than 2 per cent.

We have at times drained a well-marked accumulation of pus in the pelvis either through the vagina or through the rectum as a preliminary, or first step, and then immediately after have opened the abdomen and dealt with the intraperitoneal pathology according to ordinary surgical rules. Our experience has been that quantity, as well as quality of pus, is an important factor in the danger attending this operation, so, if by pelvic drainage we can reduce the quantity of pus in a certain case, we have by that amount lessened the danger of the succeeding laparotomy.

After pelvic drainage we have usually found that there was, at least, one other abscess aside from the accumulation in the cul-de-sac, and this was, as a rule, next to the perforated appendix. This is the reason why it is not wise to rely upon pelvic drainage alone. If the patient, often a child and in bad physical condition, is seen several days after perforation, it may be wise to drain through the rectum one day and postpone the opening of the abdomen until the next day, but not much longer (see Case XII).

The secret of success in these cases is eternal vigilance. Watch them with great care; make frequent rectal examinations; palpate the left side of the abdomen, and be prepared to explore under local anæsthesia. If there is a return of pain and rigidity, or a marked rise in temperature and pulse, early opening and drainage of secondary abscesses will save the patient, later opening of this same abscess will not always help. We have had two deaths within the first twenty-four hours; after finding and draining the large, late abscesses (Cases III and XI) in the 255 cases which we are here reporting, there have been thirteen deaths, or a general mortality of 5.09 per cent. In securing these results vaginal drainage of pelvic abscess was used ten times; rectal drainage was used 33 times; occasionally before operation, but usually some days after laparotomy. In complicating intestinal obstruction the formation of fecal fistula, and drainage of the intestine with a Paul's tube has been at times a great help. This has been done ten times.

In this paper we are reporting in detail the thirteen deaths which have occurred in 255 acute appendicitis cases, hoping they may be of interest and furnish some instruction. These 255 cases are all consecutive cases operated upon personally at the St. Paul, Minneapolis, and Stillwater hospitals. A few other cases operated upon in the country where it was not possible to keep close watch and make frequent examinations have not been included.

This list extends back some eight years, and during that time we have materially changed our views regarding treatment, so that we now feel that some of the cases which have died have been properly treated, and the deaths could not, in our present judgment, have been avoided. Others were not given as good a chance as they would have to-day, and we think that some of them should have been saved.

CASE I.—*Morphine poisoning.* No. 2994. Child, aged six years, sick five days, evening of fifth day became distended. Temperature 103°, acute gangrenous perforated appendix; accumulation of serum in the cul-de-sac. Abscess opened and drained. That night very restless, nurse had difficulty in keeping her in bed. At 10 P.M. nurse gave hypodermic of morphine 1/12 gr.; two hours later (because of no relief) second hypodermic 1/12 gr. morphine. Died 3 A.M., morphine poisoning, pin-point pupils, and respiration of six or less.

OPERATIONS PERFORMED IN FIRST FORTY-EIGHT HOURS

CASE II.—No. 3465. In this case perforation occurred forty hours before seen. Diagnosis: General septic peritonitis, gangrenous perforated appendix. Appendix removed: Drain through stab, just outside cross muscle incision. On the eighth day was very sick from extensive carbuncle-like infection of skin of side and back. Died on the eighteenth day. General septicæmia with enlargement of all glands everywhere. Abdomen, no accumulation of pus.

CASE III.—No. 3717. Young man, aged twenty-seven years. First attack commenced thirty-six hours before seen. Took long auto ride day previous. Vomiting at night. Temperature, 100°; pulse, 85; abdomen rigid; operation St. Luke's Hospital, septic peritonitis; acute gangrenous perforated appendicitis. Three ounces of thick pus with dense adhesions about appendix. One pint of thin serous pus in cul-de-sac, split rubber tube into pelvis through stab opening. Two days later tube out and catheter drain put in. Quite well until ninth day; pelvic distress. Temperature 101° and vomiting. On the twelfth day rectal section. Three pints of serous pus let out and

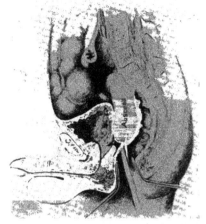

FIG. 1.—Abscess behind bladder pressing against the anterior wall of the rectum.

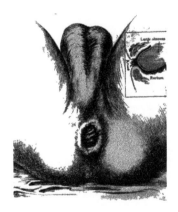

FIG. 2.—Abscess anterior to rectum bulging through the dilated anus.

tube put in. Patient died same night. Post-mortem: No pus in pelvis, but large amount of pus in upper abdomen.

CASE IV.—No. 4368. W. C., care of Doctor Humphrey, of Stillwater, several attacks before, last attack three months ago. This attack commenced eighteen ,hours before seen; operated in Stillwater Hospital. Acute gangrenous perforated appendix. Pint of thin serous pus all through lower right abdomen, not much pus in the cul-de-sac. Drain through the suprapubic stab. A second drain into the right loin. Died on the fourth day. Septic peritonitis. Post-mortem: Mesenteric thrombosis. Several intestinal perforations. One in transverse colon, two or three in lower ileum.

CASE V.—No. 4671. Man aged forty-three years. Two previous attacks. This attack commenced five and one-half hours before operation, rapidly growing worse. Septic peritonitis. Gangrenous perforated appendix. Pocket of sero-pus about appendix, also a large accumulation in cul-de-sac. Wound left opened strapped. Died twenty-four hours after operation.

CASE VI.—No. 4759. N. W. T., care of Doctor Humphrey, of Stillwater. Operation, Stillwater Hospital. One previous attack eight months ago. This attack commenced forty hours before seen with very severe pain, running into the pelvis and right testicle, and general rigidity. Gangrenous perforated appendix, enterolith in perforation. Eight ounces of sero-pus, with marked intestinal distention. Appendectomy: Two cigarette drains, one into pelvis and one into right loin. On the fourth day sudden vomiting of a very large quantity of black liquid. The man strangled during vomiting and died at once, drowned in his own vomit. Post-mortem: No peritonitis, but acute dilatation of stomach.

OPERATIONS PERFORMED AFTER FIRST FORTY-EIGHT HOURS

CASE VII.—No. 3057. Care Dr. Kerr Martel, aged forty years. Perforation five days before seen. Temperature, 102°; pulse, 100. Not doing well, abscess opened and drained through cross muscle. (Free peritoneal cavity not opened.) One pint of thin serous pus. Died of general septic peritonitis twenty-four hours later on the sixth day. Post-mortem: General peritonitis and perforated gangrenous appendix.

CASE VIII.—No. 4255. M. L., care of Doctor Perrin, Star Prairie, aged thirty-five years. Perforation six days before seen. Temperature, 103°; pulse, 120. Had colicky pains several days before perforation. Acute septic peritonitis. Large accumulation of fluid in right abdomen up into right kidney pouch and large accumulation in culde-sac. Appendix gangrenous and perforated, leaking pus; small incision outside of right rectus. Appendix removed and pus sponged out. Pelvis drained. Tapped with tube. Pus spurted two inches above abdominal wall, when the tube was put into the cul-de-sac. Felt much better that night. Died the second night after operation. Post-mortem: Septic peritonitis.

CASE IX.—No. 4804. C. A., care of Doctor Epley, of New Richmond. Man aged forty-five years. Several attacks before. This attack commenced five days ago. Acute perforation four hours before, evidently due to rupture of abdominal abscess. Septic peritonitis, perforated, gangrenous appendix. Appendix removed: Two drains, one tube in right loin, one into cul-de-sac through wound. On the seventh day on account of intestinal obstruction rectal section. On the ninth day intestine drained with Paul's tube. Died of exhaustion on the twentieth day. Post-mortem: Large abscess; two pints of serous pus in left side of abdomen.

CASE X.—No. 5028. R. B., care of Doctor Paxton, of St. Paul. Young man, aged twenty-one years. First attack commenced four days before seen. Not very sick until 2 A.M. on fifth day, when gave first symptoms of perforation. Immediate operation. Acute septic peritonitis. Small intestine coils red and distended. Ruptured appendiceal abscess with gangrenous perforated appendix. One pint of serous pus. Appendix removed. Cæcostomy and drainage of intestine with Paul's tube. Died on the eighth day of septic peritonitis.

CASE XI.—No. 4376. A. S., boy, aged twelve years. First attack commenced four days before seen. Gangrenous perforated appendix, abscess outside of cæcum. Gangrenous spot on cæcum size of quarter of dollar. Appendix removed. Stab drain into pelvis, second drain into right loin through wound and tube drains. On the fifth day fecal fistula discharged through wound. On the twentieth day another abscess opened. Died on the twenty-first day of exhaustion.

OPERATIONS ON OR AFTER EIGHTH DAY

CASE XII.—No. 3116. Little girl, aged seven years, sick five days. Temperature, 104°; pulse, 130. Diagnosis: Acute gangrenous perforated appendix, large pelvic abscess. Rectal section: Pint of pus. Should have had laparotomy on the second day. Eight days after rise of temperature and pulse with vomiting. Laparotomy abscess in the right loin, gas and much pus. Two days later (or tenth day) died of exhaustion.

CASE XIII.—Last case seen with Doctor DuBoise, Sauk Center. Brought to St. Paul on a cot in baggage car. General abdominal rigidity. Temperature 102°; pulse, 125; some vomiting. Deep pelvic abscess present in rectum. Rectal section on fourth day. One pint of sero-pus let out. On the eighth day laparotomy. Gangrenous perforated appendix removed and small right loin abscess opened and drained, wound left open strapped. On nineteenth day sub-diaphragmatic abscess ruptured with return of rigidity and temperature, 103°; pulse, 140. Very sick. Abdomen opened under local anæsthesia. Large left seropurulent accumulation opened and drained. Cæcum opened and tube put in. Died on the thirty-third day of exhaustion.

REFERENCES

Lund, F. B.: Enterostomy, Value of in Selected Cases of Peritonitis. Journal American Medical Medical Association, July 11, 1903.

Hagenboeck, A. L., and Kornder, L. H.: Enterostomy as an Emergency in General Peritonitis Following Operation Acute Appendicitis. Journal American Medical Association, April 12, 1919.

Acute Appendicitis: 822 Patients with Acute Appendicitis, Operated at Cook County Hospital. Appendectomy with Drainage, 312—32 deaths. Mortality, 10 per cent. Journal American Medical Association, March 24, 1917.

Coffey: 13,445 Collected from Various Hospitals in This Country. Mortality, 7.4 per cent. New York Medical Journal, August, 1906.

Irwin, S. T.: Acute Appendicitis. London Lancet, January 18, 1919.

Molat: London Hospital, 1900–1904, 17.2 per cent.

Mutch: 545 cases at Guy's Hospital, 13 per cent.

Beatson: 73 cases, 9 deaths, 12.3 per cent.

Billington: 360, 48 deaths, 13.3 per cent.

Burgess: 365, mortality 10.6 per cent.

Paterson: 56, mortality 8.9 per cent.

Richardson: 350, mortality 13.7 per cent.

Irwin: 84 cases, mortality 11.9 per cent.

Rullison, E .T.: 263 cases from Presbyterian Hospital, New York. Mortality of 9.1 per cent. No cases of vaginal or rectal drainage. ANNALS OF SURGERY, December 19th.

OPERATION FOR CURE OF LARGE VENTRAL HERNIA *

By Charles L. Gibson, M.D.

of New York, N. Y.

SURGEON TO THE FIRST (CORNELL) SURGICAL DIVISION, NEW YORK HOSPITAL

A brief description of this operation was made in my article on " Post-operative Intestinal Obstruction," Annals of Surgery, April, 1916. My experience in this particular procedure now numbers eight cases and the results have been very gratifying. This operation is not intended to supplant the customary operations for repair of incisional hernia or cure of umbilical hernia. It is intended for those cases for which the ordinary operations are not applicable and, in fact, usually quite impossible. The bulk of these cases would have been denied operative relief or subjected to some procedure of doubtful value, such as the implantation of a filigree.

The first operation in 1914 was done on the spur of the moment in an effort to give the patient a competent abdominal wall which was necessary to her profession as physical training instructor. It was felt at that time that the particular procedure used was somewhat hazardous, and it was a source of surprise and gratification that the operation succeeded perfectly, and at the end of six years there are no signs of any recurrence and the functional result is perfect.

Encouraged by this original result, similar operations were performed in cases of increasing magnitude, some of them apparently too great to be overcome. Success, however, attended all cases except the last (Case VIII), which showed that the limit of operative possibilities had been attained. This was a recurrent case (see photograph) with enormous prolapse and a conservative estimate was made at the time of the operation that the abdominal gap would easily correspond to the size of an adult head.

Operation.—The main principle of the operation is to close the gap chiefly by approximating the refreshed edges of the sheath of the rectus, tension being relieved by releasing incisions parallel to the line of suture on either side. This procedure is exactly similar to the operation for closure of cleft palate, according to Langenbeck, by double pedunculated flaps.

The operation is long and tedious. Before the abdominal incision can be closed the herniated contents of the sac must be properly separated and reduced. The closure is made in layers: first, peritoneum, which usually does not present any great difficulty. The next layer is usually quite deficient, as the muscles have disappeared, either from the original suppuration and sloughing or from atrophy. However, as much tissue as can be sutured under the fascial layer is secured. The releasing incisions

---

* Read before the American Surgical Association, May 4, 1920.

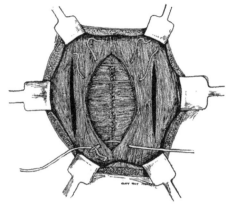

FIG. 1.—Releasing incisions in the fascia of the rectus muscle parallel to the line of suture.

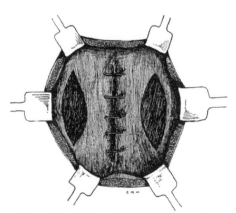

FIG. 2.—Edges of fascia reunited in midline without tension.

2.14

can be made before or after the suturing of the refreshed fascial edges. In extreme cases it must be made before. The width and length of the fascial flap can be determined by the conditions of tension. One must have the courage of one's conviction and extend the releasing incisions sufficiently to take off all undue tension. Ordinarily the flap of fascia would be about two inches wide. The greatest difficulty in making these flaps is in cases of hernia through the upper mid-abdomen, where the releasing incisions have to be carried on to the costal arch. Chromic catgut, mostly interrupted sutures have been used for the fascial closure. These sutures may be sometimes reënforced to advantage by passing some silkworm gut sutures through all the layers superior to the peritoneum.

Experience has shown that most of these wounds do not heal by primary union and a certain amount of discharge, usually non-purulent, is to be expected. It is possible that this accident is caused by spots of necrosis due to too great tension on the fascial sutures. Therefore, the superficial wound should be appropriately drained. Notwithstanding this complication in wound healing, none of these cases seem to have been injured as far as regards curative results.

My experience comprises eight cases. The ninth case, done according to the technic described here by one of my colleagues in my service, did not survive, succumbing to operative shock and paralytic ileus. Of the remaining eight cases only Case VIII, the severest, has shown any signs of recurrence. Case V is particularly interesting, as the patient had been subjected to numerous operations for an abdominal hernia which developed sixteen years prior to my intervention and had worn a filigree for five years which had successfully overcome the hernial protrusion for four years.

The surprising feature in the after results of these cases is the lack of weakness of the abdominal wall where the fascia gapes as the result of being pulled away. I had feared originally that there would be more trouble of possible protrusion at this point than of recurrence of the hernia, but with the exception of the case noted no trouble has developed.

CASE I.—I. F., aged thirty-four years, female.

First Operation.—February, 1912. Operation for appendicitis.

Second Operation.—April 14, 1913. Resection of 20 inches of ileum and anastomosis with Murphy button for intestinal obstruction. At discharge, June 14, 1913, wound was closed save for small spot at lower angle.

Third Operation.—February 24, 1914. Hernia appeared three months previously (November, 1913). Operation for ventral hernia complicated by chronic adhesive peritonitis. Several feet of intestines unravelled. Wound healed by primary union save where hæmatoma had formed, broken down, and discharged. Discharged March 20, 1914.

Follow-up Notes.—June 10, 1914: Abdominal wound firm. No

suspicion of bulging in the wound or elsewhere in the abdomen. February 1, 1920: Excellent condition.

CASE II.—N. W., aged thirty-nine years, male.

First Operation.—Cholecystostomy for cholelithiasis. February 13, 1915. Complicating operation, patient had an acute bronchitis and in coughing stitches yielded. Large hernia formed in scar.

Second Operation.—October 9, 1915: On ninth post-operative day wound was found infected. On tenth post-operative day free discharge of bile, probably all coming out of sinus in midline. Union of fascia and muscle for the most part seems firm, bulk of wound having escaped infection. On twenty-third post-operative day still profuse biliary discharge. Hernia operation seems to have held; condition excellent. On thirtieth post-operative day discharge markedly decreased. Abdominal repair seems to be firm. On thirty-ninth post-operative day patient discharged (November 17, 1915). Wound healed by primary union save at upper angle where wound opened to allow escape of biliary discharge, now slight in amount.

Follow-up Notes.—January 3, 1916: Discharge has returned. No impairment of abdominal wall. May 16, 1917: Wound firmly healed. Excellent condition. May 31, 1919: Excellent condition. No recurrence.

CASE III.—L. P., aged nineteen years, male.

First Operation.—June 12, 1913: Appendectomy and drainage for acute appendicitis. Hernia developed two weeks after discharge. Has gradually increased in size until protrusion is now the size of two fists.

Second Operation.—April 3, 1916: Convalescence delayed by superficial hæmatoma. Discharged thirty-eighth post-operative day. Skin edges still separated. No impulse on coughing.

Follow-up Notes.—October 26, 1916: Wound firmly healed. No impulse. January 10, 1917: Excellent condition. Gaining flesh. Scar firm. February 27, 1919: Excellent condition.

CASE IV.—J. F., aged sixty years, male. Hernia not post-operative. Has had ventral hernia for over four years. Came out gradually. Is now about size of fist. Strong impulse on coughing.

Operation.—July 26, 1918: Discharged August 13, 1918. Wound healed primarily.

Follow-up Notes.—March 6, 1920: No recurrence.

CASE V.—C. S., aged fifty-one years, female.

First Operation.—October 16, 1902: For epigastric hernia.

Second Operation.—August 15, 1912: Repair of ventral hernia.

Third Operation.—September 8, 1913: Repair of ventral hernia with insertion of wire filigree (local anæsthesia).

Fourth Operation.—Readmitted October 29, 1918. One year ago patient noticed bulging to left of old ventral hernia repair scar. Wire broke through skin about ½ inch about six weeks before this admission. Some of the wire was removed. Has pain at site, especially on coughing. Filigree removed under local anæsthesia October 31, 1918. November 23, 1918: Operation for repair of ventral hernia. Thirty-eighth post-operative day wound explored under ether. Skin

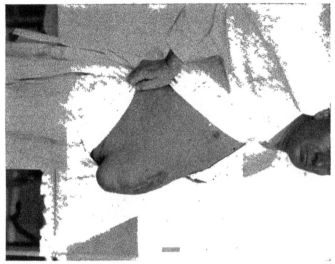

FIG. 3.—Case IIA. Taken September 28, 1915.

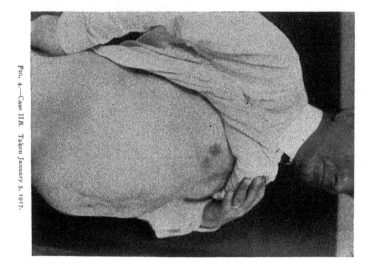

FIG. 4.—Case IIB. Taken January 5, 1917.

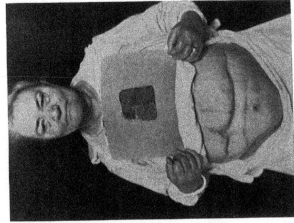

Fig. 6.—Case V. Taken March 30, 1920, showing filigree removed at fourth operation.

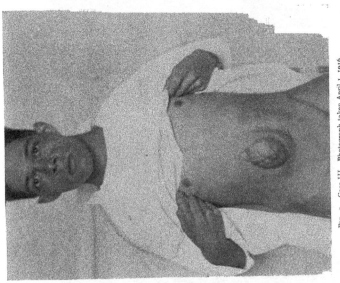

Fig. 5.—Case III. Photograph taken April 1, 1916.

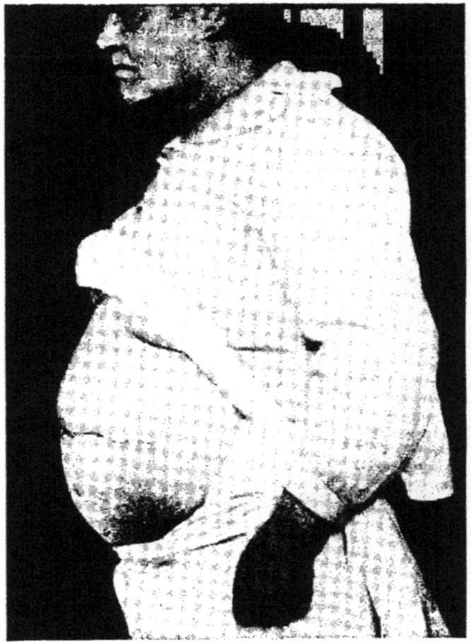

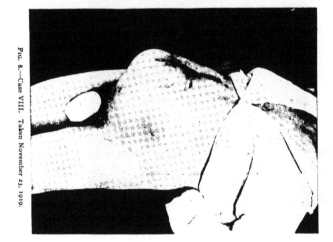

FIG. 7.—Case V. Taken March 30, 1920.

FIG. 8.—Case VIII. Taken November 23, 1919.

B.
2 6

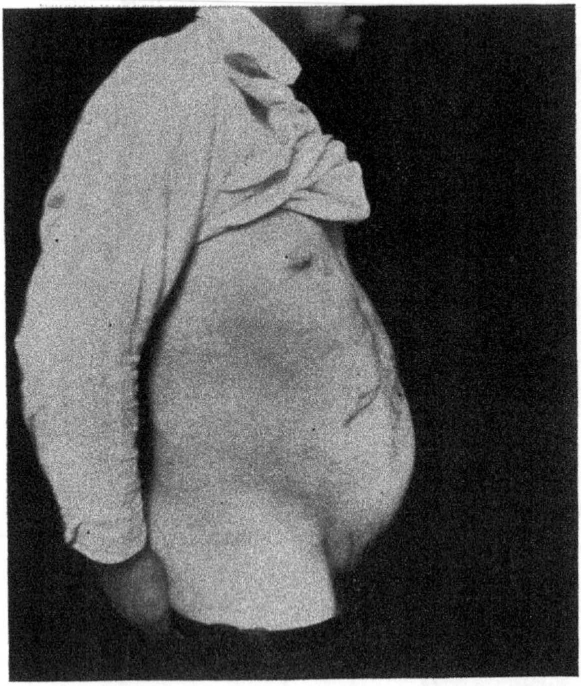

FIG. 9.—Case VIII *BJ*; Taken April 15, 1920.

tunnelled along line of incision. Involved area widely converted into one large wound which was packed open with balsam gauze. Fifty-first post-operative day allowed up. Fifty-seventh post-operative day still has a small granulating area. Hernia apparently cured. No impulse or bulging on coughing. Abdominal wall firm at site of former hernia. Patient discharged.

Follow-up Notes.—May 1, 1919: Firmly healed. Excellent condition. March 30, 1920: Excellent condition. No recurrence.

CASE VI.—M. M., aged fifty years, female.

First Operation.—December, 1901: Left salpingectomy for ectopic gestation.

Second Operation.—December, 1902: Laparotomy through old scar. Right salpingo-oöphorectomy for salpingo-oöphoritis. Convalescence complicated by fecal fistula.

Third Operation.—Readmitted July 7, 1919. Hernia appeared eight or nine years after last operation (1910 or 1911). Two lumps, size of orange, one at each end of incision. Has worn belt ever since she first noticed them. Operation July 8, 1919. Discharged August 10, 1919. Wound healed by primary union.

Follow-up Notes.—June 1, 1920: Excellent result. No bulging.

CASE VII.—B. W., aged fifty-eight years, male.

First Operation.—One year before second operation. Extensive operation for cholelithiasis. Wound broke down and hernia developed two months later.

Second Operation.—Examination: Very large individual. Ventral hernia size of child's head at term through scar in midline, reaching from umbilicus to ensiform. Operation May 23, 1919. Operation attended with much difficulty, lasting two hours and a half.

Follow-up Notes.—August 1, 1919: Patient writes that he is exceedingly well. Later but indirect reports indicate continuance of good result.

CASE VIII.—M. Z., aged forty-eight years, male.

First Operation (1914).—Operation for gall-stones.

Second Operation (1916).—Operation for ventral hernia which appeared six months after last operation.

Third Operation (1918).—Operation for recurrent ventral hernia. Hernia appeared three months after last operation.

Fourth Operation (November 26, 1919).—On twenty-sixth post-operative day considerable discharge. There is a sinus which extends upward and to the left. Counter incision made. Drainage. Fortieth post-operative day discharge stopped. Small sinus at either angle. Forty-sixth post-operative day: Discharged.

Follow-up Notes.—February 26, 1920: General bulge, but apparently not recurrence. March 22, 1920: Little recurrence in midline and some bulging without protrusion at site of releasing incision on left side.

CANCER OF THE OVARY INVADING THE SIGMOID FLEXURE *

By Philemon E. Truesdale, M.D.
of Fall River, Mass.

Approximately 3 per cent. of cancer deaths in females result from malignant disease of the ovaries. This is about one-tenth as many deaths as are recorded from cancer of the uterus, but Taylor[1] observes that it does not correctly indicate the frequency of malignant disease of the ovaries because many more of these cases are cured than of cancer of the uterus.

From the Annual Reports of the Massachusetts General Hospital for six years (1914–1919) it was found that there were 29 cases of cancer of the ovary among 758 cancers in females, and approximately 5500 laparotomies performed on females for all causes. Of these 29 cases 16, or 55 per cent., were found to be inoperable when examined by laparotomy.

In the reports from the Mayo Clinic for a period of five years (1914–1918) there were 150 operations for cancer of the ovaries and 26 " exploratory " operations for the same cause among 5175 laparotomies for diseases of the uterus, tubes, and ovaries.

Among 1700 abdominal sections for diseases of the female organs in our clinic at Fall River, 30 cases of cancer of the ovary were found. During the same period there were 250 cases of cancer in women, making the relative frequency of ovarian cancer 12 per cent. in our records. Of the 30 cases examined by abdominal section 17, or 56.6 per cent., proved to be inoperable.

The average duration of illness, i.e., discovery of a tumor or complaint of pelvic trouble, in our series was nineteen months.

Twenty-one of the patients were married and 9 were single. The relative ages were as follows: Twenty to thirty, 3; thirty to forty, 6; forty to fifty, 9; fifty to sixty, 5; sixty to seventy, 7.

The important feature in the study of these records is the high percentage of cases of cancer of the ovary found inoperable when examined by laparotomy. Add to these figures the number of cases classified as inoperable upon physical examination, on account of palpable metastatic nodes and ascites, and it becomes clear that the disease is more common than present statistics show. Occurring, as it does, most frequently within the period of the menopause, the moderately discomforting symptoms of the early or midperiod of the disease are too frequently ignored.

Ovarian cysts are sign-posts of cancer and their dangers will continue to be disregarded until the frequency of their inoperability is given wide publicity. The root of the difficulty lies in the unwarranted fear of operation, the false sense of security enjoyed by women carrying painless

---

* Read before the American Surgical Association May 4, 1920.

tumors, and occasionally an almost entire absence of symptoms in the early stage of ovarian cancer.

A pelvic tumor in a woman of cancer age cannot be " watched " with impunity any more than a tumor of the breast. " Watching " tumors until there was abundant evidence of malignancy resulted in an increase in cancer deaths from 66.9 per 100,000 in 1900 to 92 per 100,000 in 1915. Fewer women and fewer doctors now make a business of " watching " tumors, and the percentage of cancer deaths has not increased since 1915. Yet the fact that in the average hospital more than 50 per cent. of the cases of ovarian cancer are found to be hopeless at the time of operation opens up a small field, at least, in which a reduction can be made in the total deaths from cancer. This can be done if every easily palpable pelvic tumor, especially the ovarian cyst, is looked upon as potentially cancer and extirpated without inordinate delay.

Origin.—The precise origin of cancer of the ovary is still a mooted question. The subject is so intricate and so laden with theoretical dogma that the authors of gynæcologic pathology frequently record their observations and allow the reader to make his own interpretation.

Goodall has made an intensive study of the origin of ovarian tumors, publishing the results of his investigations in 1911[2] and again in 1920.[3] From his contributions a more intelligent understanding of the genesis of ovarian cancer is obtainable. In his study of the comparative embryology, histology, and function of the cow's ovary which bears a close resemblance to the human, Goodall expresses the belief that epithelial tumors of the ovary do not spring entirely from fetal rests, but that they do arise from postnatal structural defects as well. In nearly every ovary in women over thirty-five years of age he observed a dipping of the germinal epithelium into the deep crevices over the whole surface of the ovary owing to the cicatrization of the corpora lutea; and in this same class he demonstrated the resolution of the corpora to be less rapid and less complete, and marked by fibrosis and scar. On the contrary, in the child resolution is complete without shrinking or mutilation of the ovary or its surface. Therefore it seems fair to assume that, while cancer finds its origin in the primordial follicles deep in the ovary, many tumors arise from the intractions of the germinal epithelium in the cicatrization of the corpora lutea. When the cells of the corpora lutea proliferate they occasionally lose all signs of epithelial arrangement, and when they give rise to neoplasm they develop an interstitial cell growth histologically sarcoma rather than carcinoma.

A striking feature in connection with the malignant tumors of the ovary is the mixed character of the tissue growth. Several types may exist in the same specimen. The tissues may change almost imperceptibly from carcinoma to perithelioma and then to sarcoma, a process which in itself indicates the complexity of its birth cells. In the fœtus and child the ovary is frequently found lobulated, and the sinking of the

219

germinal epithelium into the primitive deep clefts gives rise to cysts which sometimes degenerate into cancer in later life. What the agent is that provokes this change remains an enigma. One thing is clear—that the defense against cancer growth possessed by the tissues of early life is lost and a local irritation only is needed to produce a cell activity in structures which are prone to take on aberrant growth.

The cystic carcinomata commonly arise in cystadenoma or the papillomatous varieties. They do not attain a very large size, and before removal they frequently are not recognized as malignant unless the papillomatous growth has extended through the wall of the tumor to invade the peritoneum. When this happens the true character of the growth is revealed by its exuberant vegetation giving rise to peritoneal and other metastases.

The attempt to classify ovarian neoplasms has proved so difficult that the older writers were content to divide cancer into two forms, the cystic and the solid. This is a practical arrangement from a clinical point of view, though it fails to indicate the embryological or developmental origin of these tumors.

Adami[*] has classified the malignant tumors of the ovary in three types:

1. New growth of epithelial type $\begin{cases} a. & \text{Cystic carcinoma.} \\ b. & \text{Solid carcinoma.} \end{cases}$

2. New growth of connective-tissue type $\begin{cases} a. & \text{Endothelioma.} \\ b. & \text{Perithelioma.} \\ c. & \text{Sarcoma.} \end{cases}$

3. Mixed tumors $\begin{cases} a. & \text{Myosarcoma.} \\ b. & \text{Adenosarcoma.} \\ c. & \text{Sarcocarcinoma.} \\ d. & \text{Cystic carcinoma.} \\ e. & \text{Cystic sarcoma.} \end{cases}$

Symptoms.—The symptoms of carcinoma of the ovary vary widely according to the size of the tumor, its rapidity of growth, and the degree of encroachment upon adjacent organs. When cancer is the result of degeneration of an ovarian cyst the symptoms may be those of the cystic tumor only, which are usually a feeling of fullness and weight in the abdomen. When carcinoma becomes superimposed there may be constitutional symptoms, such as loss of weight, interference with appetite, digestion, etc. Symptomatic evidence of cancer of the ovary may be very vague even in the mid-period of the disease. Cachexia and ascites are usually symptoms of inoperability.

Prognosis and Treatment.—The outlook for favorable results in dealing with cancer of the ovary depends upon the extent of growth before the standard operative treatment of complete removal of both ovaries is adopted. Since ovarian cyst is a known precancerous condition, this type of tumor should be removed when found, and its extirpation should

220

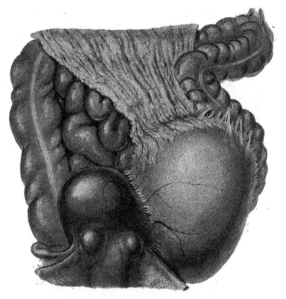

FIG. 1.—Case No. 2170. Showing large ovarian tumor adherent to fibroid uterus, omentum and bowel. Blood-vessels from the adjacent structures are seen entering the periphery of the rapidly growing tumor.

2204

be accomplished always without rupture of the cyst wall. Peritoneal metastasis, proving rapidly fatal, may result from spreading the excrescences of malignant papillomata over the peritoneum. Prompt examination of an apparently benign cyst should be made for malignant changes while the abdomen is open. Whenever new growth is found the other ovary, potentially cancerous, should also be removed, because it is common knowledge among pathologists that when fetal rests occur in one of the bilateral organs they are always present in the other.

The papillary type is often of a low grade of malignancy, and although it is found disseminated over the peritoneum, the use of radium and X-rays after the removal of both ovaries will retard, if not cure, the condition.

The prognosis in solid carcinomas of the ovary, which are also unilateral or bilateral, is not so good, inasmuch as they frequently metastasize before they are discovered. Graves[5] describes this form as genuine idiopathic carcinoma which develops directly from previously unchanged ovarian tissue. They are rare and frequently found to be inoperable. This form is usually of the medullary type, but may be scirrhous or myxomatous. According to Nicholls,[6] the ovarian tissue is frequently diffusely infiltrated or destroyed or the main mass of the organ may be pushed to one side in the course of growth. The solid tumor, though usually small, may attain the size of a child's head. On account of the rapid growth, blood supply at the periphery of the tumor may become inadequate and the vitality of its tissue is sustained by adhesions to the parietal peritoneum, intestine, and omentum. Such a condition was found to be the condition in the following case:

CASE I (No. 2170).—Admitted to our hospital in Fall River, Mass., March 7, 1915, aged forty-nine years, single.

The patient had known for years that she had a tumor in the lower abdomen. From this she had suffered no special discomfort until October, 1914, when there developed a feeling of fullness and pressure in the lower abdomen. Indigestion supervened in the form of distress at varying intervals after eating, anorexia, flatulence, sour stomach, and obstipation. During the last three months she noticed a rapid increase in size of the tumor in the left side of the lower abdomen. Her physician had advised operative treatment several months ago and, suspecting malignant disease, he now prevailed upon her to report for operation. She had lost 40 pounds in weight in six months.

Physical examination revealed no disease other than a tumor occupying the lower abdomen. It consisted of multiple solid growths arising in the pelvis, apparently uterine fibromata. On the left side an oval, smooth, solid tumor had reached the umbilicus. The entire mass had a very narrow range of mobility.

The operation revealed multiple fibroids of the uterus crowded to the right side by a solid tumor of the left ovary about the size of a cocoanut. This tumor was the fixed portion of the entire mass.

It was involved in adhesions to the parietal peritoneum, descending colon, omentum, and loops of small gut. The picture presented did not invite interference except for the reason that the ovarian tumor had the appearances of malignancy. There was very little free fluid and no metastatic nodes were discovered within the abdomen or elsewhere. Therefore, a considerable operative risk for the eradication of the disease was deemed justifiable. A sub-total hysterectomy was done. The adhesions to the ovarian tumor were unusually vascular, indicating the proliferation of numerous small vessels to sustain the vitality of the tumor. For a distance of 10 cm. the growth had invaded the descending colon, destroying the coats of the bowel. About 30 cm. of the colon was excised with the tumor. The distal stump of the bowel was infolded with a purse string of fine silk. An artificial anus was made with the proximal end. Aside from the troubles incident to a recent colostomy, the convalescence was uneventful.

Two years later, in March, 1917, the patient's general state was very satisfactory. There was no evidence of recurrence and she requested that the normal outlet of the colon be restored.

On March 19, 1917, the second laparotomy was done. After opening the abdomen no return of the disease was discovered and the field surveyed with the purpose of making an end-to-end anastomosis of the colon. This seemed impracticable owing to the wide separation of the opposing ends of the colon and the firm adhesions in the left upper quadrant of the abdomen. A workable alternative was in plain view by the juxtaposition of the head of the cæcum and the blind end of the rectum. Between the two a lateral anastomosis was made. Under these conditions the function of the large bowel became a source of interest. In spite of a competent anastomotic opening between cæcum and rectum, the normal one-way passage of intestinal contents continued by evacuation of the bowel through the artificial anus. This could not be considered extraordinary while there was the resistance at the anus of a closed sphincter muscle; but the result was the same when a tube of large calibre was placed in the rectum. An enema given through the artificial anus returned in the presence of a closed rectal sphincter, but passed out through the indwelling rectal tube. A little later enemas given by the artificial anus returned, and it seemed probable that the anastomotic opening had closed. An examination with the sigmoidoscope revealed the communication adequate. Therefore it was deemed wise to resect the colon. This was done, leaving the cæcum with its sutured end suspended in the lower angle of the abdominal incision. An indwelling rectal tube was employed to relieve back pressure. This tube was removed in ten days. About a week later a fecal fistula developed which closed spontaneously after two months.

The patient is now well, five years after removal of the growth, and the result makes justifiable an occasional excision of wide proportions in the presence of an extension of cancerous growth by contiguity.

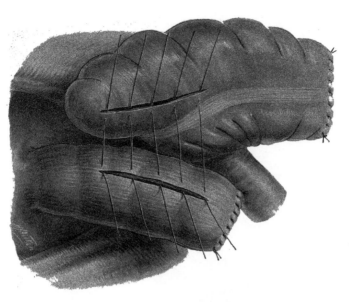

FIG. 2.—Case No. 2170. Anastomosis between the cæcum and the severed end of the rectum.

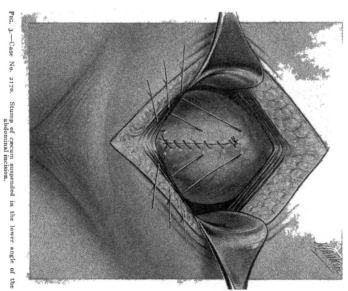

FIG. 3.—Case No. 2170. Stump of cæcum suspended in the lower angle of the abdominal incision.

222

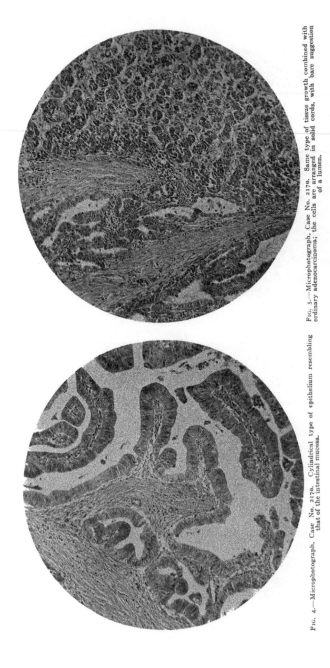

Fig. 4.—Microphotograph. Case No. 2170. Cylindrical type of epithelium resembling that of the intestinal mucosa.

Fig. 5.—Microphotograph. Case No. 2170. Same type of tissue growth combined with ordinary adenocarcinoma; the cells are arranged in solid cords, with bare suggestion of a lumen.

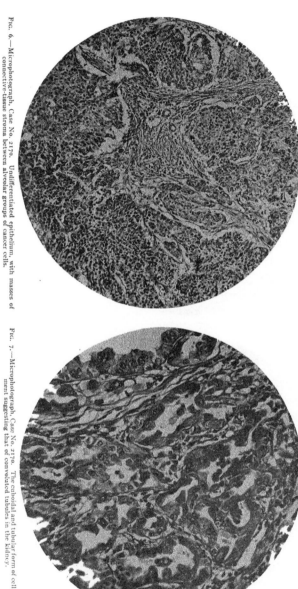

Fig. 6.—Microphotograph, Case No. 2170. Undifferentiated epithelium, with masses of connective-tissue stroma between alveolar groups of cancer cells.

Fig. 7.—Microphotograph, Case No. 2170. The cuboidal and tubular form of cell arrangement suggesting that of convoluted tubules in the kidney.

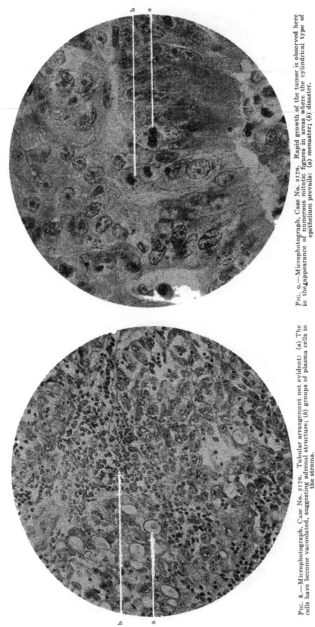

Fig. 8.—Microphotograph, Case No. 2170. Tubular arrangement not evident: (a) The cells have become vacuolated, suggesting adrenal structure; (b) groups of plasma cells in the stroma.

Fig. 9.—Microphotograph, Case No. 2170. Rapid growth of the tumor is observed here in the appearance of numerous mitotic figures in areas where the cylindrical type of epithelium prevails: (a) monaster; (b) disaster.

CANCER OF THE OVARY AND SIGMOID FLEXURE

It is hoped that the report of a case of this character, with its complications and hazards and the suffering entailed with good luck in pursuit, will serve as a reminder that " a stitch in time will save nine," and that the average woman, even of the intelligent class, is not yet aroused sufficiently to the importance of early examination for pelvic disorders and the wisdom of adopting prompt surgical measures for the removal of pelvic and abdominal new growths.

REFERENCES

[1] Taylor: Bulletin 6, Oct., 1915, Amer. Soc. for Control of Cancer.
[2] Goodall: Transactions Amer. Gynecological Soc., vol. xxviii.
[3] Goodall: Surgery, Gynecology and Obstetrics, March, 1920.
[4] Adami: Adami and Nicholls, Principles of Pathology, p. 854.
[5] Graves: Graves' Gynecology, p. 339.
[6] Nicholls: Montreal Med. Journal, vol. xxxii, 1903, p. 326.

THE RADICAL TREATMENT OF X-RAY BURNS *

By John Staige Davis, M.D.
of Baltimore, Md.

X-ray burns were quite common when long exposures were necessary to secure satisfactory plates, and before the methods of protecting patient and operator were understood. They are now comparatively rare, but during the last ten years I have had a number of them referred to me, and can recall several occasions when I have had three or four such cases in the hospital at one time.

These burns are usually caused by the use of X-rays in the treatment of skin lesions, such as psoriasis, eczema, and superficial epithelioma; by frequent exposures extending over a long period of time in the treatment of inoperable or incompletely removed carcinoma; by the reckless use of the apparatus in the hands of unskilled operators, and by long fluoroscopic exposures.

I have had under my care burns situated in almost every region of the body.[1] Some of them have been of the first degree, where the skin is reddened; a few of the second degree, where blisters formed; but the vast majority have been of the third degree, where the full thickness of the skin and often the underlying tissues were involved. It is the latter group in particular that I wish to consider in this paper.

A peculiarity of an X-ray burn is that considerable time may elapse (several weeks or months) before the extent of the damage done becomes apparent. Some very severe burns have followed single exposures, others have been the result of multiple exposures. One patient in my series had been given more than 450 treatments scattered over several years; another had fifteen-minute exposures every day for nine months, and several others had more than 100 treatments. Some of the deeper burns had existed from a few weeks to as long as fifteen years before coming under my care.

On inspection the burned area may be considerably hollowed out. The skin is hairless and atrophied, smooth, dry and shiny, with or without a blotchy brownish pigmentation. In the majority of cases there are characteristic telangiectases which may be discrete, or occur in reddish patches. Punctate hemorrhages due to rupture of dilated capillaries may be present.

On palpation the tissue is hard and board-like. Its outline where it merges into surrounding skin may be quite irregular. Occasionally the entire area is covered with a sharply differentiated brown mummified tissue.

The ulcers may be superficial, or may involve the full thickness of the skin, with a considerable depth of the underlying soft parts.[2] The history

---

* Read before the American Surgical Association, May 4, 1920.

[1] Scalp, face, neck, chest, back, shoulder, arm, forearm, hand, abdominal wall, penis, thigh, leg and foot.

[2] I have seen the entire thickness of the abdominal wall involved in a burn.

of many of them is that they heal slowly and then break down, this process being repeated over and over. Some of the ulcers never heal without operative interference.

There is usually an irregular-shaped patch of tightly adherent necrotic tissue occupying the central portion of the ulcer. The edges are thickened and grayish-red in color; are very hard, and are often everted. In fact, the clinical appearance is suggestive of malignancy. From the edges outward to normal skin we find the tissues more or less infiltrated with scar.

Exquisite sensitiveness is characteristic of the deep burns. The pain in an ulcerated area may be due to irritation caused by infection, which is always present; to changes in the nerves themselves, or to pressure on the nerves by scar tissue. Any one or all of these conditions may exist. Addiction to narcotics is not uncommon, as the burning pain, even from a tiny ulcer, may be severe and continuous. There may be intense pain, making operative interference necessary, after spontaneous healing has taken place. This pain in a healed burn may be due to nerve changes, to pressure by scar tissue, or to both conditions.

There is said to be a marked tendency to malignant degeneration in chronic X-ray burns, but my experience has been that this tendency is no more marked in these burns than in any other chronic ulcer.

Microscopic examination of the excised tissues in all my cases, where the full thickness of the skin was involved, has been negative for malignancy.

Dr. J. C. Bloodgood sends me the following report after study of the excised tissues: " The characteristic features in an X-ray burn as compared to a leg ulcer, or any other type of simple ulcer are: X-ray keratosis at the edge of the ulcer with atypical down-growth of epithelium, with or without pearly body formation; a very superficial zone of cellular granulation tissue; unusual scar tissue formation which, as a rule, extends to the muscle; thickening of the walls of the blood-vessels with endothelial obliteration, and minute abscess formation beneath the surface of the ulcer."

There is, however, a distinct tendency toward malignant degeneration when chronic ulceration follows the breaking down of a patch of keratosis, such as we find on the hands of the pioneer röntgenologist. Two such cases have been under my care. In both, the axillary glands are involved and were removed. In one case, too short a time has elapsed to predict the ultimate result, but in the other there has been no recurrence after the lapse of a number of years.

Treatment.—Recent X-ray burns of all degrees should be treated as ordinary burns, but unless there is a fairly prompt response to such treatment it is a mistake to continue it.

Palliative measures should be used in burns of the first degree. Paraffin films are often comforting; painting with collodion, or the application of sterolin,' or some bland ointment, are useful procedures.

' FORMULA.—Balsam of Peru, 4 c.c.; castor oil and Venetian turpentine, of each, 2 c.c.; alcohol (95 per cent.), 100 c.c.

Burns of the second degree, where there is blistering, have been quite rare in my series, although I have in mind one case in which both hands had been treated several times for localized sweating of the palmar surfaces. Blistering began about one week after the last exposure, and the entire skin of each hand came away like a glove after about two weeks.

It is difficult to tell at first the depth of such a burn, as one which seems to be merely blistered will turn out to be much deeper in places after the blisters have been removed. I have found that wet dressings have been more comfortable in these cases than paraffin or ointments.

In burns of the third degree which do not heal promptly and permanently by the usual methods, we must adopt a more radical procedure. The ulcer and surrounding area of induration should be excised with a wide margin out to and down to healthy tissue. It is impossible to tell the depth of the destructive process until excision is done.

The tissues are of extreme hardness and will often turn the edge of a scalpel. The subcutaneous fat may be completely destroyed, but if present is a deep yellow color and is very firm and resistant due to scar tissue involvement. In deep burns the muscle may be entirely replaced by dense scar tissue, or there may be varying degrees of infiltration with scar. The bleeding is always marked after excision and is often difficult to check as there is general oozing from all portions of the wound.

After excision, the defect should be grafted immediately if the base of the wound is of normal tissue, but if doubtful tissue is left (owing to the impossibility of complete excision), grafting should be deferred until granulations form. The type of graft used should depend upon the situation. I use "small deep grafts" in the majority of instances, but have used with satisfaction Ollier-Thiersch, or whole-thickness grafts in selected positions.

Pedunculated flaps from neighboring tissues, or from a distant part, have been of great use in situations where a pad of fat, in addition to whole-thickness skin, was necessary.

The best method of relieving the pain, aside from the excision of the affected area, is to divide the nerves supplying the area.

X-ray or radium have been used in the treatment of X-ray burns, and several patients have come under my care who had been treated in this way. I have seen no benefit follow such treatment.

Patches of keratosis which exist on the X-ray operator's hand, following frequent exposures without protection, may be successfully treated by freezing with carbon dioxide ice. This is a tedious and painful process. Radium may be used with success, but the reaction is also painful. In my opinion it is less safe than the carbon dioxide ice. Should the patches of keratosis ulcerate, neither of the methods just mentioned should be employed. Complete excision with immediate or subsequent grafting is then the method of choice.

Comments.—X-ray burns often cause complete loss of function of a part.

In more severe burns of the hands, one is struck by the rigidity of the fingers due to involvement of the tendons and overlying soft parts, and even of the joints themselves.

In those instances in which tendons have been destroyed it is advisable to fill the defect with a pedunculated flap of skin and fat, and later to restore the tendon by the method best suited to the particular case.

Where large areas are involved we seldom excise sufficient tissue, and I have noticed that infection sometimes occurs in the margins of these wounds. Occasionally there is sloughing of the entire margin of the wound, although the excision has been apparently complete, and for this reason alone it may be wise to defer grafting, or the transference of a flap.

Fulminating infections occur in areas of skin which have been burned by X-rays. Prompt excision with a generous margin is indicated, or even amputation of the part may be necessary to control the rapid spread of the infection.

The after-results of excision with grafting, or flap shifting, have been most gratifying. I have no record at the present writing of a case in which a breakdown has followed the thorough application of the method. Furthermore, function is restored in many instances and patients who have been incapacitated for years have been returned to their former activities.

ETIOLOGY, PATHOLOGY AND CLINICAL FEATURES OF BENIGN EXOSTOSES *

By Ellsworth Eliot, Jr., M.D.

of New York, N. Y.

Nutritive disturbances and traumata have long been recognized as important factors in the etiology of exostoses. In the former, exostoses, occasionally multiple, spring from those epiphyses which are chiefly concerned in the growth of the bone and not infrequently disappear when the nutritive disturbance is relieved or corrected. Exostoses due to trauma include chiefly those resulting from the irritation of long-continued friction such as may be observed in a persistent horseback rider, either at or near the inner surface of the lower epiphysis of the femur. The clinical features of these two groups of exostoses are so well known as to require no further consideration, although, in passing, it may not be amiss to call attention to the fact that exostoses arising from the epiphysial line, in the subsequent growth of the bone, gradually become separated from it, in that the actual point of origin of the growth remains stationary while the epiphysial cartilage proper recedes.

The study of the effect of acute trauma at a distance from the epiphysial line, and even at a time when the full growth of the bone has been attained, is not without considerable interest.

.Contusion of the bone, like that of the overlying soft parts, causes a variable rupture of blood-vessels with the escape of blood in the direction of. least resistance. In contusion of bone this extravasated blood collects beneath the periosteum, usually in such small quantities as to cause no perceptible swelling. Subsequently, as in the soft parts, the clot is usually absorbed, although more slowly, and at times not without leaving slight permanent irregularities in the contour of the bone due to the calcification of its unabsorbed portion. A gradually subsiding tenderness with, in exceptional cases, a distinct though slightly elastic swelling, are its only symptoms, and ordinarily there is little interference with locomotion or other use of the extremity.

Rarely, however, as in the case herewith reported, after a more or less localized trauma, a tender swelling develops, involving a considerable portion of the bone, which is very sensitive to the touch and deeply elastic in consistency. While this swelling does not usually suppurate, the absorption of the extravasated blood may not readily take place, and its persistence together with its gradual calcification may cause such a degree of discomfort that the patient is impelled to seek relief. In the absence of suppuration a permanent thickening of the bone, corresponding to the extent of the

---

* Read before the American Surgical Association, May 5, 1920.

hæmatoma, may ultimately be expected, differing only in degree from what ordinarily takes place in the mild type of this lesion. These permanent bony irregularities, of variable size, can in no wise be classified with pointed exostoses, although resembling at times the so-called ivory variety, commonly seen in the skull, which by some is considered to be of a traumatic origin.

It is quite possible, however, for a subperiosteal hæmatoma of the smallest size to prove the starting point of a more or less actively growing pointed exostosis that can not be differentiated either pathologically or clinically from the classic pointed exostosis, the result of continued and repeated friction. The rapidity of growth of an exostosis from such an origin even though based, as in the present instance, upon a single case, is particularly worthy of mention. As a class benign tumors, especially those of bone, are of slow growth. In the case referred to, however, the pointed exostosis reached a length of two inches within thirteen months, an extremely rapid growth, and the fact that friction played no part in this unusual phenomenon is demonstrated by the statement of the patient as well as by the failure of any bursa to develop over its pointed apex. While a rapid increase in size is the rule in malignant growths and may be expected in those exceptional benign tumors which undergo malignant change, the benign character of the exostosis in question was positively demonstrated by a subsequent careful microscopical examination.

Male, aged twenty years, December 15, 1915. Two and one-half months ago, while playing football, patient was kicked in the right thigh. This was immediately followed by swelling involving the entire thigh and knee and confining patient to bed for one week. At the end of that time the acute pain and disability had subsided and there remained of the swelling only that part in the middle of the thigh on its outer and anterior aspect which, about four inches long, persisted up to the present time with only slight decrease in size, although it became gradually of firmer consistency. During this interval patient has suffered from considerable pain and discomfort, especially on walking and on attempting to flex the knee. The pain has been worse at night. For the first part of this period patient walked with crutches and latterly with a cane, there being a perceptible limp.

All attempts to relieve the pain and bring about the absorption of the swelling by massage and various forms of counter-irritation having proved futile, the patient insisted on operation. Under ether, through an incision four inches long on the outer anterior aspect of the thigh, the periosteum was exposed. It was considerably thickened and on division of its outer layer an oval cavity filled with a mass of rather friable calciferous tissue and about three-quarters of an inch thick, gradually becoming thinner at either extremity, was disclosed. The demarcation between the inner layer of the periosteum and the superficial surface of this mass was well defined and easily separated with the finger. The same condition was found to exist between its deeper sur-

229

face and the adjacent layer of compact bone, so that the removal of the mass was accomplished without difficulty and in a satisfactory manner. After suture of the divided periosteum the muscular layers were closed with chromic gut, a small rubber drain being left *in situ* for twenty-four hours. Primary union was obtained and the patient was completely relieved of all discomfort.

Pathological examination of the removed tissue showed a trahecn-lated formation calciferous tissue, attached to which were strands of dense connective tissue. Between the trabeculæ there had been extensive hemorrhages. No evidence of infection.

Ten months after this operation patient first noticed intermittent burning sensations in the thigh and as these became more frequent an X-ray was taken three months later. This disclosed a typical pointed exostosis about two inches in length projecting from the outer aspect of the femur opposite the lower extremity of the scar. This was found on operation to arise from the femur at a point corresponding to what had formerly been the lower end of the organized subperiosteal clot and was easily removed. There was no bursa over its irregularly pointed extremity and the bone directly above and the site of the former clot presented a normal appearance.

A microscopical examination of the exostosis differed in no particular from that ordinarily found in that condition.

The patient was relieved of all discomfort and has had no trouble since.

While clinical observations of an unusual character are necessarily void of scientific application, they are not, however, without a certain interest, and perhaps, in the present instance, the possibility of such a clinical history in a bony exostosis may prove of some value in adding another type of benign tumor to those of vascular character which, although they may exceptionally show a rapid growth, must still be retained in the benign class.

SARCOMA OF THE CLAVICLE—END-RESULTS FOLLOWING TOTAL EXCISION *

By William B. Coley, M.D.

of New York, N. Y.

In a paper read before the meeting of the American Surgical Association in Washington, May, 1910, I reported a case of total excision of the clavicle together with ten other cases of sarcoma of the clavicle that had come under my personal observation. Adding to these the cases which I was able to find in the literature, I reported a total of 63 cases, nearly all of which had been treated by total or partial resection. In many of the cases the end-results were not known. Only 2 were traced that had remained well beyond the four-year period.

In 1912 Johansson (*Deutsche Zeitschr. f. Chir.*, vol. lxviii, 1912) found 32 cases in the literature that had not appeared in my list of previously collected cases, and, in addition, he published 3 cases that had come under his own observation.

Kalus (*Inaugural Dissertation,* Royal Univ. of Greifswald, 1912) has also reported two cases since the publication of my earlier paper on the subject.

In addition to these, I have had under my own observation since that time 5 other cases of sarcoma of the clavicle.

Only 5 of my own series of cases have a direct bearing upon the question at issue : the end-results following total excision of the clavicle. In 2 of these cases the operation was performed by myself, and in the remaining 3 by other surgeons, *i.e.,* Dr. Maurice Richardson, Dr. Huntington, and Doctor Freeman. For a fuller history of these 3 cases I would refer you to my earlier paper on the subject, published in the ANNALS OF SURGERY, December, 1910.

CASE I.—*Periosteal round-celled sarcoma of the clavicle.* J. V., male, aged sixteen years, noticed pain and swelling of the left clavicle shortly after a severe strain. The tumor was of rapid growth and involved two-thirds of the inner portion of the clavicle. The diagnosis was established by physical signs and X-ray photographs, without an exploratory operation. On November 22, 1909, I performed a total excision of the clavicle, from which the patient made an excellent recovery. A few days later he was put upon the mixed toxins of erysipelas and bacillus prodigiosus, which were kept up for a period of three months. Almost no deformity resulted from the operation and the patient retained complete functional use of his arm. He served in the Army in France during the war, and at the

---

* Read before the American Surgical Association, May 5, 1920.

time of my last examination, in February, 1918, nearly nine years later, he was in good health with perfect functional use of the arm. Microscopical examination made by Dr. James Ewing.

CASE II.—*Periosteal round-celled sarcoma of the left clavicle.* J. W. H., male, aged thirty-four years, injured the left clavicle in January, 1908, shortly after which a local swelling appeared which grew rapidly. A total excision of the clavicle was done by Dr. Maurice H. Richardson, of Boston, on May 18, 1908, the tumor being so large that the operation was very difficult. As soon as the wound healed the patient was referred to me by Doctor Richardson for prophylactic toxin treatment. The treatment was begun in New York and carried out under my direction by Dr. H. L. Trulock, of Dixmount, Maine, for a portion of two years. Doctor Richardson believed the prognosis so grave from operation alone that he stated in his letter if the man made a permanent recovery he was willing to give the entire credit to the toxin treatment. According to a letter received from the patient at the present time (April, 1920), he is still in good health without the slightest trace of a recurrence, twelve years later. Microscopical examination made by Doctor W. F. Whitney, of Massachusetts General Hospital, Boston.

CASE III.—*Periosteal round-celled sarcoma.* I have performed one other total excision of the clavicle since my former paper, the history of which is briefly as follows: T. M., male, twelve years old, entered the Hospital for Ruptured and Crippled in December, 1912, and was referred to me by Doctor Whitman. The patient had always been well until five weeks previously, when he fell from a step-ladder, the inner portion of the right clavicle striking upon the corner of a wooden box. Two weeks later a swelling appeared at the site of the injury, apparently arising from the bone; no pain, but very rapid increase in size. On December 17, 1912, or three weeks from the time the swelling was first noticed, physical examination showed a large tumor about the size of a hen's egg, markedly protuberant in the region of the sternum and right clavicle, occupying the inner half of the right clavicle and apparently involving the suprasternal region. It was very soft, almost fluctuating in consistence, some areas being denser than others; the superficial veins were markedly dilated. The X-ray photograph showed almost complete destruction of the inner third of the right clavicle. Clinical and X-ray data made the diagnosis so clear that no specimen was removed for microscopical examination. I performed a total excision of the right clavicle on December 20, 1912, with practically no loss of blood, and the patient suffered very little shock. Clinically, the tumor was definitely of periosteal origin. Doctor Ewing's full report of the whole specimen is as follows:

Specimen consists of clavicle which fractured about the middle point, where it runs directly into the tumor mass. Periosteum strips easily, shaft of bone is eroded beneath it. The outer end of clavicle is largely destroyed by tumor growth which has split up layers of periosteum and bone shaft and invaded the

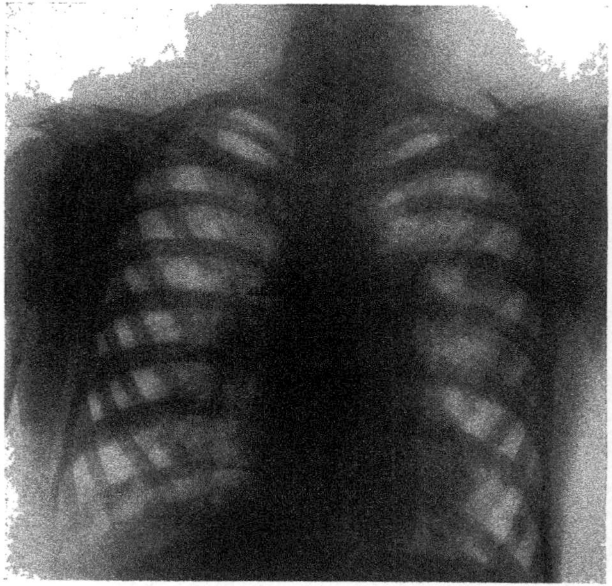

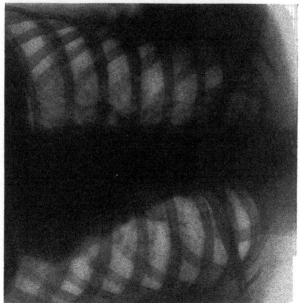

FIG. 1.—Case VI. Two and one-half months after treatment. No evidence of lung involvement at time treatment was begun.

FIG. 2.—Case VI. One month later.

232

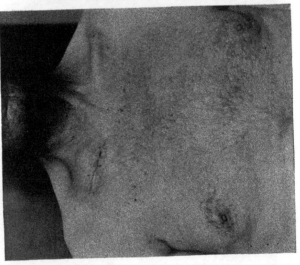

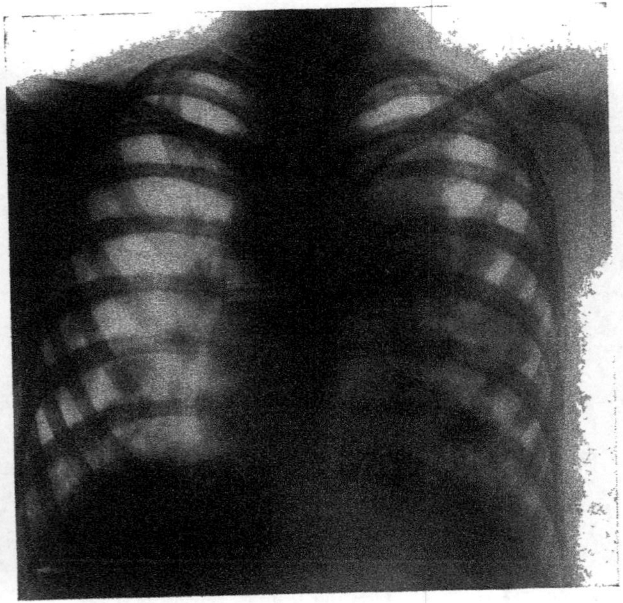

FIG. 4.—Case VII.

FIG. 3.—Case VII.

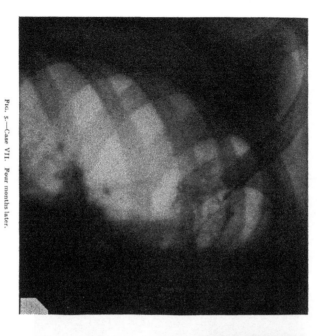

FIG. 5.—Case VII. Four months later.

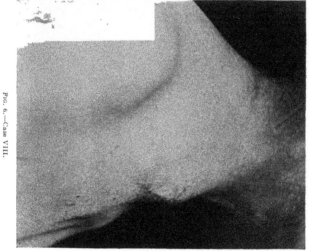

FIG. 6.—Case VIII.

232 B.

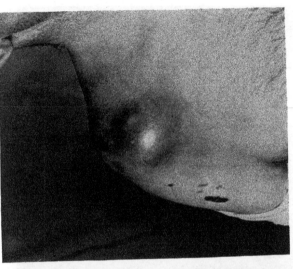

Fig. 8.—Case X.

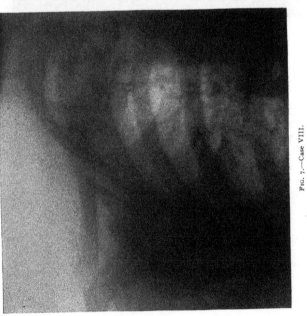

Fig. 7.—Case VIII.

surrounding muscle for a distance of ½ cm., producing a rounded tumor in this region. The gross appearance is not distinctive of either central or periosteal sarcoma. The outer end of the bone is much thickened and the bone is irregularly absorbed. Through the centre of the globular mass of tumor runs a sharp white line indicating periosteum, beyond which the tumor infiltrates muscle and fat.

Histology.—The tumor belongs in a class commonly called small round-celled sarcoma. Cells are small, 10-12 micr. in diameter, with poorly defined cytoplasm, hyperchromatic vesicular nuclei. The shape where preserved is polyhedral, cell bodies are clear, arrangement is diffuse, the cells often sheathing numerous · small blood-vessels. Size of cells remarkably uniform. One large artery is filled by mural tumor thrombus. Muscle is extensively invaded and destroyed by a diffuse focal growth of tumor cells. Histological indications are highly malignant. Exact source of the cells undetermined.

Ten days after the operation there was a marked swelling at the site of the old tumor having every appearance of a local recurrence. The patient was then put upon the mixed toxins which were continued daily until a reaction of 102°–103° was obtained. At the end of two weeks the swelling had disappeared and the patient regained his lost weight. The treatment was kept up for two months, after which he returned home for several weeks and had no treatment. He was readmitted for another course of toxins, lasting about a month. However, in the interval in which the treatment had been discontinued a local recurrence appeared just below the site of the clavicle, in the pectoral region, and also in the neck. The recurrent tumor was soft, almost semi-fluctuating and grew with great rapidity. Although the toxins were resumed and the patient was treated with radium by Doctor Abbe, nothing was able to check the rapid progress of the disease. Metastases developed in the chest shortly after and proved fatal. The total duration of life from the time the trouble was first noticed was about five months.

In this case I believe a great mistake was made in stopping the toxin treatment too soon.

CASE IV.—The case of Dr. Thomas W. Huntington, of San Francisco, Cal., although published in full in my earlier paper, is worthy of special note here, inasmuch as the patient was still in good health when last traced, seven years later. A brief history is as follows: Periosteal, spindle-celled sarcoma of the right clavicle, operated upon on September 8, 1908. Immediately after the operation Doctor Huntington wrote me inquiring as to the advisability of using the mixed toxins as a prophylactic against recurrence, and I replied that I would strongly advise their use. The treatment was begun two weeks after the operation and continued for a period of five months. When last seen by Doctor Huntington in 1915 the patient was still in good health, seven years later. (This case was one of periosteal sarcoma (spindle-celled).)

CASE V.—*Round-celled inoperable periosteal sarcoma of clavicle and scapula becoming operable under treatment.* The history of the case as contained in a personal letter received from Doctor Freeman is as follows: H. L. S., male, twenty-three years of age. First seen by Doctor Freeman July 17, 1908. The patient had sustained a fracture of the scapula and clavicle eighteen months before; enlarged glands had appeared above the clavicle three months before. One month before he came under Doctor Freeman's care he had another injury, falling upon his back. Shortly afterward a rapidly growing tumor appeared over the right clavicular region. At the time of Doctor Freeman's examination there was a large tumor, involving the upper scapular and clavicular region and extending nearly to the spine; there also was a glandular tumor in the neck, as large as a fist, and another of equal size in the deltoid region. The glands of the left side of the neck were also enlarged and had been enlarged for four weeks; the patient had lost 14 pounds in weight. A specimen of the tumor was removed for microscopical examination and pronounced large round-celled sarcoma with some spindle-cells. The case was regarded as entirely inoperable, even as regards an interscapulo-thoracic amputation. The patient was therefore put upon the mixed toxins of erysipelas and bacillus prodigiosus combined with X-rays. On September 1st, or six weeks later, marked improvement had occurred; the tumor had decreased to half its original size and was much softer. Soon after the patient returned to his home in Oklahoma. Shortly after he had a severe hemorrhage and an interscapulo-thoracic amputation was performed.

Doctor Freeman has kindly written me from time to time, giving the after-history of the case. In his latest letter he stated that the patient was well in 1918, ten years after the treatment.

The only case in my series which was operable at the time of observation, but in which it was decided to try radium instead of operation, is as follows:

Case VI.—S. L., female, aged twelve years. Family history negative. No trauma.

Patient was admitted to the Memorial Hospital in August, 1919, with a history of, one month ago, having first noticed a small nodule, the size of a marble, in the sternal portion of the right clavicle, which grew very rapidly until it had reached the size of a small hen's egg. Physical examination at this time showed a smooth, rounded swelling of the right clavicle, symmetrical in outline, moderately firm in consistence, about 2 inches by 1½ inches in diameter. The skin was normal in color, not adherent, and there was no marked dilatation of superficial veins. An X-ray picture taken on August 7, 1919, showed the inner third of the clavicle involved by a rarefying process extending outward from its inner end; space between end of bone and sternum is abnormally wide; suggests beginning in clavicle; chest negative.

Although in the opinions of the surgical staff the case was clearly operable, it was decided to try the effect of radium alone with no other treatment. Accordingly, the radium treatment was begun on August 10, 1919, and given as follows by Dr. Douglas Quick:

August 8, 1919: Radium pack, 9279 mc. hours at 6 cm. distance over the clavicle.

August 14, 1919: Bare tubes containing 17 mc. of radium emanation were inserted.

August 29, 1919: A lead tray, 8000 mc. hours, at 5 cm. distance over the tumor.

October 4, 1919: Radium pack, 10,087 mc. hours at 6 cm. distance over the tumor.

November 16, 1919: Lead tray, 3000 mc. hours, at 3 cm. distance over the tumor.

In addition she received seven X-ray treatments over the anterior chest in November, 1919.

On August 20, 1919, the patient was discharged from the hospital with a decrease in the size of the tumor. Examination on September 2d showed improvement.

An X-ray picture taken on October 7, 1919, showed very little change in the condition of the clavicle. Physical examination November 7, 1919, showed the patient to be improving slowly. An X-ray examination was made on the following day, a report of which is as follows: " X-ray of chest reveals numerous well-marked metastases in lungs. Process in clavicle remains unchanged." She was readmitted to the hospital on November 11, 1919, at which time examination showed no growth in the clavicle tumor, but examination of the chest revealed metastatic nodules. Her general condition was not so good; she was anæmic and had lost considerable in weight. She tired very easily and had occasional pain in the chest.

In spite of X-ray treatments over the chest the patient's general condition rapidly deteriorated and she died on January 20, 1920.

The entire duration of the disease in this case, from the time the tumor was first noticed, was a little over six months; and from the time the treatment was started five months. The very rapid generalization of the disease points to a high degree of malignancy of the tumor. No exploratory operation was made and hence we do not know the histological type of the tumor. It was undoubtedly a periosteal, probably round-celled. Whether the patient could have been saved had the clavicle been removed by total excision, followed by prophylactic treatment with the mixed toxins and radium, it is impossible to state. However, from the results that have been obtained in the other cases already reported, I believe that the chances of a cure would have been greater had such method of treatment been employed. While we have no evidence to show that the very rapid generalization of the disease in the lungs following so closely the introduction of bare tubes of radium in the clavicular tumor was due to the treatment there is a possibility that the introduction of these tubes and the rapid breaking down of the tumor cells may have favored the development of metastases. We have, however, used bare tubes in so

235

many other cases in precisely the same way without any apparent influence in the development of metastases, that it is fair to state that it may
have been only a coincidence in this case.

This, as far as I know, is the only case in which radium has been used
in an easily operable case in this country.

However, a case of periosteal sarcoma of the clavicle, treated with radium
alone, was briefly reported by Pinch, of the Radium Institute, of London,
about three years ago, and a personal communication from Doctor Pinch
received a few weeks ago, contains the following data:

Female, aged sixty-two, was sent to the Institute in June, 1913, for the treatment of a
large, rapidly growing periosteal sarcoma of the right clavicle, which had been present for four months. An attempt at its removal had been made in May, but the
surgeon found this could only be done if Berger's operation were performed, and
patient would not consent to this procedure. The growth formed a prominent tumor,
filling up the right supraclavicular fossa and measuring 10.5 x 6 x 2 cm.; it was very
firmly fixed to the clavicle. Microscopical examination of portions removed showed
it to be a round-celled sarcoma.

A 100 mgr. tube screened with 1 mm. of silver was buried in the tumor for twenty-
four hours. The growth steadily shrank, and by the end of July no trace of it remained.

The patient was examined in January, 1918. There had been no recurrence, and
all movements of the right arm could be performed fully and freely. Examination
February, 1920, showed the patient perfectly well with no recurrence.

While this case in a measure offsets the distressing result obtained in the
case I have just reported from the Memorial Hospital, it does not, in my
opinion, furnish sufficient evidence to justify one, at the present moment,
in substituting radium treatment for surgical operation in an easily operable
case of sarcoma of the clavicle.

The results of excision thus far reported enable one to state definitely
that the functional result following total excision is so good and the deformity
so slight, that one is not warranted in taking much additional risk in attempting to save the bone. Our own case observed at the Memorial Hospital shows
the great danger of general metastases developing while waiting to observe
the local effect of the radium-ray treatment upon the clavicle.

We have had two border-line cases, in which the possibility of removing
the clavicle was doubtful, and we decided to give the patients the combined
toxin and radium treatment. In both of these cases large doses of radium,
massive doses externally. and bare tubes inserted by means of a hollow needle
in the tumor itself. In addition the patients were kept for long periods
under large doses of the mixed toxins. In both these cases the improvement
following the treatment proved only temporary and metastases devoloped
within six months, ending in death.

CASE VII.—B. F., male, aged forty-nine years, referred to me on
August 5, 1918, by Dr. F. H. Albee, of New York, with the following
history: Eight weeks ago, while attempting to raise a window, felt
sudden, sharp pain in the right shoulder, which ceased on stopping

motion and recurred on active motion of the arm. The following day
he noticed a swelling over the right clavicle. An X-ray picture was
taken, which showed a fracture. Arm and shoulder immobilized. Another X-ray picture was taken four weeks later, on July 1st—inconclusive. Wassermann reaction negative. July 20th, exploratory operation
by Doctor Albee. Microscopical examination of specimen removed
showed large round-celled sarcoma. The report reads as follows:

> Gross section is a thin section of bone with hemorrhagic streaks and on
> one side are pinkish-white, semi-soft, irregular tabs of tissue. Microscopically,
> the entire picture is of sheets of rather polyhedral or large round cells staining
> darkly and frequently dividing. These sheets are held in a fibrous stroma and
> in an alveolar pattern, although frequently overrunning these trabeculæ or
> capsules as the case may be. The picture is typical of malignancy.

Physical examination at the time the patient came to me showed a firm
tumor occupying one-half of the right clavicle, beginning at the sterno-
clavicular articulation and extending 3½ inches outward. Yielding on
pressure shows a pathological fracture.

The patient grew rapidly worse, and in February, 1919, his condition
was hopeless.

CASE VIII.—C. A., male, fifty-seven years old, referred to me by
Dr. Geo. S. King, of Bayshore, L. I., on December 26, 1918, with the
following history: Patient always in good health until September, 1917,
when he strained his right shoulder while cranking a car. Shortly
afterward noticed pain in his neck and a swelling in the sternoclavicular
articulation on the right side. The pain and tenderness decreased
somewhat and there was little change for nearly a year. An X-ray
picture taken in December, 1918, showed some destruction of bone at
the inner end of the right clavicle. A month ago the swelling began
to increase more rapidly in size after slight exertion. X-ray pictures
taken then showed an extension in the destructive process of the bone,
with some crepitation. Wassermann reaction negative. Patient has
been unable to raise his arm to a horizontal position for the past three
weeks. Physical examination December 26, 1918, showed a swelling
occupying the inner two-thirds of the right clavicle, extending to, and
involving, the sternocleidoclavicular articulation. The tumor measured horizontally 5 inches and vertically 4 inches; it was firm, almost
bony, in consistence and very tender on pressure, particularly over the
central portion, and extended up to the cervical region several inches
above the normal clavicular line. Just above the upper margin is a small,
movable cervical gland, one-third inch in diameter. There is slight
dilatation of superficial veins. Patient had lost 15 pounds in weight
during the past year. After consultation with Doctor Downes and
other members of the staff, the condition was believed inoperable, and
it was decided to use the combined toxin and radium-ray treatment.

On December 31, 1918, bare tubes containing 3986 mc. hours of
radium emanations were introduced into the clavicle; and on January 1,

1919, a radium pack of 9864 mc. hours at 10 cm. distance was placed over the right clavicle for 9 hours.

At first there was marked diminution in size of the tumor and great improvement in the patient's ability to use the arm. After about two months, however, the swelling began to increase in size and the patient's general condition to deteriorate. In spite of continued treatment, pushing the radium to the point it was thought safe, it was impossible to gain control of the disease. The patient continued to decline and died on March 27, 1919.

The following case, like my own second case of total excision, shows the extreme malignancy of some cases of sarcoma of the clavicle. The history of this case was kindly furnished me by Dr. Walter B. James, who showed me the X-ray pictures and consulted me as regards treatment:

CASE IX.—A. L., male, forty-eight years of age; always strong and well until September, 1913, when he fell, while playing golf, striking upon the shoulder and injuring his left clavicle, but not apparently sustaining any fracture. The arm was put in a splint for several weeks. A short time after the injury, a swelling developed in the region of the clavicle, which was first believed to be tuberculous. All tests for tubercular and specific disease proved negative. An X-ray picture taken in December, 1913, showed marked destruction of the inner end of the clavicle with apparently some involvement of the mediastinal glands. Rapid decline in general health. The patient's physician, Dr. E. R. Baldwin, of Saranac Lake, on February 26, 1914, said: " The patient is now dying of slow collapse with every evidence of a dissemination of sarcoma." Death occurred two days later, making the entire course of the disease from the time of the injury to death, less than five months.

In the following case the disease ran nearly as rapid a course as in the preceding:

CASE X.—A. T. B., forty-seven years of age, was referred to my service at the Memorial Hospital, on April 3, 1917, with a history of having had an attack of influenza followed by pleurisy; was in bed for ten days. At the end of this time he first noticed symptoms in the right shoulder and outer part of clavicle, tenderness, swelling and some limitation of motion; was treated for rheumatism for a number of weeks. In the meantime the tumor of the clavicle rapidly increased in size. On April 3, 1917, the radiograph showed almost complete destruction of the right half of the clavicle, with extensive involvement of the roots of both lungs by metastatic nodules. He was treated for a brief period of two to three weeks with the mixed toxins of erysipelas and bacillus prodigiosus with no appreciable effect. In view of the marked generalization of the disease, it was thought unwise to continue the treatment. He died a few weeks later, the entire course of the disease being less than six months.

CASE XI.—H. K., male, aged thirty-one years. In May, 1897, carried heavy piece of steel on right shoulder; one month later noticed lump directly over clavicle at the point where the steel rested. July, 1897, removal of gland below clavicle by Doctor Mayer, of Buffalo. Three weeks later a nodule appeared in the axilla. When seen by me in February, 1898, the patient's neck and shoulder were occupied by an enormous tumor extending to sternum in front and nearly to the vertical column behind. No treatment advised. Prognosis: Six weeks to two months' life.

CASE XII.—Mrs. L. C., adult, was referred to me on July 19, 1912, with the following history: In June, 1911, she had had a strain in the region of the right clavicle. Two months later a small swelling was noticed in the sternal end of the clavicle, which gradually increased in size. She was treated for rheumatism for six months. The clavicle was excised by Doctor Trout, of the Jefferson Surgical Hospital, Roanoke, Va., in May, 1912, and a pathological examination showed it to be an angio-sarcoma involving the sternal end. As much of the surrounding tissue as possible was removed and X-ray treatment given; but in spite of this, a recurrence developed in a few weeks.

Physical examination, in July, 1912, at the time of my first observation, showed an inoperable recurrent mass just above the sterno-clavicular articulation. The patient complained of pain and numbness in the arm. The end-result in this case has not been traced.

CASE XIII.—D. B. A., male, adult. The patient first noticed a swelling in the sternal end of the right clavicle in November, 1909, for which an operation was performed in January, 1910. A second operation was performed in 1911, at which time the glands were removed. In August, 1914, a total excision was made, and in the beginning of the following year, 1915, the patient noticed œdema of the right arm and forearm. He was referred to me by Dr. J. B. Hulett, of Middletown, N. Y., in November, 1915, at which time physical examination showed an inoperable mass above the site of the right clavicle, extending over to the sterno-mastoid insertion and two inches backwards. The mass was firmly fixed and quite inoperable. The patient had lost slightly in weight. I was unable to get a pathological report in this case, but the tumor was undoubtedly a malignant one. It has been impossible to trace the final result.

CASE XIV.—*Round-celled periosteal sarcoma of the left clavicle.* Patient was referred to me by Dr. J. Collins Warren, of Boston. Specimen removed in October, 1903, was pronounced round-celled sarcoma. The tumor almost entirely disappeared under X-ray treatment, but later started to increase in size and was no longer controlled by the X-rays. In October, 1904, the patient was referred to me by Doctor Warren. At this time a pear-shaped tumor occupied the sternal portion of the left clavicle; there was glandular involvement above and below the clavicle and slight enlargement of left arm. From October 6 to November 26 the mixed toxins were given in conjunction with X-ray treatment, with slight temporary improvement only.

CASE XV.—H. B., male, aged twenty-two years. No single trauma, but in habit of carrying iron pipes upon left shoulder. Pain in shoulder

239

more than a year before tumor appeared. Small mass in outer portion of left clavicle noticed in January, 1910. Removed by Doctor Stewart, Newport, R. I., in March. Microscopical examination showed tumor to be round-celled sarcoma, periosteal. Recurrence three weeks later; rapid growth. Patient seen by me in September 15; toxins started immediately and continued to October 20, 1910, with little or no effect in controlling growth.

Patient died three months later.

CASE XVI.—E. S., male, aged twenty-one years. Patient broke his left clavicle in May, 1893; one year afterward a swelling appeared at the site of the fracture and grew rapidly. Partial removal of clavicle. recurrence soon after, involving scapula. Mixed toxins tried for a short period, without success. Excision of remaining portion of clavicle; entire scapula and upper extremity removed by Dr. W. W. Keen, of Philadelphia. Death eight months later from recurrence.

CASE XVII.—G. M., male, nineteen years of age. Tumor had existed for two years; first treated for rheumatism. No trauma. Came to New York Hospital in April, 1909, where Dr. Frank Hartley did a total excision. Microscopic examination made by Doctor Elsner, who reported the disease to be spindle-celled sarcoma. Three months later, local recurrence above and below the former site of the former clavicle. Patient referred to me in September, 1909, with numerous recurrent masses over the whole upper portion of the right chest. The mixed toxins were given, and while at first there was considerable decrease in the size of the various nodules and increased mobility, the improvement was temporary only and the toxins failed to control the further growths of the tumors. Patient died a few months later.

CASE XVIII.—*Periosteal sarcoma of clavicle. Partial resection. Death one year, in Case LXI, tables.*

Three cases reported by Dr. H. B. Delatour, which, by an oversight, were not included in my former paper, are worthy of note.

CASE I.—A. H., male, aged thirty-seven years; operated upon July 21, 1896, at the Long Island College Hospital. Antecedent trauma, May, 1894; injured left clavicle while wrestling; three months later tumor appeared at about the middle third of the bone. This grew slowly until November, 1895, when it suddenly ruptured while patient was walking on the street; hemorrhage profuse. The following day the tumor was removed. Hemorrhage during operation very severe, controlled with difficulty. Four months later, local recurrence; second operation in July, 1896; the tumor was the size of a hen's egg; veins dilated; no enlarged glands. Patient made a good recovery. The report states that 33 months after operation there was no evidence of a return. According to a personal communication received, the patient was alive five years later, since which time he was lost track of. The patient was able to perform the same type of work (porter in a rubber factory) as before operation, without any inconvenience. Pathological diagnosis: Type of tumor not stated, apparently of central origin.

CASE II.—Female, aged twenty years; no trauma; history of swelling and neuralgic pain in the right arm for two months. There was also a tumor in the posterior surface of the clavicle. Pathological diagnosis: Osteo-sarcoma (Dr. Van Cott). Patient lost sight of shortly after operation.

CASE III.—Sarcoma of the clavicle, involving sternum and first rib. Male, aged fifty-five years. History of a tumor of two months' duration which appeared shortly after a local injury, three months before; very rapid growth. Operation August 14, 1897. Complete extirpation of clavicle; division of rib and sternum from the left sternoclavicular articulation to the second chondrosternal articulation. Removal of a triangular portion of the sternum and inner portion of the first rib; several enlarged glands were removed from the anterior mediastinum. Patient discharged six weeks later in good condition. On December 7, 1897, the patient was admitted to the same hospital suffering from a fracture of the base of the skull, from which he died. No evidence of a return of the growth.

Case reported by Dr. George Tully Vaughan (*Med. News*, January 8, 1898).—W. S., male, twenty-eight years of age. Symptoms of seven months' duration before operation; considerable pain; tumor occupied the inner two-thirds of the clavicle. Operation at the German Hospital, Philadelphia, October 22, 1895; ether anæsthesia. The entire right clavicle with tumor removed; troublesome hemorrhage, requiring 20 ligatures. Primary wound healing, except at two points. Discharged 41 days after operation. Microscopical examination showed the tumor to be a mixed-celled (round and spindle) sarcoma. (Dr. Alfred Stengel.) One year after operation absolutely no deformity, except the absence of the clavicular prominence; patient is performing his work as fireman on a steamboat, without any inconvenience from the loss of the clavicle. Arm is free from pain and strong as ever.

A recent communication from Doctor Vaughan, dated April 16, 1920, states that the patient was perfectly well when last heard from, eighteen years after removal of the clavicle. At that time he had what his physician in the West believed to be a mild form of tuberculosis of the lung; he did not think it was metastatic or a recurrence.

Case Recently Reported and Not Included in Previous Collections.— Dodd (*Ohio State Med. Jour.*, March, 1918) reports a recent case of sarcoma of the clavicle: Female, aged thirty-five years, first noticed a swelling in the right clavicle in March, 1916. This gradually increased in size until October, 1916, when it began to grow more rapidly. In February, 1917, it had reached the size of a grapefruit. The patient was seven months' pregnant. Operation was performed in February, 1917; there was some sloughing of the flap; on the fifth day the patient developed septicæmia and died on the fourteenth day after operation. Microscopical examination showed the tumor tissue rich in cells: osteo-sarcoma with some mucoid in the cellular substance, round and spindle-celled; no giant cells were found; tumor of periosteal origin.

In view of the great size of the tumor and the extent of the involvement, I believe this case should have been considered an inoperable one.

WILLIAM B. COLEY

Myeloma of the Clavicle.—Dr. James M. Hitzrot, before the New York Surgical Society (Transactions, ANNALS OF SURGERY, 1918, vol. lxviii, p. 92), reported a case of myeloma of the clavicle in a male, forty years of age. The patient fractured his right clavicle near the sternal end in January, 1917. Shortly after noticed a small swelling at this site, which slowly increased in size. He was admitted to the New York Hospital on February 20, 1918; Wassermann test negative. Total excision of the clavicle was performed by Doctor Hitzrot. A microscopical examination of the tumor by Doctor Ewing showed it to be a myeloma. Five X-ray treatments were given in the region of the clavicle after operation as a prophylactic.

Trauma.—In my own series of cases of sarcoma of the clavicle there is a history of antecedent local injury in such a large proportion of the cases that it is very difficult not to believe that trauma is an important etiological factor in the disease. The nature of the injury varies between a strain and a blow: Case I, Severe strain, tumor developing in three weeks. Case IX, Fall; local injury to the clavicle; tumor in three weeks. Case VIII, Shortly after a severe strain of the shoulder from cranking a car. Case VI, no trauma. Case III, Is a good example of acute traumatic malignancy, inasmuch as the tumor developed two weeks after striking the clavicle upon the sharp corner of a wooden box. Case VII, Severe strain, tumor two months afterward. Case VII, Carrying a heavy steel bar directly over the clavicle, some distance. One month later a tumor developed at the exact site. Case XVIII, Severe strain from swinging off a trolley car while in motion; tumor one month later. Case XVI, Tumor at site of a fracture which had occurred one year before. Case V, Injury to shoulder (fracturing clavicle and scapula) two months before. Case XI, Severe bruising of shoulder while carrying steel bar, due to helper's dropping the other end. Tumor two to three weeks later, at the site of the injury. Case II, Plank fell over and struck patient on left clavicle six to seven years previously. Case X, No history of trauma, but tumor developed ten days after an attack of acute influenza.

Johansson states that the great majority of these tumors are sarcomata. A very rare but interesting group of bone tumors, from a pathologico-anatomical point of view, are the so-called endotheliomata. Howard and Crile, in 1905, had collected 23 such cases, and Johansson's statistic includes two additional cases probably belonging to this group.

The so-called strumametastases form another very rare type of bone tumors. Four of these are known to have occurred in the clavicle and were treated by extirpation. Histologically, they present the characteristics of adenoma. The primary tumor may be a carcinoma, Johansson states, or more rarely, also an adenoma. In a few instances no struma at all could be found; the thyroid gland was atrophic. I do not believe there has been reported a single undoubted case of primary carcinoma of the clavicle—in some cases the primary tumor was not.

SARCOMA OF THE CLAVICLE

Johansson reports the following three cases of malignant disease of the clavicle, two of which were operated upon at the Sabbatsberg Hospital:

CASE I.—A. J., female, aged sixty-eight years, 1903. In March, 1901, patient fell and sustained a supracondylar fracture of the left humerus. In February of the following year she again fell and fractured the arm immediately above the old fracture. X-rays at the time had shown no suspicion of a tumor. Good union of fracture within normal time. Good apposition and function of arm. Toward the end of the same year, patient noticed swelling at the site of the fracture, accompanied by some pain. Readmitted to the hospital on February 5, 1903. Examination at this time showed a large tumor occupying the lower half of the left humerus. Diagnosis: *Osteosarcoma*. Exarticulation of humerus. Primary union. Two weeks later, swelling of right shoulder. Examination shows a tumor, nearly half the size of a hen's egg, at the acromial end of the right clavicle. Microscopical examination: Spindle-celled sarcoma, small cells. Patient discharged from hospital March 28, 1903. Death five years later, March 2, 1908, of catarrhal enteritis. The report states that she was able to use her right arm perfectly well, and that there was no sign of a recurrence. No autopsy.

CASE II.—U. F., female, sixty-seven years of age; 1911. Patient ascribes trouble to trauma, a friend having repeatedly struck her with a board—in fun. Examination at time of admission, July 12, 1911: Firm tumor palpable over outer third of right clavicle, size of a hen's egg, attached to the bone. Diagnosis: peripheral sarcoma. July 15, extirpation of clavicle; no enlarged glands. Microscopical examination, spindle-celled sarcoma. About five months after operation, marked loss of weight, considerable coughing and pain in chest. Death of cachexia January, 1912.

CASE III.—O. B. (Military hospital, Seraphim), male, fifty-eight years of age, 1888. Slight injury to clavicle a year ago; sensitiveness at site of injury three weeks later, swelling within one month. This grew slowly at first, then increased more rapidly in size until at time of operation, beginning of August, it had reached the size of a fist, attached to the bone; no enlarged glands. Total extirpation of clavicle plus upper right points of sternum; discharged November 19, 1888. Not traced. Microscopical examination: Chondrosarcoma.

Johansson gives a brief résumé of 32 cases of tumor of the clavicle previously reported but not contained in any of the lists of collected cases so far published (see table). He also gives the references of six additional cases, stating that the respective journals were not available.

Only 3 of a series of 62 cases of bone sarcoma observed at the Sabbatsberg Hospital from 1879 to 1911 were sarcomas of the clavicle.

Age and Sex.—Of 84 cases regarding which statements as to age and sex were found, 51 were males, 33 females, or about 60 per cent. of males.

Sarcoma of the clavicle is most frequently observed at the age of puberty, the eleventh to twentieth year of life. Nearly 60 per cent. of the cases occur in patients below the thirtieth year.

Localization.—Statistics show the cases of malignant tumor of the clavicle to be about evenly divided between the right and the left side. Thirty occurred in the sternal end of the clavicle; 18 in the acromial end; 10 in the middle portion, and 4 involved the entire clavicle.

Three cases of metastatic sarcoma of the clavicle are on record, namely, Besson's case, in which nine years before a resection of the upper jaw had been done; Johansson's case here reported, in which the primary

243

tumor originated in the humerus, and Jones' case, in which the original tumor started in the tibia, causing a fracture.

The desire to know whether we are dealing with a comparatively benign or a highly malignant tumor in a given case has become more pronounced since the conservative treatment of bone sarcomas, as first proposed by Mikulicz, has been gaining ground. That histological examinations are not always reliable in this respect no doubt most surgeons have had occasion to observe.

Johansson states that Ribbert and Borst have greatly advanced the study of the histology of bone sarcoma by their recent contributions to the subject. The former considers all sarcomas of the bones as originating in the spongiosa of the diaphyses, which theory seems to find support in the great significance of the X-rays as regards determining the degree of malignity of the tumors.

Borchard, on basis of Borst's investigations, distinguishes between a central group—from which he excludes and forms into a separate group the so-called myeloid tumors—on the one hand, and an inner or outer periosteal group—according to whether they start from the inner or outer layer of periosteum—on the other hand. In the former case they are surrounded by a bone shell.

Of the 30 cases of sarcoma of the clavicle compiled by Johansson, 9 were resections, 15 total extirpations. Of the remaining 6 cases of malignant tumor of the clavicle, 5 were treated by total extirpation, one by resection.

Mortality.—Delatour gives the operative mortality as 18 per cent. (40 cases); Caddy, 16 per cent. (42 cases); Johansson's collection of 31 cases operated upon (25 sarcomas) shows no mortality. The mortality on basis of 87 cases would, therefore, be 11.5 per cent. Johansson believes, however, that this percentage is too high an estimate, inasmuch as at least 3 of the cases should be excluded, namely, v. Langenbeck's and Heath's cases in which death was due to a brain tumor; and Segond's case in which visceral metastases were the cause of death. Deducting these, the above figure would be reduced to 8 per cent. Then also allowance should be made for the fact that a number of these fatal results occurred in pre-antiseptic times.

Accepting the time limit of four years, which is the latest period at which recurrences have been observed, Johansson states that only 4 cases were found to have remained free from recurrence, one of these (Mott's famous case) fifty-five years, another ten years, and two others upwards of five years. Three of these were central sarcomas. To these should be added the Vaughan case well eighteen years, which makes 5 cases cured by total excision in a series of 90 cases.

Functional Result.—Experience has shown that the functional value of the arm after extirpation of the clavicle is but little impaired in most cases. In 21 of Johansson's 36 collected cases mention is made of the

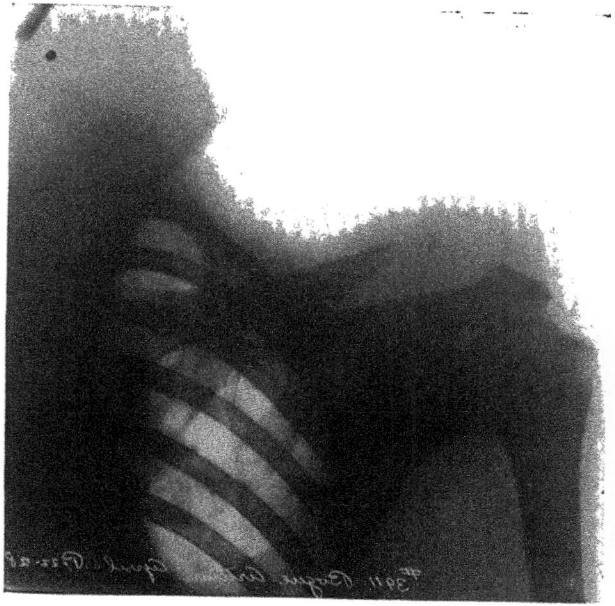

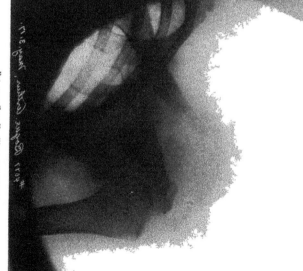

FIG. 9.—Case X.

FIG. 10.—Case X. Three months later.

functional result, and of 20 this is stated to have been good or very good. The deformity, also, is generally given as slight.

Kalus made a careful study of the literature up to 1912, which showed a total of 98 cases, 92 of which were stated to be sarcoma. He reports two cases operated upon at the Greifswald Clinic, one an osteosarcoma, the other an adenocarcinoma, which was considered to be metastatic, although the seat of the primary tumor could not be determined at the time of the operation.

In the first case (osteosarcoma of right clavicle) resection of a piece 7 cm. long was done, with Gigli's saw and bone transplantation from tibia added. The patient, a woman forty-seven years of age, was operated upon on September 18, 1910, and discharged on the 24th of October. Six months later she returned complaining of severe pain in the right clavicle. Examination showed the presence of pseudoarthroses at the junction of clavicle and transplanted bone. The pain is apparently due to the wire sutures. A second operation is done and the patient is dismissed on the 10th of April, 1911, with free use of the arm, although the pseudoarthrosis persisted. There is no deformity at the site of operation. A report obtained from the local physician nine months after the second operation, states that the patient complains of pain at the site of operation and inability to use the arm for any length of time. There are no enlarged glands; no signs of a recurrence; general condition good.

In view of the splendid results obtained after resection or total extirpation of the clavicle, without bone transplantation, Kalus believes this an entirely unnecessary procedure.

CASE II.—Male, aged sixty-two years. In August, 1911, laid a heavy beam upon his left shoulder in order to lift a wagon; pain and swelling followed. Was treated by physician with salve. In September was able to resume his work as mill worker. Two weeks later return of swelling, little pain, but limitation of motion of left arm. Later some loss of weight. Admission to the Greifswald Clinic November 1, 1911; operation on the 7th. Removal of tumor which was the size of a man's fist; considered metastatic; primary tumor not found. Uninterrupted wound healing. Discharged December 16, 1911. Head of humerus prominent on account of absence of clavicle; active abduction in shoulder-joint; active elevation anteriorly greatly limited; rotation around axis of brachium but little interfered with. The patient was reported to have died of cachexia in the middle of September, 1912 (opening of œsophagus into the stomach). Autopsy had shown a primary carcinoma of the cardia with numerous metastatic nodules in the liver.

Kalus believes this to be the first reported case of carcinoma of the clavicle which was recognized as metastatic at the time of the operation, the seat of the primary tumor (cardia) being revealed later at autopsy. I have observed two cases of secondary carcinoma of clavicle but did not operate upon either. Aimes and Delord (*Progrés Medical,* Paris, April 24, 1920, xxxv, No. 17, p. 81) found 98 cases of sarcoma in 126 cases of tumors of the clavicle.

In view of the case already referred to, that of Pinch of the Radium Institute of London, complete disappearance and apparent cure of a sarcoma of the clavicle by a single treatment with radium alone, the patient remaining well for five years—a very important question naturally arises, *i.e.,* shall we

245

TABLE OF REPORTED CASES OF SARCOMA OF CLAVICLE.

No.	Reporter	Date	Reference	Sex	Age	Side	Site	Duration	Description	Operation	Type	Result	Final report	Remarks
1	Mott	1829	Amer. Jour. Med. Sci., 828, iii, 110	M	19	L	Beneath and adherent to clavicle	......	Size of two fists	......	Osteo. with ulceration	Recovery	Well 50 years	......
2	Warren	(1832)1837 1838	Surg. Va. of ..., p. 405 Med. and Surg. Trans., xxi, 135	M	24	R	Inner end	1 year	......	Total excision	Pulsating	Recovery	Well 6 mos.	Died of pleurisy 4 weeks after Trauma
3	Travers	1838	Med. and Surg. Trans., xxi, 135	M	10	L	Inner end	1 year	......	Total excision	Osteo.	Recovery	Well 6 mos.	......
4	Liston	1844	Lancet, p. 361	M	..	..	Outer	......	......	Total excision	Soft	Recovery	Recurred in 3-4 months	......
5	Chaumet	1849	Gaz. Md. de Paris	F	18	L	Outer	9 months	Size of fist	Resection of external four-fifths	Soft	Recovery	......	......
6	Gallardon	1847	Gaz. de Hop.	F	45	..	Middle, sternum, 1st rib	......	......	No operation	Vascular pulsating	......	......	Died of bronchopneumonia
7	Rigaud	1850	Gaz. Md. Strasbourg. A. X., p. 103	F	15	L	Inner	7 years	Size of fist	Resection of inner two-thirds	......	Recovery	......	Final results not traced
8	Owens	1854	New ... M. and S. J., vol. ii, p. 164	F	35	L	Inner	1 year	Egg	Excision, one-half	Osteo-sarcoma	Recovery	Well on tenth day	......
9	Langenbeck	1855	... Klinik	F	11	L	Both ends	......	......	......	Osteo. Spindle-cell	Died on 6th day	......	......
10	Syme	1857	Ed. Md. J., iii, Pt. I, 192	F	20	..	Outer end	......	3½ x 4½ cm.	Total excision	Osteo.; myeloid cells; cystic	Recovery	......	......
11	Cooper	1858	Gaz. de Hop.	..	..	L	......	......	-	Total resection	....	Recovery	......	......
12	Esmarck	1859	...den. Diss. de reset. Kiliae ... de Paris	M	33	R	......	......	Size of a hen's egg	......	Myeloid	Recovery	Recurrence; died in 4 yrs.	......
13	Nélaton	1860	...den. ...	F	46	R	Inner end and sternum	2 years	......	......	Myeloid	......	......	Died of bronchitis
14	Gosselin	1861	Bull. Soc. de Chir., 2d series, ii	M	37	R	Inner third	......	Size of a lemon	Resection of inner third	Fibrous elements Spindle-cell	......	......	Fracture
15	Pean	1861	Gaz. de Hop., p. 419	M	37	..	......	......	Size of a citron	......	Spindle-cell	......	......	......
16	Nélaton	1863	Bull. Soc. Anat., 2d series	F	30	..	Middle	......	:	......	Fibrous and fibroplastic	......	......	......
17	Richet	1864	Dict. de Md. et de Chir. Pratiq., viii	M	65	R	Inner third	2 years	......	Resection of inner third	Myeloid	......	Recurred 18 months after in scar	......
18	Paquet	1867	Bull. de la Soc. Anat., p. 634	M	21	..	Inner end, sternum, 1st rib	6 months	12 x 8 cm.	No operation	Embryonic sand myeloid	......	......	Died
19	Delore	1868	Gaz. Md. de Lyon, iii, 93	..	Child	..	......	......	......	......	Medullary carcinoma	Recovery	......	Doubtful
20	Morin	1868	Ib.	..	..	..	......	......	......	......	......	......	......	Doubtful
21	Meyer	1868	Gaz. Md. de Lyon, N. 8, p. 93	..	Child	..	......	......	......	......	......	......	......	Doubtful

No.	Name	Year	Reference	M/F	Age	L/R	End	Duration	Size	Operation	Pathology	End (result)	Recurrence	Remarks
22	Sean and Eve	1869	Chicago Med. Exam., x, 653	M	12	L	....	14 mths	....	Total excision Vein injured at operation	....	....	....	Cervical glands enlarged; died from exhaustion
23	Gy	1870	St. Louis Med. and Surg. Jour., p. 62	M	30	L	the	....	....	....	....	Recovery	....	....
24	Britton	1870	Brit. Med. Jour., i, 518	M	35	L	ther end	2 years	Size of an i ego	Resection of all except acrom. end	....	Recovery	....	....
25	Be	1871	Nashville Jour. Med. and Surg., i, 68	M	13	L	....	7 mths	Size of an rary	....	Enchondroma (red, flesh-like)	Died	....	Doubtful; spontaneous fracture
26	Robat and Demondre Tausini	1873	Paris Thesis	F	51	L	ther end	3 months	Size of an orange	Resection of outer end	....	Healed in 15 days	....	....
27		1883	Gaz. degli Ospitali, Milano, No. 30, p. 306	F	30	..	inner end		Size of an egg	....	Myxœdema	....	....	....
28	Depris	1885	Bull. de Soc. de Chir., pp. 143–226	F	14	R	ther end	....	Size of an orange	....	Central	In hospital 31 days	....	....
29	Segond	1885	Ibid.	M	66	..	....	....	....	....	....	Died on 8th day of visceral involvement	....	....
30	Polleaillon	1885	Bull. de Soc. de Chir., p. 146	M	16	R	Outer end	18 months	Size of fist	Resection of external three-fourths Total resection	....	Recovery	Well 3 mos. died of sarcoma of femur	....
31	Kronlein and Ritter	1885	Inaug. i. Zurich	F	17	L	Central part	....	....	....	Periosteal; round cell	....	Prompt recurrence; well 10 yrs.	....
32	Wheeler	1885	Trans. Ac. M. of Ireland	M	43	L	....	....	....	....	....	....	....	Slight blow; ph... well 10 yrs later
33	Sloan	1887	Am. Jour. M. Sci., p. 485	M	14	R	....	....	....	....	Carcinoma (?)	....	....	....
34	Heath	1888	Lancet, i, 721	M	30	L	Outer end	3 years, 10 months	....	Excision	Spindle and round cell	Seven days after operation developed br. symptoms	Recurred 6 mos. after Died on 11th day	Dou.ful
35 36	Khe Wber	1888 1889	Hosp. Tiden de Kopenhagen, Feb., i, 310	F M	15 18	.. ..	....	....	....	....	....	....	....	....
37	Rouse	1889	Lancet, i, 575	M	20	..	Inner end	6 weeks	Size of an egg	Excision Resection of inner two-thirds	Myelogenous	Died of sepsis	Soon recurred	Vein injured
38	Jesset	1889	Lancet, p. 1077	F	18	R	Inner end	....	....	....	....	Healed in 2 months	....	....
39	Harlam	1863	Brit. Med. Jour., p. 848	M	31	..	....	....	....	....	Periosteal; round-cell	Primary union	Well 5 mos.	....
40	Garre-Norkus	1893	Beitrag. sur klin. Chir., ii	F	31	R	Outer end	1 yar	2 inches long	Total excision	Myeloid; pulsating	Immediate recovery	Well 5 years	....
41		1893	Am. Jour. Med. Sci., xxxiv, 350	F	20	L	....	5 y ars	....	....	Osteosarcoma	Recovery	....	Probably syphilitic

247

TABLE OF REPORTED CASES OF SARCOMA OF CLAVICLE—*Continued.*

No.	Reporter	Date	Reference	Sex	Age	Side	Site	Duration	Description	Operation	Type	Result	Final report	Remarks
42	Legueu	1895	Bull. Soc. Anat.	F	24			3 months	Nut	Total excision	....	....	....	Pulmonary tuberculosis
43	Courtin	1897	Gaz. Hbd. des Sc. Med. de Bordeaux, xviii.	F	Birth	L	Middle and inner end	....	....	....	Osteo.	....	Lived 1 mo.	
44	Verstraete (Operator Duret)	1898	Jour. de Sc. Med. de Lille, i	M	46	R	Middle and inner end, 1st and 2d ribs	7 months	Size of an orange	Total resection	Subperiosteal; encapsulated	Recovery	Traced one month	
45	Besson (Operator Duret)	1898	Ibid. Page 466	M	39	R	External end	7 months	Size of an egg	Total excision	Myeloid; periosteal Round and spindle myeloplexus	Recovery	Traced only 3 weeks	Operated on 9 years before for sarcoma of superior maxillary
46	Flament	1898	Ibid., ii	M	10	R	External two-thirds	1 month	Size of an egg	Resection of external two-thirds	....	Recovery	Well 1 month	
47	Bourg	1902	Paris Thesis	M	45	R	Middle and inner end	2 years	Size of an orange	Total resection	....	....	....	
48	Jonnesco	1903	Bull. et Mem. Soc. de Chir. de Bucarest, vi., 53			L	....	....	....	Total resection	Geo.	Recovery		
49	Degonville	1904	Paris Thesis	M	50	L	Middle third	2 years	....	....	Myeloid and ducell			
50	Kryukoff	1904	Rbk. Vrach., St. Petersburg, iii, 775	P	12	R	....	....	....	Total resection	Round-cell			
51	Buteanu	1905	Bull. Soc. de Md., et Nat. de Jassey, xix.				....	....	....	....	do.			
52	Coley	1909	Am. Surg., 1910 (Coley)	M	16	L	Middle portion, myelogenous, round-celled	6 weeks	Size of an English walnut	Total resection followed by toxins	Periosteal	Recovery	Well at present, 1910; one year later	Toxins diet immediately after operation
53	Huntington, Thos. W.	1908	Ibid.	M	39	R	Outer and middle third	2 years	English walnut in size	Total resection followed by toxins (Coley)	Spindle-celled periosteal	Recovery	Well 2 years	Followed a blow
54	Gilbert Barling, Birmingham, Eng.; personal communication	1889	Unpublished Ibid	M	33		Inner half	Several months	....	Resection total	Spindle-celled	....	Died on 4th day from suppuration of mediastinum and pleurisy	Fracture through middle of bone

248

No.	Reference	Year		Age/Sex	Side	Location	Duration	Tumor size	Operation / Treatment	Pathology	Result	Outcome	Notes
55	Ibid.	1901	Ibid	F 10	L	Middle and inner portion	......	......	Total excision	......	......	Recurred 9 months after, in ear; died a few mos. later	Plank fell over striking patient on left clavicle
56	Richardson, M. H.; personal communication (Coley)	1908	Ibid	M 34	L	Middle and inner third	4 months	......	Total excision followed by toxins (Coley)	Small round-celled	Recovery	Well 3 years and 3 mos.	Toxins then used; temporary; imprv. only
57	Hartley, Frank	1909	Ibid	M 19	L	......	2 years	......	Total excision	......	Recovery	Recurred in 3 months in side of chest	Received blow Oct. 1905
58	Keen, W. W. (Coley)	1898	Ibid	M 21	..	......	......	......	First operation, incised, interscapular thoracic amputation; toxins; Pott, lancing of abscess; second, partial [removal] of tumor	......	Recovery	Died 8 mos. later, fem recurrence	
59	Bodine (Coley)	1906	Ibid	M 8	R	......	3 months	......		Periosteal; round-celled	......	Death in a few months	
60	Warren, J. Collins (Coley)	1902	Ibid	M 40	L	......	6 months	......	No [operation]; toxins; X-ray	Periosteal; round-celled	......	Died 1 year later	Trauma; dislocation of shoulder
61	L. L. College Hospital (Coley)	1909	Ibid	M 38	L	Inner third	1 week	......	Operation wk later; Partial removal of [tumor]	Rapid growth	Recurrence in 1 sternal fossa; toxins then given with but little benefit	Died in 1 year	Strained shoulder
62	Stewart (Coley)	1910	Ibid	M 20	L	Outer third	2 months	Tumor size of English walnut, outer end of clavicle	Operation; Dr. Stewart, Newport, R. I., 1910 March. (E skin)	Periosteal; round-celled	Recurrence 3 weeks; very rapid growth	Mixed toxins (Coley) Sept. 15 to Oct. 15, 1910; no effect on very large tumor	
63	Coley	1898	Ibid	M 31	R	Outer end	9 months	Tumor of enormous size	General condition very bad; prognosis, few wks of life	No operation	No treatment		No single trauma, but habitually carried iron pipes and heavy material on left shoulder. Died

249

TABLE OF REPORTED CASES OF SARCOMA OF CLAVICLE—*Continued.* (Most of the following cases were collected by Johansson.)

No.	Reporter	Date	Reference	Sex	Age	Side	Site	Duration	Description	Operation	Type	Result	Final report	Remarks
64	Johansson	1903	Deutsche Zeitschr. f. Chir., 1912	F	68	L	Acromial end secondary to osteosarcoma of humerus	Few weeks after extirpation of humerus f. osteosarcoma	Size of half a hen's egg	Extirpation of clavicula	Spindle-celled sarcoma small cells	Good	Death 5 yrs. later of enteritis—no sign of recurrence	Fractured humerus twice. Osteo-sarcoma exarticulation of humerus
65	Ibid.	1911	Ibid.	F	67	R	Outer third	6 months	Size of a hen's egg hard trauma	Extirpation of clavicle	Spindle-celled sarcoma	Fair	Six months later death cachexia	
66	Ibid. (military hospital)	1888	Ibid.	M	58	R	Sternal end		Trauma swelling 1 month later	Total extirpation	Chondro-sarcoma	.....	Not followed up	
67	Smith J. W.	1902	Brit. Med. Jour., 1902, I, p. 720	M	18	L	Outer two-thirds	5 months	Trauma	Total Excision	Chondro-sarcoma	Good	Recurrence 1 year later	Death
68	Barton	1874	Dublin Med. Jour. of Med. Science, 1874, I, p. 92	F	24	L	Below left clavicle near sternal end	Little over a year	Size of cocoanut	Inoperable	*Medullary cancer	No operation	Death duration of life, 2 years	Autopsy showed metastases of lung and right humerus
69	Jones	1880	Trans. Path. Soc., London, 1880, vol. 32, p. 242	F	45	L	Primary in tibia, metastases in parietal bone and clavicle, sternal end		No trauma	No operation	Sarcoma			
70	Sansom	1884	Lancet, 1884, I. p. 563	M	40		Supraclavicular fossa, extending into axillary cavity	5 months	First noticed swelling of right shoulder and arm, started in middle of clavicle	No operation	Mixed-celled sarcoma periosteal	.....	Death	Autopsy showed metastases in kidney
71	Lunn	1886	Trans. Path. Soc., London, 1886, Vol. xxxviii, p. 287	M	64	R	Right clavicle	2 weeks	Large tumor starting in periosteum	No operation (inoperable)		.....	Death	Autopsy showed nodules in surface of liver
72	Sutton	1890	Lancet, 1890, II, p. 821	F	26	R	Acromial half			Resection of acromial half	Myelogenous	Excellent		Not traced
73	Other	1891	Traité des Resections, 1891, Vol. III, p. 895	F	42	..	Sternal end		"Pulsating tumor"	Resection of sternal end		Only fair	Death after 2 years	Nothing stated recurrence

*Almost certainty sarcoma from description of case.

74	Caddy	1892	N. Y. Record, 1892, Vol. xliii, p. 586	M 26	R	Sternal end	10 mths	Large tumor sternal end	Resection of inner two-thirds	Periosteal spindle-celled	Good	6 mos. later no recurrence	Death
75	Gibb	1895	Glasgow Med. Jour., 1895, Vol. xliv, p. 301	F 16	L	Sternal end	mths	Trauma	Resection of inner third	Spindle-celled	Good	Local recurrence 15 mos. after operation	
76	Baur	1896	Annals of Surgery, 1903, Vol. xxxvii,	M 37	L	Me of lunicle	mths	Trauma	Excision of clavicle after recurrence	"Osteosarcoma"	Very good	No recurrence three years later	
77	Baur	1897	Ibid.	F 20	R	Acromial end	2 months	No trauma	Excision of entire clavicle	Osteosarcoma	Good	Not known	
78	Delatour	1897	Ibid.	M 55	..	Sternal end	3 months	Trauma	Excision of sternal end of clavicle plus piece of sternum and of first rib	Sarcoma	Complete use of arm	4 mos. later fracture of base of skull	No evidence of return of tumor
79	Vaughan	1898	Med. News, Jan. 8, 1898	M 28	R	Inner two-thirds of clavicle	7 months	Large hard tumor	Removal of entire right clavicle with tumor	Mixed-celled round and spindle	Excellent	Perfectly well 18 yrs. later	Personal report from Doctor Vaughan
80	McBurney	1898	Annals of Surgery, Vol. xxviii, p. 259	M A	L	Sternal end	18 months	....	Total excision	Osteosarcoma	Almost normal Gd	Not known	Further history not known
81	Curtis	1898	....	M 37	L	....	Trauma 9 years ago	abt 9 years ago	Total excision	Osteosarcoma	Gd	1 year later operation for metastasis in 7th rib of left side	
82	Beatson	1902	Brit. Med. Jour., 1902, I, p. 129	F 16	..	Sternal end	7	No trauma	Gd excision	Angiosarcoma round-celled	Almost normal	No recurrence 2 yrs. later	
83	Smith	1902	Brit. Med. Jour., 1902, I, p. 720	M 35	R	Sternal end	5 n onths	Bra	Tal excision	Chondrocma	Gd, little deformity	Free from recurrence when last seen, 13 mos. after operation	
84	Carson	1904	Am. Pract. of Surg., Vol. vi, p. 420	F 18	R	Sternal end	6 months	No trauma	Total excision	Sarcoma	....	Not known	
85	Vogel	1908	Med. Klinik, 1908, I, p. 286	M 27	R	Outer half	2 months	Trauma 7 mos. before; size half of hen's egg	Resection of outer two-thirds bone transplanted from tibia	ed sarcoma	Good	Well 2 yrs. later, no recurrence	Transplanted bone was soon pushed off

251

TABLE OF REPORTED CASES OF SARCOMA OF CLAVICLE—*Continued.*

No.	Reporter	Date	Reference	Sex	Age	Side	Site	Duration	Description	Operation	Type	Result	Final result	Remarks
86	Jordan	1908	Deutsche med. Woch-enschr., 1908, I, p. 175	F	8	L	....	....	....	Total excision of left clavicle, piece of scapula and 1st rib	Round-celled sarcoma	Good	Well and free from recurrence 7 mos. later	....
87	Roith	1908	Deutsche med. Woch-enschr., 1908, I, p. 175	F	17		Medial portion	....	Size of goose egg	Total excision	Cysto-sarcoma	Good	....	Cause not stated
88	Piperata	1909	Deutsche Zeitschrift f. Chir., 199 Bd. 102, p. 195	M	74	L	Sternal portion	3 months	....	Resection of sternal end	Chondro-sarcoma	....	Death after 3 years	Partly local recurrence, partly metastases
89	Piperata	1909		M	19	L	....	7 months	....	Resection of left clavicle with tumor	Spindle-celled sarcoma	....	Death within a few mos.	
90	Piperata	1909	Ibid.	F	23		...	5 months	Inoperable	No operation	Sarcoma	....	Died within 10 months	
91	Ganducheau et Masson	1909	Bull. et Mém. Soc. Anat. de Paris, 1909, p. 61	M	54		Mie portion	6 mths	No trauma—size of walnut	Type of operation not stated	Periosteal round-celled sarcoma	Not stated	Not stated	
92	Patel	1910	Lyons Med., 1910, p. 715	M	24	L	Middle portion of left clavicle	3 months	Size of hen's egg	Total excision	Sarcoma osteides	Excellent, hardly pr-fect	Not stated	Wassermann positive Hg. J. R. treatment; tumor increased in size steadily
93	Wilson	1911	Lancet, 1911, I, p. 1422	F	11		Inner half	....	No trauma	Resection of inner half	Sarcoma probably periosteal mixed celled	Good	Free from recurrence 7 mos. later	
94	Schmidt	1906	(Ref. Annual Rep.)	F	57		....	....	Grown into deltoid muscle, thyroid structure	Excision of clavicle	Tumor of thyroidal at-ture	Good result	....	Thyroid not enlarged
95	Halperine	1908	(Ref. Guibe)	M	54		Outer end	20 years then trauma	More rapid growth after trauma; size of fist	Total excision	Thyroidal structure; struma present	....	....	Grew rapidly after trauma

252

No.	Author	Reference	Year	Sex/Age	Side	Location	Duration	History / Symptoms	Operation	Pathology	Result	Recurrence	Thyroid gland
96	Guibé	Bull. et Mém. Soc. Chir. de Paris, 1909, p. 117	1909	F 51	R	Outer third	......	No trauma pulsating tumor, size of a hen's egg. No glands. Struma and struma metastases	Exarticulation of inner and then outer half		Very good	No recurrence a little over a year later	Thyroid gland atrophic
97	Jaboulay	(Ref. Annual Rep., 1909)	1909	M 60		......			Extirpation of clavicle; 2 weeks later partial removal of struma	Struma, metastases in clavicle. Spontaneous fracture of bone	Good	Not known	
98	Suchard and le E.	Rev. de Chir., 1883, Vol. 3, p. 618	1883	F 62	R	Sternal end	6 months	No trauma, size of hen's egg; pulsating	Total excision	Malignant tumor cystic epithelioma		No recurrence, abs. 10 months later	
99	d'Estar and A. F. Bock	Rev. de Chir., 1908, Vol. 39, p. 343; St. Louis Med. Jour., 1894, p. 347	1908	F 50		Outer two-thirds	......		Almost total resection	Lymph-angioma	....		Author > epits wry tile benefit from operation 6 mos.,
100			1894	M 55	R	Sternal end	3 months	No trauma, pain severe	Removal of tumor large size	Large round-celled sarcoma	Survived operation		amputation of arm at lder joint for osteo-sarcoma
101	A. T. Bristow	Blyn. Med. Jour., 1898, p. 306	1898	M 22	L	Lower border	2–3 weeks	Painful, size of duck's egg	Removal of clavicle	Fascial sarcoma later, osteo-sarcoma mixed, small round-cells, no spindle cell	Excellent recovery	2 wks. observation O. K.	
102	Jas. Thorburn	Canadian Practitioner	1883	M 43	R	Above sternal half	9 weeks	Trauma carried holes size of orange	Removal of tumor	Spindle-celled sarcoma, some round-cells	Good	Recent observation	No a tumor in ... region found—to be ... on ... since ... hood
103	Küttner	Allg. Med. Centralztg. p. 198	1909			Sternal end	.	Size of fist, spontaneous fracture	Exarticulation sternoclavicular joint	Spindle-celled sarcoma	Good functional result		
104	Ibid.	Ibid.	Ibid.			Ibid.	......	Size of hen's egg	Total excision	Osteo-chondro mixed sarcoma	Good functional result		
105	Pinch	Personal communication		F 62	R	......	4 months	10 x 6 x 2 cm.	Inoperable except by Beiger shoulder joint amp. Patient refused	Round-celled sarcoma	Treated by radium only	Complete disappearance	Well 5 years

253

PERSONAL CASES OBSERVED BY THE WRITER SINCE THE TIME OF HIS LAST REPORT IN 1910.

No.	Name	Year	Sex	Age	Side	Site	Duration	Trauma and other data	Operation or treatment	Type	Result functional	Final result	Remarks
1	B. P.	1918	M	49	R	Sternal half	8 weeks	Strain of shoulder, patholog. fracture	Exploratory by ther surgeon. ller toxin and radium treatment	Large round-celled sarcoma	Temporary improvement only	Death in 6 mos.	Borderline case as regards operability
2	C. A.	1918	M	57	R	Inner two-thirds	1¼ year	Strain of shoulder	...ed inoperbl. ... tons and radium (Giley)	....	Temporary improvement nly	Death, March 27, 19, a year and 5 mhs after the injury	Borderline case
3	T. M.	1912	M	12	R	Inner half	5 weeks	Trauma; size of hen's egg	Total mn, recurrence; then toxins 2 months	Periosteal small round-celled sarcoma	Recurrence after 10 days	Temporary improvement; death 5 ms. after first noticed	
4	S. L.	1919	F	12	R	Sternal portion	1 month	Size of hen's egg	Radium	Periosteal	Local improvement, but generalization of disease	Death within 6 months from the tmor was first noticed	This case was ble wh a sen, but it was decided to use dim treatmnt alone

give radium treatment or toxin treatment, or a combination of both, before excision, or, shall we excise the clavicle and use the treatment, singly or combined, after operation as a prophylactic against recurrence? I have never used the toxins in operable cases of sarcoma except in such cases where operation meant the sacrifice of the limb. In sarcoma of the clavicle, the loss of the clavicle cannot in any sense be regarded as analogous to the loss of a limb. The single brilliant success of Pinch, in which no operation was performed, is offset by the Memorial Hospital case, in which radium was tried in preference to operation, with rapid generalization of the disease and a disastrous end result. Personally, I would strongly hesitate to use radium alone, or with toxins, in any operable case of sarcoma of the clavicle, for fear that early metastases of the lungs might develop while watching the usual rapid and remarkable local disappearance of the tumor. If the clavicle were of great importance to the patient, like one of the bones of the arm or leg, I would take the chance of trying to save it by the use of toxins and radium before operating; but, our own results as well as those that have been reported by other men, show that the functional use of the arm is practically normal after total excision of the clavicle and the deformity is so slight as hardly to be regarded.

In 87 cases of sarcoma of the clavicle in which the sex was noted, 49 occurred in the male, and 38 in the female, the greater number in the male being probably accounted for by the fact that the male is much more exposed to injury than the female.

As regards the age of the patient at the time the sarcoma was first noticed, our statistics show that by far the greatest proportion occurred in youth or early adult life, e.g.: 1 at birth; 5 between the ages of one and ten years; 29 between the ages of eleven and twenty years; 17 between the ages of twenty-one and thirty years; 16 between the ages of thirty-one and forty years; 12 between the ages of forty-one and fifty years; 10 between the ages of fifty-one and sixty years; 6 between the ages of sixty-one and seventy years; 1 over the age of seventy years.

As regards the site, as far as known 39 occurred on the right side and 33 on the left; in 41 cases at the sternal end, 16 at the middle, 18 at the outer, and in 1 case both clavicles were involved.

Regarding the duration of the disease, our statistics show in 9 cases less than one month; 2 cases less than one month; 4 cases less than two months; 9 cases less than three months; 1 case less than four months; 3 cases less than five months; 7 cases less than six months; 6 cases less than seven months; 2 cases less than nine months; 4 cases less than one year; 2 cases less than one year and two months; 2 cases less than one year and six months; 7 cases less than two years; 1 case less than four years; 1 case less than five years; 1 case less than seven years; 1 case less than nine years; 1 case less than twenty years.

My own series of cases show a definite history of trauma in 12; no trauma in 3; and not stated in 3 cases.

WILLIAM B. COLEY

In the total number of tabulated cases, 108, the disease was too far advanced for operation at the time of observation in 10 cases; and in 56 cases total excision, or practically total excision, was performed.

It is worthy of note that only 5 patients out of 80 treated by total or partial excision of the clavicle are known to have remained well beyond four years. While 3 out of 4 patients treated by the mixed toxins of erysipelas and B. prodigiosus as a prophylactic after total excision are alive and well from six to twelve years.

CONCLUSIONS

1. Malignant tumors of the clavicle are comparatively rare, only 16 cases having occurred in upwards of 275 cases of sarcoma of the long bones personally observed. The greatest number belong to the sarcoma group, the few cases of carcinoma being metastatic developments from some recognized or unrecognized primary focus.

2. Sarcoma of the clavicle occurs more frequently in men than in women, probably due to the fact of the greater liability of the clavicle to injury in the male than in the female.

3. Sarcoma of the clavicle in the great majority of cases is associated with recent, antecedent, local trauma, either in the form of a direct blow or severe muscular strain.

4. *Diagnosis:* A clinical history of pain and localized swelling of the clavicle usually following recent injury, with rapid increase in size, supplemented by a fairly characteristic X-ray picture, will usually make an early diagnosis comparatively easy without the necessity of an exploratory operation.

5. *Treatment:* Local removal of the tumor or even a limited, partial resection should be avoided. The treatment of choice, while the tumor is in an operable stage, should be:

    a. Total excision of the clavicle as soon as the diagnosis is made.

    b. As soon as possible after operation, a course of systemic treatment with the mixed toxins of erysipelas and bacillus prodigiosus should be begun and continued for a period of at least six months. When possible this should be supplemented with local or regional treatment with radium or X-rays.

6. The mortality of total excision of the clavicle under modern technic is so small as to be practically disregarded and the functional use of the arm remains unimpaired.

To Contributors and Subscribers:

All contributions for Publication, Books for Review, and Exchanges should be sent to the Editorial Office, 145 Gates Ave., Brooklyn, N. Y.

Remittances for Subscriptions and Advertising and all business communications should be addressed to the

ANNALS of SURGERY
227-231 S. 6th Street
Philadelphia, Penna.

ANNALS of SURGERY

| Vol. LXXII | SEPTEMBER, 1920 | No. 3 |

SOME OF THE THINGS THAT SURGEONS AS A PROFESSION STAND FOR*

By WILLIAM WILLIAMS KEEN, M.D.

OF PHILADELPHIA, PA.

EMERITUS PROFESSOR OF SURGERY IN JEFFERSON MEDICAL COLLEGE

IT is trite, but profoundly true, for me to say that the distinguished honor you conferred upon me six long and fateful years ago, in April, 1914, in New York City, is deeply appreciated. How ignorant we were as to what was then " in the lap of the gods!" How little we dreamed that in three months' time the dogs of war would be loosed on faithful Belgium and heroic France; that when Britain's honor was touched, she, too, would spring to arms in defense of the Rights of Humanity, of the sacredness of what the whole civilized world recognized as solemn binding treaties, but which Germany deemed only " scraps of paper!"

The heart of the people of America was with you then and is with you to-day. Many of us tugged at the leash when the Louvain Library was given to the flames, when Rheims was ruined by the representatives of Kultur, and still more when the *Lusitania* was torpedoed without warning and went to the bottom in twenty-one minutes. Eleven hundred and fifty-four men, women, and children, including one whom we all loved— a gracious woman on an errand of mercy—were thus murdered by the pitiless Huns. I have seen the coarse, misdated medal struck by the Germans to commemorate forever this hideous crime.

Many of us are also tugging at the leash to-day, longing to help you in your hour of peril. We resent the sinister influences at work, even in some high places, to create dissension between us and our " Allies," as I love to call you. We would gladly throw in our lot with you all—Belgium, Britain, France, Italy, Portugal, and Japan.

What amazing courage and steadfastness you have shown. What impossible things you have done on plain and on mountain peak, in trench and in hospital, on land, on the sea, under the sea where you were comrades of the fish, high in the air where you outstripped and were the envy of the eagle.

We were lost in admiration of your prowess, and suffered with you

---

* The presidential address at the Fifth International Congress of Surgery, July 19, 1920.

in your sacrifice of those that were dearest to you. Even in your hours of defeat instead of yielding to despair you showed what the inspiration of adversity could do, and plucked victory from the Hun.

Finally, when we Americans were allowed to come to your aid, how exultantly our young men and old men, young women and old women sprang to your help and were at least of some aid, though at the eleventh hour. It will always be a joy to us that Château-Thierry was the nearest approach of the Huns to Paris—a perilous nearness of but half a hundred kilometres. There, with uplifted and forbidding hand our message ran: "Thus far and no further," "and it was so," as saith the Scriptures of the Creative Week.

How prophetic, though all unconscious, was the presidential address of that noble Belgian, Professor Depage, in April, 1914! How he turned words into deeds of great pith and moment at La Panne! What lessons in the surgery of wounds he taught us!

How splendidly all of you wrought not only for humanity, but for science! In the four years of the war, how you have transformed surgery! A new era dates from 1914 to 1918!

For me to attempt to discuss any surgical subject before you would be presumptuous. It is for me to sit at your feet and learn how you have acquired your present affluence of surgical knowledge.

In this address, therefore, I venture to recall to your minds some of the things which we as a profession should stand for.

I regret that I can only give a brief paragraph or two to each topic. As to some, you will not all be in accord with me. I can only state my own belief as to what is, or ought to be, the attitude of our guild.

1. *Education.*—I need only to point you to one so lately rapt from us, Osler the scholar, who taught us all what we should study; not only practical medicine in its various branches, among which we may have a chosen one, but the history of medicine, the biographies of our past heroes; nor yet only medicine, but the humanities representing the "Literature of Power" as contrasted with the "Literature of Knowledge"; not only solid prose, but cadenced poetry, with its wings to lift us towards the stars; not only modern literature, but we should also drink of the old, old fountains of inspiration from Judea, Greece, and Rome. Medical education, strictly so called, has made great strides in the last thirty years due to the persistence of the leaders in medical thought and influence. It must still progress *semper et ubique.*

2. *Research.*—I need only pronounce the word to awaken in your minds the contrast of the last years of the great war with the first year when you were groping your way to the light. The absolutely proved conquest of typhoid, typhus, tetanus, smallpox, and perhaps above all the victory over unparalleled infection, are eloquent witnesses to the value—the medical, military, and economic value—of research. This is the greatest of the great achievements of the war.

The savant in the laboratory and the clinician in the hospital have been wedded at the bedside in the bonds of a scientific fellowship, never before so welcome and never before so fruitful for the good of mankind.

Fortunately, in our medical schools, our institutes of research, and the new Red Cross laboratories at Geneva, this wonderful work will be still further developed.

3. *Professional Uprightness.*—In one respect, I have an exultant pride in the honor and uprightness of our ancient guild. With our women patients, our honor is always at stake. We see them alone and we trust them with that which we hold as dear as life itself. On the other hand, they give their honor into our hands with many and unusual temptations. Yet, how rare it is that a medical man is even accused of wrongdoing! Among the hundreds of thousands in many lands (and there are black sheep in every flock), the lapses from honorable and upright conduct are so few that even its possibility scarcely ever occurs to any woman as the door of the consulting room is closed.

The wonder is that among so many women patients there are not more adventuresses who would endeavor to blackmail us. The community trusts us as no other class of men is trusted, and we, God be thanked, have proven ourselves worthy of their trust.

We are a profession, as distinguished from a trade. In the latter there is always a ready means of fixing values by the pound or the yard or by number. The services of our guild can never be weighed in the balance or be measured by length or breadth or number. We should never lower our standards.

A new remedy, a new splint or brace, or a new method of treatment, therefore, should be as free as the air we breathe, a new splint devised in Philadelphia should be as available in Paris, in Tokio, in Cape Town, or in Buenos Aires as in Philadelphia. A new remedy should be available for all doctors and all patients in all parts of the world. They should not be compelled to wait till they could get either the one or the other from Philadelphia or Paris or London, especially when, as often may be the case, to wait even a day may mean death or disability.

4. *Venereal Diseases.*—Never before has this menace to the health and general welfare of the community been so generally appreciated by the public as well as by our profession as during and because of the war. What injures the individual injures the state. Hence the most extraordinary and extraordinarily successful campaign against venereal diseases inaugurated by the war should be zealously continued, now that the war is over.

Ever since the fifteenth century, increased and disseminated by war, syphilis has always been a scourge both to armies and to the population among whom they were encamped. But in the great war the incidence both of syphilis and of gonorrhœa immediately dropped to a startling degree the moment that the men came under army discipline and with the safeguards which surrounded each camp. By these same means the health of the community was protected. The incidence of venereal diseases in the Army was far below that in the civil community.

Now that the armies have been demobilized, the lessons taught the men by lectures and especially by the cinema films, it is hoped, will not be forgotten but will still act as deterrents.

But after all, the only sure and permanent deterrent will be a change in our moral attitude, our moral standards. There must be a " change of heart " to make permanent a change of conduct.

Our young men must be convinced that at the marriage altar where a new family is founded, the bridegroom should be as clean and as pure as the bride. He should realize his responsibility in the conservation of his wife's health and in the creation of strong and healthy children.

A single standard of sexual morality is the only righteous and just standard. It should be just as disgraceful in the judgment of the men and women in the community for a man to have a mistress, as for a woman to have a privileged lover. Social ostracism, now visited only upon the woman, should be meted out equally to the man.

We—we doctors, I mean—who especially well know all the evils not only to the husband, but to the wife and to their children—would not willingly give our daughters to men who are victims of gonorrhœa or of syphilis. Surely, those of us who have sons would be unwilling for them to marry young women already besmirched. Shall our daughters be less jealously guarded than our sons? You know what it would be for your son or your daughter to have wretched, syphilitic children, doomed to a life of misery, to whom death would be a blessing and the tomb a welcome relief.

In the United States, impressed especially by the gravity of the venereal peril, eleven states of the forty-eight have passed laws to safeguard the community from the perils of transmissible and especially of venereal diseases in the marriage relation, in order to safeguard the health of the wives and children. The requirements vary all the way from a medical certificate, after a physical examination, made shortly before marriage, to a mere affidavit of one or both parties that they are free from any venereal or other communicable disease which would impair the health of the children born of such a union. The penalty is fine or imprisonment or both.

I have made a number of personal inquiries from lawyers of the best standing as to how these laws really are working. Some have been enacted too recently to enable any reliable judgment to be formed as to their value; some are ineffective, or ineffectively enforced; some are evaded by marriage in an adjacent state having no such law. Those that are really enforceable and also enforced are of value, in the judgment of health officials and lawyers, partly because their penalties act as deterrents but chiefly because of their moral and educational value.

This movement is sure to grow. I venture the opinion that as the facts as to these diseases and the requirements of the laws become more widely known, especially among young women about to marry, they will be more and more insisted upon by the young women themselves or by their parents.[1]

Proper education in sexual matters should be given to young boys and girls by their parents or by physicians. They should be taught the facts of reproduction in a clean and pure way before they acquire such knowledge by the often filthy teaching from boys and girls a little older than themselves.

5. *Our Altruism.*—We are the only *self-destructive* profession. In unselfish devotion to the welfare of the community, in the battle royal against disease, in the fight for pure water and pure milk and wholesome housing—in a word, in preventive medicine, I glory in the fact that we doctors are always the leaders.

Every disease that is abated, such as smallpox, typhoid, typhus, diphtheria, dysentery, and such like, has had its chief adversary in our profession. A single epidemic of smallpox in a single city will bring more actual revenue to the doctors than a quarter of a century of vaccination, but we are the vanguard in insisting upon vaccination in order to stop this procession of death. We lead the fight for pure water and pure milk to prevent epidemics of typhoid—again wholly to our own financial detriment.

This twentieth century will be only a few years older when yellow fever, one of the former great scourges of the Western Hemisphere, will be actually entirely blotted out of existence. This will be the first instance ever known of such a wonderful miracle in the history of the human race. The glory of it belongs to our profession—to Carlos Finlay, to Walter Reed and his associates, and to that prince of sanitarians, General William C. Gorgas, of the United States Army, whose world-lamented death has occurred since these lines were written.

All honor, then, to the men of our guild for unselfish devotion to the health of the state.

6. *Abstention from Alcohol.*—I have no doubt there will be a greater diversity of opinion on this point than on any other. I can only state my own opinion and give the reasons why I hold it. What I shall say has no relation to the use of alcohol as a medicine but wholly to its use as a beverage.

Without doubt, the least prejudiced conclusion, based upon the results obtained by the most scientific and most rigid experimental investigation, is that

---

[1] The best two publications to be consulted are, " American Marriage Laws in Their Social Aspects," by Fred. S. Hall and Elizabeth W. Brooke, Russell Sage Foundation, New York, 1919, and in a careful study in the Social Hygiene for April, 1920, 105 West 40th Street, New York City, by Mr. Bernard C. Roloff, Executive Secretary of the Illinois Social Hygiene League.

of Dr. Raymond Dodge and Dr. Francis G. Benedict, head of the Carnegie Nutrition Laboratory in Boston. His conclusion is tersely stated in these words: "Any use of alcohol, even though it be occasional, must be regarded as contrary to scientific teachings."[2] Miles,[3] experimenting on doses of 30 c.c. of absolute alcohol, suitably diluted, says that 27 cases out of 30, *i.e.*, 90 per cent., showed inferior functioning after this dose. Kraepelin[4] and Mitander[5] demonstrated greater or less losses of efficiency in the target practice of experienced marksmen after small doses, such as 30 to 40 c.c., of alcohol.

While these results are attained by scientific experiments of great accuracy in a small number of men, the results of prohibition in the United States and later of the adoption of the Prohibition Amendment to the Constitution, demonstrate the extraordinarily beneficial results even within the few months since its adoption. The fact that private stocks of liquor are not yet exhausted, and that the machinery for the effective enforcement of the law is as yet incomplete, and therefore that liquor can be obtained if one can pay the higher prices now charged only add to the strength of the argument from these results.

For actual conditions in New York City I have to thank Mr. Bird S. Coler, Commissioner of the Department of Public Welfare, and Dr. John Fitzgerald, temporarily in charge of Mr. Coler's office. They have most courteously given me complete information covering nine large municipal hospitals, and one even more valuable source of information, a large municipal lodging house.

Of course, I can only epitomize the facts and opinions of the medical officers in charge.

In the lodging house the admissions for January, February, and March, 1919, under license numbered 22,350. In the corresponding months for 1920 under prohibition, they were 4607.[6] Not only were the results so remarkable in numbers, but "the applicants were better, cleaner, and healthier than formerly." Intoxicated applicants were rare, while "formerly we were obliged to call a policeman nightly to have the drunks removed." The employees were giving better care to their personal appearance and were saving money. "I have met men on the street," writes the superintendent, "who were formerly regular lodgers and was surprised at their neat and clean appearance. They are working steadily and buying clothes instead of drink."

Among the hospitals the general result was a largely decreased num-

---

[2] Scientific Aspects of Moderate Drinking, Boston Med. and Surg. Journal, Feb. 18, 1904.

[3] Effect of Alcohol on Psycho-Physiological Functions, Carnegie Institution Publication No. 216, 1918.

[4] Münch. med. Wochnr., 1899, No. 42.

[5] Bericht des 10. Int. Kongr. gegen den Alkohol, Budapest, 1905, pp. 193–204.

[6] The report for March being rendered on the 16th, I added the average for the remaining five days.

ber of admissions, especially for intoxication and delirium tremens. Also, again, among the employees there was great improvement. One report says of them that some of the former worst offenders were opening bank accounts.

The Psychopathic Ward at Bellevue Hospital, of New York City, handles more alcoholics of the vagrant and poor class than any other hospital. Dr. M. S. Gregory, the Director of that ward, writes that in January and February, 1920, instead of 400 to 500 cases a month, there were only one or two a day so that the ward was *abolished!* As soon as the lax administration of the law set in, the number increased to five or six or even ten a day. This, however, was a much smaller number than before prohibition.

In Philadelphia, the House of Correction, in which the most of the cases of vagrancy and alcoholism are treated, instead of a population of over 2000 before prohibition, has a population of only about 400 to 500 since prohibition became effective. In the first four months of 1920, the savings by reason of fewer employees, less wages, less food, and other expenditures, were sufficient to pay all the expenses of the entire Department of Public Welfare for the remaining eight months of the year.[7]

A similar diminution of the number of inmates in the County Prison in Philadelphia has raised the question whether the House of Correction and the County Prison could not be combined with consequent large economies. Four adjoining counties in Massachusetts are about to abolish three jails as the one remaining jail can accommodate all the prisoners of the four counties.

In Philadelphia in the first six months of 1919, under license, there were 17,114 arrests for intoxication. In the last six months under war prohibition, the number was 6509, a decrease of 62 per cent.

In the alcoholic department of the Almshouse (Philadelphia City Hospital) the admissions in the last six months of 1917 and 1918, *i.e.*, before war prohibition, were 1470 and 1184, respectively. In the same period in 1919 under war prohibition, there were only 276, a decrease of 77½ per cent.

In Massachusetts, Mr. H. C. Parsons, Deputy Commissioner for Probation for the whole state, as a result of the first year of prohibition, reports that during the first five months of 1919, under license, there were 34,176 arrests for drunkenness. In the corresponding months of 1920, under prohibition, there were only 10,324—a diminution of practically 70 per cent.

Judge Cabot, of the Juvenile Court, states that the family relations are greatly improved. The parents, instead of neglecting their homes, are trying to make them attractive to live in, and instead of spending their time and money in the saloons, are taking their children to the cinema ("movies") and to church.

---

[7] Personal statement to me by Hon. E. L. Tustin, Director of Public Welfare, in Philadelphia.

Many rural courts have no culprits before them for days and even weeks.

During the war the great improvement in social conditions following the prohibition of vodka in Russia told the same story.

I need not urge on this audience the argument that alcohol is the most powerful and most frequent cause of sexual immorality and its attendant venereal diseases, to say nothing of the evil effects of the alcohol itself.

Whatever may be the conclusions of scientific experiment on the effects of alcohol, the huge experiments on the millions of human beings in the United States as shown above and in Russia seem to me to be conclusive that total abstention from alcohol results in less drunkenness, less poverty, less crime, less disease, fewer accidents, and smaller expense to the city and the state. If so, is it not our duty as a profession to urge total abstinence from the standpoint of the health and the general welfare of the entire community?

As the Supreme Court of the United States has decided that the Eighteenth, the Prohibition Amendment, is constitutional, and is, therefore, the supreme law of the land, it is proper to call attention to the serious effect that prohibition will have upon industry and trade.

Under prohibition undoubtedly fewer hours are lost by workingmen and fewer industrial accidents occur, since both are largely due to alcoholic excesses. In the modern keen competition for the markets of the world, a drinkless nation will thus have a most important economic advantage over a drinking nation, both in the better character of its workmen and in the more uninterrupted hours of labor. Hence the output of its products will be greatly increased and the cost lessened.[1]

7. *Bravery.*—In combating great plagues, when and where have the doctors been cowards? Where have they run away to gain safety for themselves, leaving the victims of disease to suffer and die unattended?

Let Serbia and Poland respond. Let the southern cities in the United States—Norfolk, Memphis, New Orleans—so often devastated by yellow fever, reply. In Europe and America, let the cities which have been decimated by cholera give answer.

The case needs no argument. It is confidently committed to the jury of the world without instructions from any judge. The verdict is and has always been, " Guilty of the highest bravery known among men." Without the gorgeous trappings of war, without the beating of drums and the blare of trumpets, with only " Duty " as a watchword, and Godlike compassion as a motive, they have ministered to the sick and dying and only too often have been among the slain.

8. Finally, we stand for pure and undefiled religion as the surest guide for the present and the surest hope for the future. Observe, I say, not theology, which is a separating, a sundering force, but religion, which is even etymologically that which binds together, and morally is the supreme hope of the world.

---

[1] By accident this and the preceding paragraph were omitted in the French translation in the Gazette des Hôpitaux of July 17, 1920.

THINGS THAT SURGEONS STAND FOR

BE STRONG

Be strong!
We are not here to play, to dream, to drift;
We have hard work to do, and loads to lift.
Shun not the struggle; face it. 'Tis God's gift.

Be strong!
Say not the days are evil—who's to blame?
And fold the hands and acquiesce—O shame!
Stand up. speak out, and bravely, in God's name.

Be strong!
It matters not how deep intrenched the wrong,
How hard the battle goes, the day, how long;
Faint not, fight on! To-morrow comes the song.

—Maltbie D. Babcock.

THE TREATMENT OF CHRONIC EMPYEMA *

By TH. TUFFIER, M.D.

of Paris, France

By chronic empyema is meant a suppuration of the pleura with no tendency to spontaneous cure. This chronic character in itself is always grave. The frequency of the condition has diminished since our better knowledge of the manner of treating acute infections. From the month of August, 1914, to the month of December, 1919, I operated upon 91 acute and chronic suppurations of the pleuræ.

I. TREATMENT OF ACUTE SUPPURATIONS—PREVENTIVE TREATMENT OF CHRONIC SUPPURATION

1. One must first determine the bacteriologic nature of the effusion. Exploratory puncture is here of value. It is, in fact, of the first importance. Pneumococcic pleurisies are usually mild and are often cured by simple aspiration, while streptococcic pleurisies are grave and most often require thoracotomy.

2. If repeated punctures leave a residuum as shown by radioscopy, thoracotomy is done at the point of election in the posterior axillary line under local anæsthesia.

3. Evacuation of effusions and disinfection of the pleura follow. In certain cases the pleura can be closed, *completely and immediately*. Example, 3 cases (2 pneumococcic with cure, 1 staphylococcic with return of suppuration and secondary disinfection with Dakin solution, secondary closure and cure). In most cases we prefer drainage by siphon after thoracotomy. This is the most simple procedure. Radioscopic examination shows progressive diminution of the pleuritic process. For bad conditions persisting in spite of drainage (as to pulse, temperature, and general condition), and a continued large infected cavity in the pleura we proceed thus: Extensive thoracotomy and pleuroscopy under local anæsthesia permitting a view of the form and dimensions of the pleuritic cavity; disinfection by the Dakin method, numerous Carrel tubes placed in all corners of the cavity. If a broncho-pleural fistula exists, discontinuous injections of oxygen are substituted for the Dakin solution. When the culture curve has reached zero and a dry compress placed at the opening of the cavity remains dry for twenty-four hours, complete closure is made of the surgical orifice, resection of the edges of the fistula, tamponing of the pleura to avoid discharge of blood into the interior, and complete suture of the wound. One thus transforms the former pyothorax into an

---

* Read before the American Surgical Association, May 3, 1920.

aseptic pneumothorax which is spontaneously cured by bringing back the parietal pleura into contact with the lung.

The volumes of the operated cavities were as follows: 6 had a content of 2 to 3 litres; 5 had a content of 1 to 2 litres; 7 cases showed enormous cavities, exact size not given; 2 cases showed rapid cure; 7 cases were lost, all of acute pleurisy medically treated, this variety being always more grave than suppurating and operated pleurisy.

With regard to the time of thoracotomy, of the 7 patients succumbing after intervention 5 were operated early after the pleural effusion ·had

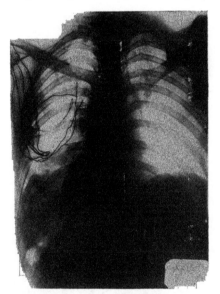

FIG. 1.—Use of armed rubber tubes for exploratory purposes.

occurred, when suppuration had scarcely begun and *general* evidences of infection were intense. All 5 cases were streptococcic. Case XII was cyanosed, with arterial hypotension of marked degree. Case XX after a three-months pregnancy presented the same symptoms with intense dyspnœa and oliguria. Case XXIII added to these symptoms an œdema of the thoracic wall. Patients affected with purulent pleurisy recent in origin or with post-grippal or originally purulent pleurisy were ill but a few days (eight to fifteen at most). Onset was sudden and all cases presented the septicæmic type characterized by more or less cyanosis of the face and extremities, dyspnœa whose intensity was more in relation to the toxæmia than with the quantity of pleural effusion, and pharyngo-laryngeal

267

symptoms. To these phenomena of intoxication were added in three of the cases (XXII, XXIV, XXV) external evidences of the general infection (facial erysipelas, diffuse phlegmon, erysipelas of the costal wall on the side affected) which developed with the greatest rapidity.

Thoracentesis done before operation brought no relief to these cases. The abundant effusion, invading the entire pleura, was an ill-looking, dirty-yellow, sero-sanguineous liquid, often of putrid odor and associated with adhesions of greater or less density.

In Case XXIV we were able to verify the septicæmic character of the

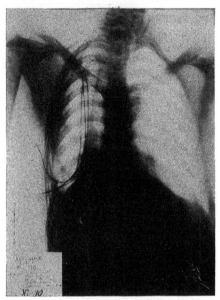

Fig. 2.—Use of armed rubber tubes for purposes of exploration.
(Gagneux.)

infection by spleen changes (enormous size and doughy consistence), the pleurisy being thus but a local manifestation of the general condition. In these five cases the blood culture was positive for streptococcus. Another of the cases (Case XXII) cured, is of the same kind. In these the operative intervention was later, and we repeated several times before and after operation intravenous injections of antistreptococcic serum.

Analysis of the events following intervention at the height of the infection prove that the pleural effusion was only an epiphenomenon and that it was the general infection which was in no wise modified by the evacuation of the effusion which brought these patients to us. I will not venture to draw the conclusion that one must temporize in the treatment of suppurating pleurisies and to wait until they play the rôle of operation abscess before being incised. At all events, these facts plead against immediate thoracotomy in the non-surgical pleurisies which concern us. If the effusion causes untoward conditions, remedy of it by puncture is better than a more complete operation.

Notwithstanding other treatment, *four acute cases became chronic,* causation being as follows:

Pleural diverticula and broncho-pleural fistulæ rendered disinfection im-

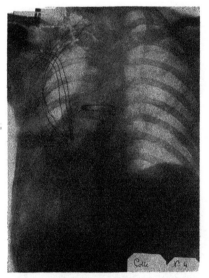

FIG. 3.—Use of armed rubber tubes for purpose of exploration. (Cotte.)

possible. One could easily locate the seat of a chronic infection by seeking out the situation of the microbic attack. When in a pleural cavity that appeared to be aseptic one sought in various regions for the microbic focus, one found a single and persistent septic cavity. By means of electric pleuroscopy one thus diagnoses a diverticulum of the pleura which is not reached by the antiseptic solutions injected and which empties itself very completely.

Bronchial fistulæ are equally factors in producing chronic conditions because of the septic features which they entail. I have noticed two effects of this sort of infection, the first being a necrosed bronchial cartilage, the course and termination of which were followed under conditions described below, *viz.:*

CASE XI.—The patient before entering our service had spent a month being treated, and several thoracenteses had been made. Some days before operation injection of methylene blue was made into the pleura, with the production of attacks of a minor grade of vomiting (" spitting blue "). After operative intervention disinfection of the pleura by Dakin's solution was very badly borne and induced incessant coughing. Pleuroscopy then revealed, on the pulmonary pleura at the level of the interlobular fissure, a little

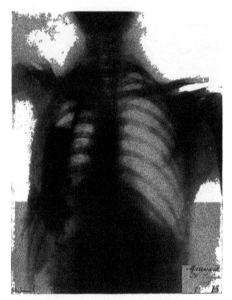

FIG. 4.—Empyemic cavity filled with bismuth for purposes of exploration.

sphacelated plaque, grayish-green in color, irregular, and about the size of a dime. It could not be detached by the forceps and contact with it provoked pain and cough.

Instillations of Dakin's solution at this point determined diagnosis of an eschar and probable bronchial fistula (cough and discharge of Dakin's solution from the mouth). From December 18, 1918, to January 22, 1919, discontinuous insufflations of oxygen were resorted to in order to disinfect the pleura, the Dakin's solution not being tolerated. The bronchial eschar becoming then more and more limited by granulating pleura, disinfection with Dakin's solution was resumed. By February 9th the eschar was reduced to the size of a pea and no further signs were caused by it.

There are also anatomic or pathologic diverticula which one can diagnose *de visu* by electric illumination of the pleura. Such diverticula are described in Case XII.

When bronchial fistulæ are recent and without necrosis of cartilage, they do not embarrass closure of the pleura. I have operated two broncho-

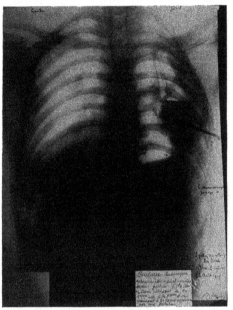

FIG. 5.—Empyemic cavity filled with bismuth for purposes of exploration.

pleural fistulæ of some weeks' duration only and after the opening of a pleurisy into the bronchi before operation. The cavity was asepticised, the costal orifice closed, and the patient cured as simply as if he had never had a fistula.

There is another variety of chronic fistula especially grave, ending generally in gangrenous processes, following pulmonary injury. Here the orifice is located at the bottom of the pleural cavity, and one clearly sees a suppuration which nothing can control. Cough is frequent, expectoration of pus more or less abundant, no disinfectant can stop the infection. In such cases I have tried to close the costal wall only to fail.

271

The second effect referred to is that of broncho-pleural fistula with
bronchial ectasia around the fistula. In removing adhesions about the
fistula in a case of this kind I found a series of cavities varying from the
volume of a large pea to that of a filbert, containing pus and constituting
areolæ-like veritable honeycomb. In short, such a case shows a bronchial
focus, localized, and with pulmonary sclerosis. Incision and opening of
these cavities are indicated, but are unsatisfactory. In one case still under
treatment bronchial suppuration persisted. One must resort to extirpation of the pulmonary nidus by incision (partial pneumectomy) into

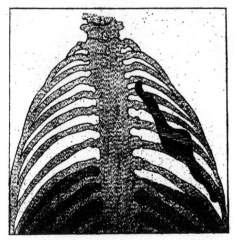

Fig. 6.—Showing empyemic cavity filled by an injection of bismuth.

healthy tissue. The bronchial fistula may become permanent by direct
continuation with the thoracic wall of a small orifice which closes during
expiration. An example is seen in a case which I operated during childhood, twenty-five years ago, the fistula persisting without the least embarrassment from infection. It has always resisted every freshly
attempted treatment.

Small abscesses may be remarked in the visceral pleura, visible by
electric pleuroscopy and being capable of retarding cure. At their site
the serous membrane was markedly thinned, having the appearance of
onion skin, ready to break, and consequently leaving an ulceration or
perhaps a bronchial fistula, splendid avenue of communication for the
transfer of infection between the pulmonary tissue and the pleura.

In Cases XXVI and XXVIII we diagnosed, by pleuroscopy, similar
ulcerations located at the middle of the median lobe of the lung. In fact,
they were multiple intrapleural abscesses as in Case XXIII.

Whatever the cause of chronicity, once induced it requires a long and difficult treatment. The cavity may be indurated, fixed, fibrous, inelastic, or completely calcareous, with thick walls. I have operated cases lined with calcareous plaques like oyster shells (Tuffier and Gy, *Revue de Chirurgie,* 1907, pp. 329-346). To fill this cavity the lung must return to its contact with the pleural membrane or the pleura must advance to a contact with the retracted lung. The ill-advised operation of Estlander consisted in obliterating the costal opening, which permitted the skin and muscles to heal before the lung was in good condition; it meant abolition of pulmon-

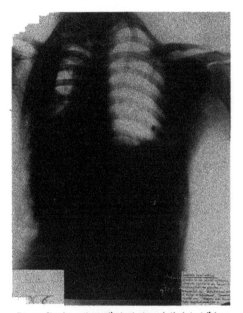

FIG. 7.—Showing radio-opacity in the lower half of the left lung.
(Cotte, June 2, 1917.)

ary function in the affected region, with all the trouble incident to it. Our object is precisely the contrary. It consists in every case where possible in removing the pleural shell to permit the lung to return to its proper position in the thoracic cage, intact or nearly so, continuing a nearly normal function.

II. TREATMENT OF CHRONIC EMPYEMAS, RECENT AND OLD

Cases are those of pleural fistula. Treatment should always be preceded by a methodical exploration of the cavity, which includes noting its extent and form and examining the pulmonary mobility during expiration

19

and inspiration and the effort necessary, the degree of pulmonary expansion being thus ascertained. The resulting information indicates application of one of two methods, *viz.:* Disinfection of the cavity and respiratory exercise; or, closing of the surgical wound by the method of Depage and Tuffier. If the cavity is intractable, pleuro-pulmonary decortication, partial or total, may be practised.

Exploration.—(*a*) Radioscopy and radiography. The pleural fistula is often narrowed, leading to a cavity; radiography permits exact knowl-·edge of its form and extent. By introducing several rubber tubes carry-

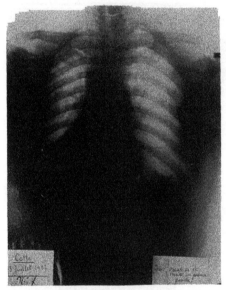

Fig. 8.—Showing radio-opacity in the middle of the left lung.
(Cotte, July 8, 1917.)

ing wire, one ascertains extent, direction, and form (Figs. 1, 2, and 3). If this method is insufficient, injection is made of a paste of bismuth or barium (Figs. 4, 5, and 6). Radioscopy (Figs. 7 and 8) should show the extent of the cavity during inspiration and expiration, and the degree of effort. It permits thus a study of pulmonary expansion, one learns the minimum volume of the cavity and the play of the lung antero-posteriorly and laterally, and therefore one knows the location of points of adhesions which must be attacked. I have noticed cases where the cavity during forced expiration disappeared completely, prognosis being especially favorable.

Radioscopy permits at the same time to follow the involution and diminution of the cavity during disinfection. Respiratory exercises with forced expiration are continued during the entire term of exploration and disinfection.

(*b*) Pleuroscopy. This enables investigation of the obstacles to contact of the lung with the thoracic wall. If the fistula is large, one does pleuroscopy through the orifice as in cystoscopy. Essentials to be noted are color of the cavity, surface of its walls, irregularities, diverticula, bronchial fistulæ, and the regions suppurating.

(*c*) Bacteriologic and microscopic examination. This establishes the

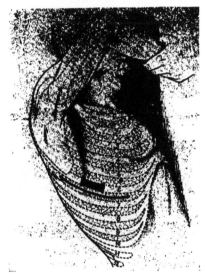

FIG. 9.—Incision in the intercostal space.

number and nature of the bacteria, their location, and gives the base of the culture curve during disinfection.

(*d*) Surgical exploration. This may be followed immediately by the surgical treatment. Method: Local or general anæsthesia; lighting by the forehead lamp; wide thoracotomy following along the intercostal space (Fig. 9) corresponding to the fistula, resection of its borders and of the bony callus which surrounds and results from the fusion of the ribs; removal of adhesions; separation of the edges of the cavity by means of a special instrument (separator). One thus learns the extent of the cavity and the consistence of its walls in different regions. Three forms of pathology may be found: (1) A fistulous tract sometimes very long, extending

275

from the base of the thorax to the upper ribs; (2) a regular cavity with considerable retraction of the lung, always difficult to cure; (3) a fissured cavity, narrow but with a very long principal diameter, often directed from above downward and backward, which diminishes considerably during respiratory effort. These cases may present diverticula of which the most difficult of cure are those which form pockets, bilobed or multilobed, with constrictions between each lobe. If the cavity is small and not greatly infected, one can attempt immediate pleuro-pulmonary decortication or the resections necessary to a cure. We thus treated eight cases (two acute, six chronic), but this exploration should most often be followed by chemical disinfection of the cavity.

(e) Disinfection of the cavity. I prefer the Carrel-Dakin method when

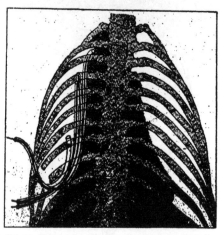

Fig. 10.—Rubber tubes, armed, introduced into the fistula for purposes of disinfection.

possible. Rubber tubes are armed with silver wire, very fine and pliable, and placed in such a fashion as constantly to irrigate the cavity and all diverticula (Figs. 10 and 11; see also Figs. 1, 2, and 3). This procedure is indispensable and the essential of the method. It is necessary to have several tubes and to place the patient in a position permitting the antiseptic liquid to have access to the diverticula. Disinfection may be more or less rapid, but it is often very slow. Its progress is mapped by curves (Figs. 12, 13, 14, and 15). This series shows some of these difficulties.

This procedure may be impracticable if there is a broncho-pleural fistula. Irrigation produces cough and a chlorine taste in the mouth which cannot be borne. Therefore, before placing the tubes, introduce into the pleural cavity a wick of gauze to tampon the bronchial orifice and prevent flow of the liquid to the mouth. At the time of injection one can also place the patient in lateral decubitus, lying upon the fistula. These means are often insufficient at the beginning of treatment; later the liquid no longer passes into the bronchi, probably as a result of spontaneous narrowing of the broncho-pleural orifice, and disinfection becomes easy.

When all these means fail, I replace them by continuous or discontinuous aëration with oxygen gas, passed into all the recesses of the cavity as the Dakin liquid is distributed. This method was applied in five cases. Bacteriologic examination of these cases showed three with

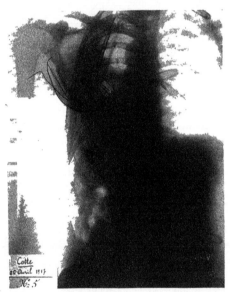

FIG. 11.—Use of armed rubber tubes for purpose of disinfection.
(Case of Cotte, see figs. 3, 7, 8.)

streptococcus alone, one associated staphylococcus, diplococcus, streptococcus, coccidia, and a mononucleated organism, and one with no bacterial finding. All five patients were cured.

Naturally this disinfection is often difficult and stubborn. The cause must be sought. The location of the bacteria explains in certain cases the resistance of the septic process to treatment, for example, in case of a pleural diverticulum not reached by the disinfectant solution and which must be located and treated, or again, with a bronchial fistula demanding oxygen or tampon with a compress before employing the Dakin solution; the culture curve may be irregular, as may be readily noted. Two cases were operated in two stages; I first closed off the aseptic region and later instituted disinfection of infected locations. During the stage of disinfection respiratory exercises were continued as the cavity grew smaller. Extent of the treated cavities:

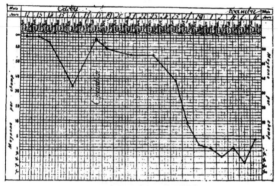

FIG. 12.—Microbe curve: showing progressive diminution of infection under treatment.

Content before operation .... 360 c.c.	Content at time of closure .... 150 c.c.
Content before operation .... 141 c.c.	Content at time of closure .... 70 c.c.
Content before operation .... 45 c.c.	Content at time of closure .... 8 c.c.
Content before operation .... 360 c.c.	Content at time of closure .... 60 c.c.
Content before operation .... 125 c.c.	Content at time of closure .... 25 c.c.
Content before operation .... 65 c.c.	Content at time of closure .... 20 c.c.
Content before operation .... 175 c.c.	Content at time of closure .... 15 c.c.

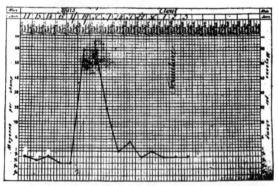

FIG. 13.—Microbic curve, showing effect of drainage and disinfection.

Early disinfection is essential; pulmonary decortication formerly done by Delorme's method nearly always failed. Before closure two conditions are important: (1) The culture curve must read zero, streptococci being absent; (2) the pleura, without further application of Dakin solution and dressed only by sterile gauze, should not secrete. One can then

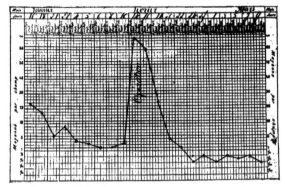

FIG. 14.—Microbic curve, showing effect of drainage and disinfection.

close the *parietal orifice* with no further concern about the cavity (Depage-Tuffier) or perform pleuro-pulmonary *decortication*. In cases where decortication alone is applicable, I operate before securing total disinfection.

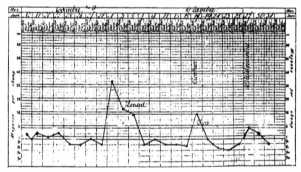

FIG. 15.—Microbe curve, showing average number of organisms in the microscopic field.

The Depage-Tuffier Method.—The culture curve reading zero and the cavity no longer secreting, the surgical incision is closed.

1. Introduce aseptically into the pleura a narrow wick, in order to prevent entrance or stay of blood within the pleural .cavity during the operation.

2. Under local anæsthesia the edges of the orifice are resected throughout its depth and down to healthy tissue, all incisions are tamponed and

perfect hæmostasis of the wound is secured. Closing is done either in one plane with silkworm gut, or in two planes, the deeper with catgut and the superficial with silkworm. Closure is complete with aseptic dressing applied.

This method is indicated in all cases where the cavity is reducible by the respiratory effort, even in recent cases with uninfected bronchial fistula. Sutures are removed on the seventh day.

Should there be a bloody effusion into the pleura during or after the operation, I insert a bundle of silkworm threads to drain the cavity for twenty-four hours. One can follow the regression of the cavity by radios-

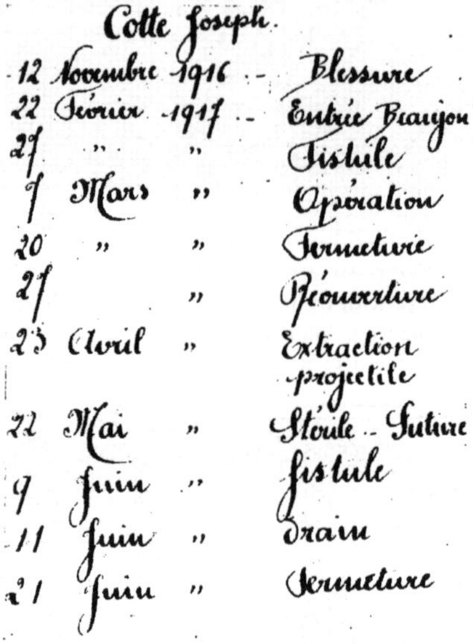
Cotte Joseph.
12 Novembre 1916 .. Blessure
22 Février 1917 .. Entrée Beaujon
27 " " Fistule
7 Mars " Opération
20 " " Fermeture
27 " Réouverture
23 Avril " Extraction projectile
22 Mai " Stérile .. Suture
9 Juin " Fistule
11 Juin " Drain
21 Juin " Fermeture

FIG. 16.—Syllabus of the various stages in the treatment of a case of chronic pleuritis and fistule following a perforating gunshot wound of the thorax.

copy and auscultation. Usually resorption appears complete when the dressing is removed on the eighth day. If suppuration again complicates, I open the cavity anew.

Pleuro-pulmonary Decortication.—This operation was made in nine intractable cases, seven with total decortication and two with partial decortication. The fistula had been present two hundred and eighty days in the non-surgical cases and ninety-three days in the traumatic cases. Cavities invariably contained streptococci. The period of disinfection averaged thirty-three days for the non-surgical cases, forty-three days for the surgical cases. The method is the method of election in old and obstinate cases with cavities indurated and not reducible by respiration. It includes two stages: (1) Thoracotomy with wide exploration, and (2) decortication, complete or incomplete, total or partial.

Exploration is made by thoracotomy. Resection is made of the edges of the fistula and of the osseous plaques often due to the fusion of the ends of sectioned ribs. Wide separation, always difficult, of the surgical in-

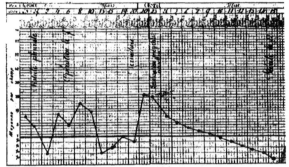

Fig. 17.—Microbic curve in the case of Cotte. (See Fig. 16.)

cision and the laying bare of all recesses and the entire cavity, are practised. If prior disinfection of the cavity is thus obtained, one continues with the decortication. If pulmonary decortication by Delorme's method has not been successful, it is only because it was not preceded by disin-

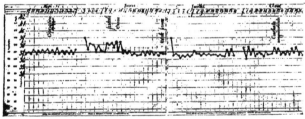

Fig. 18.—The later microbe curve in the case of Joseph Cotte (see Figs. 16 and 17), gunshot wound of lung.

fection of the pleural cavity, and in my early operations I always saw decortication followed by a new infection.

Operative Method—Total Decortication.—(1) Wide incision of the pleura is made to open the entire cavity thoroughly. (2) The cicatrix and osseous plaques about it are resected. Wide thoracotomy is done, beyond the limits of the cavity. Separation, by a separator, is made of the lips of the wound (Fig. 19). One ascertains the plane of pleuro-parietal cleavage at the level of the wound,.this plane being often difficult to find.

Stripping of the pleuro-parietal region leading to the sinus of the cavity is done, here again amid grave difficulty in passing from the pleuro-parietal entrance to the pulmonary site. Adhesions are often intimate and·thick at this level. The false pulmonary membrane is stripped off¨and here the difficulties are especially great. If, in some cases, the plane of pleuro-pulmonary cleavage is easy to find and follow, adhesions are usually so intimate that stripping of the false membrane results in penetration into pulmonary tissue with consequent bleeding. Total decortication has been successful with me only for cavities limited to the size of the two fists,

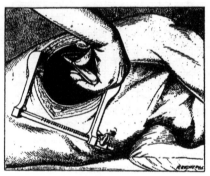

FIG. 19.—Dividing pleuro-parietal adhesions at the bottom of the cavity.

and I have never decortified an entire pleural cavity. Sometimes the process remains incomplete because of diverticula which cannot be reached or on account of deep adhesions involving the pericardium. Immediately after the removal of the false pulmonary membrane one sees the lung resume its expansion and again fill up the pleural cavity.

Pulmonary Decortication Alone.—In three cases, after wide pleural incision, I liberated the cavity at the level of the pleuro-pulmonary adhesion by attacking the false pulmonary membrane, which permitted the lung to expand. I did not trouble about the pleuro-parietal membranes. All these cases were cured.

Partial and Segmented Decortication.—Adhesions between the pulmonary false membrane and the lung are such that one can extirpate them only in sections. The periphery is incised at the union of the parietal and the pulmonary pleuræ to liberate the lung (Figs. 20 and 21). One then attacks the false membrane in different places where it appears likely to yield more readily, leaving it untouched where the fusion is especially intimate. Islands of adhesions are thus left, of greater or less thickness, on the surface of the lung. One then thins out, by dissection, the thickness of the adhesions up to the pulmonary surface. I do not

282

like to penetrate the pulmonary tissue, which always bleeds abundantly and thus constitutes an obstacle to cure.

In all these methods it may be necessary to resect one or two ribs more or less extensively. But in all cases preference is given to liberating the lung, so that it may fill the pleural cavity. One resects the skele-

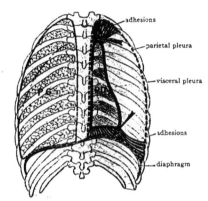

FIG. 20.—Points along which the incision should be carried at the periphery of the cavity.

ton only when expansion is absolutely impossible. If the raw surface left by decortication bleeds but little, I completely close the surgical wound in one or two planes. If there is a slight bloody oozing, I introduce a bundle of silkworm sutures to insure drainage for twenty-four hours. If

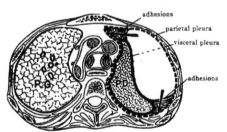

FIG. 21.—Diagram showing where the incisions should be carried in order to liberate the lung.

the oozing is very abundant, I apply to the bleeding pulmonary surface a large wick to drain it, suturing completely at the end of twenty-four hours.

Complications of Operating Chronic Empyemas.—In eleven cases the wound had to be reopened because of secondary suppuration, but the accumulation was much reduced in proportion to the original cavity.

TH. TUFFIER

In two cases the wound had to be opened twice. All of these were cured. Two other cases had to be reopened, one for an osseous fistula, the other for hæmoptysis. Slight thoracic deformity was mentioned in nine cases and considerable deformity in a case of seven months' duration.

Content after operation	15 c.c.	Content at closure	3 c.c.
Content after operation	120 c.c.	Content at closure	45 c.c.
Content after operation	17 c.c.	Content at closure	4 c.c.
Content after operation	37 c.c.	Content at closure	4 c.c.

In three cases the pleural site was disinfected *de novo* and cured.

Subsequent medical treatment consisted in exercises for inspiration and expiration, the effect being watched by means of a registering pneumograph.

Final Results and Conclusions.—All my cases have been seen six months to three years after operation. Thoracic deformity was slight. The radiographic reading was an interesting evidence of the thickness of former adhesions or of cicatrices shown to have almost completely disappeared. The costo-diaphragmatic sinus alone was visible at its inferior portion.

To summarize, chronic pleurisies are exceptional when acute effusions are well treated. Chronicity depends on a chronic pulmonary infection or on special anatomic peculiarities. Costal resection in the treatment of chronic empyema should be reduced to the minimum. Closure of the surgical incision and pleural decortication should be preceded by disinfection of the cavity and then gives success which was formerly unknown.

(I have to thank Dr. Merrill A. M. Cross, Paris, for the translation of this article.—THE AUTHOR.)

THE TREATMENT OF CHRONIC EMPYEMA

STATISTICAL TABLE *

RECORD OF 91 CASES FROM THE MONTH OF AUGUST, 1914, TO THE MONTH OF DECEMBER, 1919

46 cases of medical purulent pleurisy.
43 cases due to wounds of the lungs.
2 cases due to infection of a hæmothorax.

I

A. Out of the 46 medical cases 29 were opened by myself and treated by the Depage-Tuffier method.

The microscopic examinations showed:

15 cases streptococci only.
5 cases pneumococci only.
7 cases association of staphylococci-diplococci and streptococci.
1 case streptococci and pneumococci.
1 case streptococci and leukocytes.

I practiced the operation at the first sign of:

Pleurisy in 9 cases from 8–22 days.
Pleurisy in 13 cases from 2½ months.
Pleurisy in 4 cases from 2⅛ months.
Pleurisy in 1 case from 4 months.
Pleurisy in 2 cases from 6 months.

The duration of the sterilization was:

7 cases from 6 to 24 days.
3 cases from 1 month.
9 cases from 1½ to 2½ months.
4 cases from 3 to 4 months (case dating from several months).
In certain cases the record was incomplete.

The volume of the cavity was about:

80 c.c. in 1 case.
200 c.c. in 2 cases.
300 c.c. in 2 cases.
700 c.c. in 1 case.
1100 c.c. in 2 cases.
1600 c.c. in 1 case.
1 litre in 1 case.
1 litre in 2 cases.
Total in 4 cases.

In another case the cavity contained about 3 litres at the opening and more than 1½ litres at the closure of the pleura.

Six patients died almost immediately after the operation, 3 were streptococci and 3 were without record of any kind.

One case was opened and treated solely by oxygen, the microscopic examination showed streptococci and dated from 3 months.

Three were opened; they recovered, but they were treated by simple drainage.

Three were opened and closed immediately. Two pneumococci (success), 1 diplococcus (failure).

* Translated by Miss Carrie Patterson.

B. Two cases were sent to me already opened and had been already treated by Dakin; they had been opened for over a month and showed streptococci; 1 dated from 4 months and had been sterilized in 10 days, the other dated from 3 years ½ and had been sterilized in 4 months. Both recovered.

C. Two cases were decorticated, 1 showing streptococci and the other was without record. One dated from 3 months, the other from 1 month. The sterilization was complete in 11 days. Result—recovery.

II

Consecutive purulent pleurisy from wounds of the lung—43 cases.

Out of these 43 cases 19 were opened by myself and treated by the Depage-Tuffier method.

The microscopic examination on the 19 cases showed 14 times association of staphylo-diplo-cocci, strepto once and distryptococci in 4 cases were not mentioned.

In 4 cases when I operated, the wound dated from 20 days.

In 2 cases it dated from 1 month and a few days.
In 5 cases it dated from 2 months and a few days.
In 2 cases it dated from 3 months.
In 2 cases it dated from 4 months.
In 2 cases it dated from 5 to 7 months.
In 2 cases there were no records.

The duration of the sterilization was:

In 5 cases 15 days.
In 8 cases 1 month and a few days.
In 2 cases 2 and 3 months.
In 2 cases 4 months.
In 2 cases without record.

In 1 case the closure took place the day of the operation. There was no sterilization. This dated from 5½ months.

B. Seventeen cases were sent to me *chronic*, 14 from 1 month. (Eleven closed Depage-Tuffier method and 3 decortications.)

The microscopic examinations showed: Ten times associations staphylo-diplo-cocci, batonnets-strepto. Once pneumococci and bacillus of Friedlander. Three cases are not mentioned.

When I practiced the operation the wound dated:

2 cases 2 months and a few days.
3 cases 3 months.
3 cases 4 months.
3 cases 5 months.
3 cases 7 months.
1 case 8 months.

The duration of the sterilization was in:

2 cases 15 days.
4 cases 1 month and a few days.
3 cases 2 months and a few days.
1 case 3 months and a few days.
1 case 6 months and a few days.

In 3 cases the pleural site was reopened, disinfected anew and the result was recovery.

286

Three in less than a month. The microscopic examinations showed:

    I pneumococci et bacillus of Friedlander.

I associations of perfringens, anaërobes, staphylococci, vibrion septique.

    I without record.

All these cases except 2 actually recovered. The 2 failures were 2 bronchial fistulæ with ectasia of the bronchiæ.

THE TREATMENT OF CHRONIC EMPYEMA*

By Carl A. Hedblom, M.D.

of Rochester, Minn.

Definition.—The word empyema is from the Greek signifying a collection of pus in a cavity. This was the sense in which the word was used by Hippocrates, Galen, Ætius, and others. Ætius, in fact, defined the term much as it would be defined to-day: he stated that those persons are called "empyici" in whom an abscess in any part of the pleura has ruptured into the pleural cavity. Aretæus *Cappadox* wrote: "Those persons in whose cavities above, along the region of the chest, or in those below the diaphragm, abscesses of matter form, if they bring it up they are said to be affected with empyema, but if the matter pass downwards they are said to labor under Apostemes." Later, Cælius *Aurelianus* and others called a collection of fluid anywhere in the body empyema. Guy de Chauliac, 1363, defined the word as follows: "Empyma or empyema in Greek signifies a collection of pus in whatsoever part of the body it may be, but more properly used meaning a collection of suppurative matter in the testes, thorax, or abdomen. In a more restricted sense it means pus in the thorax: this is the most proper and common significance. Following it one calls those who have pus in the thorax 'empyes' or 'empyiques' in Greek, and suppurants or purulents in Latin."

Later a difference of opinion developed as to whether the term empyema should be limited to collections of pus or what other effusions should also be included. Boerhaave wrote: "Whenever there is a collection of pus between the lungs and the pleura in the cavity of the chest it is called an empyema." De Sauvages, Cullen, and others, restricted the term to pus only. Kisnerus also wrote that when the fluid is not pus but serous (aquosa simplex) it should be called hydrops of the chest. It was argued by others, on the contrary, that what was blood in the thorax may have changed to pus and that therefore collections of fluid of any kind and collections of air should be included.

The drainage operation was also called "empyema" (Dictionnaire des Sciences médicales). The expression "the operation of empyema was performed" was of frequent occurrence.

Leonus *Lunensis* (Dominicus), 1597, used "empyemate" and "purulentia" as synonymous for fluid occupying sometimes all, sometimes part, of the empty cavity of the thorax (cavitate vacua pectoris).

In the modern use of the term the word may still be defined as a col-

* Thesis submitted to the Faculty of the Graduate School of the University of Minnesota in partial fulfillment of the requirements for the degree of doctor of philosophy in surgery, May, 1920.

Abstract read before the Cleveland Academy of Medicine, February, 1920, and before the American Association for Thoracic Surgery, May, 1920, New Orleans.

lection of pus in the pleural cavity, although an interlobar empyema might be construed to fall outside this definition. In the transitional stage between acute empyema and a preceding serous effusion the distinction is a matter of definition. In the chronic condition the effusion is always frankly purulent.

It is also difficult to make an inclusive definition of what constitutes chronicity. Certain types of empyema, those with large bronchial fistulas, those with cavities at the apex, and some of uncertain duration at the time they were first recognized are often potentially chronic from the onset, in the sense that they do not progress to a cure by simple drainage treatment. Perhaps the most generally accepted criterion of chronicity, however, is the duration of the process. A great many writers consider an empyema of six weeks' duration to be chronic. For the purpose of this discussion, with the exceptions noted, three months are taken as the time limit between the acute and chronic condition.

HISTORICAL REVIEW

The history of empyema up to the last three decades is essentially that of chronic empyema. To what ancient period its recognition and drainage treatment date we do not know. It seems probable that incision for drainage of empyema necessitas was done by the Chinese and Egyptians. The earliest known direct references to the condition, now extant, are those of Hippocrates. His teachings as to etiology, symptomatology, prognosis, and treatment contain much that is fundamental to our present-day conception. The symptoms and signs, as he stated them, were pain in the chest, high fever, cough, distress when attempting to lie on the sound side, and œdema of the feet and of the eyes. After an illness of fifteen days the patient was examined for fluid. This examination consisted of shaking him by the shoulders and diagnosing the presence and site of fluid by the splash. If no splash could be elicited the side in which the pain and swelling was most marked was considered the one affected. Hippocrates taught that the matter should be let out either by knife or cautery. If there was a swelling externally, he directed that an opening should be made in it, if not, the opening should be made at the level of the third rib from the last, and rather behind than in front. He made the incision superficially with a large bistoury, then continued with a lancet wrapped in linen, the point only being free, or used a trocar or trephine or the cautery throughout. After some of the pus had been let out he closed the opening with a tent of lint attached to a thread. Every day it was removed and pus evacuated. On the tenth day he injected warm wine and oil. When the discharge became clear and glairy, he introduced into the opening a hollow metal tube.

He observed that patients who became affected with empyema after pleurisy recovered if they got clear of it in forty days after the time it ruptured; but if not, it passed into phthisis. As to prognosis he stated that if pure and white pus flowed when empyema was treated either by cautery or incision, the patient recovered; but if the pus was mixed with blood and was stringy and fetid, he died.

Euryphon, a contemporary of Hippocrates, treated empyema with the actual cautery. Celsus, who practised at the beginning of the Christian era, is the author of our next most ancient reference. He wrote on the symptomatology and prognosis much as did Hippocrates. He stated: " 'Tis common for fistulæ to extend beneath the ribs. When this case occurs, the ribs in that part must be cut through on both sides and taken out lest anything corrupt be left within," and, " Fistulæ of the chest are very difficult of treatment, so that sometimes physician, sometimes patient, giving up hope, leaves the case to Nature herself."

Pliny related the story of a soldier with empyema whose life was despaired of by his physician. Seeking relief by death in battle, he was wounded in the thorax; the pus escaped and he recovered.

Leonidas *Alexandrinus*, a Roman physician of the second century, recommended the actual cautery for effecting drainage. He remarked that his contemporaries feared less to open the chest by the cautery than by the knife.

Aretæus *Cappadox*, of uncertain date, probably a contemporary of Galen, said concerning the pathology of empyema: " It is a wonder how from a thin, slender membrane having no depth, like that which lines the chest, so much pus should flow; for in many cases there is a great collection. The cause is an inflammation from redundancy of blood, by which the membrane is thickened; but from much blood much pus is formed immediately. But if it be determined inwards, the ribs being the bones in that region * * * I have said above that another species of phthisis would naturally occur. But if it points outward the bones are separated, for the top of the abscess is raised in one of the intercostal spaces, when the ribs are pushed to this side or that."

Cælius *Aurelianus*, who lived in the early part of the fifth century, according to Haller a contemporary of Leonidas, wrote on abscess and empyema. Buck credits him with being familiar with ascultation of the chest.

Galen in his writings emphasized the importance of providing for the escape of pus in the thorax in order to avoid the ravages, especially of phthisis, of which it might be the cause. He removed portions of carious ribs, injected warm wine into the cavity (pectore), and urged the patient to cough while leaning toward the affected side. If the pus and injected fluid did not thus escape, aspiration was done.

Two Greek physicians of the early middle ages who wrote on empyema are Ætius and Paulus Ægineta. Ætius, besides giving a very clear definition of the pathologic condition, stated that in certain cases empyema is formed without fever. He approved of the cautery in its treatment. Paulus Ægineta wrote a compend of medicine which later was translated into Arabic and Latin. His writings on empyema were based on the teachings of Hippocrates and Galen but showed some originality. He is quoted by Marcellus Donatus to the effect that cautery or incision of the thorax, by allowing vitality to flow out with pus, causes immediate death or an incurable fisula results.

During the latter part of the middle ages some of the earlier medical literature was preserved by the Arabs. Their most notable contributor to surgical literature was Albucasis. He recommended incision or cautery operation for drainage of empyema. Avicenna and Avenzoar also approved of paracentesis and the cautery. Zacchias, however, said that the Arabian physicians feared the operation for empyema. Lelorraine said that the Arabs disagreed as to the advisability of operation. Nicolaus Massa, while granting that incurable fistulæ might be left after operation, maintained that a fistula is vastly better than certain death. He recorded a case of draining sinus following a stab wound that closed after seven years. He cited the case of a girl who for six days coughed up eight pounds of pus daily, and ultimately recovered.

Guy de Chauliac, besides giving a definition of empyema which very closely agrees with our present conception of the disease, mentioned that the operation was performed by his contemporaries.

Smetius, 1574, reported a case of empyema following a dagger wound of the thorax. An incision was made between the tenth and eleventh ribs and much foul pus was evacuated. The cavity was then irrigated with honey and water.

Vesalius taught that incision should always be made for empyema and that no one should die of the disease. Certain persons would die because of their wounds and not because of the operation. He referred to several cases in which he operated successfully. He wrote also on thoracic fistulæ.

Amatus *Lusitanus* was one of the first of a considerable number of physicians of the Renaissance period who wrote on empyema. His is also one of the most original and independent expositions on the subject. He outlined in detail the teachings of Hippocrates on the treatment of empyema and discussed the relative advantages of the incision and the cautery. With regard to the site for drainage, he pointed out that Hippocrates ordered that the drainage should be made as near as possible to the septum transversum (diaphragm) without injuring it. As to which interspace this should be, he said that rather than rely on the authority of Hippocrates, he determined it for himself on the cadaver. He wrote:

"At one time a brother of Andreas Vesalius, the renowned anatomist, in my presence was carefully cutting up a human body. Snatching the knife with which the excellent youth was dissecting, I made an opening between the second and third ribs on the left side, and after the knife itself had been thrust in I discovered that the 'septum transversum' could draw no harm from it. However, the madness of physicians reaches this point that they do not cut between the second and third ribs (counting from below), but rather between the fourth and fifth, or if it pleases the gods, between the fifth and sixth, although they cannot draw the corrupt matter easily without loss of the patient, since the pus is held in a bag and they cannot do away with it even when the legs are raised and the head is hanging down."

He cited a successful case in which he drained between the third and fourth ribs.

Marcellus Donatus had a case of empyema necessitas that progressed to a spontaneous cure; he remarked that almost all empyema patients and many suffering from a wound penetrating into the chest died because physicians feared to cut in the right region, an operation which he advised. However, if pus would not drain through the mouth, he believed that the opening should be made between the third and fourth ribs (counting from below) rather than lower down, on account of the danger of injury to the diaphragm. He added that the incision should be made wherever pus had collected, and cited many authorities for the statement that pus might drain through the urine. He spoke also of perforation of the diaphragm by the abscess.

Leonus *Lunensis* (Dominicus) gave detailed directions for the medical treatment, internal and external, and referred briefly to the use of incision and cautery in cases not cured by such treatment.

Castellus, in his treatise on the diseases of the thorax, discussed at great length the external and surgical treatment, but did not add anything original.

Fabricius *ab Aquapendente* systematically discussed the subject and described the instruments used by Hippocrates and by Paulus Ægineta. He stated that most persons who had received a penetrating wound in the thorax had to wear a silver tube for life and that he knew of patients who had carried tubes for twenty or thirty years. Fistulæ persist, he wrote, because of the constant motion of the chest, because the pleura is sinewy and bloodless, and because of the tortuous course of the fistulous tract. To avoid the motion, patients should be in bed and refrain from work and all speech, from wrath, and any repressed breathing whatsoever; second, the hard skin of the fistula should be removed either by softening or corroding or burning or by drug or by instrument. The pleural cavity could also be closed by the scar. Furthermore, all corruption must be removed and the fistulous tract straightened by cutting the curves with a knife. Fabricius thought that the rib resection operations recommended by Celsus were very difficult, dangerous, and cruel. He was of the opinion that a rib could not be removed without tearing the pleura and so causing the death of the patient. He recommended a curved silver drainage tube and treatment of the fistula as though it were a spring and not an ulcer.

Zacutus *Lusitanus* published records of three cases. In the first, pus drained by the urine; in the second, in which there was much purulent sputum, the patient recovered spontaneously on a milk diet; in the third, after great fear and misgiving as to the result should operation be undertaken, it was decided to be guided by the dictum of the "old man" (oraculum senis). An incision was made and the patient recovered.

Cases were reported by Horstius, by Tulp, and by Jalon, in which pus is said to have drained by the urine, and in Tulp's case, also by the umbilicus. Cures following operations were described by Kisnerus and Riedlinus. Operative treatment was discussed by Zacchias, Camerarius, Scultetus, Fienus, and Fliccius. Scultetus' article is the earliest accessible reference in the French. He discusses indications, time, site, technic, and instruments to be used in the operation of paracentesis. He stated that the "temperament" of the air must be considered and cited Hippocrates' recommendation that the winter and summer should be avoided if possible on account of the sudden changes in the air at these seasons. He also mentioned that a purulent effusion is in need of earlier drainage than a hydrops on account of the rapid increase in amount and the ulceration produced by the latter. He believed that of all sites for drainage the seventh interspace, recommended by Hippocrates, is the best because it furnishes the most dependent drainage. He recommended injections of wine and oil after operation.

Fienus wrote on paracentesis for empyema. This is the earliest available article in the German. He defined paracentesis as a cut through which an opening is made into the body cavity (Hole des Leibes) whether by a cold iron or cautery. He discussed in a most interesting manner the problems involved in pneumothorax produced by this operation.

Fliccius, after citing the authorities with regard to suitable location for drainage, decided that the best place is between the fifth and sixth ribs. Kisnerus wrote that venesection, generally a most excellent remedy, is almost supreme in cases of empyema.

Kinner refers to blistering (ustiones) and cites Ætius, who directed that empyema patients should be burned about the neck, back, and sides in eight places in all. Kinner stated that this treatment should be shuddered at and that it was easy to believe Ætius was made a physician from a hangman or a tormentor rather than from a goldsmith.

Wilhelm ten Rhyne is quoted by Riedlinus as stating that Japanese surgeons inserted the leaves of India fig trees in empyema patients.

The available literature from the eighteenth century is essentially a repetition of the foregoing; that is, citation and discussion of authorities and a few isolated case reports. Ingram is the author of the earliest available treatise in the English. He reported a case successfully drained and took issue with Sharp, who in his "Operations of Surgery," Chapter XXIV, says that the operation "should be discarded as unnecessary when blood or matter is fluctuating in the thorax," and confines the necessity of it to "cases of water." A few other successfully operated cases were recorded by Springsfeld, Valentin, Gädücke, Carboué, and others. Koelpin reported a case of pulsating empyema proved at operation. A few spontaneous cures and many post-mortem findings are recorded by Warner, Fürst, and Morin.

Lapeyre said that while the operation for empyema is known to all persons of the art, it is rarely practised because of the uncertainty of diagnosis and lack of assurance as to success of the operation. He believed, however, that the operation should be done oftener. He reported one case of empyema pointing in the chest wall which was opened and drained.

The greatest impetus to advance in surgery of the thorax since Hippocrates was the marked improvement in diagnosis by the art of percussion of the thorax described by Auenbrugger in 1761. It was only after several decades, however, that this new method was appreciated. The great clinician, van Swieten, who was Auenbrugger's teacher, ignored it. Stoll was the first to mention its great value in detecting pleurisy and especially empyema, in order that operation might be performed. Corvisart and Laennec[106] were among the first outside of Vienna to emphasize its importance. Corvisart translated Auenbrugger's treatise into the French.

The literature of the first eight decades of the nineteenth century is full of discordant notes with regard to the treatment and citations of patients with empyema necessitas. In some cases the cavities ruptured spontaneously; others were opened by simple incision. A great number of necropsy protocols were published.

Hourelle, 1808, wrote that in the advanced stages of empyema, internal medication is at best useless and that blistering, scarification, and fomentations are not much better. He stated that the danger is not in operation, but in the difficulty of applying it with certainty.

Burin d'Aissard stated that the operation had been feared because of the misapprehension that air in the chest will almost always kill the patient. He was of the opinion that when a fistula results it should be left to time and a good regimen.

The pessimistic note is again sounded in 1825 by Dumont, who said that there is always a possibility of cure by spontaneous absorption, by thickening of the pleura, by sclerosis, by absorption by way of the urine and bowels, or by absorption into the blood. He recommended mercury, purgatives, bleeding, and a rigid diet. He added that the most common termination is death.

Rullier, in speaking of the difficulties of diagnosis, points out that Dionis, Baffos, and Corvisart all opened the chest without finding pus and that several of their patients died.

Putegnat laid down as indication for operation acute and chronic dyspnœa, local and general œdema, and emaciation, for the relief of which all medical remedies had failed.

294

Colson, writing on empyema following a perforated wound of the thorax, mentioned the professional " sucer " present at every duel ready to draw out the blood from the wound. So successful was this treatment that it was thought to be of the devil; and in one case a priest refused the last sacrament to a wounded man thus treated. Bache states that the cause of chronic empyema is the failure of lung expansion.

In 1834 Faure reported before the Academy of Medicine in Paris a series of eight cases in which operation had been performed. Two patients were cured and all the others improved. This report precipitated a prolonged discussion, for many physicians held operation in disfavor. Thus Barlow stated that Andral and Louis regarded empyema as necessarily fatal. Laennec is quoted as saying that the operation for empyema is rarely successful. Of fifty patients treated by Dupuytren, only four were cured. When he himself developed empyema he refused operation and is quoted as having said that he would die at the hand of God rather than with the help of the surgeon.

The unsatisfactory status of the treatment of purulent pleural effusions is strikingly reflected in results obtained. The greater number of case reports up to 1834 were those of empyema necessitas; some patients recovered spontaneously after draining (Malin and Salomon, Shortridge, Steinheim), others after incision (Heyser, Claessens, Cleland, and Tourtuel). A few cases were recognized and treated before the chest wall was perforated (Colegrove, Martini, Wolfly). A large number of operated cases ended fatally (Kilgour, Cayol, Bonnet, and many others). Small series of cases were reported by Chambers, Oke, Hartshorne, Niese, and in 1841 a series of forty-three collected cases by Sédillot.

Colson, 1876, stated that the use of syringes, cannulas, and other aspirating devices employed by Dionis, Anel, Scultetus, Bruer, and others, had fallen into disfavor. After the work of Bowditch, in 1852, the aspiration method again came into vogue.

Gimbert reported a case in which seventy-four aspirations and lavages were done, followed by a cure. Bouchut, in 1872, told of one patient tapped fifty-eight times during sixteen months and another one hundred and twenty-two times during eleven months. In one instance 50 gallons of " matter " is said to have been aspirated during four and one-half years without any diminution in the daily amount. Simmonds found that in forty-eight collected cases treated by aspiration forty-two were unimproved.

Although the ancients, following Hippocrates' teachings, probably diagnosed and operated in many cases of empyema in the acute stage, the later operative treatment was largely for empyema pointing in the chest wall. Besides the cutting and cautery operation the use of caustic stone was also described. Some practised burning a deep hole and palpating the bottom of it for pus. In 1810 Aupepin described a " new " technic for performing thoracotomy by making the opening in the skin and intercostal tissue at slightly different levels. The valve-like arrangement so produced was designed to prevent pneumothorax after the withdrawal of the aspiration tube.

In 1881 Homén published a series of ninety-one collected cases of patients treated by incision and published by seven different authors between 1868 and 1876. Of this group, 47.25 per cent. of patients were cured, 23.08 per cent. had residual fistulas, and 29.67 per cent. died. Fifty per cent of 52 of these patients who had irrigation in addition to incision were cured, 17.31 per cent. developed fistulas, and 32.69 per cent. died. In a larger series of 141 patients the mortality was 33.33 per cent.

Rib Resection for Drainage.—Rib resection in empyema is mentioned by Galen, who states that he removed pieces of rib that were necrosed in a case of empyema necessitas. By other physicians they were cauterized, removed, or let alone. No mention is found of resection of a sound rib until 1860, when Walter resected the eighth rib for drainage of a chronic empyema caused by a knife stab between the ribs. The fibrous membrane was removed with finger and spatula. " The cavity was so large as readily to admit the head of a child a year old." The cavity was washed with tincture of iodine, zinc sulphate, and decoctions such as of white oak bark. The chest wall retracted and the cavity was completely obliterated in the course of a year. Roser is said to have been the first to propose resection, but it was not until 1865 that he performed the operation. Peyrot, Billroth, Fraentzel, Koenig, Ewald, and others, were among the first to perform the operation. Weissenborn, 1876, reported a series of five cases.

Plastic Operation for Obliteration of Chronic Cavities.—According to Peitavy, Simon first recommended rib resection in order artificially to reduce the size of the cavity in chronic empyema. Peitavy published the case in which Simon made the observation that the cut ends of the resected ribs approximated. Simon taught this idea in his clinic in 1869. Heineke first published these observations in 1872, in his " Compendium der Chirurgischen Operations und Verbandlehre." Küster, in 1877, wrote that in chronic cases he resected one or two ribs in front of and behind the fistula. Létiévant reported a cure in a chronic case and emphasized the fact that not only drainage but collapse of the cavity was promoted by rib resection.

To Estlander, however, is generally accorded the credit of having directed attention to the principle of multiple rib resection for obliteration of chronic cavities. He resected a sufficient number of ribs completely to unroof the cavity. In his first communication,[63] in 1879, he reported six cases. In a later report[64] he emphasized that each case should be dealt with according to the condition found and that in cases with large cavities it might be necessary to repeat the operation a second or even a third time. Five of his eight patients were cured, two died, and one was still convalescing at the time he wrote.

Gallet collected the first 100 cases in which operation was performed by the Estlander method. In 9 of the 18 patients who died, necropsy showed large cavities with collapsed lungs. Voswinckel reported the results in 129 collected and 6 personal cases of multiple rib resection. Fifty-six per cent. of these patients were cured; 20 per cent. had improved; 4 per cent. were not improved; and 20 per cent. had died. In one case the results were uncertain. Of 14 tuberculous patients included in this series, 8 died, 2 were cured, 3 improved, and 1 did not improve.

The plastic operation was variously modified. Resection of segments of the ribs at the borders of the cavity through parallel incisions was made by Tietze and others. Wilms strongly advocates this method, especially for tuberculous empyema. He calls it the " Pfeiler Resection." Jaboulay and Leymarie resected the sternal ends, and Boiffin[22] the vertebral ends of the ribs. Tietze resected the ribs as for a Schede operation, but instead of excising the pleura, tamponed it against the lung. He stated that it produces a concentric pull on the lung and diaphragm.

In 1890 Schede described the extensive resection that bears his name. After turning up a skin and muscle flap of larger extent than the cavity, the whole of the chest wall underneath was resected, the skin muscle flap being then allowed to fall against the collapsed lung. He stated that in case the cavity extends to the pleural dome, it is also necessary to resect the first rib. He reported 10 cases with 2 deaths, and later 389 collected cases with 87.7 per cent. cures and 12.3 per cent. mortality. Bergeat collected 134 cases in which 56.5 per cent. of the patients were cured; 4.5 per cent. were improved; 14.3 per cent. had residual fistulas; 1.5 per cent. were not improved, and 23.2 per cent. died. Sudeck, Depage, Beck, Helferich, Friedrich, Sauerbruch,[156] and others, attempted to lessen the duration and shock of this formidable operation by dividing it into stages by various modifications. Sudeck, Depage, Friedrich, and later Melchior and Goebel made use of the thickened parietal pleura to help in obliterating the cavity.

In 1892 Delorme enunciated a new principle in the treatment of chronic empyema cavities, namely, that of their obliteration by reëxpansion of the lung. Previous to this time attention had been consistently centred on the chest wall, the collapse of which was considered the only means of obliterating the cavity. This new method was foreshadowed by Cornil, Oulmont, Ehrmann, and others. In several post-mortem cases in which the empyema had been of three months' to a year's duration, Oulmont was able to double or treble the size of the collapsed lung by gentle insufflation. Laennec[107] also expressed the opinion that the reason the lung remained collapsed in these cases is because of the limiting membranes and not because of the condition of the lung. Others, on the contrary, were of the opinion that sclerosis in the lung tissue or inseparable adhesions on its surface preclude any possibility of reëxpansion of the lung. It remained for Fowler and Delorme to prove the point on the living patient. Fowler performed his first operation October 7, 1893, and reported the case December 30th, of the same year. He considered the operation adapted to non-tuberculous cases, and concluded the article as follows: " The case suggests a method of dealing with some of the instances of old empyema with persistent sinus which resist all means usually employed for their cure."

In May, 1892, Delorme dissected off the parietal pleura more than 1 cm. thick in a patient with a small empyema cavity. The expansion of the lung that resulted suggested to him the possibility of obliterating large cavities by a similar procedure. In June of the same year (1892), before the Academy of Medicine, and in April, 1893, at the Surgical Congress, he proposed the method. January 20, 1894, Delorme first performed the operation in a case of empyema of four and one-half months' duration, and obtained complete expansion of the lung. To Delorme, therefore, belongs the credit of first having enunciated the principle and to Fowler the credit of first having performed the operation. In 1896 Delorme published the results in 18 cases; 5 patients were completely cured; 2 were improved; and 8 were not benefited. Delorme recognized no contraindication to operation except a poor general condition of the patient. He wrote that tuberculosis is not a contraindication, but that in its presence it is almost impossible to secure complete obliteration of the cavity.

Modifications of the decortication operation as first described by Delorme and Fowler have been numerous. The most important one designed to conserve the chest wall was the introduction of rib-spreading exposure. Roux found that by retracting at the anterior angle of an intercostal incision good exposure was secured. Sauerbruch[157] described an improved technic with subsequent suture around the ribs for air-tight closure. Friedrich and others have used rib retraction. Lilienthal[118] sectioned the ribs in addition to spreading them. Boiffin[23] used a posterior incision to secure access to the paravertebral space. Quénu and Soubottin sectioned the entire thickness of the chest wall anteriorly and posteriorly, but without removing the ribs. Krause, Jordan, Goullioud, and others did extensive resection, practically combining the Estlander and Delorme operations. Ringel and others combined the Schede and Delorme procedures. After decortication Lambotte proposed insufflation of the lung through a preliminary tracheotomy.

Successful case reports have been published by Bazy, Battle, Newton, Cotte, Meyer, and Kümmell. Lund reported seven cases with two deaths, neither due to shock. Mayo and Beckman reported seven cases, with one death. They expressed the opinion that the operation has not received the consideration it deserves. Dowd reported fifteen cases; fourteen of them were in children whose average age was five and one-half years. There was one operative death. Dowd wrote that in extreme cases there are many disappointments and that it is easier to secure expansion of the lung than to maintain it. Lilienthal[117] reported twenty cases with three deaths, Whittemore fifteen cases with eleven complete cures and no mortality. In twenty-nine cases mentioned by Binnie, seventeen patients were cured; nine were not improved, and three died. Violet collected seventy-nine cases. Forty-eight and one-tenth per cent. of the patients were cured; 7.7 per cent. were improved; 31.7 per cent. were not improved, and 11.4 per cent. died. One case was not completed. Kurpjuweit reported fifty-six collected cases. Thirty five and seven-tenths per cent. of the patients were cured; 19.7 per cent. were improved; 33.9 per cent. were not improved, and 10.7 per cent. died.

In a case in which it was impossible to separate the thickened pleura from the lung, Ransohoff found that by making gridiron incisions about 0.6 cm. apart, a considerable expansion of the lung was obtained owing to wide separation of the cut edges of the pleura. This procedure has been used since quite extensively in conjunction with the various modifications of the plastic operations.

Lambotte recommended suturing the lung to the parietal pleura after decortication, if the lung failed to expand.

Kurpjuweit advised extensive rib resection to bring about expansion.

Souligoux proposed cutting the thickened membrane at its reflection to the parietal pleura, thus securing mobilization *en masse* if the lung failed to expand. The method appears to be practical, however, only if the lung also expands at least in part.

Robinson described a plastic operation for closure of chronic cavities posteriorly, making use of the muscles of the thoracic wall to help fill the cavity. Taddei obliterated a cavity by transplanting a lipoma. Beck obtained very good results by the use of skin flaps after radical excision of the roof of the cavity. He has also reported 80 per cent. of patients cured in 150 cases of chronic empyema sinuses in which bismuth paste was used.

Irrigation of Chronic Cavities.—The use of irrigation for chronic cavities dates back to Hippocrates. He directed that wine and oil should be injected on the tenth day. Galen and Rhazes, the Arabian, used water and honey. Guy de Chauliac employed various decoctions. Evacuants and detergents were used by Fabricius ab Aquapendente, Ambrose Paré, Dionis, Willis, and others.

Lamotte, according to Massiani, was the first to reject all irrigations. Opinions have differed on the subject ever since. Van Swieten, Ravaton, Maraud, and Pelletan used various fluids. Bell, Chopart, Desault, and Lassus condemned the practice as dangerous.

Velpeau advised irrigation in encapsulated cavities. Boinet and Boudant recommended chlorides and iodides, and Sedillot, a caustic solution, as the therapeutic agent. Since that time a great variety of solutions have been used, such as methyl salicylate, phenol, creolin, iodine, saline solution, hydrogen peroxide, boric acid and carbolated iodine, corrosive sublimate, and "purefied air." After the use of intrapleural antiseptics fell decidedly into disrepute, it was renewed again by J. B. Murphy, who was a staunch advocate of the use of formalin in glycerine.

In the available literature, the first mention of the use of chloride of lime was by de Brabant in 1837. Townsend in 1845 recommended a " weak solution of chloride of lime as an antiseptic."

Since the work of Dakin and Carrel with the hypochlorite solution, intrapleural injection has come into favor again. Its use, however, has been largely limited to acute cases.

From the foregoing historical review it is found that, although empyema has been recognized and treated for twenty-six centuries, it is only sixty years since a sound rib first was resected for drainage. During the next thirty years attention was directed solely toward collapsing the thoracic wall for obliteration of the cavity. The most radical stage was reached in the complete Schede resection. Since that time the trend has been toward increasing conservatism, the first real contributions in this direction being those of Delorme and Fowler. It has also become more clearly and generally recognized that there is a considerable variability in the pathologic and clinical aspects of the disease.

The first essential to a consideration of treatment is a clear conception of the cause of chronicity and of the pathology involved. Since chronic cavities and residual sinuses are often but different stages in the same case, the two conditions are considered together. It should be recognized, however, that each may exist independently.

The most common causes of persistent fistula, apart from chronic cavities, are osteomyelitis of the rib, bronchocutaneous fistula, extreme sclerosis of the walls of the sinus, foreign bodies, and, occasionally, tuberculosis. The common causes of a persistent cavity are inadequate drainage; pneumothorax, whether from early open drainage or from a ruptured subpleural abscess resulting in more or less complete collapse of the lung not yet fixed by adhesions; too late drainage after the lung has become fixed firmly in a collapsed position; persistent bronchial fistulas; the presence of foreign bodies; reinfection; and tuberculosis. Of all these factors insufficient drainage is the most common. As a result of the prolonged suppuration a pyogenic membrane which may be 1.25 cm. or more thick is formed. This membrane tends to prevent expansion of the lung even after the primary cause is removed. Treatment should naturally be designed, so far as possible, to remove the cause. Dependent drainage and removal of necrosed rib or foreign material are simple procedures, yet they often bring about a cure after years of chronicity. If a bronchial fistula is present its closure is usually a prerequisite to healing.

The pathologic condition often can be recognized only in part. Conditions of the lung with respect to tuberculous and other sclerotic changes

300

are ften difficult to determine. If an extensive pulmonary tuberculosis is present, or if the bacilli are demonstrated in the pleural exudate, or the typical microscopic picture is found in the sectioned pleura, the diagnosis is established. A history of a primary pleurisy with serous effusion, later becoming purulent, is also at least very suggestive. Often, however, the history and findings are indefinite and uncertain. Primary tuberculous empyema, secondarily infected by injudicious drainage or from within, may present a typical picture of the ordinary suppurative pleurisy.

Whether or not the lung is capable of expansion is difficult to decide with any certainty. Various methods to ascertain this have been described, mostly based on a decrease in the size of the cavity during forced expiration. Obviously such a determination may be more a measure of the relative rigidity of the thickened pleura than the elasticity of the lung. Reineboth's ingenious method, depending on the changes in pulmonary circulation that result in increasing the intrapulmonary pressure in a lung that is still expansible but in which changes do not occur if expansibility is lost, unfortunately has not so far proved of practical value. The mechanism by which a collapsed lung expands is of much practical importance and the subject of much difference of opinion. The presence of an intrapleural pressure less than atmospheric and the reason for this so-called "negative" pressure is an elementary fact in physiology. It is also recognized that if an opening is made into the pleural cavity, the lung collaspses from equalization-pressure on the two sides of the lung alveolus. Other factors of the first importance to the clinical application of these fundamentals until recently have received but scant attention. Among such factors are the size of the opening in the chest wall in relation to the size of the glottis, the presence of adhesions between the lung and the chest wall, the mobility of the mediastinum, and the vital capacity. The importance of the relationship between the opening in the chest wall and the glottis was recognized by Houston. He asked van Swieten if a person wounded in both sides of the thorax would die. On being answered in the affirmative Houston produced a small normal dog on which he had opened both pleuras three days before. This astonished van Swieten, who repeated the experiment and was persuaded that when air entered the two pleural cavities the wounds were fatal only if the two openings combined were larger in area than that of the glottis. Later Cruveilhier repeated these experiments. It remained for Graham and Bell, however, to point out the great importance of the relationship to the treatment of acute empyema. They showed that in acute cases, owing to the mobility of the mediastinum, the two pleural cavities react as one to changed intrathoracic pressure. Lowering or neutralizing the negative pressure on the one side changed the pressure the same on the other side. Graham showed that the absolute size of an opening in the chest wall, compared with that of the glottis, depends on the vital capacity at the time. Thus a man with healthy lungs can withstand a much larger opening than one with pneumonia or poorly developed lungs.

These considerations are of fundamental importance in the treatment of empyema. The large number of variables involved explains, at least in large measure, the apparently divergent experiences and opinions on the subject of acute pneumothorax. In chronic empyema, because of the fixation of the mediastinum and the presence of pulmonary adhesions, the two pleural cavities function independently. For this reason a wide opening on the affected side does not produce respiratory insufficiency.

The mechanism by means of which the lung reëxpands has been variously explained. Roser held that it was by the progressive growth of adhesions along the margins of the cavity, the contraction of which pulls out the lung. Weissgerber, on the other hand, held that lung expansion is due to increased intratracheal pressure during expiration, resulting in a summation expansion of the lung. The different conceptions are reflected in the variety of devices for increasing the intratracheal tension, on the one hand, and for decreasing the tension in the pleural cavity, on the other. More recent opinion is also divided. Physicians still use pleural suction. Perhaps the majority, however, are of the opinion that the lung, when free, expands essentially because of the increased tension from within the bronchi, during coughing, straining, or other effort involving closure of the glottis, and that closed drainage, valve action, a pus-soaked dressing, and the like are used chiefly in helping to hold the amount of expansion gained. There is much clinical evidence also indicating that progressive adhesions help to hold the lung out, once it is expanded.

Some surgeons believe that adhesions are always detrimental. Thus Lloyd, on the principle that the adhesions tend to prevent expansion, routinely separated them at operation. He reported cases of 225 patients treated in this manner, but with less than 50 per cent. complete cures and 20 per cent. mortality. Homans has expressed the belief that adhesions in the early stage, are often the cause of chronicity, but that fixation of the lung to the diaphragm favors expansion.

In chronic empyema the greatly thickened membranes prevent the action of the mechanism which brings about expansion of the lung. If these membranes are removed, incised, or disintegrated, the same mechanism again comes into play, provided the lung has retained its elasticity.

At operation it is often observed that when the patient coughs or strains the liberated lung expands in response to the increased intratracheal pressure. In the after-treatment, as in the acute condition, the same factors favor permanent expansion. In the cases in which cavity obliteration occurs following the liberating action of Dakin's solution, it can be determined when operation is performed for a small residual cavity, that the lung is adhering progressively at the periphery of the cavity. Dunham observed at necropsy, in cases in which Dakin's solution was used, that the walls of the cavity were covered with granulations favorable for adhesions, while in those in which there was no treatment a shaggy fibro-purulent deposit was found. In case of reinfection these adhesions tend to break down and the cavity enlarges.

Tuffier, Stevens, and others have reported series of cases in which, after sterilization, the tubes were withdrawn and the pneumothorax left to itself, but this method has resulted in many recurrences. If the treatment is successful, the lung apparently expands in proportion as the air absorbs, but in some instances cavities have persisted for months. It seems reasonable to believe that such treatment is more suitable in recent cases than when the condition has persisted for years. To what extent an increasing pulmonary circulation, incident to deep breathing exercise and other effort, aids in bringing about expansion, can not be stated, but some experimental evidence has been found to indicate that an increased circulation in the capillaries tends to expand the lung alveolus.

In cases of tuberculous empyema a large cavity may persist for years without any tendency toward lung expansion. At operation in some such cases it is found that the pleura is not appreciably thickened; the failure to expand is probably due to a fibrosis of the lung by which it has lost its expansibility. Fibrosis seems to occur also in long-standing pyogenic empyema.

Aside from considerations of etiology and pathology, the guiding principle in the choice of treatment should be conservatism. Chronic empyema is not necessarily incompatible with years of life and usefulness. In such cases it may be questioned whether radical treatment involving considerable loss of function is ever indicated. It would certainly seem difficult to justify a high mortality, particularly if a safer and more effective method is available. Shortening convalescence is often mentioned as one of the arguments for a radical procedure, but it seems that shortening convalescence does not justify an increased mortality. In the choice of a method of treatment the first consideration, therefore, should be the life of the patient, the second, the preserving of function, and the third, the shortening of the convalescence.

CLINICAL STUDY OF CASES AT THE MAYO CLINIC

In 49 of 150 cases of empyema at the Mayo Clinic prior to 1910 the Estlander operation was performed; in 9 the Schede resection, and in 1 the Delorme decortication. One death occurred following a Schede operation. The 210 patients with empyema treated between 1910 and November, 1917, had more or less extensive rib resections. A Schede operation was done in six instances, a decortication in seven, and Ransohoff's discission of the pleura in one. There were fourteen deaths; one followed a decortication.

During a little more than two years beginning November, 1917, 150 patients with chronic empyema have been treated in the clinic, with a few exceptions, by the writer. Eight of these patients had sinuses only, some of which, however, were fairly extensive. The others had chronic cavities varying in capacity from 50 to 2500 c.c. One hundred and seventeen of the series had been operated on elsewhere. Most of the others came with large accumulations of pus, variously diagnosed. One boy presented himself for the treatment of an extreme scoliosis due to unrecognized empyema of probably eight years' duration. One had been given up as a hopeless case of malignant disease. Unresolved pneumonia and abscess of the lung were diagnosed in many of these cases. Fifteen had tuberculous empyema. Judging from the history, clinical findings, and course, thirteen others may also have been tuberculous. One case of actinomycotic empyema is not included.

It may be noted that three months are taken arbitrarily as the time limit between acute and chronic empyema. In some patients in the series, not previously operated on, the date of onset had to be approximated from the history. In many of the others, in which the duration was calculated from the date of a late operation, it was probably considerably longer than stated. The duration of the empyema by periods and the number of cases in each is indicated in Table I.

TABLE I

Duration of Empyema

	Cases
3 to 5 months	38
6 to 12 months	47
13 to 24 months	30
2 to 3 years	12
3 to 5 years	7
5 to 10 years	11
10 to 15 years	3
15 to 20 years	1
More than 20 years	1
	150

TABLE II

Age

	Patients
Less than 5 years	6
6 to 10 years	5
11 to 15 years	6
16 to 20 years	24
21 to 30 years	58
31 to 40 years	34
41 to 50 years	9
51 to 60 years	7
66 years	1
	150

Only eleven were children under ten, yet five of the unrecognized cases were in this age group. In one of these the diagnosis had been first diphtheria, then scarlet fever, and finally typhoid fever.

TABLE III

Occupation

	Cases
Farmer	54
Business man	23
Laborer	11
Housewife	9
Student	10
Carpenter	6
Machinist	5
Soldier	3
Miner	3
Railroad man	9
None	6
Not stated	2
Miscellaneous	9
	150

The occupation seemed to bear no obvious relation to incidence.

In nineteen cases there was a fairly definite family history of tuberculosis. Alcoholism in moderation was noted in thirty-seven, and in excess in three. A past history of pneumonia was given in 105, in several of which there had been more than one attack. Pleurisy had been present in association with pneumonia in sixty-four, and was primary in sixteen. A serous effusion followed pneumonia in two definitely tuberculous cases. In eight instances of primary effusion a definite diagnosis of tuberculosis could not be made, but several of these cases ran a clinical course characteristic of a tuberculous empyema secondarily infected.

TABLE IV

Chief Complaints

	Cases
Draining sinus	87
Pain in chest	22
Weakness	11
Fever	7
Cough	9
Abscess of lung	6
Œdema	4
Arthritis	4
	150

The history of onset was given as sudden in 108 cases, insidious in thirty-two, and not stated in ten. The etiologic factors stated in the history were as follows:

TABLE V

Etiologic Factors

	Cases
Pneumonia	65
Pleurisy	15
Influenza	38
Trauma	8
"Cold"	6
Not stated	7
Miscellaneous	11
	150

Pain was a definite symptom in sixty-five; it was localized in the thorax in fifty-seven, and in the joints in four, and associated with respiration in six. Marked weakness was noted in fifty-five; cough was present in seventy, absent in twenty-eight, not stated in thirty-two, and was associated with sputum in sixty. The sputum was profuse in eleven; 500 c.c. in three, and 1000 c.c. in two, these being cases of bronchial fistula. Dyspnœa and pallor were noted in thirty-six and weakness in fifty. Hæmoptysis was noted in four. Loss of weight was a fairly prominent symptom.

TABLE VI

Loss of Weight

	Cases
Less than 10 pounds	6
11 to 15 pounds	7
16 to 20 pounds	14
21 to 30 pounds	14
31 to 40 pounds	12
41 to 50 pounds	2
51 to 60 pounds	3
61 to 70 pounds	2
None	10
Amount not stated	34
No mention	46
	150

Fever was present in seventy-five cases, and associated with chills in twenty-two. There was a leucocytosis in two-thirds of the cases in which a count was recorded. The average counts were as follows:

TABLE VII

Leucocytosis

	Cases
10,000 to 12,500	28
12,500 to 15,000	17
15,000 to 20,000	20
20,000 to 25,000	14
25,000 to 30,000	5
30,000 to 40,000	2
None	45
Not stated	19
	150

A persistent high leucocyte count was frequently observed in the cases in which Dakin's solution treatment was used without fever or other symptoms of toxic absorption. A secondary anæmia was present in the majority of patients, and to a considerable degree in about a third. The averages in 126 were as follows:

TABLE VIII

Hæmoglobin

	Cases
40 to 50 per cent.	10
50 to 60 per cent.	30
60 to 70 per cent.	46
70 to 80 per cent.	36
80 to 90 per cent.	4

A low blood-pressure indicative of an asthenic condition was noted more often than a high pressure. No significant variation was found between systolic and diastolic pressures.

TABLE IX

Systolic Blood-pressure

	Cases
80 to 90	3
90 to 100	15
100 to 110	24
110 to 140	77
140 to 160	5
160 to 180	1
Not stated	25
	150

CARL A. HEDBLOM

The urinalysis indicated only a relatively small number of cases with kidney involvement, even though the average duration was more than one year in sixty-five of the cases. On the basis of the terminology used in the Mayo Clinic, "albumin 1" signifies the slightest possible trace demonstrable. The albumin content was found to be as follows:

TABLE X

Albuminuria Graded 1 to 4

	Cases
Grade 1	66
Grade 2	25
Grade 3	1
Grade 4	1
None	43
Grade not stated	14
	150

Bacteriologic studies of the exudate at operation revealed the usual bacterial flora. Except for tuberculous infection, there appeared to be no clear relationship between the type of organism and the severity or course of the process in these chronic cases.

The right side was involved in eighty cases and the left side in seventy. The most constant physical signs aside from the presence of a sinus were dulness and flatness to percussion in varying proportion and degree. Dulness was noted in eighty-three and flatness in sixty-two.

Limitation of respiratory excursion was found in the majority of cases.

Fremitus was noted in the area involved in eight cases. Clubbing of the fingers was stated to be present in nineteen and clubbing of the toes in one. The heart was displaced to the right in fifteen and to the left in nine. A palpable liver and spleen, indicative of a degeneration, was noted in five and six cases, respectively.

The clinical diagnosis of the presence of empyema presented little difficulty. A typical empyema is most apt to be overlooked in children. Occasionally an encapsulated empyema with a large bronchial fistula may be quite difficult to distinguish from an abscess of the lung. In some cases, as in one of this series, both were present. In other cases in which there is a history of cough with large amounts of sputum, the differentiation may be impossible without X-ray. Three patients in this series with such symptoms had been treated for months for abscess of the lung. In one instance an empyema had persisted for years without breaking through either lung or chest wall. One case of typical empyema necessitas simulating an acute mastitis was observed. The clinical diagnosis supported by the X-ray examinations in this series was as follows:

TABLE XI

Clinical Diagnosis

	Cases
Chronic empyema	115
Effusion or empyema with tuberculosis	9
Empyema with pneumothorax	7
Empyema with bronchial fistula	8
Empyema or abscess	3
Pleural effusion	5
Pneumonia	1
Dermoid cyst	1
Echinococcus cyst	1
	150

It will be noted that a diagnosis of tuberculosis was made clinically in nine of the cases, but the tuberculous lesion was in the lung in five; a tuberculous effusion was specified in four. A diagnosis of a pulmonary lesion was made in three additional cases by the Röntgen-ray. One of these and two others were proved microscopically. All of these patients gave a history of pleurisy with effusion. Thirteen other patients gave a similar history of a primary pleurisy with effusion. Four of these patients were later proved to have a tuberculous infection of the pleura. Three who were shown by the röntgenogram to have pulmonary involvement clinically responded very well to treatment; the other two reacted in a manner characteristic of a tuberculous empyema. From these findings it appears that while both a pulmonary lesion and a history of a preceding pleurisy with effusion are important in the differential diagnosis of a tuberculous empyema, a pleurisy with effusion is probably the more significant. A tuberculous empyema may run its course without any clinical or Röntgen findings to suggest the condition (Fig. 1).

The choice of surgical treatment for chronic empyema has been between simple drainage and some type of operation designed to collapse the chest wall or to expand the lung. In the earlier cases in this series, if a cavity of any size persisted, simple drainage was first tried, followed by a decortication. In the autumn of 1918, Dakin's solution was first used in an attempt to obtain partial sterilization of the cavity before a decortication or plastic operation was performed. It was then discovered that not only the patient's general condition was improved greatly, but the cavity showed an unmistakable tendency to reduce. The solution was then used systematically and an extensive operation performed only after the hypochlorite solution treatment had been tried. If operation was indicated for a cavity of considerable size in a non-tuberculous case, an attempt was made routinely to obtain expansion of the lung before a collapse operation was performed.

Methods of Treatment.—The methods of treatment were as follows: (1) Simple rib resection, forty-two cases; (2) Dakin's solution with or without minor drainage operations, fifty-one cases; (3) pulmonary decortication, thirty cases; and (4) plastic operation on the chest wall, twenty-seven cases.

1. *Simple Rib Resection.*—Thirty-four of the forty-two patients in this group had been operated on elsewhere. Many of them had undergone several, and one eleven drainage operations. Among those who had not had previous operations there were several with large cavities. Two had bronchial fistulæ and were emptying the contents of a large cavity through the bronchus. Two had drainage tubes in the pleural cavity, the presence of which had been unsuspected. Faulty drainage was the rule; the drainage opening had been allowed to close or narrow down to a sinus before the cavity had become obliterated, or the opening was not at the most dependent point. The capacity of the cavity in this group was less than 250 c.c. in twelve, between 250 and 500 c.c. in eight, and near 1000 c.c. in two; in one the lung was almost wholly collapsed.

The results of simple drainage operation, not counting the tuberculous cases, were: Complete recovery, twenty-six cases; persistent sinus at last report, four cases; and death, one case. Eight patients could not be traced. Of the tuberculous patients one was greatly improved, one somewhat improved, and one was not benefited. All three had been drained previously elsewhere.

2. *Dakin's Solution With or Without a Minor Drainage Operation for a Small Residual Cavity.*—There were fifty-one cases in this group. The technic employed consisted in the insertion of a catheter through the old sinus or through a trocar and cannula, aspirating the pus and irrigating with the sodium hypochlorite solution. As a rule, normal saline solution was used for the first irrigation, and if there had been cough with sputum it was used always in order to avoid the marked bronchial irritation if a bronchial fistula should be present. Irrigation was performed at intervals of from one to three hours. Once or twice each day the cavity was half filled with the solution, which was aspirated after about ten minutes. Once a week the cavity was filled by gravity and the capacity noted. In this way progress was measured. The patients were encouraged to use blow bottles and other devices to produce increased intratracheal pressure. While they were blowing the catheter was connected with a tube, the other end of which was under water in order to allow the air to escape as the lung expanded and to prevent its return. The patients were given setting-up exercises and encouraged to be outdoors as much as possible besides. A generous diet was prescribed.

TABLE XII

Results of Dakin's Solution Treatment in Fifty-one Cases

Capacity of cavity	Average number of days of treatment	Capacity of cavity at end of treatment	Average decrease in capacity of cavity per cent.	Cases
Less than 100 c.c.	35.9	10 c.c.	90.0	11
100 to 250 c.c.	34.1	11 c.c. to 27.5 c.c.	89.0	16
250 to 500 c.c.	56.4	11 c.c. to 22.0 c.c.	95.6	15
500 to 1000 c.c.	45.2	11 c.c. to 22.0 c.c.	97.8	5
1000 to 2000 c.c.	32.0	80 c.c. to 160 c.c.	92.0	4

	Cases
Complete recovery	34
Sinus at last report	6
No late report	6
Convalescence not completed	4
No benefit (tuberculosis)	1
	51

A large portion of the time spent in treatment was for the final obliteration of a cavity after it had been reduced 50 to 75 per cent. (Figs. 2 and 3).

Besides the reduction in the size of cavities of more than 90 per cent., there was a striking general improvement in all these patients. A gain in weight of from 1 to 2 pounds each day for a period of two or three weeks was frequently observed. A slight amount of bleeding and occasionally some cough were noted, but no serious complications. The hypochlorite solution was used in fifteen patients preliminary to pulmonary decortication. Six were treated for a period not exceeding three weeks, all of these showing an appreciable decrease in the size of the cavity. In the other cases, with one exception, there was also a material decrease (Figs. 4 to 12).

TABLE XIII

Result of Dakin's Solution Treatment Preliminary to Decortication in Fifteen Cases

Capacity of cavity	Duration of empyema, months	Days of treatment	Capacity of cavity at end of treatment
360 c.c.	6	9	210 c.c.
500 c.c.	20	10	200 c.c.
200 c.c.	21	12	100 c.c.
500 c.c.	6	12	180 c.c.
240 c.c.	4	19	150 c.c.
300 c.c.	4	21	240 c.c.
150 c.c.	3	27	150 c.c.
420 c.c.	15	30	390 c.c.
1000 c.c.	14	32	90 c.c.
150 c.c.	7	42	15 c.c.
1500 c.c.	3	43	100 c.c.
400 c.c.	4	46	30 c.c.
500 c.c.	6	70	60 c.c.
2000 c.c.	6	75	120 c.c.
2000 c.c.	14	150	240 c.c.

Several of the patients in this series would not have withstood an operation of any magnitude without the preliminary treatment. One was a girl with complete collapse of the lung following traumatic empyema. She was reduced from 120 pounds to 73 pounds and was brought to the clinic on a stretcher. She was completely cured with almost full re-expansion of the lung. Another patient had an almost total pneumo-thorax, a complete inhibition Wassermann reaction, and a severe grade of nephritis with œdema. His blood was rendered negative to the Was-sermann test, his lung reëxpanded about 90 per cent., and he gained about 30 pounds as a result of the preliminary treatment.

3. *Pulmonary Decortication.*—There were thirty cases in this group. The operation, except in some early cases before Dakin's solution was employed as a routine, was performed only after the antiseptic method had been used and a large cavity remained. In a few of the early cases, only, the cavity was comparatively small. In these cases in which it failed to obliterate, it had been rendered relatively sterile, and the patient's general condition was very materially improved.

Decortication was done under general anæsthesia through a rib-spreading exposure. By use of a suitable rib retractor, adequate expo-sure was obtained without cutting the ribs. In some cases in which the cavity lay very high, incision was made in the sixth or fifth interspace, cutting the scapula across and resuturing it. Possibly resection of the ribs posteriorly would have been a better procedure. The thickened visceral pleura was incised and separated by blunt dissection. In many cases the preliminary irrigation had softened it to such an extent that the separation could be done very readily. If cavities were large a complete visceral decortication was done, mobilizing the entire lung. In one case only, of primary tuberculous empyema, it was absolutely impossible to separate or satisfactorily to incise it, but partial obliteration of the cavity was secured by mobilizing the lung, as first suggested by Souligoux.

TABLE XIV

Results of Decortication in Thirty Cases

	Cases
Complete cure without further surgery	15
Complete cure after secondary plastic operation for small residual cavity	5
Persistent sinus, last report	3
Death following operation	1
Death from other causes several weeks after patient left hospital	3
Under treatment	3

Two of the three patients with small sinuses were tuberculous. In

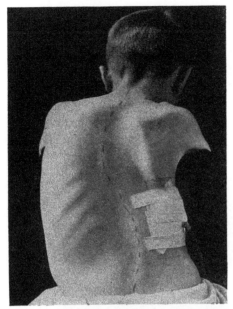

Fig. 1. (Case 269926).—Unrecognized empyema probably of eight
years' duration; cavity obliterated by Dakin's solution and minor
drainage operation.

31ª

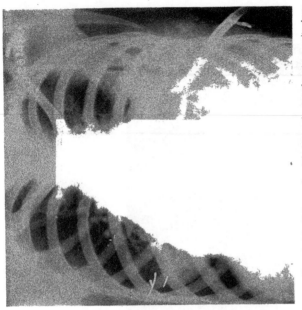

FIG. 5 (Case 261485).—Full expansion of the lung at the apex of empyema cavity shown in Figs. 4 and 5 after about four months' treatment. Complete cure followed plastic operation on residual cavity.

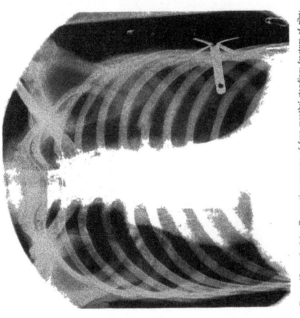

FIG. 4 (Case 261485).—Traumatic empyema of four months' standing; fracture of ribs; almost complete collapse of the lung before Dakin's solution treatment. Patient's weight, 73 pounds; normal weight, 125.

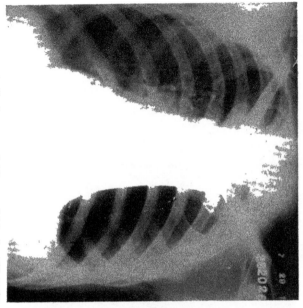

FIG. 6 (Case 282026).—Chronic empyema of eighteen months' duration; with massive collapse of lung; chronic nephritis with œdema, and complete inhibition Wassermann test.

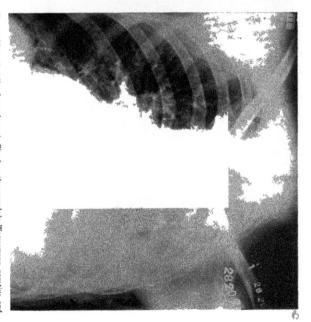

FIG. 7 (Case 282026).   Lung shown in Fig. 6 partly expanded; Wassermann negative, and patient gained 30 pounds in weight.

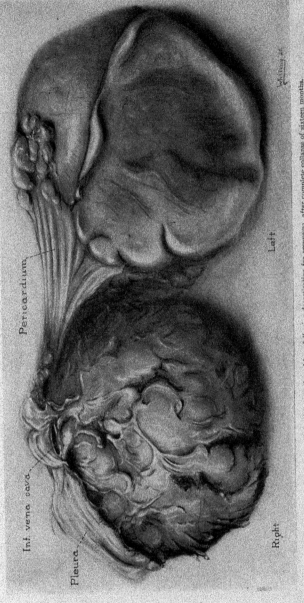

Pericardium

Inf. vena cava

Pleura

Right

Left

Fig. 8 (Case 307153).—Partial expansion of lung following decortication for empyema, after complete collapse of sixteen months.

one of these the cavity was practically obliterated. The patient gained very materially in weight and general condition following operation. The one operative death was due to a streptococcus pneumonia occurring dur‐ ing an influenza epidemic. Two of the patients who died several weeks

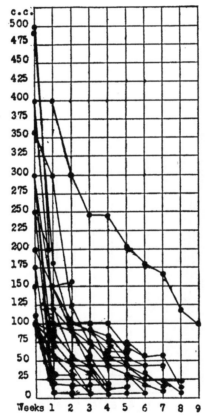

FIG. 2.—Twenty-eight cases, capacity from 100 to 500 c.c.

after operation also had epidemic influenzal bronchopneumonia. Necropsy in one of these showed one lung expanded and an empyema on the other side. The third patient, in whom the cavity had been reduced to about 30 c.c. capacity by operation, died of pulmonary hemorrhage seven months later. Tuberculosis bacilli were found in the exudate and tubercles in

313

the pleura shortly before death. At no time did the X-ray show any evidence of tuberculosis (Figs. 13 to 17).

4. *Plastic Operation Involving the Collapse of the Chest Wall.*—Twenty-
seven patients were treated by this method. The duration of the disease

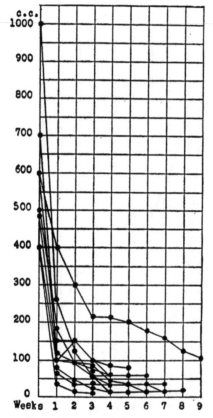

FIG. 3.—Ten cases, capacity from 400 to 1000 c.c.

was more than one year in twenty-one and more than two years in
eleven; in one it was of twenty-three years' duration. Five patients were
definitely proved to be tuberculous; two others belonged to the group of
primary pleurisy with effusion which ran a course suggestive of tuberculosis. Dakin's solution was used in eight patients in this group (Fig. 18).

TABLE XV

Results of Dakin's Solution Treatment Preliminary to Plastic Operation in Eight Cases

Capacity of cavity	Duration of empyema	Days	Capacity of cavity at end of treatment
500 c.c.	3 months	22	120 c.c.
150 c.c.	4 months	55	30 c.c.
60 c.c.	3 years	57	45 c.c.
100 c.c.	3 years	35	100 c.c.
200 c.c.	10 months	30	60 c.c.
150 c.c.	1 year	9	150 c.c.
500 c.c.	9 months	47	30 c.c.
750 c.c.	7 years	90	300 c.c.

In nineteen cases the solution could not be used on account of fistulas, or they were early cases treated before the solution was used routinely.

The operation involved resection of the ribs over the entire cavity, and with one exception, in which an Estlander operation was performed, excising the intercostal tissue and parietal pleura. A complete Schede operation was not found necessary in any case. The extent of rib resection was reduced in the majority of cases by the skin sliding method described by Beck. In a few instances a skin-muscle flap, as recommended by Robinson, was made. Resection of the lower angle of the scapula was necessary in three instances in which the cavity lay directly under it. In one case of tuberculous empyema of twenty-three years' standing, the whole chest wall was resected *en masse*, after the method recently described by Peuckert. In another, also tuberculous, the Wilms operation was performed in three stages.

TABLE XVI

Results Following Plastic Operation in Twenty-seven Cases

	Cases
Cure	15
Residual sinus at last report	3
Death	2
Convalescence not complete	4
Not traced	3
	—
	27

Two of the patients with persistent sinuses were tuberculous. In one the sinus closed after many months. In one the sinus was due to multiple bronchial fistulas with an associated bronchiectasis. The closure of bronchial fistulas, as I have mentioned, is necessary to the cure of an empyema cavity.

The cases of bronchial fistulæ in this series may, for convenience, be divided into three groups; namely, those in which the fistulæ closed spontaneously, those in which it was obliterated by operative procedure, and those in which it persisted.

CARL A. HEDBLOM

In the first group are a number of cases in which the hypochlorite solution was used. A bronchial fistula was judged to be present if the patient coughed during irrigation and at the same time tasted the solution. In some instances these symptoms were so slight and transitory that the treatment could be continued provided the cavity was not filled. In others irrigation could be done only when the patient assumed a certain posture. Occasionally it was necessary to substitute saline solution for longer or shorter periods. In a considerable number there was slight bleeding from time to time. In no case was the bleeding profuse. In a few the fistulas were observed at operation; they were uniformly small.

In the second group are the ten cases in which the fistulas were 0.7 cm. or more in diameter. They were multiple in one case only. Four were due to perforation of large unrecognized empyemas of long standing. These closed after wide open drainage was provided. In one case of ten years' duration a large fistula was found at the costovertebral angle. It was closed by an extensive resection and cauterization of the tract. In another instance the scar tissue was completely removed and the edges of the fistula sutured after preliminary cauterization. The remaining four fistulas were closed by resection of the ribs and thickened pleura followed by skin plastic.

In the group of cases with persistent bronchial fistulas were two tuberculous cases. In one an unsuccessful partial plastic operation was done; in the other no treatment was given for the fistula. A third patient had twenty or more bronchial fistulas in the same lobe of the lung, with extensive bronchiectasis. Considerable improvement in the general condition and obliteration of most of the fistulas resulted from granulation tissue proliferation after cauterization (Fig. 19).

RESULTS OF ALL METHODS OF TREATMENT

TABLE XVII

Summary of Results of Treatment in 150 Cases of Chronic Empyema

	Drainage operation Cases	Dakin's solution treatment Cases	Decortication operation Cases	Plastic operation Cases	Total Cases
Complete recovery	26	34	20	15	95
Residual sinus at last report	6	6	6	3	21
No report, or convalescence not completed	8	10	3	7	28
No relief	1	1	0	0	2
Death *	1	0	1	2	4
Total	42	51	30	27	150

Some of the persistent sinuses followed plastic operations for tuber-

* Besides the patients whose deaths were recorded as operative, four patients died after leaving the hospital, two several weeks after operation of streptococcus pneumonia; one died seven months after operation of tuberculosis, and one of " meningitis."

316

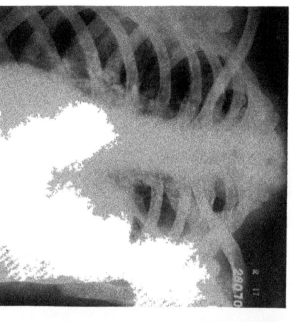

FIG. 9 (Case 266791).—Chronic empyema of four months' standing before treatment.

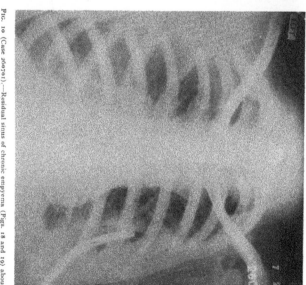

FIG. 10 (Case 266791).—Residual sinus of chronic empyema (Figs. 18 and 19) about nine weeks after decortication. Later cure was complete.

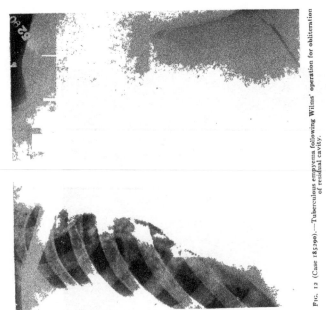

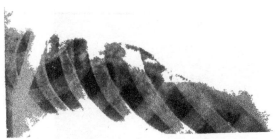

FIG. 12 (Case 185290).—Tuberculous empyema following Wilms' operation for obliteration of residual cavity.

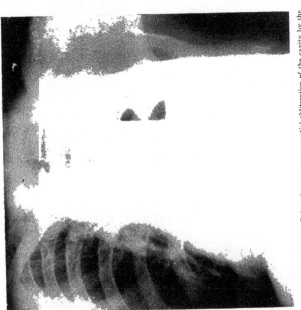

FIG. 11 (Case 185290).—Tuberculous empyema; partial obliteration of the cavity by the use of Dakin's solution treatment.

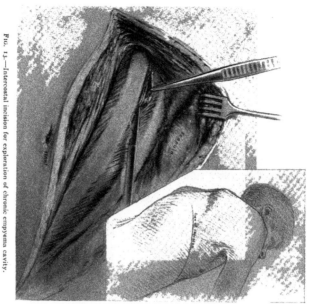

FIG. 13.—Intercostal incision for exploration of chronic empyema cavity.

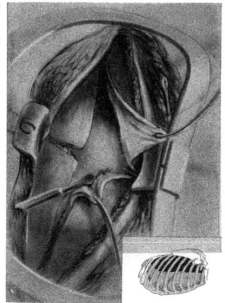

FIG. 14.—Decortication following a crucial incision in the pleura in a case of large cavity. The apex of the scapula has been removed, the ribs being divided in the sixth interspace. Retractor devised by the writer.

316

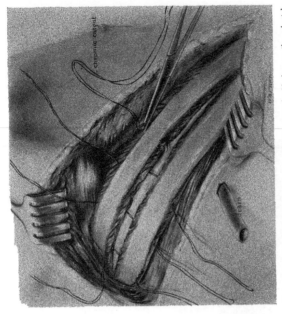

FIG. 16.—Air-tight closure of chest wall. Catheter through old sinus or through stab wound for aspiration and suction.

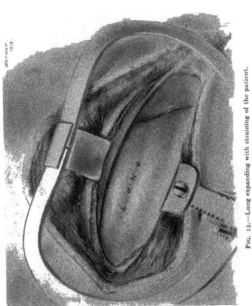

FIG. 15.—Lung expanding with straining of the patient.

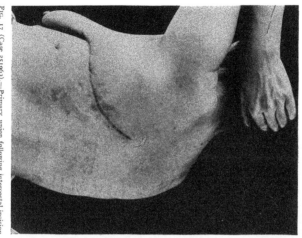

FIG. 17 (Case 251963).—Primary union following intercostal incision for pulmonary decortication. All ribs intact. The patient has free use of her arm.

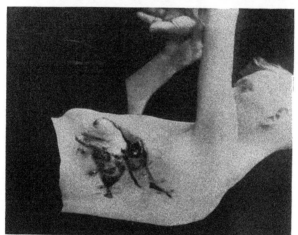

FIG. 18 (Case 214734).—Plastic operation for closure of the chronic cavity.

316

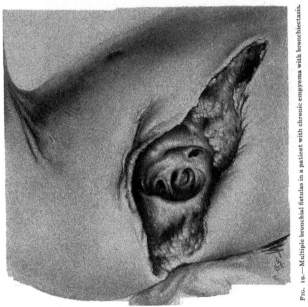

Fig. 19.—Multiple bronchial fistulas in a patient with chronic empyema with bronchiectasis.

culous empyema, others are in recent pyogenic cases giving promise of complete closure. Practically all non-tuberculous sinuses can be obliterated by plastic operation. Since, as experience has shown, however, that the majority of the sinuses heal spontaneously, expectant treatment for a limited period has been considered justified and in many cases advisable.

TABLE XVIII

Operative Deaths

Cause of death	Operation	Cases
Sepsis and inanition	Rib resection for drainage	1
Cerebral abscess	Plastic operation	1
Tuberculous meningitis	Plastic operation	
Influenzal pneumonia	Decortication operation	1

CONCLUSIONS

From the study of the literature and of 150 cases from the Mayo Clinic, the following tentative conclusions may be drawn:

1. Chronic empyema has been recognized and treated during twenty-six centuries, but it is only sixty years since the first rib resection for drainage was done. The successive stages in the progress of treatment since that time are as follows:

(a) Increasingly radical treatment, designed to obliterate the cavity by the collapse of the chest wall, involving successively more extensive operations, and culminating finally in a complete radical resection.

(b) A conservative trend manifested primarily in the modifications of the complete resection, but more in the attempt to preserve the chest wall and to restore the lung to its structural and functional relationships as first advocated by Delorme.

(c) The adaptation of the Carrel-Dakin hypochlorite solution technic to the treatment of chronic empyema cavities.

2. Chronic empyema is a disease which is not incompatible with life nor with a fair degree of health and usefulness. The principles of treatment should, therefore, be, first, the preservation of life, and second, as far as possible, the conservation of function. Shortening convalescence, while very desirable, should always be a subsidiary consideration.

3. The choice of treatment must be made with cognizance of the variable etiology and pathology of the process, and the general condition of the patient.

4. A major procedure is indicated only if non-operative or less extensive surgical treatment reasonably may be considered less effective.

5. In case of sinuses and small cavities, adequate drainage is usually sufficient to effect a cure with or without short preliminary hypochlorite solution treatment. It is at least open to question whether a radical

operation is indicated in these cases for the sole purpose of shortening convalescence at the risk of an appreciably increased mortality.

6. Dakin's hypochlorite solution treatment is the method of choice in the treatment of the ordinary type of chronic empyema cavity of any size, for the following reasons:

(a) The general condition of the patient is, as a rule, improved to a remarkable degree.

. (b) The cavity may be obliterated or greatly reduced in capacity by the liberation and expansion of the lung (resulting from the treatment).

(c) If the lung expands in part the extent of a later operation will be proportionately reduced.

(d) If the lung entirely fails to expand, the cavity will have become relatively sterile in preparation for operation, thereby lowering post-operative morbidity and mortality.

(e) Pulmonary decortication will be materially facilitated in some cases, owing to the softening action of the solution on the visceral pleura.

7. A pulmonary decortication through a rib-spreading exposure after preliminary hypochlorite solution irrigation is the most conservative treatment for cavities that are not obliterated by drainage or Dakin's solution treatment alone. If such an operation is successful, the lung is restored to its normal structural and functional relationship, thereby obliterating the cavity. If the operation is only partly successful, the magnitude of a secondary destructive operation is proportionately decreased.

8. Since it is impossible to judge with certainty before operation of the relative expansibility of the lung in every recent non-tuberculous case, a decortication should be done rather than a destructive operation, thereby giving the patient the benefit of the doubt.

9. If the lung does not expand, or if a considerable cavity persists following decortication, a plastic operation is indicated.

10. If the cavity is of considerable extent or the patient debilitated, a two- or three-stage plastic operation is to be recommended.

11. The recognition of tuberculous empyema is often difficult. A history of a primary pleurisy with effusion seems more often to signify a tuberculous condition than does a pulmonary lesion, unless the latter is active and extensive. A tuberculous empyema may be present in the absence of clinical or X-ray evidence of pulmonary involvement. The typical microscopic picture in the sectioned pleura or the demonstration of the bacilli in the exudate may constitute the only evidence in such cases.

12. A tuberculous empyema not secondarily infected should not be drained, and should be aspirated only for a considerable accumulation of fluid. For a tuberculous empyema secondarily infected, either by operation or spontaneously, drainage is necessary.

13. In the absence of bronchial fistulas and of bleeding, secondarily infected tuberculous empyema may be markedly benefited by antiseptic solution treatment. The amount of fibrosis or other pathologic change

in the lung in such cases determines the degree of expansion of the lung, whether following antiseptic solution treatment or decortication.

14. If the lung fails to expand in whole or in large part, a several-stage operation designed to collapse the chest wall is indicated. Tuberculous patients are relatively poor operative risks.

15. Adequate drainage is the first indication in cases of empyema cavities which are draining through large bronchial fistulas. The fistulas may be obliterated spontaneously following such treatment.

16. Operative closure of bronchial fistulas that persist is necessary to complete healing. It may be accomplished by decortication of the involved portion of the lung with cautery, suture, or skin plastic to cover the opening of the fistula. Occasionally healing results from simple granulation of surrounding tissue after destruction of the epithelial lining of the bronchial stoma.

17. Closing the bronchus that is draining pus from within the lung may result in a secondary lung abscess.

18. A large bronchial fistula is a contraindication to Dakin's solution treatment.

19. Sinuses of variable duration are common following more or less complete obliteration of empyema cavities; a large proportion eventually are obliterated without radical treatment; for those which persist, plastic operation is indicated.

20. Operative mortality in chronic empyema has been due largely to shock and infection. Reduction of the extent of operation and preliminary sterilization will materially lower this mortality.

BIBLIOGRAPHY

[1] Ætius (Amidenus or Antiochenus): Medici Græci contractæ ex veteribus medicanæ tetrabiblos, hoc est, quaternio, sive libri universales quatuor, singuli quatuor sermones complectentes, ut sent in summa quatuor, sermonun quaterniones, id est, sermones, sedecim, per Ianum Cornarium medicum physicum latine conscripti. Lugduni, Godefr. et Marcelli Beringer, 1549, 1032 pp. De pectore suppuratis, ex Archigene. Empyrici, Cap. lxv, 515–518.
[2] Albucasis: Quoted by Donatus.
[3] Amatus Lusitanus (Joh. Rodriguez): Curationum medicinalium centuria prima. Florentiæ, L. Torrentinus, 1551, 391 pp. De empyemate, 284–289.
[4] Anel: Quoted by Colson.
[5] Aretæus Cappadox: The Extant Works of * * * ed. and transl. by Francis Adams. London, Sydenham Soc., 1856, 510 pp.
[6] Auenbrugger, L.: On Percussion of the Chest, 117–148 In: Camac, C. N. B.: Epoch-making Contributions to Medicine, Surgery and Allied Sciences. Philadelphia, Saunders, 1909, 445 pp.
[7] Aupepin, P. C.: Sur un nouveau procédé de l'empyème. Paris, 1810.
[8] Avenzoar: Quoted by Paulus Ægineta.
[9] Avicenna: Quoted by Paulus Ægineta.
[10] Bache, E. P.: Sur l'empyème et sur l'operation de l'empyème. Paris, 1827.
[11] Baffos: Quoted by Rullier.

CARL A. HEDBLOM

[22] Barlow, G. H.: Case of Empyema and Pneumo-thorax. Guy's Hosp. Rep., 1839, iv, 339–351.
[23] Battle, W. H.: Chronic Empyema: The Value of Decortication of the Lung. Lancet, 1917, i, 371–373.
[24] Bazy: A propos de l'empyème et de la decortication du poumon. Bull. et mém. Soc. de chir. de Par., 1904, n. s. xxx, 893.
[25] Beck, C.: Zur Behandlung des Pyothorax. Berl. klin. Wchnschr., 1898, xxxv, 330–333, 353–355, 376–379.
[26] Beck, E. G.: Skin-flap Implantation as a Radical Measure to Cure Old Suppurative Lung-abscesses and Empyema Abscesses. Tr. West. Surg. Assn., 1916, xxvi, 181–186.
[27] Bell: Quoted by Massiani.
[28] Bergeat, E.: Ueber Thoraxresection bei grossen, veralteten Empyemen. Beitr. z. klin. Chir., 1908, lvii, 373–512.
[29] Billroth: Quoted by Homén.
[30] Binnie, J. F.: Manual of Operative Surgery. Philadelphia, Blakiston's Son and Co., 1916, seventh ed., 1378 pp.
[31] Boerhaave, H.: Dictionnaire des sciences médicales. Adelon, Alard (et al.). Paris, Crapart and Panckoucke, 1815, xii, 50.
[32] Boiffin: Quoted by Tuffier, T.: État actuel de la chirurgie intrathoracique. Paris, 1914, 55 pp.
[33] Boiffin: Quoted by Violet.
[34] Boinet: Du traitement des épanchements pleurétiques purulents par les injections en général, et les injections iodées en particulier. Arch. gén. de méd., 1853, 5 s. i., 277–296, 521–538.
[35] Bonnet: Observations pour servir a l'histoire des pleuresies avec épanchement, et de l'empyèma; recueillies a l'hospital Saint-Antome. Arch. gén. de méd., 1829, xxi, 86–96.
[36] Bouchut: Quoted by Schede.
[37] Boudant: Quoted by Boinet.
[38] Bowditch, H. I.: Paracentesis Thoracis. Am. Jour. Med. Sc., 1852, n. s., xxiii, 103–105. On Pleuritic Effusions, and the Necessity of Paracentesis for Their Removal. Am. Jour. Med. Sc., 1852, n. s., xxiii, 320–350.
[39] De Brabant, B.: Épanchement de pus dans la cavité gauche de la poitrine, suite de pleuresie; operation de l'empyème; guérison. Ann. Soc. de méd. de Gand, 1837, iii, 102–104.
[40] Bruer: Quoted by Colson.
[41] Buck, A. H.: The Growth of Medicine from the Earliest Times to About 1800. New York and New Haven, Yale Univ. Press, 1917, 600 pp.
[42] Burin d'Aissard, L. M.: Sur l'empyème. Paris, 1812, 29 pp.
[43] Cælius Aurelianus, In: Haller, A. Biblotheca Chirurgica. Bernæ, Haller et Schweighauser, 1774–1775, ii, 397.
[44] Camerarius, Joannes Rudolphus: Sylloges memorabilium medicinæ et mirablium naturæ arcanorum centuriæ xx. Edite altera, emendata, et quatuor centuriis postumis aucta. Tubingæ, J. G. Cotta, 1683, 1662 pp., 385–386.
[45] Carrel, A., Dakin (et al.): Traitement abortif de l'infection des plaies. Rev. d'hyg., 1915, xxxvii, 1016–1024.
[46] Castellus, Petrus Vascus: Exercitationes medicanales ad omnes thoracis affectus decom tractatibus absolutæ. Tolosæ, R. Colomerium, 1616, viii, De empyemate, 675–686.
[47] Carboué, J.: Historia morbi Lichtscheidiani (Empyema). Jour. d. chir., 1792, iv, 129–137.
[48] Cayol, J.: Pleuresie chronique; operations de l'empyème. Clin. d. hôp., Paris, 1828–1829, iii, 49.

THE TREATMENT OF CHRONIC EMPYEMA

Celsus, Aurelius Cornelius: Of Medicine. In eight books. Trans. by James Grieve. London, Wilson and Durham, 1756, 519 pp.

Chambers, R.: On Chronic Pleurisy with Effusion, or Empyema. Lancet, 1844, i, 181–183.

Chopart: Quoted by Massiani.

Claessens: Vomique survenue a la suite d'une peripneumonie aigue; guérison par une ouverture pratiqués a une tumeur formee entre les 3me et 4me fausses cotes du cote gauche. Ann. Soc. de méd. de Gang, 1839, v, 170–173.

Cleland, W.: Edinburgh Med. and Surg. Jour., 1831, xxxv, 347–351.

Colegrove, B. H.: Case of Empyema, with Successful Operation. Buffalo Med. Jour., 1847–1848, iii, 6–8.

Colson, J. F. J.: De l'operation de l'empyème. Paris, 1826.

Cornil: Quoted by Violet.

Corvisart: Quoted by Forbes, J.: Biographical Sketch of Leopold Auenbrugger, 117–119. In: Camac, C. N. B.: Epoch-making Contributions to Medicine, Surgery and Allied Sciences. Philadelphia, Saunders, 1909.

Cotte, G.: Empyème chronique de la grande cavité pleurale; thoracoplastic par le procédé de Saubottin-Quénu. Guérison. Bull. et mém. Soc. de chir. de Par., 1917, n. s., xliii, 867–868.

Cruveilhier: De empyème et de quelques expériences sur les animaux. Bull. de l'Acad. de méd., 1836, i, 280.

Cullen, W.: In: Dictionnaire des sciences médicales. Adelon, Alard (et al.). Paris, Crapart and Panckoucke, 1815, xii, 50.

Delorme, E.: Nouveau traitement des empyèmes chroniques. Gaz. d. hôp., 1894, lxvii, 94–96.

Depage: Quoted by Küttner: Operationen am Brustkorbe: Chirurgische Operationslehre, edited by Bier, A., Braun, H., and Kümmell, H. Leipzig, Barth, 1912, ii. Operationen am Brustkorb.

Desault: Quoted by Massiani.

Dictionnaire des sciences médicales. Adelon, Alard (et al.). Paris, Crapart and Panckoucke, 1815, xii, 51.

Dionis: Quoted by Colson.

Dionis: Quoted by Rullier.

Donatus, Marcellus: De medica historia mirabili libri sex. Mantuæ, F. Osana, 1586, 1–96, 185–312. Suspiciendæ thoracis collectiones, 92–95.

Dowd, C. N.: Persistent Thoracic Sinus Following Empyema. Jour. Am. Med. Assn., 1909, liii, 1281–1285.

Dumont, A.: De l'empyème. Paris, 1825, 27 pp.

Dunham, E. K.: An Application to Empyema of the Principles Underlying the Use of Antiseptics. ANNALS OF SURGERY, 1918, lxviii, 148–151.

Dupuytren: Quoted by Küttner: Chirurgische Operationslehre, edited by Bier, A., Braun, H., and Kümmell, H. Leipzig, Barth, 1912, ii, Operationen am Brustkorb.

Ehrmann: Quoted by Violet.

Estlander, J. A.: Resection des cotes dans l'empyème chronique. Rev. mens. de méd. et de chir., 1879, iii, 157–170.

Estlander, J. A.: Encore quelques mots sur la resection des cotes dans l'empyème chronique. Rev. mens. de méd. et de chir., 1879, iii, 885–888.

Euryphon: Quoted by Neuburger, M., History of Medicine. Transl. by E. Playfair, London, Frowde, 1910, i, 404 pp.

Ewald: Quoted by Homén.

Fabricius, ab Aquapendente (Hieronymus): Opera chirurgica. Francofurti, N. Hoffmannus, 1620, 1096 pp. De thoracis sectione in empyemate. Cap. xlvi, 168–190. De thoracis fistulis, Cap. xlviii, 190–195.

CARL A. HEDBLOM

[68] Faure, R.: Operation d'empyème. Jour. d. sc. méd. de Montpel., 1834, ii, 160–168.
[69] Fienus, Thomas: Zwölff Bücher von der Wund-Arzneikunst oder Chirurgia. Nürnberg, W. E. Felsecker, 1675, 71–88.
[70] Fliccius, J. H.: Diss. exhibens casum viri empyemate ex pleuritide laborantis. Heidelbergæ, Walter, 1685.
[71] Fowler, G. R.: A Case of Thoracoplasty for the Removal of a Large Cicatricial Fibrous Growth from the Interior of the Chest, the Result of an Old Empyema. Med. Rec., 1893, xliv, 838–839.
[72] Fraentzel: Quoted by Homén.
[73] Friedrich, P. L.: Die operatif Beeinflüssung einseitiger Lungenphthise durch totale Brustwandmobilisierung und Lungenentspannung (Pleuro-Pneumolysis totalis). Verhandl. d. deutsch. Gesellsch. f. Chir., 1908, xxxvii, 534–570.
[74] Fürst, J. Z.: Von einer Person, die durch einen Schnitt in der Seite von dem Eiter in der Brust, das aus dem Seitenstechen entstanden, geheilet worden, und nachher an der Wassersucht gestorben. Auserl. med.-chir. Abhandl. d. röm.-kais. Akad. d. Naturf. Nürnberg, 1771, xx, 300–304.
[75] Gädücke: Ein durch die Oefnung der Brust geheiltes Lungengeschwüre. Verm. chir. Schrift Berlin und Stettin, 1776, i, 304–306.
[76] Galen: Quoted by Homén.
[77] Gallet: Quoted by Violet.
[78] Gimbert: Pleuresie purulente chez un enfant de ans; 74 ponctions et lavages; empyème final; guérison. Lyon méd., 1875, xx, 347–355; also, Abeille méd., Paris, 1875, xxii, 437–440.
[79] Goebel, C.: Zur Frage der plastischen Füllung alter Empyemhöhlen. Zentralbl. f. Chir., 1918, xlv, 120–121.
[80] Goullioud: Quoted by Violet.
[81] Graham, E. A., and Bell, R. D.: Open Pneumothorax: Its Relation to the Treatment of Empyema. Am. Jour. Med. Sc., 1918, clvi, 839–871.
[82] Guy de Chauliac: La grande chirurgie, composée l'an de grace 1363. Restituée par Laurens Joubert. Rouen, R. du Petit Val, 1615, 711 pp.
[83] Haller, A.: Bibliotheca chirurgica. Bernæ, Haller and Schweighauser, 1774–1775, ii, 8.
[84] Hartshorne, H.: Empyema, With Perforation of the Walls of the Chest. Am. Jour. Med. Sc., 1848, xvi, 349.
[85] Heineke: Quoted by Homén.
[86] Helferich: Klinische und anatomische Beobactungen an grossen Empyemhöhlen. Arch. klin. Chir., 1892, xliii, 208–220.
[87] Heyser: Wchnschr. f. d. ges. Heilk. Berlin, 1840, 49–57.
[88] Hippocrates: Genuine Works of Hippocrates. Trans. from the Greek by Francis Adams. London, Sydenham Soc., 1849, 2 vols.
[89] Homans, J.: The Prognosis and Treatment of Empyema, With Respect to the Shape of the Cavity and the Relation of the Lung to the Chest Walls. ANNALS OF SURGERY, 1918, lxvii, 697–706.
[90] Homén, E. A.: Die Methode des Estlander durch Rippenresectionen chronische Fälle von Empyem zu behandeln. Arch. f. klin. Chir., 1881, xxvi, 151–203.
[91] Horstius, Gregorius: Observationum medicinalium singularium. III. De morbis pectoris. Ulmæ, J. Saürii, 1625.
[92] Hourelle, P. F.: Sur l'empyème et les differentes éspeces d'épanchemens qui peuvent se faire dans la capacité de la poitrine. Strasbourg, 1808.
[93] Ingram, D.: Practical Cases and Observations in Surgery. London, Clarke, 1751, 20–46. Empyemas of various kinds.
[94] Jaboulay: Drainage transthoracique pour une pleuresie purulents. Lyon méd., 1909, cxiii, 1075–1076.

[98] Jalon, P.: Empyema per urinas perfecte judicatum. Miscellanea curiosa sive ephemeridium medico-physicarum Germanicarum Academiæ naturæ curiosorum. Norimbergæ sumptibus U. M. Endteri, 1687. Decuria ii, vi, 204-205.

[99] Jordan: Erfahrungen über die Behandlung veralteter Empyeme. Verhandl. d. deutsch. Gesellsch. f. Chir., 1898, xxvii, 261-269. Also, Arch. f. klin. Chir., 1898, lvii, 546-554.

[100] Kilgour, A.: Edinburgh Med. and Surg. Jour., 1841, lv, 361-367.

[101] Kinner, D.: De thoracis empyemate. Lipsiæ, J. Georgi, 1686.

[102] Kisnerus, J. E.: De empyemate, Jenæ, Krebsianis, 1686, 24 pp.

[103] Koelpin, A.: Acta Soc. med. Havn., 1777, i, 120-137.

[104] Koenig: Quoted by Homén.

[105] Krause: Quoted by Violet.

[106] Kümmell: Gross Empyemhöhle durch Dekortikation und Entfaltung der Lungen in kurzer Zeit zur definitiven Heilung gebracht. Deutsch med. Wchnschr., 1918, xliv, 536.

[107] Kurpjuweit: Quoted by Bergeat.

[108] Küster, E. G. F.: Fünf Jahre im Augusta Hospital. Ein Beitrag zur Chirurgie und zur Chirurgischen Statistik. Berlin, Hirschwald, 1877, 315 pp.

[109] Laennec: Quoted by Buck.

[110] Laennec: Quoted by Violet.

[111] Lambotte: Quoted by Violet.

[112] Lamotte: Quoted by Massiani.

[113] Lapeyre: Observation sur l'operation de l'empyème. Jour. de méd., chir. et phar., 1775, xliii, 130-135.

[114] Lassus: Quoted by Massiani.

[115] Lelorraine, L. A.: De l'operation de l'empyème. Paris, 1846.

[116] Leonidas Alexandrinus: Quoted by Priou, J. B. E.: De l'empyème ou des divers épanchemens dans la poitrine. Paris, 1817, 65 pp. Also by Haller, A.: Bibliotheca chirurgica Bernæ and Basileæ, Haller and Schweighäuser, 1774-1775, ii, 2.

[117] Leonus Lunensis (Dominicus): Ars medendi humanos, particularesque morbos a capite, usque ad pedes. Francofurti, Wecheli, 1597, 1276 pp. De empyemate seu purulentia. Cap. x, 671-676.

[118] Létiévant: Centralbl. f. Chir., 1876, 414.

[119] Leymarie: Quoted by Küttner: Chirurgische Operationslehre, edited by Bier, A., Graun, H., and Kümmell, H. Leipzig, Barth, 1912, ii, Operationen am Brustkorb.

[120] Lilienthal, H.: Empyema; Exploration of the Thorax with Primary Mobilization of the Lung. ANNALS OF SURGERY, 1915, lxii, 309-314.

[121] Lilienthal, H.: Intercostal Thoracotomy in Empyema; an Original Method. New York Med. Jour., 1915, ci, 191-193.

[122] Lloyd, S.: The Surgical Treatment of Empyema. ANNALS OF SURGERY, 1907, xlv, 373-381; Med. Rev. of Rev., 1907, xiii, 112-122; Post-grad., New York, 1907, xxii, 144-158.

[123] Lund, F. B.: The Advantages of the So-called Decortication of the Lung in Old Empyema. Jour. Am. Med. Assn., 1911, lvii, 693-697.

[124] Malin and Salomon: Wchnschr. f. d. ges. Heilk., 1834, iii, 161-166.

[125] Malle: Observations sur l'empyème. Bull. Acad. de méd., 1836, i, 402.

[126] Maraud: Quoted by Massiani.

[127] Martini: Mag. f. d. ges. Heilk. Berlin, 1825, xix, 426-433.

[128] Massa, Nicolaus Venetus: Quoted by Donatus.

[129] Massiani: Thèse de Paris, 1851.

[130] Mayo, C. H., and Beckman, E. H.: Visceral Pleurectomy for Chronic Empyema. ANNALS OF SURGERY, 1914, lix, 884-890. Also Tr. Am. Surg. Assn., 1914, xxxii, 687.

CARL A. HEDBLOM

[128] Melchior, E.: Ueber die plastische Verwendung der parietalen Pleuraschwarte bei der Operation chronischer Empyeme. Zentralbl. f. Chir., 1916, xliii, 249–252.
[129] Meyer, W.: Chronic Empyema; Thoracoplasty with Delorme's Operation. Med. Rec., 1917, xci, 437.
[130] Morin: Jour. de méd., de chir. et de pharmacol., 1776, xlvi, 138–160.
[131] Murphy, J. B.: Empyema of Pleural Cavity—Resection of Ribs (Estlander). Surg. Clin. of John B. Murphy, 1915, iv, 885–896.
[132] Newton, A.: A Case of Chronic Empyema Treated by Visceral Pleurectomy. Med. Jour. of Australia, 1916, i, 7–8.
[133] Niese: Ueber das Empyem. Mitth. a. d. Geb. d. Med., Chir. und Pharm., Altona, 1837–1838, v. 58–59.
[134] Oke, W. S.: Three Cases of Empyema or of Pleural Abscess. Prov. Med. and Surg. Jour., London, 1842, iv, 206–208.
[135] Oulmont: Quoted by Violet.
[134] Paulus Ægineta: The Seven Books of Paulus Ægineta. Transl. from the Greek by Francis Adams. London, Sydenham Soc., 1844–1847, 3 vols., i, 494.
[137] Paré, Ambrose: Quoted by Boinet.
[138] Peitavy: Zur Radicaloperation des Empyems. Berl. klin. Wchnschr., 1876, xiii, 262–265.
[139] Pelletan: Quoted by Massiani.
[140] Peuckert: Die Technik ausgedehnter Thoraxresektionen bei veralteten Empyemen. Beitr. z. klin. Chir., 1914, xci, 482–488.
[141] Peyrot, J. J.: Étude expérimentale et clinique sur la pleurotomie. Paris, 1876, 155 pp.
[142] Pliny: Quoted by Van Rossin: De empyèmate. Paris, 1846.
[143] Putegnat: Note sur l'empyème. Ann. Soc. d. sc. méd. et nat. de Brux., 1838, 19–24.
[144] Quénu and Saubottin: Quoted by Tuffier.
[145] Ransohoff, J.: Discussion of the Pleura in the Treatment of Chronic Empyema. ANNALS OF SURGERY, 1906, xliii, 502–511.
[146] Ravaton: Quoted by Massiani.
[147] Reineboth: Quoted by Lawrow, W.: Die chirurgische Behandlung des Pleuraempyems. Beitr. z. klin. Chir., 1913, lxxxiii, 67–126.
[148] Rhazes: Quoted by Massiani.
[149] Rhyne, Wilhelm ten: Quoted by Riedlius.
[150] Riedlinus, Vitus: De empyemata sectione felicite curato: Miscellanea curiosa sive ephemeridium medico-physicarum Germanicarum Academiæ Cæsareo-Leopoldinæ naturæ curiosorum. Lipsiæ, T. Frittschium, Decuriæ iii, 1694, i, 216–218.
[151] Ringel: Beitrag zur Resektion des Thorax bei veralteten und tuberculösen Totalempyemen. Arch. f. klin. Chir., 1903, lxxi, 246–257.
[152] Robinson, S.: The Treatment of Chronic Non-tuberculous Empyema. Surg., Gynec. and Obst., 1916, xxii, 557–571.
[153] Roser, W.: Ueber die Operation des Empyems. Amtl. Ber. ü. d. Versamml. deutsch Naturf. u. Aerzte, 1864, Giessen, 1865, xxxix, 216–218. Also Arch. d. Keilk., 1865, vi, 33–43.
[154] Roux: Quoted by Violet.
[155] Rullier: Empyeme. Dictionnaire des sciences médicales. Paris, Adelon, Alard (et al.), Crapart and Panckoucke, 1815, xii, 49–142.
[156] Sauerbruch: Quoted by Binnie.
[157] Sauerbruch: Quoted by Garré, C., and Quincke, H.: Lungenchirurgie. Jena, Fischer, 1912, 2d ed., 250 pp.
[158] de Sauvages de la Croix, F. B.: Dictionnaire des sciences médicales. Paris, Adelon, Alard (et al.), Crapart and Panckoucke, 1815, xii, 50.

[159] Schede, M.: Die Behandlung der Empyeme. Verhandl. d. ix Cong. f. Innere Med. Wiesbaden, 1890, ix, 41–141. Also (abstr.) Therap. Monatsch., Berlin, 1890, iv, 275–277. Also (abstr.) Allg. Wien. med. Ztg., 1890, xxxv, 258.

[160] Scultetus, Joannes: L'arcenal de chirurgie. Mis en françois par François Deboze. Lyon, A. Collier fils, 1674, 385 pp., 163–173.

[161] Sedillot, C.: De l'operation de l'empyème. Thèse de Paris, 1841.

[162] Sharp, Samuel: Quoted by Ingram.

[163] Shortridge, S.: Case of Empyema Terminating Favorably by Spontaneous Opening. Edinburgh Med. and Surg. Jour., 1842, lviii, 426–428.

[164] Simmonds: Quoted by Schede, M.

[165] Smetius a Leda, Henricus: Durch Einschnitt geheiltes Empyem. (Transl. from his: Miscellanea medica, liber x, by G. Waltz.) Arch. f. path. Anat. (etc.), Berlin, 1886, civ, 391–392.

[166] Souligoux: Quoted by Violet.

[167] Springsfeld, G. C.: De rariore quodam empyemate pectoris; sub quo materia saniosa per singularem canalem, serpendo versus dorsi spinam formatum, ad femoris usque musculos descenderat. Acta Acad. nat. curos, Norimb, 1754, x, 296–303.

[168] Steinheim: Geschichte eines nach einer vermuthlichen Leberentzündung entstandenen Empyems mit glücklichem Ausgange. Jour. d. Chir. u. Augenh., 1830, xiv, 57–74.

[169] Stevens, F. A.: Recurrences After Operations for Empyema. Jour. Am. Med. Assn., 1919, lxxiii, 812–814.

[170] Stoll: Quoted by Auenbrugger.

[171] Sudeck, P.: Eine Modification des Schedeschen Thoraxplastik bei Totalempyemen. Deutsch Ztschr. f. Chir., 1898, xlvii, 255–259.

[172] Van Swieten: Quoted by Massiani.

[173] Taddei, D.: L'obliterazione della cavita nell'empiema cronico totale con innesto di tessuto lipomatosa. Presentazione di un malato guarito. Policlin., sez. prat. 1918, xxv, 737.

[174] Tietze, A.: Zur Behandlung grosser Thoraxempyeme. Berlin klin. Wchnschr., 1918, lv, 628.

[175] Townsend, R.: Empyema. Cyclopædia of Practical Medicine, edited by Forbes, Tweedie, et al. Philadelphia, 1845, ii, 21–39.

[176] Tourtuel: Ausserordentliche Eitersammlung in der Brusthöhle nach einer Lungenentzündung. Jour. d. pract. Heilk., Berlin, 1811, xxxii, 5 St., 31–42.

[177] Tuffier, T.: Treatment of Purulent Pleural Effusions. Med. Rec., 1919, xcvi, 464–467.

[178] Tulp, Nicolæs: Pus thoracis per umbilicum. Observationes medicæ. Ed nova. Amstelredami, L. Elzevirium, 1652, 403 pp.

[179] Valentin, M. B.: Épanchement de sange considerable causé par la lesion de l'artere, mammaire droit, guéri par l'opération de l'empyème au lieu d'election. Jour. de chir., 1702, iii, iv, 108–115.

[180] Velpeau: Quoted by Massiani.

[181] Vesalius, Andreas: Quoted by Donatus.

[182] Violet: De la décortication pulmonaire dans l'empyème chronique (opération de Delorme). Arch. gen. de méd., 1904, i, 657–678.

[183] Voswinckel, E.: Ueber die Behandlung veralteter Empyeme durch ausgedehnte Rippenresection. Deutsch Zeitschr. f. Chir., 1897, xlv, 77–109.

[184] Walter, A. G.: Case of Traumatic Empyema of Sixteen Months' Standing, with Fistulæ; Treated Successfully. Brit. Med. Jour., 1860, i, 48–50.

[185] Warner, J.: Phil. Tr., London, 1759, li, pt. 1, 194–200.

[186] Weissenborn, M.: Ueber das Heilverfahren bei Lungenvereiterung. Berlin, G. Schade, 1876, 29 pp.

[187] Weissgerber, P.: Wie entfaltet sich nach der Operation des Empyems die comprimirte Lunge bei offenstehender Pleurahöhle? Berl. klin. Wchnschr., 1879, xvi, 107–108.

[188] Whittemore, W.: The Surgical Treatment of Chronic Empyema. Boston Med. and Surg. Jour., 1920, clxxxii, 396–398.

[189] Willis: Quoted by Boinet.

[190] Wilms: Die Behandlung der Empyeme und der lange bestehenden tuberkulösen Pleuraexsudate mit der Pfeilerresektion. Deutsch. med. Wchnschr., 1914, xl, 683.

[191] Wolfly: Maryland Med. Rec., 1832, iii, 56–61.

[192] Zacchias, P.: Quæstionum medico-legalium tomus posterior quo continentur liber nonus et decimus nec non decisiones Sacræ Rotæ Romanæ ad prædictas materias spectantes a D. Lanfranco Zacchia collectæ. Lugduni, Buguetan and Rau, 1661, 552 pp.

[193] Zacutus Lusitanus (Abraham): Praxis media admiranda. Lugduni, Hugvetan, 1637, 117–122, 160 pp.

THE MORELLI METHOD OF ASPIRATION DRAINAGE FOR ACUTE EMPYEMA *

By LINCOLN DAVIS, M.D.
OF BOSTON, MASS.
VISITING SURGEON, MASSACHUSETTS GENERAL HOSPITAL

FOR many years surgeons operating for acute empyema have striven to obtain air-tight suction drainage of the chest, recognizing its importance and value in securing early re-expansion of the lung, and hence in bringing about prompt functional cure.

It is quite generally recognized that a very important factor is the institution of suction drainage at a time when expansion of the lung is still possible; that is, before the retracted lung has become bound down by tough, organized, fibrinous exudate.

There have been many ingenious and useful devices for securing aspiration drainage which have given more or less satisfactory results in the hands of their originators, but no one method has been very generally adopted. Bülau,[1] at the Medical Congress of Vienna, in 1890, advocated air-tight drainage of acute empyema by means of a catheter introduced through the canula of a large trocar, which is inserted through an intercostal space. The canula is then withdrawn, leaving the catheter held tightly in place by the closely fitting soft tissues. The catheter is connected with a rubber tube which in turn is immersed in a bottle containing an antiseptic solution. This bottle being placed at a lower level than the chest, allows of siphon drainage. This method, with various modifications for retaining the catheter and rendering its fit air-tight, together with the addition of irrigation, has been used up to the present time, and lately has received added prestige from its successful and wide application in the epidemics of empyema following influenza, by Whittemore and others. It is a simple and extremely useful method. There are, however, certain disadvantages. (1) The calibre of the catheter being necessarily restricted, it is liable to become clogged. This may be obviated to a certain extent by systematic irrigation. (2) It is extremely difficult to maintain a hermetically air-tight joint for more than a few days at the most; after this time leakage occurs about the catheter, and it is then practically impossible to restore the original air-tight condition. (3) Any adjustment or changing of the catheter is very difficult. (4) If the lung is not readily dilatable, all the pus cannot be drained from the pleural cavity by this method, so long as the apparatus remains air-tight.

Forlanini,[2] of Pavia, pointed out the latter defect in the method, and

* Read before the American Surgical Association, May 3, 1920.
[1] Bülau: Zeitschr. f. klin. Medicin, vol. xviii, p. 31, 1890.
[2] Forlanini: Policlinico, N. 100, 11, 12, 13, 1890.

advocated in 1890 preliminary thoracentesis with the introduction of air into the pleural cavity simultaneously with the evacuation of the pus, followed later by the institution of suction drainage by the method of Bülau. Fórlanini insistently urged the advantages of producing artificial pneumothorax in empyema, not only in permitting complete evacuation of the effusion in cases in which the lung is bound down and the chest walls rigid, but in doing so without change of intrapleural pressure, and without arousing the so-called pleural reflexes of pain, cough, dyspnœa, etc. He also advocated inhalations of compressed air in the after treatment to aid in re-expansion of the lung.

R. W. Parker,[3] of London, had previously in 1882 advocated pneumothorax in the treatment of empyema, but his suggestion seems to have found little favor at that time.

Eugenio Morelli,[4] a pupil and assistant of Forlànini, who had worked for many years with the latter in the development of his therapeutic pneumothorax in phthisis, recognized the applicability of artificial pneumothorax in the treatment of wounds of the lung during the war, and devised an ingenious apparatus for the treatment of war wounds complicated by empyema, which has a useful application to the empyema of civil life. Having had occasion to observe Morelli's marked success with the empyema of war wounds, and subsequently having applied the method myself in a small number of cases of civil empyéma with very satisfactory results, I feel that the method is worthy of consideration in a symposium on empyema.

Morelli has devised a pneumatic jacketed drainage tube (Fig. 1) which by inflation of the dumbbell-shaped soft rubber jacket closes the thoracotomy wound hermetically tight. This will remain tight for many days, is easily kept in place, and can readily be readjusted if for any reason the drainage is not satisfactory. It is held firmly in place by means of a spider (Fig. 2) made of thin malleable metal which fits over the pneumatic sac, the feet of the spider being adjusted to the chest wall. The drainage tube is passed through a central opening in the spider which is of slightly smaller calibre than the latter. The whole is covered with a layer of gauze and fastened by strips of adhesive. These drainage tubes were incidentally pictured in an article by Lieutenant Colonel Bastianelli on " Artificial Pneumothorax in Chest Wounds" in *Surgery, Gynæcology and Obstetrics* for January, 1919, p. 5.

The technic of the method is as follows: The diagnosis of empyema having been made, a preliminary thoracentesis is performed and the purulent exudate is withdrawn and replaced with an equal quantity of air by means of the apparatus depicted in Fig. 3.

This consists of a bottle of the capacity of a litre, closed by a rubber stopper which is perforated by two glass tubes, one of which is connected by rubber tubing to the thoracentesis needle, and the other with a three-way cock, which is in turn connected with a filter, consisting merely of a glass

[3] Parker, R. W.: Lancet, 1882, p. 689.
[4] Morelli: La Cura delle Ferite Toraco-polmonari, Bologna, 1918.

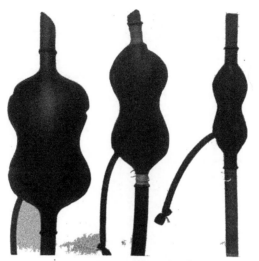

FIG. 1.—Pneumatic jacketed drainage tubes—three sizes.

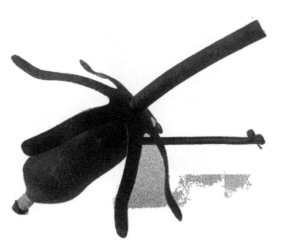

FIG. 2.—Metallic spider for holding drainage tube in place.

329ᵃ

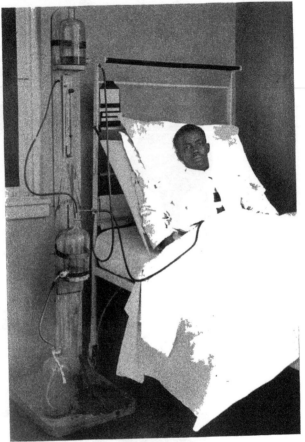

FIG. 5.—Apparatus set up.

tube filled with sterile cotton, and finally a syringe of at least 100 c.c. capacity with a perfectly fitting piston.

The apparatus is operated as follows: Having been sterilized and the joints made tight, the large thoracentesis needle is introduced into the chest and the connection between the bottle and the syringe being open, a suction stroke is made with the piston of the syringe; this produces a rarefaction of the air contained in the bottle, and results in the flow of the fluid in the chest into the bottle to replace the displaced air. When the flow of the fluid begins to subside, a reverse stroke is made with the piston of the syringe, forcing the air in it back again into the bottle, whence, finding its place taken by the fluid, it will be obliged to pass on into the pleural cavity, where it will be distinctly heard gurgling through the pleural effusion as it rises to its upper surface. When the gurgling ceases a new aspiration is made with

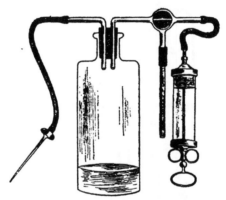

FIG. 3.—Thoracentesis apparatus.

the syringe, followed by a new insufflation of air into the pleural cavity, and so on, until all the fluid has been evacuated from the chest, or the bottle is completely filled with fluid, all the air which it previously contained having entered the pleural cavity. When one bottle is full another may be substituted, and the process repeated. The three-way cock and filter come into play when it is desired to put in a greater quantity of air than the amount of fluid extracted, or, vice versa. With this method, if the air is warmed to body temperature, there is absolutely no change in the intrapleural pressure, and no modification of the cardiac condition results. There is no danger of œdema of the lung, nor sudden rupture of pleural adhesions, no sense of constriction nor other pain, no cough nor stimulation of the pleural reflexes; in fact, no untoward disturbances of any kind.

Morelli strenuously advocates this method of thoracentesis for all pleural transudates and exudates of whatever nature, claiming, with much logic, in addition to the advantages already enumerated the much lesser likelihood of a reaccumulation of fluid, than when aspiration is done by the ordinary method, which greatly increases the negative pressure of the pleural cavity.

Having replaced the pus of the empyema with an equal amount of air, on the following day a thoracotomy with resection of a square piece of rib is done under local anæsthesia, and the previously described pneumatic drainage tube inserted and connected with the apparatus in Fig. 4, consisting of a wooden stand upon which are set three bottles. The upper bottle is for

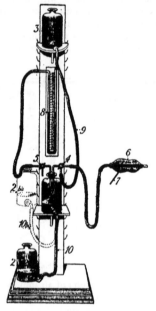

FIG. 4.—Empyema apparatus.

the purpose of irrigation. The middle bottle placed at about the level of the bed is connected directly with the drainage tube, and is partly filled with an antiseptic solution; it is connected by a tube at its bottom with a third bottle set at a lower level, and aspiration drainage is exerted by the difference in level of the fluid in the two bottles. In the case of a recent war wound of the lung complicated by empyema, Morelli maintains at first drainage with positive pressure in the pleural cavity by raising bottle (2) to the position of (2 bis) in the cut, above the level of bottle (1). For ordinary cases of civil empyema this is not necessary, and negative pressure is exerted at once by lowering bottle (2) to a point corresponding to the amount of negative pressure desired. A manometer is connected with bottle (1), by a three-way cock at (5), which registers the negative pressure in bottle (1), as well as in the pleural cavity. There is a three-way cock also at (4), which allows of irrigation, which is useful in clearing the tubes of coagula of fibrin, or inspissated pus.

This apparatus, which seems somewhat complicated, works very well in practice. It can be seen at a glance whether or not the drainage is working, and irrigation may be carried on with great ease and perfect cleanliness. For practical purposes the whole thing may be greatly simplified by merely connecting the pneumatic jacketed drainage tube with two bottles containing liquid at different levels, one standing on a chair, and one on the floor, cutting out three-way cocks, manometer, and irrigation bottle, which are unessential accessories.

The advantages of this method are, that not only can large fibrinous clots be removed directly at the time of operation, but a drainage tube of larger calibre than the trocar method permits of can be used, so that subsequent obstruction of the drainage is less likely. Furthermore, air-tight drainage can be maintained for a longer period of time, as the pneumatic jacket of the tube adjusts itself to the wound and does not tend to work loose; it causes no necrosis of the tissues, but bright granulations spring up along the tract of the wound, which heals promptly when the tube is removed. It is at all times surprisingly comfortable It is especially adapted to cases in which there are fibrinous clots which so often clog the tubes of small calibre, and in cases in which through delay in operating tough adhesions have formed which will require somewhat prolonged aspiration for the complete re-expansion of the lung.

If it is inconvenient, as is often the case, to do a preliminary thoracentesis with induction of artificial pneumothorax, in my opinion the same benefits may be obtained, with practically negligible risk, while performing the operation at one sitting. It is only necessary to exercise care in allowing the pus to escape very slowly from the chest by making at first a small opening in the pleura, which can be controlled by digital pressure, preventing at the same time the rapid and tumultuous entry of air which is as much to be avoided as is the forced expulsion of pus.

For cases in children, or in recent cases in which the effusion is thin and of a turbid serous nature, the trocar and catheter method is quick, simple, and entirely adequate; the importance, however, of replacing the withdrawn purulent exudate with air, so as to allow of the complete evacuation of the former, as insisted upon by Forlanini and Morelli, should be borne in mind. This can be accomplished by means of the thoracentesis apparatus of bottle and syringe of Fig. 3, which should be connected with the catheter as soon as the latter is introduced into the chest, and negative pressure instituted later by means of the two-bottle method. If the lung is fully dilatable no harm is done by introducing the air, which will readily be sucked out again by the apparatus. Simple siphon drainage, however, will not suffice for this, as the siphonage will be broken by the column of air in the tube, which will not affect, on the contrary, the two-bottle method.

The value of irrigation with Dakin's solution, or other antiseptic, in empyema is emphasized by Morelli, and is now generally recognized. Apart from its antiseptic value it is of special importance in all cases of air-tight suction drainage in keeping the tubes free from plugging. Care must be taken to introduce only small amounts of fluid at a time, and to make sure that as much returns from the chest as is put in.

The features of the Forlanini-Morelli method in the treatment of empyema are in brief: the systematic induction of pneumothorax, continuous aspiration drainage combined with irrigation, and an air-tight pneumatic jacketed drainage tube of great value in appropriate cases.

ABSCESS OF THE LUNG*

By John A. Hartwell, M.D.
of New York, N. Y.

There exists in the literature some confusion as to the lesions included under the term abscess of the lung. In this communication a definition is employed which it is believed accurately describes the lesion, and at the same time is comprehensive enough to include the associated necrosis which so often is a part of the lesion.

Abscess of the lung means a collection of pus within the destroyed lung parenchyma; that is, it must be outside the lumen of the respiratory tree. Dilatation of the bronchi with a purulent inflammation of the mucosa and an excessive expectoration of foul sputum is not to be confused with abscess. This lesion—bronchiectasis—may coincidently be present, but is not necessarily so. Surrounding the abscess—really a portion of its wall—there often exists a destruction of lung tissue which may be somewhat massive and approach gangrene. One must, to a certain extent, be empiric in delimiting this lesion from a true gangrene. When the condition has resulted from bacterial invasion, via the respiratory tract, and is early manifest by the suppurative process, the term gangrenous abscess is accurately descriptive. Gangrene should be reserved for a massive destruction of lung tissue, either from true circulatory disturbance, or from such an overwhelmingly virulent infection that the lung tissue is killed in mass by toxins or vascular plugging before there can be a sufficient reaction to generate pus. If this division be followed, the number of cases of lung gangrene reported will be materially lessened, and a better understanding of the pathological processes be possible.

A case of true gangrene—the only one coming to my personal attention—has recently been reported to me through the courtesy of Dr. Lincoln Davis, of the Massachusetts General Hospital. A child received a penetrating wound with a crochet needle into the upper right lobe of the lung. Two days later she began to suffer pain and marked swelling around the site of puncture which rapidly increased up to the time of her admission to the hospital, one week after the injury. She was then very sick, the manifest signs being an emphysematous cellulitis in the neck and upper chest, with evidence of a hæmo-pyo-pneumothorax. Thoracotomy was performed. Death occurred the following day. Autopsy showed the entire upper lobe of the lung converted into a necrotic sac containing brownish opaque fluid. There was neither the surrounding inflammatory zone nor the pus content of an abscess formation.

Dr. Albert Frost, of the Interne Staff, has made the following sum-

* Read at a joint meeting of the New York Surgical Society and the Philadelphia Academy of Surgery, February 2, 1920.

mary of autopsy findings from the protocols of six thousand autopsies at Bellevue Hospital for the purpose of studying the relations in this type of lesion. There have been 148 cases with the anatomical diagnosis of lung abscess and gangrene of the lung. Abscess and gangrene are included in this summary under one head, because of the fact that so many of the cases of so-called gangrene of the lung cannot be differentiated from abscess.

Of the 23 cases with an anatomical diagnosis of gangrene, only 7 could be definitely spoken of as a true gangrene from the descriptions.

Of these 148 cases there were 50 which should be regarded as clinical abscesses, in that the abscess was of such size that it could have been detected before death, either by physical examination or by X-ray. Of these clinical abscesses there were 25 situated in the upper lobes, 22 in the lower lobes, and 3 in the middle lobe.

Other interesting data are briefly summarized in the following table:

Subpleural abscesses associated with empyema .... 34 cases
Abscesses mentioned as having ruptured into the pleura in which there was
    an accompanying empyema .... 12 cases
Empyemas mentioned as draining through the trachea .... 2 cases
Abscesses mentioned as rupturing into bronchi .... 15 cases
Pus from abscess mentioned as having foul odor .... 47 cases
Abscess result of necrosis of infarcted area .... 17 cases

The etiological factor in the production of these abscesses, including both the clinical and pathological lesions, was, so far as possible, determined from the associated autopsy findings. Only those cases in which the cause was evident are included in the following:

Bronchopneumonia	29	Septic endometritis	7
Lobar pneumonia	18	Infective endocarditis	6
Pyæmia	15	Acute suppurative otitis media	5
Septicæmia	11	Thrombosis pulmonary artery	4
Thrombosis in peripheral venous channels (sinus, jugular and inferior vena cava)	8	Purulent bronchitis (cause or effect)	3
		Tracheotomy	2

In the literature the differentiation between abscess and gangrene is often made from the odor of the sputum and the pus. Exceedingly foul pus is made to connote a gangrene without regard to the pathology. This, obviously, is incorrect, as is proved by the clinical and pathological cases described. In several of these the pus was stinking, and yet the evidence is conclusive that no true gangrene was present.

While abscess of the lung may result from other sources, the great majority have as a direct antecedent some type of respiratory infection, if, in such infection, the aspiration inflammations be included. In the literature the statement is found that among these the true pneumococcus lobar pneumonia is the most common antecedent. We have not found this to be the case, either actually or relatively. Of 13 cases, associated with a pulmonary infection, observed clinically, 10 of which will be analyzed in detail, only 3 followed this type of infection. What is still more significant, in each of these three, secondary invaders were found in the abscess content, and the pneumococcus apparently had no part in abscess formation.

MacCallum, in a personal communication, says, " I am skeptical about those abscesses said to occur in the course of a pneumococcus lobar pneumonia. At least, they never look like abscesses, but like areas of more advanced destruction with no special limitation." He expresses the belief that even these are due to secondary invaders; an opinion amply sustained by our study.

In 770 consecutive cases of pneumococcus lobar pneumonia admitted to the Rockefeller Hospital, only 2 developed lung abscess, and each of these showed other infecting organisms. One of them completely recovered from the lesion in the lobe first involved, and later the abscess containing no pneumococci, formed in the other lung, in a part where the evidence of lobar pneumonia was very recent and scant. In this series there were two others showing a pneumococcus infection, but the diagnosis of a lobar pneumonia could not be substantiated by the physical signs or the radiograph. During the same period there were 140 cases of bronchopneumonia admitted, one of whom developed a lung abscess.

The entire number of abscesses observed in this hospital has been 9, the remaining 6 being divided as follows: 2 followed previous tonsillectomies with mixed infections; 1 occurred primarily with a staphylococcus aureus infection; 2 occurred primarily with a very mixed bacterial infection, and 1 resulted as a late manifestation of a staphylococcus aureus pneumonia. Our studies lead to the conclusion that the staphylococcus aureus is an important agent in abscess formation.

Great interest attaches to the subject of the pathogenesis of the abscess. In this connection the recent studies of Cecil and Blake are important. These authors found in their studies of the pathogenesis of pneumonia and other pulmonary infections that the inflammation in the lung parenchyma, following injections of virulent cultures into the trachea of monkeys, preceded by some hours the exudation in the air vesicles.

Inasmuch as the infecting organisms must sooner or later invade and break down this interstitial tissue, if an abscess is to result, this very early invasion throws light on the occurrence of a primary abscess, that is, pus formation before there is any pneumonic consolidation. In fact, in some cases, such consolidation may never appear. More often, however, the presence of a true consolidation may be demonstrated. The changes from this condition with the vesicular exudate and the interstitial inflammation to abscess formation are to some extent elucidated by the study of the pneumonic lung, particularly when there exists a mixed bacterial flora.

Many cases of pneumonia coming to autopsy exhibit areas in which

JOHN A. HARTWELL

the interstitial spaces are packed with the products of the pneumonic inflammation, the vesicle walls are more or less destroyed, and the lung substance is converted into an acutely inflamed zone showing foci of necrosis. In many instances these foci have progressed to a farther stage and liquefaction is present, *i.e.*, a beginning abscess (Figs. 1 and 2). The majority of such foci are very small, and while pathologically they are abscesses, this could not have been determined clinically. It is to be assumed that, had such cases survived, there would have occurred, in some, at least, a farther development, and clinical evidence would have been present. Chickering and Park found in the lungs of patients dying from staphylococcus aureus pneumonia, multiple abscesses varying in size from a millimetre to a centimetre. The content varied from a necrotic mass to a thick, greenish, yellow pus. In no instance was the abscess large enough to have given clinical signs.

All these studies emphasize the belief that lung abscess is a very important possibility much more often than is realized. We have no knowledge of how frequently these small focal abscesses form and undergo resolution and drainage, but this evidence is in favor of its frequent occurrence. We are not informed as to the causes which bring about their continued growth into large abscesses. One is compelled to fall back upon the unknown factor of resistance and virulence, with, in addition, the factor of a better or poorer drainage *via* the bronchioles. Study of the bacteriology yields the information already mentioned. Abscesses are encountered clinically, following all types of pneumonia, but the rule is to find a secondary invader, such as staphylococcus or streptococcus, occurring alone or in conjunction with the influenza bacillus. All these organisms have been found in the sputum of patients suffering from lung abscess. On the other hand, all types of lung infections regularly occur without the development of lung abscess. The clinical facts on which to base a belief that the ordinary pyogenic bacteria, particularly the staphylococcus aureus, are more prone than other organisms to produce a lung abscess are given above. It is to be emphasized that a staphylococcus aureus infection may produce an abscess without a true pneumonia. A well-marked abscess may occur almost with the inception of this infection, and be fully developed within a few days of the onset of the illness. Such a lesion is the primary lung abscess already mentioned.

There is, in every case of abscess, an exit for the fluid pus *via* the vesicles and small bronchioles. This drainage, however, is often inadequate, and following the law of all suppuration, the process extends along lines of least resistance. Abscess cavities, from five to ten centimetres in diameter, up to an entire lobe, may thus be formed. A fluid content of several hundred cubic centimetres is not uncommon. Ultimately, a larger bronchus is opened to it, drainage is free, and the complete pathological picture of the abscess is present. Often several large bronchial openings into the abscess are present.

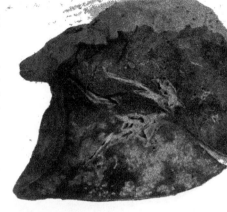

FIG. 1.—Lobar pneumonia, showing the areas of necrosis, which are the starting points of abscess.

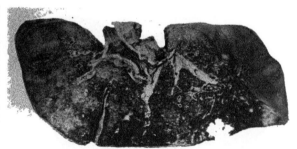

FIG. 2.—Influenza pneumonia, showing a necrosis beneath the pleura with a nearly large bronchus. This type of lesion going on to abscess formation may also produce an empyema which will drain through the abscess cavity and the bronchus.

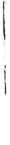

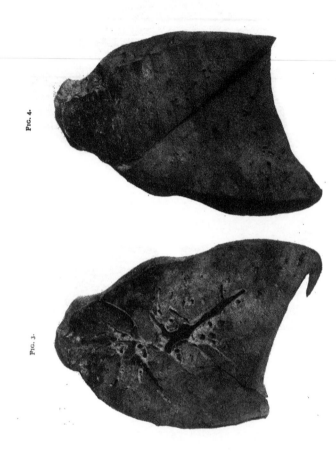

FIG. 3.

FIG. 4.

FIGS. 3 and 4.—A lung distended to the normal inspiratory extent and hardened in formalin. Fig. 3 shows the large bronchi ("drainage tubes") at the junction of the middle and deep thirds, while Fig. 4 shows the absence of these at the junction of middle and superficial thirds.

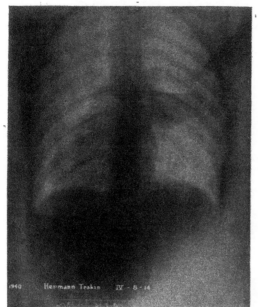

FIG. 5.—A typical shadow of an abscess cavity containing pus below and air above.

33

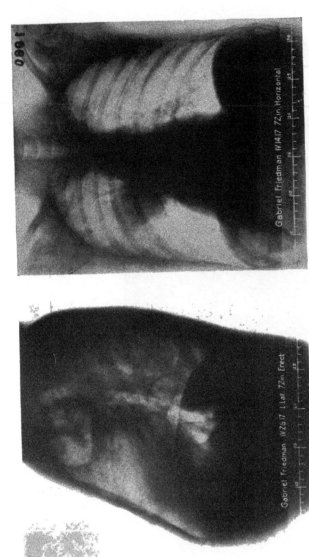

FIGS. 6 and 7.—A deep-seated staphylococcus abscess slowly working toward the anterior wall in spite of free bronchial drainage.

An abscess in the more superficial parts of the lung tends to reach a considerable size before it lies in relation to a bronchus of sufficient lumen to afford an avenue of adequate drainage. In the deeper parts, on the other hand, such bronchi are more numerous, and it is possible for drainage to be more complete (Figs. 3 and 4). This is an important fact from a therapeutic standpoint. It also has a most important bearing, as we believe, upon the occurrence of empyema and its occasional drainage through the lung and trachea.

When the abscess is fully established, as seen, for instance, at operation, its wall is a ragged surface of necrosing lung tissue around which, microscopically, are found œdema, leucocytes, dilated and thrombosed blood-vessels and bacteria, all of which pack the air vesicles as well as the interstitial space. Its outline is often irregular, giving the impression that several foci of suppuration have coalesced into one abscess. Between these diverticula the lung substance may be dead in considerable areas. When the infecting organisms are unusually virulent a surrounding gangrenous condition may supervene. Putrefactive organisms gaining entrance from the mouth to such areas produce a putrid mass. Such lesions are not uncommon, and should be designated as already discussed, as gangrenous abscess rather than lung gangrene.

Since, whatever the cause of the abscess, there exists an antecedent inflammation, the surrounding zone is always well marked. It is emphasized in abscesses secondary to the pneumonic infections, because such abscesses occur in portions where resolution has been incomplete and the interstitial inflammation is marked. In studying the physical signs of abscess formation and in reading radiographs, this zone must be given due consideration. It often acts as a very troublesome mask to a proper diagnosis.

The following case[1] illustrates the pathological and clinical development of an abscess as the sequela of a true lobar pneumonia, where the pus formation was due to a mixed infection.

On February 6, 1914, the patient, a male, aged forty-two years, developed a left upper lobar pneumonia with typical signs and X-ray findings. The sputum was rusty from the onset. On admission two days later there was isolated from the sputum a Gram-positive diplococcus, a Gram-negative capsulated bacillus, the Friedländer and the influenza bacillus. On the fourth day of the disease there was elicited a flat note over the centre of the consolidation. Resolution and deffervescence failed, and on February 21st there were made out the signs of cavity formation, but the X-ray failed to demonstrate any change in the shadow.

[1] All the clinical cases herein reported, with the exception of the last one, were observed and treated at the Rockefeller Institute Hospital. I desire to express my thanks to Dr. Rufus Cole for the privilege of having treated them and including them in the report.

On February 27th there appeared the first expectoration of pus, 250 c.c., from which the same organisms as found in the early sputum were isolated. The physical signs and the X-ray now fully demonstrated the presence of a cavity in the centre of the upper left lobe. His general condition remained excellent and operation was delayed until March 7th with the hope that sufficient drainage, *via* the trachea, might result in a cure. This failing, the surgical procedure followed in all the cases was undertaken. The exact position of the cavity was determined with the exploring needle, and under novocaine anæsthesia a portion of the underlying rib—in this case the fourth to the left of the sternum—was resected. The two pleural surfaces being found adherent, they were incised, and by blunt dissection the abscess cavity was opened. It was about 10 cm. in diameter and pathologically showed the typical lesion described above. The pus contained the organisms above named, with the exception of the pneumococcus. Tube, and later vaselined gauze, drainage was established, and healing was complete on May 8th.

The course of the abscess development is in this case sufficiently clear by reference to what has already been said. The severity of the interstitial infection produced a local inflammation which failed of resorption (Figs. 1 and 2), and in the course of two weeks pus formation was present, and a week later a bronchus of sufficient size for internal drainage was opened into.

This case contrasts quite sharply with the following, who developed a well-marked left lower lobar pneumonia on April 20, 1914. On admission three days later the sputum showed a pneumococcus and a Gram-negative bacillus. The process in this lobe went on to a normal resolution on the seventh day, with a normal temperature. On April 25th, however, pain and friction râles developed over the right upper lobe. On May 5th the temperature rose to 103.4°, and signs of consolidation developed in the right lung anteriorly. An exploratory needle puncture in the third space, 5 cm. from the right edge of the sternum, entered a pus and air cavity. Cultures from the pus gave a pure growth of hæmolytic staphylococcus aureus. Operation showed an abscess which was multilocular, each focus containing only a few c.c. of pus with an extensive surrounding zone of necrotic lung. A cure resulted in about two months.

This case illustrates the rôle of the staphylococcus aureus in abscess production. The lobe first attacked followed the normal course of a pneumococcus lobar pneumonia, but another lobe attacked by the staphylococcus promptly passed into the suppurative condition and developed an abscess.

A third case presents still another phase of the subject.

The patient, a male aged twenty years, was admitted to the hospital on April 11, 1914, with the history of having had a cold for two days and a chill and sudden pain in the right chest two days before admission. He suffered from a dry cough with occasionally the expectoration of a little mucopurulent sputum, which contained a non-hæmolytic streptococcus, a pneumococcus, and a Gram-negative bacillus, the latter predominating. There were no evident signs of consolidation made out at any time during the nine days he remained in the hospital. The temperature ranged from 100° to 102.8°, pulse about 80, and respirations 30. The X-ray on the third day following the chill showed a denser shadow corresponding to and extending immediately around the right hilus.

On the ninth day of the disease there occurred free expectoration of 100 c.c. of brownish-gray pus which contained characteristic elastic fibres arranged partly in alveolar form. These were recovered from a mouse inoculated with this pus: (1) Pneumococcus mucosa, bile soluble. (2) Pneumococcus IV. (3) Streptococcus hæmolyticus. (4) B. Influenza.

The X-ray (Fig. 5) now shows a distinct abscess cavity with a very limited surrounding zone of consolidation containing free fluid and air. This cavity was not determined by the physical signs.

An exploration needle introduced deeply into the substance of the lung through the sixth space, near the angle of the right scapula, withdrew pus of the same character and containing the same organisms. The patient declined operation and made a complete recovery.

This condition in which the abscess is an early manifestation of a deep-seated lung infection is contrasted with the more superficial abscesses. In the former the drainage may prove adequate because of the immediate vicinity of the large bronchi which act as efficient drainage tubes. In the latter extensive destruction of lung tissue must take place before such tubes are reached, and hence spontaneous recovery is less possible (Figs. 3 and 4). Not all deep-seated cases escape without operation, however, as is shown by the following:

A man, aged thirty-six years, was admitted to the hospital April 13, 1917. Two weeks prior to admission be caught cold and had a sticking pain in the *right* chest. He states there was cough and bloody sputum, but no fever. He was only absent from work for three days. A few days later there was a recurrence of illness with severe coughing, blood-tinged sputum, and sticking pain in the *left* chest. There was no chill and he states no fever until four days prior to admission. No history of having inhaled any irritating gas or foreign body could be obtained.

The physical examination revealed a soft friction rub in the left axilla, and below the angle of the scapula posteriorly there was a slight exaggeration in whisper. Elsewhere the lungs showed no abnormal signs. The remainder of the physical examination was negative. No portal of entry for infection could be found. Blood culture was sterile with 10 c.c. in 150 c.c. broth and 2 c.c. on 10 c.c. agar plate.

The patient appeared acutely but not seriously ill. Temperature, 102.8°; pulse, 95; respiration, 28; white blood-cells, 40,000. The only change in the general condition or physical signs, until the seventh day of illness, was the development of slight dullness over the left mid chest posteriorly. On that day there was severe coughing and suddenly purulent sputum was expectorated in very large amounts. It was greenish brown in color. Smears showed many varieties of bacteria. Injected into a mouse it yielded staphylococcus aureus in the heart's blood. Dullness with sonorous and sibilant râles were present over the left mid chest anteriorly.

Diagnosis of lung abscess with free bronchial drainage was made. It probably was of staphylococcus origin and lay deep within the middle portion of the left lung. The patient was kept under observation for ten days, because his general condition remained satisfactory, the abscess was draining freely and a serious question was present as to whether the better operative approach was from before or behind.

During this period the temperature ranged from 100° to 102.5°. Pulse 80 to 100. Respiration 22 to 32, and the blood count 40,000 to 50,000 with about 88 per cent polymorphonuclears. The physical signs changed only in that dullness developed anteriorly over the left mid chest and percussion here elicited tenderness. The sputum was abundant, 190 c.c. on one occasion. It was almost pure pus, greenish in color, with tinge of blood, and of very foul odor. Staphylococcus aureus was recovered from the heart's blood of the mouse on several occasions following injections of purulent sputum. No source of a staphylococcus aureus could be found anywhere in the body. No tubercle bacilli were found.

The X-ray plates showed the development of the abscess and its approach to the anterior chest wall. They gave no evidence of a pneumonia or a tuberculosis (Figs. 6 and 7). The exploring needle inserted about the eighteenth day of the disease in the third intercostal space, at the outer border of the left pectoral muscle, entered the cavity and withdrew very foul, thick, brownish pus.

Under local anæsthesia 6 cm. of the third rib at this point was resected and immediately beneath the two layers of the densely adherent pleura and a thin shell of remaining lung tissue was found an abscess cavity 15 cm. in diameter contatining about 250 c.c. of the same foul pus. Internally, the cavity seemed to be bounded by the pericardium, but on all other surfaces there was comparatively healthy lung tissue. The pleural cavity was not infected. The abscess was in the inferior portion of the upper lobe. So far as could be ascertained the post-operative behavior of the lung condition was satisfactory. Drainage continued free and there was no other evident involvement of lung tissue. The patient, however, lost weight and strength, refused to eat, and died without evidence of sepsis three weeks following operation. No autopsy was granted and the immediate cause of death was not determined.

This case is of the type of primary abscess with the staphylococcus aureus as the exciting organism. The X-ray (Fig. 6) failed to show the usual shadow of a pneumonic consolidation. The abscess ruptured into a large bronchus with a resultant expectoration of a large amount of foul pus on the seventh day of his illness which is too early for the development of the abscess through a preceding stage of consolidation. Notwithstanding the deep-seated position of the lesion, and its early drainage by the tracheal route, it continued to extend toward the pleural surface, and obviously was not destined to recover without external drainage.

From the early sticking pain in the left chest and the friction rub heard in this axilla, it is evident that the original infection involved superficial as well as deep portions of the lung, but with not sufficient lesion to cast a shadow with the X-ray.

Suppuration occurred first in the more seriously damaged central portion and later extended into the superficial part where drainage was less complete. This was proved by the fact that at operation the two pleuræ were adherent and thickened, although the abscess itself was still situated some distance below the surface.

Other organisms than the staphylococcus aureus are capable of producing a pathological condition with similar clinical manifestations to those just mentioned, as is shown in the case of a man aged twenty-eight years who was admitted to the hospital on April 6, 1914. His illness began on April 2d with a chill and pain in the right chest behind. He immediately (?) began to expectorate large amounts of foul pus.

The physical signs were not marked, though some dullness existed with diminished fremitus and breath sounds over the lower right chest behind.

Two days after admission—the sixth day of his illness—an exploratory puncture deep into the right lung yielded very foul pus. Operation revealed a markedly inflamed lung with many small abscess cavities underlying the adherent and thickened pleuræ. The whole area of disease was evidently undergoing a breaking down suppurative process. The responsible organisms in this case, as determined both from the sputum and the pus, were Gram-positive cocci, Gram-negative fusiform bacilli, Gram-positive diplococci, and a short-chained coccus. The Gram-negative organisms were obtained only under anaërobic conditions. Healing was delayed until the twelfth week, owing to the presence of an open bronchial fistula, which only closed after nine weeks.

A case of true staphylococcus aureus pneumonia, with resultant multiple abscess formation—the type described by Chickering and Park—going on to recovery without operation, is illustrated by the following. A man, aged twenty-four years, was admitted to the hospital with this history. His illness began with an ordinary cold, after three days of which the patient had a chill and severe pain in the right side of the chest. He was admitted to the hospital fifteen hours later. At this time he appeared very sick. Temperature, 105°; pulse, 124; respiration, 34; lips cyanotic. Examination showed evidence of a beginning consolidation in the right axilla. Sputum on culture yielded a pure growth of hæmolytic staphylococcus aureus. Blood cultures were negative.

On the fourth day of his disease, which followed the course of a severe pneumonia, the patient coughed up a mass of homogeneous, hemorrhagic sputum, swarming with staphylococci. The condition continued unchanged up to the eighth day. Exploratory puncture then yielded 10 c.c. of thick, grumous, chocolate-colored pus, smears of which showed only staphylococci.

On the thirteenth day the patient first began to expectorate freely pure pus, but in small quantity, after which there was a suggestion of amphoric breathing and loud râles in the posterior part of the right axilla. He remained acutely sick during this period, and developed foci of suppuration in two of his fingers and also in the chest around the site of the needle puncture. Other punctures into the lung were done on the twenty-first and twenty-seventh days, but in each instance the needle, as at the first puncture, passed into very solid lung tissue and only withdrew a few drops of pus, and in one instance entered a foul-smelling air cavity. During this period the amount of foul, purulent sputum gradually increased, but was not excessive until the thirty-fifth day, when, after coughing, there was a sudden gush of very foul-smelling pus which was projected outward like vomitus. From this time forward the progress was satisfactorily toward complete recovery, there being a gradual healing of the lung process. Complete recovery was established on the ninety-second day of his disease. Operation was deemed unwise in this case, because the process was an unresolved staphylococcus pneumonia with many small necrotic foci with which surgery would have found great difficulty in dealing. When the large abscess finally developed it promptly reached a large bronchus and a change toward recovery was immediately instituted.

Mention has been made of the relation of empyema secondary to abscess formation, and subsequent drainage of both the abscess and the pleural suppuration through the tracheal tree. I incline to the belief that this is the usual sequence of events when an empyema drains in this way. An abscess of considerable size develops in the superficial part of the lung, and failing to reach any bronchus of size, there is no expectoration of pus. Such a lesion gives no physical signs to differentiate it from the surrounding consolidation, and so is not diagnosed. In its extension it finally reaches the pleural surface, ruptures through, and produces a secondary empyema. The physical signs of the latter completely mask the abscess, and the case appears as an empyema only. The extension of the abscess, however, is also toward the deeper portion of the lung, and in this direction a large bronchus is ultimately reached, and there results a free expectoration of pus. This is interpreted as the "rupture of an empyema " into the lung which is obviously an incorrect deduction. The actual lesion is a lung abscess reaching an outlet in two directions—first, into the pleura, and second, into the bronchus. Often expectoration of pus is not a marked feature, and operation on the empyema is undertaken prior to this secondary exit. The communication into a bronchus, however, exists, and following operation, one essential for the cure of the empyema is lacking, namely, the coincident expansion of the lung as the suppuration in the pleura is overcome. The open bronchus produces a continued internal pneumothorax, the lung fails to expand, and cure of the empyema is delayed long after the proper interval. This is often one of the underlying causes of persistent sinus following an operation for what was believed to be a simple empyema.

The employment of Dakin's solution for cleansing the pleural cavity after rib resection has demonstrated the presence of these coexisting lesions not infrequently. When present, the patient promptly smells and tastes the chlorine, and in many cases violent pulmonary irritation is set up with uncontrollable coughing. This never results when this solution is used in a simple uncomplicated empyema. Its appearance is proof that one is dealing with the condition under discussion, and in my belief, the use of Dakin's solution must never be continued, no matter how efficient one may have found it in the uncomplicated cases.

This occurrence of an empyema masking completely the presence of a large abscess of the lung was illustrated by two cases in this series.

In the first the illness began with pain in the right chest and the expectoration of foul pus. He was admitted to the hospital two weeks later, during which time the later symptoms had continued.

Examination by exploratory puncture showed that the right chest contained thick, yellowish-green, foul pus, similar in appearance to the sputum. Both contained Gram-positive and Gram-negative cocci and Gram-negative bacilli. Injected into a mouse there were isolated Gram-positive diplococci with large capsule (pneumococcus mucus). The exudate agglutinated with antipneumococcus serum III. The X-ray showed the shadow of a pleural effusion. Operation revealed a large abscess containing very foul pus in the middle of the right lower lobe. There was also a very thick fibrous purulent exudate in the pleura overlying this. The patient recovered, but still had a small clean bronchial fistula when last reported.

The second case is of unusual interest. The patient, an officer, aged twenty-three years, with the A. E. F., developed an arthritis in August, 1918, while on duty in the advanced zone. At about the same time he was slightly gassed with chlorine. He was sent to a rear hospital where, on September 15th, under local anæsthesia, a tonsillectomy was done. A month later he suffered from an attack of influenza and pneumonia. There is some evidence that prior to this he was ill with a pulmonary infection and at times expectorated pus, sometimes a " half cupful in a day." He remained ill through

the winter and was finally operated upon in March, 1919, for empyema. He was told that two quarts of pus were evacuated. Dakin
solution was instilled into the pleural cavity on one occasion and he
continued to " taste it for a week," so that it was not employed a
second time. In the course of ten weeks the operative wound closed.
On June 30, 1919, the X-ray and the physical signs showed that he had a
complete pneumothorax, the lung having contracted to a small mass
near the root and along the left border of the pericardium. The operative wound was still closed and he was without constitutional symptoms.

In August, 1919, he became acutely ill and coughed up large
amounts of somewhat foul pus. There was no pus in the pleural
cavity as demonstrated by exploratory puncture, though after four
weeks the sinus opened and for a short time there was a moderate
discharge. The sinus closed, the pus expectoration ceased, and in
December an X-ray showed the lung expanded to fill almost the
entire chest. There was a recurrence of purulent expectoration in
January. At this time the X-ray and the physical signs demonstrated a cavity in the middle of the left lung posteriorly. The expectoration subsided in three or four weeks, and in April an X-ray and
the physical examination failed to demonstrate any cavity formation.

The course of the disease in this case seems to have been an abscess,
probably following the tonsillectomy, which ruptured into the pleura,
producing the empyema. This was operated upon and the opening closed,
but the lung failed to expand because of the internal pulmonary fistula
which kept up a continued pneumothorax. This condition is evidenced
by the fact that the chest wall instead of retracting, as is usual with a
collapsed lung, expanded to a marked degree, as is amply illustrated in
the X-ray by the wide separation of the ribs, a finding called to my attention by Dr. Codman, of Boston.

Subsequently the abscess discharged through the trachea, its fistulous
opening closed, and gradually the lung expanded to its full extent with a
resulting cure of the complex lesion.

The infecting organism in this case was found in every instance to be the
streptococcus hæmolyticus.

This analysis of these pathological and clinical observations is believed to fully justify the findings included in the introductory remarks,
namely, that the pneumococcus is not an important factor in lung abscess;
that the staphylococcus aureus is often responsible; that abscess of the
lung frequently is a primary lesion in that a true pneumonic consolidation as connoted by the name pneumonia does not precede it; that abscess
of the lung includes in its pathology a marked degree of surrounding
necrosis, or even massive gangrene, and that when an empyema ruptures
into the lung and discharges through the bronchus the original lesion was
a lung abscess which, by its extension, finally found two outlets for its
purulent content.

THE TREATMENT OF BRONCHIAL FISTULÆ *

By Carl Eggers, M.D.

of New York, N. Y.

A bronchial fistula, as its name implies, is a communication between a bronchus and the outer surface of the lung. It may be the only condition for which a patient comes under treatment, or it may exist in connection with an empyema cavity. According to etiology, bronchial fistulæ may be divided into those due to: (1) Intrapulmonary suppuration. (2) External violence.

1. *Intrapulmonary Suppuration.*—Lung abscess and bronchiectasis are the two conditions that come into consideration, the former more often than the latter. An abscess may be the result of aspiration, or it may occur in connection with streptococcus or staphylococcus pneumonia. Whether it ruptures spontaneously into the pleura, producing a pyopneumothorax, or whether it is operated on, a bronchial fistula may result. If it ruptures spontaneously, a broncho-pleural fistula usually develops, while after operation we are more apt to find a broncho-cutaneous fistula.

2. *External Violence.*—Gunshot wounds of the lungs are the most common cause of bronchial fistula due to violence. This is particularly true of injuries with shell fragments which cause laceration and destruction of lung tissue, and which may produce an infection that delays early healing.

Anatomically bronchial fistulæ may be divided into: (a) Broncho-pleural fistulæ; (b) broncho-cutaneous fistulæ.

a. *Broncho-pleural Fistulæ.*—The diagnosis of broncho-pleural communication is frequently made in empyema patients, especially since the introduction of Carrel-Dakin treatment. While in some cases a fistula undoubtedly exists, as evidenced by violent cough with strangulation and cyanosis, and the statement of the patient that he tastes the solution as soon as Dakin is introduced, the only evidence advanced in the majority of cases is that the patient coughs whenever Dakin solution is allowed to run into the empyema cavity. That in all these cases a real bronchial fistula exists, is questionable. In many of these patients, especially in those in whom simple cough is induced by the introduction of Dakin solution, we are probably dealing with a reflex or a superficial injury of the lung parenchyma. Such an injury may have been produced by the point of an aspirating needle, or the point of a trocar used for catheter drainage. In favor of this assumption is the simple fact that one sees only a few cases of pyopneumothorax as compared with those cases in whom a broncho-pleural fistula is diagnosed. If a bronchial communication existed, and if this communication were the result of the rupture of an abscess, air should be found in the empyema cavity of all these cases. It is also noteworthy that one only infrequently encounters a broncho-pleural fistula when operating for chronic empyema, even in those cases in whom a fistula had previously been diagnosed.

However, if a lung abscess has ruptured into the pleura, producing a pyopneumothorax, a real broncho-pleural fistula may develop. Such a fistula often heals, but sometimes it may be responsible for the persistence of a chronic empyema cavity and under these conditions treatment is demanded.

b. Broncho-cutaneous Fistulæ.—They may exist in connection with an empyema cavity, but usually they come under treatment alone and constitute the principal condition requiring attention. They are most often due to operative interference in case of lung abscess or to a gunshot wound. The fistula may be small, or so large that the patient is able to carry on retrograde breathing through it with his mouth and nose closed. The fistula opens directly on the skin and is continuous with it.

TREATMENT.—I. *Broncho-pleural Fistulæ.*—As stated before, the diagnosis is frequently made, but not so often corroborated. In case a small communication exists in a patient with an acute empyema, no special treatment is necessary. The routine treatment applicable in that particular case of empyema is all that is required. As the empyema gets well, the fistula usually closes. Even in those cases in whom cough and cyanosis are produced by the introduction of Dakin solution, the treatment, as a rule, does not have to be discontinued. These patients will stand the treatment quite well if the solution is injected slowly and in small amounts, with the patient in a sitting position. A good-sized outlet tube or safety valve should be provided. If Carrel-Dakin treatment is not well borne, simple drainage should be used.

In empyema cases that have passed into the chronic stage, and in whom a broncho-pleural communication clinically persists, the fistula as such does not often require treatment. As a matter of fact, it is rarely found during operations for chronic empyema. In only a few instances of a large series of chronic empyema operations was a fistula demonstrated. In all these cases one does not have to operate for the fistula, but for the chronic empyema. Obliteration of the cavity by mobilization of the chest wall and the lung with decortication of the latter will bring about healing of both conditions. The fact that the lung is mobilized and able to contract and expand, makes it possible for the edges of the fistula to unite.

2. *Broncho-cutaneous Fistulæ.*—Patients with this condition come under treatment for the fistula itself. In order to get satisfactory results, it is necessary to take into consideration the etiology of the fistula, the length of time it has existed, and any special point that may have bearing on it. As long as a bronchial fistula is a safety valve for pus coming from some intrapulmonary focus, it must not be interfered with. If the

suppuration persists too long, the cause must be looked for and removed. It may be found to be a lobulated cavity or a sinus too narrow to carry off secretions properly. One must wait until the suppuration within the lung has cleared up, before considering means to close the fistula. It will be found that the fistula narrows down as the suppuration diminishes and often closes spontaneously. Cauterization of the tract may favor such a result. However, a few cases will refuse to heal after suppuration has ceased and the fistula has taken on a healthy appearance. The two common causes for this are: (a) The formation of a rigid ring at the mouth of the fistula, holding it firmly to the chest wall and preventing collapse and union of its walls. (b) Epithelialization of the entire tract. Knowing the causes of the persistence of a bronchial fistula, suggests its treatment, which is surgical. All cases should not be treated alike, however, and I shall therefore endeavor to bring out important points on the basis of six broncho-cutaneous fistulæ on whom I operated during the last year.

CASE I.—H. G. D. The patient had a large bronchial fistula below the angle of the left scapula, with infection of the surrounding tissue. Retrograde breathing was possible. There was no empyema cavity present. The fistula was probably the result of a spontaneous rupture of a lung abscess, producing a pyopneumothorax, for which he had been operated in December, 1917. He had been in a hospital sixteen months. Unsuccessful attempts to close the fistula by operation had been made, the last in December, 1918. There was slight unproductive cough and his general condition was good. On account of the extensive scarring of the chest wall with infection, and the peculiar position of the fistula, running up under the tip of the scapula, it was decided to do the operation under general ether anæsthesia and to divide it into two stages.

April 28, 1919: Operation. First stage. Excision of old scars which radiated in several directions. Skin and muscle flaps liberated. New bone formation arising from the ends of formerly resected ribs presented quite some difficulty. A portion of the fourth, fifth, sixth, and seventh ribs had to be removed. The thickened pleura and scar tissue was dissected away and the lung then mobilized. The wound was packed with gauze without inserting any sutures.

The after-treatment consisted in daily cleaning of the wound and then packing it with gauze soaked in Dakin solution. This caused a rapid débridement of all infected tissue. The granulations became bright red and epithelium began to spread from the mouth of the fistula over these granulations.

May 19, 1919: Operation. Second stage. The skin and muscle flaps were mobilized. An elliptical incision was made around the fistula, a short distance from its mouth, and the epithelium lining it then cauterized with the paquelin. A single row of catgut sutures was then inserted to close the fistula. After this a muscle flap was laid over the suture line and fastened in place. This was followed by closure of the rest of the muscles and skin. Two small rubber drains were inserted.

A few days after operation there was a temperature rise to 103°, accompanied by cough and followed by the expectoration of a slough. The fistula reopened temporarily, discharged necrotic material for a few days, and then closed. Except for an obstinate subcutaneous infection, the convalescence was uneventful and the final result was very good.

A review of this case would seem to show that the division of the operation into two stages was well chosen on account of the infection lodged in the tissue. The temperature and the casting off of slough was due to too deep cauterization of epithelium. This is not a good procedure, as the cases done later have proved. Cauterization should be done lightly to just destroy the epithelium, but not enough to produce a slough. The temperature might also have been avoided had the secretions had free exit early. In those cases in whom a fistula is the result of an old lung abscess, it should not be sutured, but left open to allow drainage.

CASE II.—J. A. C. R. This patient presented a small bronchial fistula of the lower right chest, posteriorly. A piece of the ninth rib had been resected in November, 1918, for an empyema following influenza. Drainage had been continuous, but at the time he came under observation it was very slight, and the empyema cavity had entirely healed, leaving only the bronchial fistula.

May 6, 1919: Operation. Resection of 3 inches of the eighth and ninth ribs, under local anæsthesia. The thickened pleura was excised and the lung mobilized. After cauterization of the fistula its outer opening was sutured. The muscles and skin were then closed, inserting one small rubber drain. On account of a subacute infection the fistula reopened a week later. As soon as the wound had cleaned up, adhesive plaster strapping was applied and an early closure of the fistula obtained.

CASE III.—C. V. M. Patient was admitted May 1, 1919, with a large bronchial fistula of the left upper chest, anterior axillary line, just below the inferior border of the pectoralis major. His history showed that he had a Vincent's angina in November, 1918. This was followed by what was diagnosed as either a lung abscess or an empyema that had ruptured into a bronchus. On January 17, 1919, a portion of the eighth rib had been resected posteriorly, but no pus was found. On January 24, 1919, an intercostal incision had been made in the third left interspace anteriorly, and pus was evacuated. A bronchial communication was noted at that time. At the time of admission he was still discharging thick pus, which made us suspect a cavity. In order to outline this, bismuth oil mixture was injected. The patient immediately spit up much of the injected material, but a certain amount entered the cavity. The X-ray showed a narrow sinus running backward and upward into the upper part of an empyema cavity extending downward posteriorly along the inner border of the scapula.

June 5, 1919: Operation. To establish drainage at the dependent part of the cavity, about 2 inches of the fifth, sixth, and seventh ribs were resected posteriorly to the inner side of the scapula. A thick-walled cavity was entered, containing pus and bismuth. The thick-ened wall was excised and the lung decorticated. One gauze strip and two rubber drains were inserted, and the muscles and skin partly closed.

The bronchial fistula anteriorly was blowing air freely. Its margins were completely excised and it was then closed with three rows of sutures, without doing any cauterization. This wound healed by primary union. There was no escape of air at any time.

The posterior wound had entirely closed on July 2, 1919, about one month after operation.

CASE IV.—B. M. N. Bronchial fistula of posterior right chest. This fistula was the result of a two-stage lung abscess operation performed September, 1918. Repeated cauterizations had failed to bring about healing. His general condition was good, there was no temperature, only slight unproductive cough, and the secretion was normal in amount.

The X-ray showed a resection of part of the ninth rib with new bone formation in the shape of a ring at the site of the former opera-tion. A tube entered the upper portion of the lower lobe.

August 19, 1919: Operation. Incision surrounding the fistula. Resection of about 3 inches of the tenth, ninth and eighth ribs under local anæsthesia. Mobilization of lung and excision of mouth of fistula. Lining of fistula lightly cauterized. No suture of the sinus was attempted on account of the danger of setting up a pneu-monic process by retention. The upper and lower muscle flaps were then sutured together, turning the cut surfaces inward for attach-ment to the lung. A small tube drain was inserted through this muscle suture at some distance from the sinus to act as a safety valve. Skin closed.

The wound secreted considerably for a few days and then cleared up. The sutures were removed six days after operation, and on September 6, 1919, two and one-half weeks after operation, the wound was firmly healed and has remained so. At no time did any unusual amount of cough or expectoration develop.

CASE V.—S. M. This patient had a large bronchial fistula of the right upper chest, just below the clavicle. It was the result of a gunshot wound received in action September 7, 1918. The history showed that he had been operated on two days after receiving his injury, and that the bullet was removed through the wound of entry. A hæmothorax developed which became infected and was drained posteriorly by rib resection. This empyema cavity closed in March, 1919, but the bronchial fistula showed no tendency to heal.

When he came under observation he had a depression of the right upper chest with a rigid opening the size of a penny in the region of the second rib, under the middle of the clavicle. There was considerable scar tissue about the fistula. Retrograde breathing was possible. The secretion was slight in amount.

The X-ray showed a cavity of the right upper lobe. Part of the second rib was missing, the first was intact, and the third showed an area of periosteal thickening. There was no foreign body visible.

August 21, 1919: Operation. Local anæsthesia (½ per cent. novocaine). Horizontal incision along second rib, surrounding the sinus. The pectoralis muscle was bluntly dissected back, above and below, and the entire second rib then resected. The dense scar surrounding the fistula was removed and the lung mobilized for a considerable distance above and below. We then found that we were dealing with a smooth cavity in the lung, the size of a pigeon's egg. Two large bronchial openings were visible in this cavity, one above and the other below, evidently the retracted ends of the main bronchus. There were also several smaller bronchial openings. The entire cavity was very lightly cauterized with a paquelin, not paying any especial attention to the bronchi. A transverse lung suture was then done by one row of continuous chromic catgut sutures, which brought the divided ends of the bronchus into apposition, and gave a tight closure. In order to cover this suture line and to fill in the defect occasioned by the resection of the second rib, it was decided to use a muscle flap. The entire pectoralis major muscle was liberated under local anæsthesia, retaining its attachment to the humerus as a pedicle. It was then divided in the direction of its fibres and the upper half laid directly onto the lung, filling in the space between the first and third ribs. This flap was then sutured into place, and in addition sutures were placed between its upper border and the clavicular portion, and its lower border and the upper border of the lower flap. A small safety drain was inserted at some distance from the lung suture and brought out through a stab wound. The skin was closed entirely.

On the third day the patient was out of bed. There was at no time any escape of air.

On September 6, 1919, sixteen days after operation, the wound was firmly healed, the patient had no symptoms, and there was no deformity.

CASE VI.—J. F. A. The patient presented an exposed area of lung with several small bronchial openings in the posterior right chest. The condition was the result of a gunshot wound received in action September 29, 1918. He was operated on five days later and again in December, 1918, January, 1919, and May, 1919.

There was considerable scarring of the chest wall due to former operations. The empyema cavity had healed.

August 27, 1919: Operation. General anæsthesia. Incision surrounding exposed area of lung with its bronchial openings. Muscles pushed back. Resection of part of tenth, ninth, eighth, and seventh ribs, which proved very difficult because a complete bony ring had formed. Intercostal tissues removed. The lung was mobilized over a large area which was necessary to relieve tension and allow a suture of normal lung over the affected area. Some difficulty encountered. Muscles of chest wall then united over the lung and skin finally closed. Drain inserted in lower part of wound.

The convalescence was somewhat prolonged because for a while there was an escape of air and bronchial secretions. Some of the difficulty was due to the fact that we were dealing not alone with one fistula, but with an area of lung containing several openings. However, the wound healed and the final result was very good.

CONCLUSIONS

Observations made on this series of cases, and the results obtained, lead me to make the following statements:

1. Broncho-pleural fistulæ usually close spontaneously.

2. In the few cases in whom a fistula is responsible for the persistence of a chronic empyema, treatment favoring the obliteration of that cavity will result in a closure of the bronchus.

3. Broncho-cutaneous fistulæ must be carefully studied and their etiology and the present condition of the lung taken into consideration.

4. As long as the fistula acts as a safety valve for intrapulmonary suppuration, it must not be interfered with.

5. Mobilization of the lung and fistula, allowing it to recede from its fixed position, is the most important factor in bringing about closure.

6. Muscle flaps are very valuable to cover the bronchial sinus after the necessary preparation has taken place. They aid in the closure and obviate deformity.

7. Cauterization of the fistula should always be done very lightly, to simply destroy the epithelium, never so deep as to produce a slough.

8. In case the wound is clean, suture of the bronchus should be done.

9. In cases due to lung abscess, in which it is feared that closure of the bronchus may result in damming back of secretions with the danger of pneumonia, the bronchus should not be sutured, but a muscle flap simply laid over it, placing a drainage tube at some distance to act as a safety valve.

10. Whenever possible the operation should be done under local anæsthesia.

PENETRATING WAR WOUNDS OF THE CHEST

A CLINICAL STUDY OF ONE HUNDRED AND SIXTY CASES

By George J. Heuer, M.D.
of Baltimore, Md.,

George P. Pratt, M.D.
of Omaha, Neb,.

AND

Verne R. Mason, M.D.
of Baltimore, Md.

At the time of America's entrance into the war, surgical opinion among the French, British, Germans, and Italians regarding the treatment of penetrating thoracic wounds had only in a measure crystallized. It had been clearly demonstrated that patients with sucking thoracic wounds did not respond well to expectant treatment, and unless immediately operated upon, died, in the large percentage of cases, either from shock, hemorrhage, and traumatopnœa, or from later infectious complications. But this was perhaps the only point in the surgical treatment of thoracic wounds upon which there was general agreement. It was emphasized by some (Duval and others) that at forward hospitals acute hemorrhage was a factor which contributed toward, or was responsible for, a certain mortality, and constituted a positive operative indication. The necessity for controlling active hemorrhage was admitted, but that it occurred in actual war experience and that it therefore constituted an operative indication, was denied by others (Hartman, *et al.*), who stated that under existing war conditions patients arrived at forward hospitals either moribund, in whom no operation was justifiable, or with hemorrhage spontaneously checked. It was asserted by some (Duval and British observers) that a large foreign body—over 1 cm. in diameter—should be removed at a primary operation in both open sucking wounds and closed wounds; and for the reason (infectious complications) that the removal of foreign bodies was generally admitted to be necessary in the treatment of wounds elsewhere. There was, however, no unanimity upon this point. A number of surgeons (among them Tuffier) were of the opinion that foreign bodies were well tolerated by the lung; that therefore in closed wounds and in open sucking wounds—unless at operation they lay directly at hand—they should be left alone until some complication directly attributable to them demanded their removal. It had been observed that the tangential and other wounds associated with extensive rib fractures, even though the parietal wounds were not open, were prone to develop infectious complications under expectant treatment; and in the opinion of some should therefore be subjected to immediate operation in order to avoid these complications. Upon this point, however, there

352

was no general agreement. These were the larger questions which were still being discussed. Among the minor questions were those referring to the treatment of small open wounds and the method of approach and closure of thoracic wounds. The question of approach was whether this should be through the wound of entrance or exit or at a point of election. The question of closure of thoracic wounds was whether this should be complete and without drainage; partial, that is, closure of the pleura leaving the parietal wound open; or with drainage of the pleural cavity.

In regard to the less serious injuries there was quite general agreement. The through-and-through bullet wounds, if without open pneumothorax or extensive rib fractures, and the penetrating bullet and small shell wounds of similar character, were generally admitted to do well under expectant treatment and were treated medically. The more important questions still being discussed were the time and method of aspirating hæmothorax and the time and method of treating infected hæmothorax.

Evacuation Hospital No. 1, the first of the forward hospitals to be established in the American Expeditionary Forces, began its activities with a fairly definite routine in the treatment of thoracic injuries;[1] namely, to treat expectantly or medically the through-and-through bullet wounds without open pneumothorax or extensive rib fractures, and the penetrating bullet and small shell wounds of similar character; and to operate immediately or as soon as possible upon (a) those with open sucking pneumothorax, at the time of the primary operation removing foreign bodies, controlling hemorrhage, and suturing or resecting the lung when indicated; (b) those with an acute continuous hemorrhage threatening life; (c) those with large intrapleural or intrapulmonary foreign bodies; and (d) those with extensive rib fractures. The question of complete tight closure of the thoracic wound was left for the time being an open one, but primary drainage of the pleural cavity was not contemplated. With the exception of one period, this outline for the treatment of thoracic injuries was consistently carried out. During a period of activity in September, 1918—a period of great stress of work, during which there was an influx of new surgical teams inexperienced in thoracic surgery—we in part failed to carry out this routine, and erred, if of necessity we did so, on the side of conservatism. This circumstance, although unfortunate, we believe, from the standpoint of the patient, enables us to offer a comparison of results which we otherwise could not do.

What have been the results of this more or less consistent line of treatment of thoracic injuries? Is it from the standpoint of immediate results the best immediate treatment of thoracic injuries in the army zone? Should it be modified toward radicalism or conservatism under

[1] Dr. John Gibbon, of Philadelphia, then surgical consultant to Evacuation Hospital No. 1, was responsible for this routine treatment of thoracic injuries; and to his good judgment and his many helpful suggestions are largely due the results obtained in the treatment of thoracic wounds at Evacuation Hospital No. 1.

varying circumstances? Our study may throw some light upon these questions and upon the unsettled points mentioned in our introductory paragraph.

The material which forms the basis of this study includes the following:

(a) One hundred and nineteen cases of penetrating thoracic wounds which were entirely under our care at Evacuation Hospital No. 1.

(b) Twenty-two cases in which the primary operation was performed by a number of surgeons at Evacuation Hospital No. 1 during September, 1918. These cases were seen and examined on admission by one of us (Heuer) who then acted as *triage* officer. After operation they came under our care, and such secondary operations as were necessary for post-operative complications were performed by us.

(c) Twenty-four cases observed at Base Hospital No. 18 at a time when it functioned as an evacuation hospital. These cases were most carefully studied and are of value in comparing the results of treatment instituted early with that instituted late.

It should be emphasized that we have unusually good records of all the cases included in this report; and because of the active coöperation of internists (Pratt and Mason), röntgenologist[2] and surgeon.

For convenience in discussion we may divide the cases into two groups—(1) those not primarily operated upon, and (2) those subjected to immediate operation.

GROUP I. ONE HUNDRED AND FIFTEEN CASES NOT PRIMARILY OPERATED UPON

A summary of this group may be given as follows: Of the 115 cases there were 53 bullet wounds and 62 shell wounds; 47 were perforating with a wound of entrance and exit; 68 were penetrating with retained missiles either in the chest wall, pleura, lung, or upper abdomen. Six were small (1–2 cm.), open sucking wounds; 109 were closed wounds. Of the perforating wounds, all, with one exception, were due to bullets.

The patients arrived at Evacuation Hospital No. 1 in the majority of instances within twelve hours after their injuries; at Base Hospital No. 18 in from one to seven days after their injuries. In the evacuation hospital series a slight or moderate grade of shock was the rule on admission; but in addition to these moderate grades, profound shock was not uncommon and was observed in twenty-one cases. Eleven of these cases recovered after vigorous shock treatment; 10 cases, practically moribund on admission, died within an hour or two after their arrival. Eighteen cases entered Evacuation Hospital No. 1 with normal pulse and blood-pressure, in whom all signs of shock were absent; and this was practically true of the base hospital series.

It would require too many pages to comment at length upon the physical findings in this group of cases, and we shall therefore but men-

<hr>

[2] We are indeed indebted to Dr. Ira M. Lockwood, of Lincoln, Neb., at the time rontgenologist at Evacuation Hospital No. 1, for his coöperation in the study of these cases. His painstaking localization work especially was invaluable to us.

tion some of them. *Cough, hæmoptysis,* and *dyspnœa* were extraordinarily common and would appear to occur almost invariably when the pleura and lung are penetrated. *Acute primary hemorrhage* threatening life was not seen in a single instance in this series. In the ten cases moribund on admission, hemorrhage, if that was the chief cause of the serious shock, had spontaneously ceased. As will be noted later, secondary hemorrhage occurred in two cases. *Mediastinal compression symptoms* (dyspnœa, cyanosis, tachycardia) due to a high grade of hæmothorax were noted in twelve cases; but in none were they so urgent as to require immediate aspiration for their relief. *Extensive subcutaneous emphysema* was present in twelve cases, a slight degree in many cases. *Pure hæmothorax* occurred in 94 of the 115 cases, or in 81 per cent. In thirty-eight cases the fluid level reached well above the angle of the scapula (hæmothorax large) ; in twenty-nine cases reached the angle of the scapula (hæmothorax moderate) ; in twenty-seven cases did not reach the angle of the scapula (hæmothorax small). *Hæmopneumothorax,* exclusive of seven cases subsequently developing an anaërobic infection with gas formation, was demonstrable in twelve cases. In six cases it occurred in open wounds, in six cases in closed wounds. A *pure pneumothorax* occurred in three cases. *Hemorrhagic consolidation of the lung,* not the common type occurring about the wound tract, but involving the lung at some distance from the wound, was demonstrable at autopsy in four cases; in three it involved the lung on the side of the injury; in one the lung contralateral to the injury. *Collapse of the lung,* that interesting condition emphasized especially by British observers, was seen in only one case, but may well have frequently escaped detection. *Elevation and immobility of the diaphragm* upon the side injured was observed, although its frequency, due to the difficulty of recognizing the exact position of the diaphragm in the presence of hæmothorax, cannot be accurately stated. *Pleural and pericardial friction rubs* occurred in a few cases. *Mild abdominal signs and symptoms* were rather common in the low thoracic injuries; were marked in four cases in which a board-like retracted abdomen with hiccup and vomiting strongly suggested the perforation of a hollow abdominal viscus.

The position and course of the parietal wounds may be seen in the accompanying diagrams (Figs. 1 to 4). The wounds involved almost every part of the thorax; the missiles penetrated in almost every direction. In general the wounds were small punctured wounds without extensive laceration of tissue. Only 6 of the 115 were open wounds and these could be converted into closed wounds by a pressure dressing. Only two wounds of the entire series were obviously infected at the time of admission. The incidence of *associated rib fractures* cannot be accurately stated, for the chipping of a rib so easily escapes detection. Extensive rib fractures, however, were noted in eight cases, fracture of the clavicle in one case, of the sternum in two cases, and of the scapula in five cases. In the vast majority of cases the *foreign bodies* retained within the thorax were small (1 cm. in diameter or less). In eight cases the shell fragments measured over 1 cm., but not over 2 cm. in diameter; in seven instances machine-gun or rifle bullets were retained.

The *clinical course* in these cases was either normal for thoracic wounds or complicated by infection or hemorrhage. Dismissing the ten cases moribund on admission and dying a few hours after their arrival, 80 cases pursued a normal clinical course, 25 developed some complications with reference to their thoracic injuries.

What we may term a normal uncomplicated course may be briefly outlined. The patients, admitted in a condition of shock, often with dyspnœa, cyanosis, and anxiety, and with a varying amount of pain, cough, and bloody expectoration, present the picture of a serious injury. With complete rest in a heated bed and with morphia in adequate doses to induce quiet, the whole picture, as a rule, changes within a few hours, and, with the exception of the very seriously shocked, almost invariably by the following day. Their general appearance improves, their color returns, their pulse becomes stronger, their blood-pressure rises; dyspnœa and cyanosis become less marked; and their anxiety disappears. Cough with bloody sputum varies; it may be slight or it may be troublesome for days. Their striking change for the better is a source of astonishment, and gives rise to the impression that their previous apparently serious condition was out of all proportion to the injury or the amount of blood lost. In the seriously shocked the response to treatment is not so marked, and, as in eleven cases of this series, the condition of shock may give rise to anxiety for from twenty-four hours to three days. Fever in cases progressing normally is the rule and may vary within wide limits. In our series of cases the temperature soon after admission rose to 100° to 101°, sometimes to 103° to 104°, and showed either a continued elevation over several days or daily slight remissions. Most frequently the temperature began to decline on the third to the fifth day, but showed a daily rise to 99° to 100° for from ten days to two weeks. A relatively high fever may, however, persist for two weeks and may not completely disappear for three or four weeks. In a relatively few the temperature may be normal and remain so throughout the course. With the exception of cough, bloody sputum and fever, which are common to these injuries, no untoward symptoms appear; and within two weeks the patient's strength has returned and he is able to be up and about.

Complications.—Unlike that in many institutions in forward areas in which prompt evacuation of patients was imperative, it was our policy not to discharge patients with thoracic injuries until the danger of all complications had passed. We believe, therefore, that the complications to be enumerated represent practically the total incidence of complications in this series.

Infected Hæmothorax.—This, the most frequent complication of penetrating thoracic wounds, occurred in 18 or 17 per cent., of the 105 cases which survived the immediate effects of their injuries. Three of the 15 cases in the base hospital series, or 20 per cent., developed this complication; 15, or 16.5 per cent., of the evacuation hospital series. The predominating infecting organisms were the gas bacillus of Welch in seven cases, the streptococcus hæmolyticus in three cases, the streptococcus viridans in one case, pyogenic staphylococci in five cases, and unknown in two cases. When we critically examine the cases which developed infected hæmothorax, we find that seven cases had neither open wounds, large retained foreign bodies (in two of these cases the size of the foreign body is not known), nor extensive fractures; in other words, did not present the conditions which we had learned predisposed to infectious complications. The remaining eleven cases, however, presented one or more of these conditions. It is interesting to note that four of the six cases with small open wounds developed infected hæmothorax; seven of the eight cases with retained shell fragments larger than 1 cm. in diameter developed this complication; as did three of the eight cases with extensive rib fractures. Eleven of the cases which developed infected hæmothorax were wounded by shell fragments which were lodged within the thorax; seven were wounded by bullets, of which six perforated the thorax and one penetrated and lodged within the thorax. While too small a series from which to draw any positive conclusions, the evidence from it supports the view that open sucking chest wounds, large retained foreign bodies, and extensive fractures of the bony thorax are conditions which favor the development of infectious complications.

The clinical course in cases developing an infected hæmothorax is usually quite different from those progressing normally. We can distinguish two groups of cases: those in which infection develops early and those in which it appears late. In the instances of early infection the temperature, which in cases progressing normally begins to fall on the third to the fifth day, fails to do so; rather it shows each day a little higher elevation or may assume a septic curve. In addition, the patient does not feel well nor look well, as in uninfected cases, but complains of thoracic pain and dyspnœa, has tachycardia, is restless, and has disturbed sleep. Such relatively benign symptoms should give rise to the suspicion of infection and warrant aspiration for cultural purposes. In the single case of streptococcus viridans infection, no more alarming symptoms developed; but the streptococcus hæmolyticus, gas bacillus, and some of the pyogenic infections were accompanied by high fever, tachycardia, signs of toxæmia, and thoracic pain. In the instances of late infection (developing from one to three weeks after the receipt of the wound) a normal course with a falling temperature was rather suddenly followed by a sharp elevation of temperature and by the symptoms and signs we have just enumerated. The physical signs in both groups may remain as before; or show an increase in the fluid level. Most striking in their symptomatology and physical signs are the infections with anaërobic organisms (Welch

357

bacillus), whether occurring early or late. Within twenty-four hours the patient, previously progressing normally, becomes seriously ill, with a temperature of 104°, with a pulse of 120 to 140, and with dyspnœa, cyanosis, toxæmia, and delirium. Physical examination shows a marked change due to the gas formation. A pneumohæmothorax has replaced the hæmothorax, and the intrathoracic pressure has increased, as shown by the cardiac displacement.

Pneumonia.—Pneumonia occurred in two forms—as a septic bronchopneumonia occurring about the seat of the lesion, or as a lobular or lobar pneumonia. Obviously, it is difficult to form any accurate estimate of the frequency of pneumonia upon the side wounded; for the presence of hæmothorax, of hemorrhagic consolidation, of congestion, and of the symptoms of fever, cough and blood-stained sputum, so common in all chest wounds, makes a proper interpretation of the physical signs almost impossible. By autopsy examination pneumonia was demonstrated in seven cases, four of which were associated with infected hæmothorax. In two cases an extensive broncho-pneumonia of the usual type occurred in the lung contralateral to the injury; in two cases a widespread septic bronchopneumonia surrounded the pulmonary wound; and in two cases a bilateral septic broncho-pneumonia was present. In only one case did we observe a pneumonia of the lobar type; and in the lung contralateral to the injury. By physical examination four other cases which recovered were considered to have had a broncho-pneumonia on the side of the injury.

Pulmonary abscess and gangrene were exceedingly rare in this series. In one case included under the cases of infected hæmothorax above, pulmonary gangrene with secondary abscess formation was recognized by the fetor of the breath and the offensive expectoration, and was confirmed by autopsy examination. In a second case a lung abscess, unsuspected clinically, was found at autopsy. The patient, with two penetrating thoracic wounds and multiple wounds of the extremities, developed gas gangrene of one leg necessitating a thigh amputation. He died with all the symptoms of gas intoxication. At autopsy a lung abscess 7 by 5 cm. was found along the wound tract in the middle lobe of the right lung, lying freely in which was a fragment of rib driven into the lung by the missile. The missile itself was embedded in the liver with no reaction about it.

Septicæmia, pyæmia, and *purulent pericarditis* occurred in association with other infectious complications of thoracic wounds in three cases.

Infection of the parietal wound, as previously noted, was observed in but two cases on admission, and in these was of no moment. The single serious infection which occurred in this series was a gas infection (Welch bacillus) which developed in a bullet wound and spread rapidly in the tissues of the thoracic and abdominal walls. In spite of the most radical incisions, the patient promptly died of gas gangrene. At autopsy there was no other cause of death.

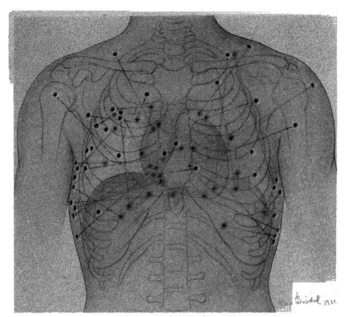

FIG. 1.—Composite picture of forty of the penetrating wounds of the ventral surface of the thorax of which we have accurate records. The wound of entrance is represented by a black dot, the course of the missile by a dotted line, and the point of lodgment of the foreign body by a shaded dot.

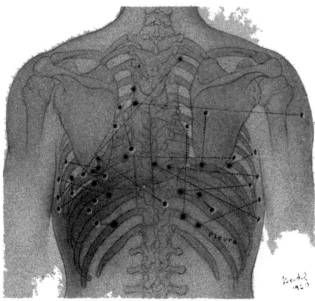

FIG. 2.—Composite picture of twenty-three of the penetrating wounds of the dorsal surface of the thorax. The same technic for representing the wound of entrance. the course of the missile, and the point of lodgment of the foreign body is used as in Fig. 1.

358

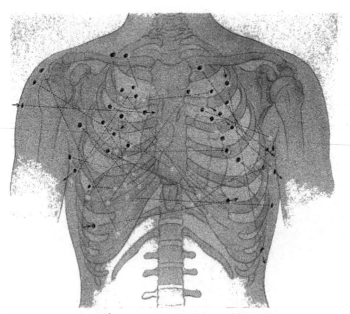

FIG. 3.—Composite picture of thirty-nine of the perforating wounds of the ventral surface of the thorax of which we have accurate records. The wound of entrance is represented by a black dot, the course of the missile by a dotted line, and the wound of exit, if upon the dorsal surface of the thorax, by a white dot. The wounds which perforated the ventral surface of the thorax alone are represented by black dots and arrows.

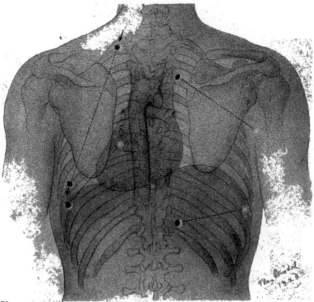

FIG. 4.—Composite picture of the perforating wounds of the dorsal surface of the body. The same technic for representing the wounds of entrance and exit is used as in Fig. 3.

Secondary or late intrapleural hemorrhage occurred in two instances. One patient was wounded by a shell fragment posteriorly, the missile traversing the right thorax obliquely and lodging under the skin just to the right of the sternal margin. For six days he pursued a normal uncomplicated course; then suddenly after violent coughing complained of weakness and went into collapse. When seen he was pallid, cold, and sweating, and had a scarcely perceptible pulse at the wrist. The signs of hæmothorax had increased. Although recognizing the hemorrhage, thoracotomy to control it was out of the question. In spite of our usual measures to combat shock the patient died. At autopsy the right thoracic cavity was completely filled with blood, and the heart markedly dislocated toward the left. An open wound of the right internal mammary artery was found and it was supposed that a clot had been dislodged from the vessel during the paroxysm of coughing. The other patient was wounded in the left supraclavicular space, the foreign body lodging in or upon the left diaphragm. In addition to a high grade of hæmothorax he had abdominal pain, marked abdominal rigidity, and hiccup. Twice in the early days of his injury he vomited blood. On the tenth day after the injury, following an effort to sit up in bed, he suddenly complained of left thoracic pain and almost immediately went into collapse. Pallor, sweating, air hunger, imperceptible pulse, and a mounting hæmothorax, all indicated a secondary hemorrhage. The day of and the day following the accident 2700 c.c. of bloody fluid were aspirated because of pressure symptoms. The cultures from the fluid, previously sterile, showed a hæmolytic streptococcus, and therefore a rib resection with drainage of the infected hæmothorax was done so soon as the patient's condition warranted it. Subsequent sterilization of the cavity by Dakin's solution was followed by secondary closure of the sinus tract.

Treatment.—The treatment in this group of cases may be briefly outlined. Absolute rest in a warm bed and morphia in sufficient doses to induce quiet were the first and important steps in the treatment. Shock was immediately and energetically treated by the usual methods. As previously noted, all our efforts in the treatment of shock were unavailing in the ten cases practically moribund on admission. In the lesser degrees of shock, blood transfusion, intravenous gum acacia (Bayliss's solution), intravenous saline, hypodermoclysis and salt and coffee per rectum, together with elevation or bandaging of the extremities were used. Our success in treating shock depended upon its degree and duration. The profoundly shocked in our experience did not respond to the various methods which we employed, excepting to blood transfusion when hemorrhage was the factor in the production of shock; nor did those who had been seriously shocked for from twelve to twenty-four hours before coming to us. It is indeed difficult in such a small series of cases to form any just estimate of the value of various measures in the treatment of this condition. Through the efforts of our " shock teams " we have accurate records of pulse and blood-pressure determinations before and after the use of various measures; and we may summarize our experience as follows: (a) That marked beneficial effects follow the use of external heat, rest, and morphia in the lesser degrees of shock; (b) that blood transfusion is of the greatest value in those in whom hemorrhage is the factor in the production of shock. Yet we observed patients profoundly shocked in whom there was no evidence of serious hemorrhage and in whom blood transfusion had but slight, if any, effect upon the pulse or blood-pressure. In these cases Bayliss's solution failed to have any more effect. (c) That in profound shock of *long duration* neither Bayliss's solution nor intravenous saline, hypodermoclysis, nor salt and coffee per rectum had any appreciable effect upon the pulse or blood-pressure. In the few cases which recovered it cannot be said, however, that these measures did not have some beneficial effect. (d) That in the lesser degrees of shock intravenous saline or salt and coffee had about as marked an effect upon the pulse and blood-pressure as did gum acacia. Our poor results in the treatment of profound or serious shock we feel were due to the fact that the condition as we saw it at an evacuation hospital was not comparable either to the *recent* shock produced in the laboratory or to that seen in civil life following operations. It had persisted for hours and sometimes for twenty-four hours before treatment could be instituted.

The subsequent treatment of this group of cases consisted in the treatment of mediastinal compression symptoms, of hæmothorax, and of infectious complications. Mediastinal compression symptoms were treated by aspiration. In the majority of the twelve cases requiring this procedure, one aspiration of 500 to 800 c.c. sufficed; in two cases as many as three aspirations on successive days were necessary. The treatment of hæmothorax was along well-established lines. Aspiration was done for two purposes—for diagnosis and for treatment. Knowing that every thoracic wound was potentially infected, and fearing the consequences of unrecognized infected hæmothorax, a small syringeful of blood for cultural purposes was aspirated either daily or every other day in all cases which were not progressing perfectly normally. Aspiration for treatment was performed because the large collections of fluid are absorbed very slowly, and when not removed give rise to a thickened pleura and adhesions obliterating the costodiaphragmatic sulcus; conditions which impair pulmonary function and give rise to many post-traumatic subjective complaints. In the series of 105 cases, aside from the removal of small amounts of blood, aspiration of from 200 c.c. to 3000 c.c. of blood was performed in thirty cases, and chiefly in those with large collections of fluid. Two methods of aspiration were used—an early aspiration of from 200 c.c. to 500 c.c. on the fourth or fifth day, repeated if necessary on succeeding days until all the blood was removed; or a late aspiration, usually on the tenth to the twelfth day, removing at one sitting all the blood that could be obtained. A third method—early total aspiration combined with artificial pneumothorax, used with especial success by Italian observers—was not employed by us. Of the two methods used by us, early aspiration was used in twenty cases, late aspiration in ten cases. To have used aspiration in the treatment of hæmothorax in but 30 per cent. of our cases would appear to indicate that we were not enthusiastic in its use; but this is not true. In the earlier period of our experience, we, as many others previously inexperienced in the treatment of thoracic wounds, failed to aspirate many cases which later would have been subjected to this treatment. In the large and moderate collections of fluid, aspiration is an aid in the treatment of hæmothorax, for it permits a more rapid expansion of the lung, and, when done early, probably prevents the deposition of a thick layer of fibrin upon the pleural surfaces. We have no evidence, however, that aspiration prevents the obliteration of the costodiaphragmatic angle nor the formation of adhesions between the diaphragm and costal pleura. A study of the X-rays of our cases shows that practically all cases previously having a large or moderate hæmothorax had at the time of their discharge (a month or more after their injury) adhesions obliterating the costodiaphragmatic angle; and to practically the same extent whether aspirated or not. Pleural thickening was a much less conspicuous finding; nor was retraction of the thorax very evident. If we can judge from our own series, obliteration of the costodiaphragmatic angle is the most constant and conspicuous of the abnormalities following hæmothorax.

The treatment of the eighteen cases developing infected hæmothorax consisted, with one exception, in rib resection and drainage so soon as the diagnosis was established by cultures of the aspirated fluid. We cannot see any justification for delaying operation and resorting to aspiration until a frank empyema has developed, for only too often a delay is followed by septicæmia, purulent pericarditis, pyæmia, and death. Operation was followed by sterilization of the pleural cavity by Dakin's solution; with subsequent excision and closure of the sinus so soon as the cavity was sterile. In the single exception to this form of treatment—an instance of streptococcus viridans infection—we resorted to repeated aspiration. The patient eventually recovered, but his convalescence was prolonged beyond that of those treated by rib resection, and we are certain that he would better have been treated as the others.

Of these 18 patients, 11 recovered and 7 died. An examination of the autopsy records of the 7 dead shows that in only one was death due to a simple infected hæmothorax. Four cases showed an extensive bronchopneumonia; one case, pulmonary abscess and gangrene associated with a bronchial fistula; and one case showed a healed sterile cavity, death being due to septicæmia and pyæmia, the result of a purulent knee-joint. In the cases which recovered, the cavities were sterile and closed at the time the patients left the hospital. We know the late results in only two cases, and both of these are of great interest. Due presumably to firm adhesions preventing the expansion of the lung, the cavity persisted in one case for four months, in the other for eight months. Yet during all this time the sinus tracts, closed over the sterile cavities, remained healed and the patients suffered in no way because of the presence of their unobliterated pleural cavities. Subsequently both cavities became obliterated; and since their return to this country we have X-rays of these patients showing the complete obliteration of these long-standing cavities.

The treatment of the other infectious complications requires no further comment.

Results.—Of the 115 cases included in this group 10 were admitted in a moribund condition and died within a few hours after their arrival, untreated excepting for measures to combat shock. In the 105 cases which survived their primary injury, there were 11 deaths, 7 of which occurred in the group of cases which developed infected hæmothorax. Of the 4 other deaths, one followed hemorrhage from the internal mammary artery; one, gas infection of the thoracic wall; one, gas gangrene of the leg; and one, lobar pneumonia. In two cases death was wholly due to causes unrelated to the thoracic wounds. The total mortality in this group was, therefore, 18 per cent. If we exclude the cases moribund on admission and those dying from other injuries, the mortality in the 105 cases is 8.5 per cent. As previously noted, 80 cases pursued an uncomplicated course. These were kept in bed, as a rule, for from ten days to two weeks; were discharged in from three weeks to one month. They were comparatively free from symptoms and apparently well, and we have the feeling that few could have developed later complications. In the 11 of the 18 cases which survived infected hæmothorax, the pleural cavities were sterile and the sinus tracts closed before the patients were discharged.

Discussion.—When we review this series of cases in the light of our study, could we have improved our treatment? The group of 10 cases moribund on admission were clearly beyond our help, and if any treatment could have benefited them, it should have been and perhaps was carried out at the dressing station. With the exception of one case of fatal secondary hemorrhage, all the 11 deaths not occurring immediately from shock and open thorax were the result of infectious complications, and it is to these that we should particularly devote attention. Seven deaths followed infected hæmothorax; one death was due to an uncomplicated pneumonia, 2 to gas infection and gangrene. Granted that the surgeon is skilled in thoracic work, it would seem in the light of subsequent events that we could have done better had we excised and closed the open wounds, removed the large foreign bodies, and repaired the extensive rib fractures, for these conditions were obvious factors in the causation of infected hæmothorax. We should, in other words, have taken these cases from the non-operative group and placed them in the operative group.

GROUP II. FORTY-FIVE CASES SUBJECTED TO IMMEDIATE OPERATION

These cases include: (1) Twenty-two operated upon by a group of surgeons at Evacuation Hospital No. 1 during September, 1918; they were seen and examined by one of us (Heuer) who then acted as *triage* officer, and after operation came under our care; (2) 8 cases operated upon at Base Hospital No. 18 at a time when it functioned as an evacuation hospital; and (3) 15 cases operated upon by one of us (Heuer). Ten were bullet wounds and 35 shell wounds; 9 were perforating with a wound of entrance and exit; 36 were penetrating wounds with retained foreign bodies. Thirty-three were large open " sucking " wounds; 12 were closed wounds.ᵃ These figures show the preponderance of shell wounds over bullet wounds in these more serious injuries.

Time Interval.—In the evacuation hospital series the time interval between receipt of the injury and admission to the hospital varied between six and twenty-four hours, in the large majority being about twelve hours. In the base hospital series it varied from twenty-four hours to eight days.

Shock.—In the evacuation hospital series a profound degree of shock was the rule in those with open sucking chest wounds. The patients arrived pale, cold, and pulseless, with a low blood-pressure and with dyspnœa, cyanosis, and anxiety. Undoubtedly, open pneumothorax is one of the most important contributing factors in this serious grade of shock, and it was often noted that the patient's condition improved after the thoracic breach was closed. Moreover, it seemed clear that the large open wounds were associated with greater shock than the smaller wounds. In those with closed thoracic wounds, shock was a less conspicuous feature, and in at least five cases the appearance and clinical signs of shock were absent. In the base hospital series shock, with one exception, had been recovered from at the time of the patient's admission.

Cough, hæmoptysis, and *dyspnœa* were more troublesome in those with open sucking wounds than in those with closed wounds. While in the latter, cough can usually be controlled by sedatives, in the former it cannot be satisfactorily checked until the thoracic wound is closed. Dyspnœa, relatively uncommon in our series with closed wounds, was invariable in open wounds, was sometimes most distressing, and was always accompanied by a varying degree of cyanosis. It persists so long as the thorax is open, and indeed tends to become progressively worse.

Acute primary hemorrhage threatening life did not occur in those with closed wounds; was in no instance the indication which led to thoracotomy in those with open wounds. Yet upon opening the thorax in four of the cases the lung was found to be actively bleeding, the continuation of which would undoubtedly have caused a fatal termination.

ᵃ In the Base Hospital No. 18 series the original condition of the wounds at the time of admission is not positively stated. In the absence of a definite statement it is assumed that they were closed wounds, and are counted as such.

Character of Wounds.—With the exception of the twelve closed wounds, the character of the wounds in this group of cases was in marked contrast to those in the preceding group. They were large, varying in size from 2 to 5 cm. in diameter, and showed extensive laceration of the skin, subcutaneous tissues and muscles. In practically every case, from one to three ribs were extensively fractured, and in addition there occurred fractures of the scapula, sternum, and spinous processes of the vertebræ. Six of these extensively lacerated wounds with comminuted fractures of the bony thorax were caused by bullets, the remainder by shell fragments.

In the open wounds the retained foreign bodies varied in size from 1.5 to 3 cm. in diameter; in the closed wounds they were small.

Hæmothorax in pure form occurred in all but one of the twelve cases with closed wounds. The amount of fluid in those with open wounds varied with the position of the open wound, for the blood escapes from the wound with respiratory movements and coughing.

Abdominal signs were noted in eight cases. These consisted chiefly of upper abdominal tenderness and rigidity. In no case was there hiccup, and in only one case was vomiting noted. At operation the diaphragm was perforated or lacerated in all cases which showed abdominal signs; in one case which showed perforation of the diaphragm no abdominal signs were present.

Clinical Course.—The clinical course in this group of cases cannot be discussed, for all the cases were within a short time after their arrival subjected to operation. Yet we know from our observation of the ten cases included in Group I as moribund, and from the literature of French, British, German, and Italian observers during the early period of the war what the clinical course of these cases is when treated expectantly. In those with large open wounds, shock is not recovered from, but rather becomes more profound and death occurs in the majority of cases in from twenty-four to forty-eight hours. Should life be prolonged for several days, infection invariably occurs and terminates the course. The mortality in the early period of the war was practically 100 per cent. In those with small open wounds life may be prolonged, but infection is almost certain.

Operative Treatment. (a) Indications. Before taking up our operative procedures let us for a moment discuss our operative indications. As noted in our introductory paragraph, our routine operative indications were open pneumothorax, large retained foreign bodies, extensive rib fractures, and acute primary hemorrhage threatening life. To these we must add our inability to positively diagnose the presence or absence of an intra-abdominal injury. When we analyze our cases these operative indications occurred as follows:

1. Open sucking thoracic wounds occurred in thirty-three of the forty-five cases (73 + per cent.), and was the urgent operative indication. In twenty-six of these cases we have records of extensive fractures of one to

three ribs combined in some instances with fractures of the scapula, sternum, and vertebral spines. In twenty-three of these cases a large foreign body was retained. In the shell wounds of the thorax, therefore, the combination of three of our operative indications presented itself in the large majority of cases (70 per cent.). Open thorax alone without extensive fractures or retained foreign bodies was the indication in two cases. Large retained foreign body alone was the operative indication in only one case. Extensive fractures alone was the indication in but two cases, but from our experience in Group I should have been the operative indication in others.

2. Acute hemorrhage threatening life was not the prime indication in any case, but as previously noted, in four of our personal cases active hemorrhage from the lung was found at operation. Active bleeding from the thoracic wall was not observed.

3. Our inability to diagnose the presence or absence of an intra-abdominal injury was the indication for thoracotomy in six cases, but in two there was the additional indication of a large retained foreign body. Had we felt sure of the absence of an abdominal injury, four of these cases might well have been treated expectantly.

Operative Procedures.—Contrary to the outline given in our routine that operation in thoracic injuries should include excision of the wounds, removal of foreign bodies, control of hemorrhage, treatment of the wounded lung when indicated, and subsequent complete closure of the thoracic wound, this complete operation, if we may so term it, was not consistently carried out. Rather, three more or less distinct procedures were carried out, and it will be of interest to compare the results obtained in each.

1. The simplest procedure employed was the excision or *débridement* of the wound of the soft parts and the removal of bone fragments. The thoracic cavity was not opened widely, the hæmothorax not evacuated, the foreign body not removed, and the lung not examined. The pleura or intercostal muscles were closed, and the skin either closed or left open. The procedure, then, consisted simply of *débridement* with closure of open wounds, or *débridement* with opening and reclosure of closed wounds. This type of procedure was employed in seven of the base hospital cases and in one of the evacuation hospital cases—eight cases in all. It is evident from the histories that these were the least seriously injured. Shock had been completely recovered from in the base hospital series and was absent in the single case in the evacuation hospital series. The wounds were small, the rib fractures not so extensive as in the more serious injuries. The results in this group of cases were as follows: Three of the eight patients died; one from presumably a valve pneumothorax, one from pulmonary gangrene, and one from lung abscess. The death from valve pneumothorax was due to faulty technic and should have been avoided. An incomplete closure of the pleura was followed by symptoms of pressure pneumothorax which were recognized too late to save the patient. At

autopsy nothing to account for death excepting a pneumothorax was found. Two additional cases which recovered developed post-operative complications. In one the wound, not completely closed at the primary operation, became infected, with the subsequent development of pyopneumo-thorax; in the other an infected hæmothorax developed requiring a subsequent rib resection and drainage. Fifty per cent. of these cases, therefore, developed post-operative infectious complications following incomplete operations, of which 37.5 per cent. died. It should be remembered, however, that operation in these cases was performed late—at a time when infectious complications are more prone to occur.

2. The second procedure consisted in the *débridement* of the wounds, an exploratory thoracotomy, the evacuation of the blood in the thorax, the *débridement* and suture of wounds in the lung when feasible, and the removal of foreign bodies when possible. The pleura was closed, but the overlying muscles and skin were left open because of the presumed danger of infection. This procedure was carried out in twelve cases. Six patients recovered without complications and were discharged well. Four patients developed infections in the wounds which had been left open, the infection resulting in the reopening of the pleura and the development of a pyopneumothorax. Three of these four cases died, their death being due to infection; one recovered after a secondary rib resection and drainage at a point of election. Two additional cases died within twelve hours of the operation from shock. The mortality in this group was, therefore, 41.6 per cent. Infectious complications occurred in 33.33 per cent. In contradistinction to the first group of cases these were operated upon early; that is, within eighteen hours from the receipt of their injuries. It is interesting to note that none of these cases developed pulmonary abscess or gangrene. How much a complete operation had to do with it is difficult to determine. Bone fragments embedded in the lung, if of any size, were certainly removed. Foreign bodies were removed in three cases; were not removed in five cases. In three perforating wounds foreign bodies were not present.

3. The third procedure consisted in the careful excision or *débridement* of the wound, the careful removal of all bone fragments from the pleura, the evacuation of the hæmothorax, the removal of foreign bodies and bone fragments from the lung whenever possible, the excision of the wounds in the lung when feasible, followed by suture, and the complete air-tight closure of the thoracic wound. This so-called complete operation was carried out in twenty-five cases. Twenty-one patients recovered, all but one without any complications whatever; one case developed a post-operative infected hæmothorax but recovered following a rib resection with drainage. Three cases died of shock within twelve hours of operation; one case died of a post-operative streptococcus empyema. The mortality in this group, therefore, was 16 per cent. Post-operative infectious complications occurred in 8 per cent. In this series foreign bodies were removed in

fifteen cases, not removed in three cases, and not stated in three cases. In four cases of perforating wounds no foreign bodies were present.

Discussion.—When we compare the results obtained by these three procedures the most striking dissimilarity is in the frequency of post-operative infectious complications. Following the first procedure, 50 per cent. of the cases developed such complications; following the second, 33.33 per cent.; and following the third, 8 per cent. The condition of the patient may be eliminated as a factor in these results. Shock was absent in the first group, present in equal degree in the second and third groups. The time interval is a definite factor in the results in the first group, for the operations were performed late, when infectious complications are more prone to occur. Time is not, however, a factor in the results in the second and third groups. The difference in the results appears to be due to the type of operation which was performed. In the first group the operation was totally inadequate. Lacerated wounds of the lung and large collections of blood in the presence of infected missiles and bone fragments—wound conditions which are prone to give rise to infection—were left untreated. In the second group, although a relatively small number of foreign bodies were removed, the obvious great mistake was the failure to completely close the thoracic wound. As a result the parietal wound became infected, the pleura reopened, and a pyopneumothorax developed—conditions which were responsible for all the deaths not due to shock. The third procedure as outlined above, and including the complete air-tight closure of the thoracic wound, gave by far the best results and would appear to be the operation of choice in cases requiring immediate operation. That it is adequate when carefully performed is indicated by the fact that in fifteen cases operated upon by one of us (Heuer) there was not, aside from a single stitch abscess, a single complication of any sort.

Results.—The results in this group of forty-five cases have been in part indicated above. The total mortality in the series was twelve, or 26.6 per cent. Of the thirty-three cases which survived, thirty recovered without complications, and three developed infected hæmothorax which required a secondary rib resection and drainage. In the thirty cases which recovered without complications, the immediate and presumably also the late results, were most satisfactory—much more so than in cases treated expectantly. The lung was completely expanded in ten days, pleural thickening did not occur, and adhesions fixing the diaphragm in a high position were absent. Subjective complaints of thoracic pain, dyspnœa, and tachycardia were quite uniformly absent. The results were so much better than in cases treated expectantly that one is almost tempted to suggest thoracotomy in the treatment of hæmothorax. Of the twelve cases which died, five deaths were due to shock, six to post-operative infectious complications, and one to post-operative pneumothorax.

To sum up the entire series of 160 cases: There were 127 recoveries and 33 deaths, a general mortality of 20 per cent. If we exclude the 10 cases moribund on admission and dying untreated and the 2 deaths due to causes unrelated to their thoracic wounds, the mortality is 13 per cent. Eighty cases in the non-operative group recovered without complications; 25 developed complications, with one exception of an infectious nature. Of these 11 died. Ten patients died of shock, untreated except for measures to combat shock. Thirty cases in the operative group recovered without post-operative complications; 10 developed post-operative infectious complications, of which 7 died. Five cases died of shock within twenty-four hours after operation.

As a result of this study we may offer what evidence we have bearing upon the treatment of penetrating thoracic injuries. Our experience confirms what had already been established, that a large open thoracic wound constitutes a positive operative indication, and tends to show that the small open wound as well should be immediately closed. That the large retained foreign body is an operative indication is not so evident from our study, but it is quite apparent that it is prone to give rise to infectious complications and should, therefore, in our opinion, be removed. In the absence of all other operative indications, however, should we deliberately perform a thoracotomy in order to remove a large foreign body from the lung? Only rarely in our experience (one case in our series) will this question arise, for, as we have shown, the large foreign body is most frequently associated with open wounds and fractures of the bony thorax. In the absence of all other indications, however, the large foreign body in our experience should or should not be an operative indication, depending upon the experience and skill of the surgeon in thoracic surgery. Our experience shows that extensive rib fractures also are prone to give rise to infectious complications, and sufficiently often to warrant operation. As an isolated condition, however, extensive rib fractures are uncommon, and occur most frequently in conjunction with open wounds or large foreign bodies. Acute continued hemorrhage was never in our experience, either in the non-operative group or in the operative group, an isolated operative indication, yet in four cases operated upon because of other indications, active hemorrhage was found. Our experience, therefore, is similar to Hartmann's that in practice acute continued hemorrhage is rarely an indication, yet its possibility must always be remembered.

As a good working basis in the treatment of penetrating chest wounds we feel that the operative indications we have discussed should stand, but realizing that while stated as single indications, they rarely occur alone. When operation is indicated our experience shows that as complete an operation as the wound conditions demand, with removal of the foreign body and complete closure of the thoracic wound, is the operation of choice.

Should we be content with the medical, or non-operative, treatment of those penetrating wounds which do not present the above indications? If we exclude from our 105 cases the relatively few with small open wounds, with large retained missiles and with extensive rib fractures, but 7 of the entire series developed infectious complications and but 5 died. When it is remembered that these results were obtained in the army zone, where the mortality from thoracic wounds is highest, we must at the present time be satisfied with this method of treatment. From the standpoint of functional end-results it leaves much to be desired, for, as we have found and as the literature indicates, retraction of the chest, thickened pleura, adherent diaphragm, and subjective complaints are common sequelæ. It is clear that operative measures prevent these sequelæ and might prevent some of the infectious complications, yet it seems certain that an added mortality due to indiscriminate operative measures would more than counterbalance the benefits derived.

From a survey of the entire literature on war wounds of the thorax, and from a study of our cases, we feel warranted in saying that the treatment which has been outlined is the best immediate treatment of thoracic injuries which has thus far been suggested. Should it be modified toward radicalism or conservatism under varying circumstances? We have no evidence to show that even under the best conditions more radical treatment would yield better results. On the other hand, our own series of cases shows the bad results of conservatism; that is, of treating expectantly those with open chest wounds, large retained foreign bodies, and extensive rib fractures. We felt compelled during one period, because of stress of work and the inexperience of surgeons in thoracic work, to include the less seriously wounded, showing these conditions among the non-operative group; with the result that our percentage of infectious complications and our mortality were greatly increased.

THORACO-ABDOMINAL INJURIES: SOME TECHNICAL PROCEDURES DEVELOPED BY THE WAR *

By Chas. Gordon Heyd, M.D.
of New York, N. Y.
PROFESSOR OF SURGERY IN THE NEW YORK POST-GRADUATE MEDICAL SCHOOL AND HOSPITAL

Introduction.—It became a surgical axiom among chiefs of surgical teams in the A. E. F. that the mortality of war injuries was directly proportional to the multiplicity of wounds. Approximately 10 per cent. of all chest cases were associated with an injury to the diaphragm and the contents of the upper abdomen, while 12 per cent. of all abdominal cases were combined with injury to the chest or diaphragm. The right and left side were about equally proportioned and in about 10 per cent. were combined with an injury to the kidney. The lethal factor within the first twenty-four hours in the thoraco-abdominal type of wound was invariably shock or hemorrhage. In the type of case in which the abdominal lesion predominated there was in addition to the peritoneal penetration the visceral penetration with hemorrhage from liver, spleen, kidney, and mesentery, and the effusion of intestinal contents from the intestinal canal.

Every surgeon adopted a personal classification of the surgical indications for thoracotomy or for laparotomy, depending upon which injury was considered to be most likely death producing in its character. It was early recognized that combined thoraco-abdominal injuries passing from side to side through either the right or left hypochrondriac region were relatively benign—the projectile passing through both sides of the costo-phrenic sinus, traversing the liver on the right side or the spleen on the left, and producing a variable amount of damage. As the traject of the projectile approached the midline the greater the incidence of death. This fact was brought to our notice by observing that more cases arrived at the hospital dead from midline injuries than from side-to-side injuries through the hypochondriac regions. Examples of peculiar types of combined thoraco-abdominal wounds were as follows: (1) Penetrating wound involving the right lung, diaphragm, liver, and gall-bladder. (2) Penetrating wound involving the liver, stomach, and duodenum. (3) Penetrating wound involving the pericardium, diaphragm, stomach, and duodenum. (4) Penetrating wound involving left lung, diaphragm, spleen, stomach, transverse colon, and pancreas. (5) Penetrating wound involving right kidney, diaphragm, and liver. (6) Penetrating wound involving diaphragm, spleen, omentum, and pericardium.

---

* Read before the American Association for Thoracic Surgery, May 1, 1920.

Anatomical Classification of Thoraco-abdominal Injuries.—Thoraco-abdominal injuries may be classified anatomically into six types. (1) The perforating wound through the costo-phrenic sinus with minimum degree of damage to diaphragm and which was characterized usually by slight, if any, visceral lesion. (2) Penetrating wound with orifice of entry high on the thorax, perforating the lung and penetrating the diaphragm with moderate or severe visceral injury. (3) A wound low down in the axillary line, usually in the seventh, eighth, or ninth intercostal space, with injury to the liver, spleen, and stomach, with gross hemorrhage into the abdomen, and rarely perforation of the colon or small intestine, and in which the entire picture was dominated by the abdominal injury. (4) A wound low down in the axillary space with considerable loss of lateral chest wall and diaphragm, resulting in herniation or prolapse of the omentum and abdominal viscera into the thoracic cavity or externally. (5) A wound in the lumbar region with injury to the kidney and associated with injury to diaphragm and abdominal viscera. (6) Tangential wounds of the chest and abdominal wall with a concussion hæmothorax and suspected chest and abdominal injury, but which upon operation proved to be superficial and without injury to either thoracic or abdominal viscera.

When the perforation in the diaphragm was of fair size or associated with gross loss of substance, herniation or prolapse of the omentum from below into the negative chamber of the chest was common, the first organ to pass through being usually the left gastro-splenic fold of the omentum. Peculiar combinations were found—omentum and spleen; stomach and spleen; stomach and transverse colon; stomach, transverse colon, and spleen. The stomach, as a rule, was only partially herniated and the herniation usually of small size.

In the group in which the abdominal injury was of major proportion the chest injury was, as a rule, of secondary or slight importance. When the injury was low down in the axillary region the lung was free from injury in more than 50 per cent. of cases.

Visceral Injuries—Liver, Spleen, and Stomach.—When the liver was injured three types of hepatic wounds were observed: (1) The tangential wound through liver substance, trench-like in character and usually with the hemorrhage arrested at the time of operation. (2) A seton with a complete clear-cut tunnel through liver substance and rarely with radiating fissures. (3) Fragmentation or pulpefaction of a lobe or portion of the liver. The initial hemorrhage from liver injuries was severe, but regardless of the type of injury it had invariably stopped at the time of operation, except when the injury was in the nature of fragmentation where the hemorrhage was continuous in type and uniformly fatal.

The search for foreign bodies in the substance of the liver was comparatively easy and they were usually located at the end of the traject or lying free in the neighborhood. Pulpefaction or fragmentation of liver substance when it occurred involved the right lobe in over 90 per cent. of cases. The projectile in this type was, as a rule, a large shell fragment and the resulting hemorrhage progressive and continuous. The same injury on the left side brought about the same type of injury to the spleen as to the liver, with the general exception that most splenic injuries were associated with continuous and persistent hemorrhage and a much greater tendency to fragmentation. As an example of a very extensive injury inflicted on the left side by a comparatively small foreign body the following is reported: A penetrating wound due to small shell fragment, orifice of entry the left chest in the eighth interspace, in the midaxillary line, penetration of the diaphragm, tunnelling of the spleen, lateral laceration of the stomach, the projectile continuing its course through both sides of the transverse colon and lodging in the head of the pancreas. The man died at the end of twenty-four hours from suppurative, gangrenous pancreatitis.

Mortality.—The mortality in the forward area from abdominal injuries was approximately 50 per cent.; from chest injuries with extensive operative procedures approximately 50 per cent.; from thoraco-abdominal injuries usually 60 per cent., but not infrequently 75 per cent.

Technical Procedures.—It is interesting to note that in our earlier work injuries to the diaphragm were repaired through the abdomen and it was only when chest surgery was established upon a rational technic that it was found easier to repair the diaphragm through a thoracotomy than by way of the abdomen.

It was during the development of chest surgery that it was found technically satisfactory to repair the diaphragmatic wound by way of the thorax, and furthermore it was determined that quite a large tear or rent or loss of substance of the diaphragm, with protrusion of the abdominal viscera and omentum, could be easily sutured or the diaphragm approximated to the lateral margin of the chest wall. The one essential to either thoracic or abdominal technic was that the diaphragmatic injury should be sutured, for if left unrepaired death was the inevitable consequence irrespective as to the degree of abdominal injury.

The operative approach varied with the type of injury and its location. The mechanical factors involved were in brief:

(a) Injuries to diaphragm only—usually in costo-phrenic sinus.

(b) Injuries involving penetration of diaphragm with damage to subjacent viscera and with or without gross loss of diaphragm substance.

It followed logically that to either of the above there was added a technical repair of chest and lung injury, of any renal lesions or a preliminary or secondary laparotomy according to the anatomical findings. When adequate exposure of the diaphragm could be obtained by enlarging either the orifice of entry or exit the operative procedures were carried out through the wound. If the wound was not in a suitable position six to eight inches of the sixth or seventh, rarely the eighth, right rib were resected subperiosteally, the rib space spread by a rib spreader, the pleural cavity carefully cleansed of all blood and temporary packing off of pleural cavity by pads instituted.

The repair of injuries to the diaphragm was immediately carried out or the diaphragmatic injury was enlarged so as to deal with intra-abdominal complications. There were obviously well-defined limits to the amount of work that could be performed upon the viscera of the upper abdomen, for with reduction of herniated viscera and repair of injuries to the liver, spleen, portions of the cardiac end of the stomach and occasionally the colon, very little further operative manipulation could be carried out. For injuries lower down in the abdomen it was necessary to supplement the thoracic technic with a laparotomy to deal specifically with the abdominal condition.

The suturing of the diaphragm was a matter of comparative simplicity, and after the first suture was tied it was utilized as a traction suture and the remaining portion of the diaphragm was readily sutured with a lock-stitch of No. 2 chromic catgut.

In the type of injury involving the seventh to the ninth rib in the axillary line there was usually a loss of the marginal portion of the diaphragm; and it was relatively easy to suture the parietal portion of the diaphragm to the parietal pleura and so hermetically seal off the chest leaving the wound entirely beneath the diaphragmatico-pleural suture the diaphragm to the parietal pleura, and so hermetically seal off the chest, wall—the so-called method of De Page—was not, however, carried out unless the parietal attachment of the diaphragm was torn away from the chest wall. We had recourse to this method a number of times, and it is surprising how readily the level of the diaphragm can be elevated and applied to a relatively high location on the chest wall. We never had occasion to do pneumopexy either to fix the lung or to be used as a secondary means of closing a diaphragm or chest-wall defect.

The two cases of pericardial injury were repaired through enlarging the orifice of entry in the first patient and by major thoracotomy through the seventh interspace in the second patient.

If the wound of the chest involved the midportion of the axillary space in an oblique manner it almost uniformly injured the lung and perforated the diaphragm with injury to the abdominal viscera. In this type of injury an intercostal thoracotomy was done from the midscapular line to the mammary line with removal of six inches or more of the seventh rib. By enlarging the rib space with a rib spreader it was comparatively easy to reduce herniated viscera or to enlarge the diaphragm aperture and eviscerate portions of stomach, colon, omentum, small intestines and spleen into the chest cavity for inspection or repair. In one case a splenectomy was performed through the thoracic cavity. Likewise through this incision the lower portion of the lung could be delivered and such necessary surgical procedures as were indicated carried out. In every case the laceration and traject in the lung was cleansed and closed. The mechanical cleansing of the traject was ofttimes incomplete, but it was early established that the lung tissue itself, by reason of its peculiar vascularity, was quite able to take care of a considerable degree of infection. As evidence pointing to this contention one recalls the extreme rarity of gas gangrene of the lung tissue itself. The handling of the lung was not associated with marked fall in blood-pressure, and was not associated with the same degree of shock as would be induced by similar manipulations of the intestines. When the injury was low on the chest wall with compound, comminuted fracture of the sixth, seventh, or eighth rib in the axillary space, or if the wound was of a type known as " cave-in " or " stove-in " chest, the entire wound was enlarged, the soft tissues débrided and both ends of the fractured ribs resected, and by separating the edges of the entire wound the injury to the diaphragm was readily repaired. In these cases an element of greater importance than the injury itself was the innumerable indriven bone particles scattered through lung and diaphragm, occasionally penetrating the diaphragm and being imbedded in the liver or omentum.

In liver wounds involving the superior surface or where the projectile injured the liver laterally through the costo-phrenic sinus, the traject was swabbed out, lightly débrided and cleansed with a Volkmann spoon. Trench wounds accessible to suture were occasionally coapted or omentum sutured into the gap and once the round ligament of the liver was so utilized. In wounds characterized by fragmentation of the liver the thoracotomy was supplemented by a laparotomy for the purpose of mass gauze packing in the attempt to arrest hemorrhage.

In injuries to the diaphragm and associated with a wounded kidney it was an invariable rule to do the posterior surgery first, as it was soon discovered that to do a thoracotomy or laparotomy and then turn the patient over upon the abdomen carried with it a greater shock-producing element and mortality than the same procedures carried out in the reverse order. It was also an invariable rule to catheterize all suspected kidney injuries or to have the patient void on the table, for it was not an infrequent occurrence to be quite surprised at finding a bloody urine from a patient which from the location of the wound could hardly be suspected of having a kidney injury.

The wounds to the kidney with diaphragmatic injury were, as a rule, clean-cut tunnels through the upper pole of the kidney; and only once did we see complete fragmentation of the upper half of the kidney. We lost one case eleven days post-operatively from secondary hemorrhage due to a lateral tear in the vena cava. In one case the injury to the chest was discovered quite accidentally during an exploratory operation on the kidney, when in the course of débridement of the wound of entry there was an insucking of air. A single suture applied to the costo-phrenic sinus closed this orifice and the case was practically considered as one without injury to the chest.

A rather surprising example of a foreign body passing through the abdomen without any injury to the viscera was as follows: A gunshot wound perforating the right costo-phrenic sinus, the right kidney, entering the abdomen, passing to the external side of the ascending colon and imbedding itself in the peritoneum on the anterior abdominal wall. After débriding the kidney wound and introducing a drain down to the kidney traject a laparotomy was performed and foreign body removed. Complete exploration of the abdomen revealed absolutely no injury to the abdominal viscera. Patient made an uneventful recovery.

A critical review of thoraco-abdominal injuries and the surgical procedures adopted to deal with them, together with the immense collective experience derived from battle surgery, would seem to suggest a wider technical application of major thoracotomy to deal with lesions involving the diaphragm and the viscera immediately subjacent to it.

One of the surprising features in connection with thoraco-abdominal surgery was the facility with which the diaphragm could be elevated and sutured and the comparative ease with which the parietal diaphragm could be approximated to the parietal pleura even after great loss of substance.

It would seem that these experiences in thoraco-abdominal injuries point the way to a better technical consideration of diaphragmatic hernia, for with positive pulmonary anæsthesia and distention of the lung it should not be dangerous to do a major thoracotomy in the seventh or eighth interspace and approach the reduction of a diaphragmatic hernia from within the chest and by suture of the diaphragmatic hiatus from the thoracic side accomplish a much better technical result. Lesions of the liver, superior cardiac portion of the stomach and some spleen lesions might offer a wider application for transthoracic laparotomy with better results than are now obtained by any classical methods of approach through the abdomen.

The treatment of heart wounds through a transpleural exposure and by means of an intercostal incision under differential pressure anæsthesia offers a quick, technical exposure with ample room and obviates the dangers of pneumothorax and would seem to indicate a better technic than any type of extrapleural operation.

TRANSACTIONS

OF THE

NEW YORK SURGICAL SOCIETY

Stated Meeting held March 10, 1920

The President, Dr. WILLIAM A. DOWNES, in the Chair

TUBERCULOUS TENOSYNOVITIS

Dr. WILLY MEYER presented a man twenty-seven years of age, who came under his care two years ago, March, 1918. He was a strong young man who complained of stiffness in his left hand which had lasted for some time and inability to lift heavy objects. On examination, there was the picture of involvement of the extensor sheaths of the forearm. A large swelling covered more or less the radial aspect of the forearm. One could feel small rice-like corpuscles in the tendon sheath. The patient was advised to have the tuberculous tissue totally extirpated, leaving no focus of diseased tissue. Doctor Meyer stated that he had had a few such tuberculous tendon cases and had learned that the entire tuberculous mass must be removed in order to effect a permanent cure. At operation he was successful in removing the entire mass from tendon to tendon completely in one piece thus leaving the bare tendons exposed. The wound was wiped with a 5 per cent. iodoform ether solution, thus combining antiseptic with aseptic surgery, and the wound was completely closed without drainage, with a few silkworm-gut sutures. Rubber tissue was used to cover the line of the incision, and the dressing and splint applied.

The patient had a high temperature at first which soon came down. The dressing was left on for two weeks when primary union was found. To-day the man had an absolutely perfect functional result and was in good health. To show the rapid return of good function, it might be mentioned that the operation was performed on May 18, 1918, and in October of the same year he entered military service in the Coast Artillery, having free use of his arm and hand.

DUODENAL FISTULA AFTER CHOLECYSTECTOMY, CLOSED BY THE MEANS OF INTESTINAL FEEDING

Dr. WILLY MEYER presented a man fifty years of age who came under his care for recurrent attacks of cholecystitis. On the Medical Division he had just passed through a severe acute attack. On May 26, 1919, Doctor Meyer performed a cholecystectomy by Perthes' incision, which was lengthened up to the xiphoid. The operation was technically difficult because of firm adhesions around the gall-bladder and appendix in a rather stout man. On trying to separate the peritoneal cover from the gall-bladder, as usually done, he found that all the layers of the gall-bladder wall formed a firm unit. It, therefore, became necessary to shell out the bladder from the liver. In doing this a portion of the liver tissue came off with the bladder. The result was a very alarming venous hemorrhage, which evidently came from a branch of the portal vein. Three gauze tampons with prolonged firm compression were required to control the bleeding.

Following the operation, the patient was put to bed in the Sims's posture for twenty-four hours, as he usually did after cholecystectomy. Having done the operation just before the association meetings, the removal of the tampons had to be left to the assistants; he feared that it was done piecemeal. Soon after the removal of the tampons, it was noticed that bile came from the fistula, and at times a considerable amount of tissue was discharged. Doctor Meyer said he saw the man again in October, when he had gained twenty pounds, but he still had the fistula, from which at times a large amount of fluid escaped, which, however, had not macerated his skin. Examination of stomach and duodenal contents with the Finhorn tube proved the discharge to come, not from the upper, but from the lower part of the duodenum. Radiographs corroborated this conclusion. Having had one case in which after a secondary operation on the bile ducts a duodenal fistula was cured by feeding through a long tube, a long intestinal tube was introduced in this case. The tip of the tube soon slipped into the jejunum, where the X-ray showed the metal tip near the left anterior superior spine. Of course, no food was allowed by mouth. Improvement was soon noticed. There was a temporary discharge off and on, but on December 4th the fistula was closed. At about the middle of the same month a piece of a gauze tampon was passed through the rectum.

In connection with this case, Doctor Meyer said there were a few points of interest. One of these was with reference to the systematic examination of the duodenal contents. This had been done in addition to radiography in every case of suspected gall-bladder disease in the course of the last four to six years, making a chemical, microscopical and bacteriological examination. The X-ray had shown positive results in gall-stones in about 15 to 20 per cent. of the cases. In cases of cholecystitis without stones they were of no assistance in establishing the diagnosis. Here examination of the duodenal contents was of very great value; in fact, it was the best diagnostic means we had at present. The finding of turbid green-brown bile determined where the incision should be made, namely, on the gall-bladder. If aspiration during operation showed the same condition of the bile, cholecystectomy was done. This bile would quite frequently be reported to be sterile, but clinically the patients got well. Bacteria were often found in the gall-bladder wall on tissue culture.

What was the color of healthy bile in a healthy gall-bladder? If surgeons could get the permission to aspirate the bile from normal gall-bladders, a relation between the presence of black-green bile and gall-bladder disease

NEW YORK SURGICAL SOCIETY

could soon be established. At the present time we did not know much about the contents of the gall-bladder in the normal living person. He believed, however, that green bile, or green-brown turbid bile, in the presence of positive clinical symptoms was an indication for the extirpation of the gall-bladder. Physiologists taught that normal bile was golden-yellow in the hepatic duct as well as in the gall-bladder.

Doctor Meyer stated that he had seen five cases in which the gall-bladder was tightly adherent to the duodenum, and when the gall-bladder was extirpated a hole was found in the latter. In several cases there was a combination of gall-bladder disease and duodenal ulcer. Where the gall-bladder was tightly adherent to the duodenum, great care should be exercised at operation in stripping it off. It was wise rather to leave a patch of gall-bladder attached to the duodenum. Nature, in cases of need, made the gall-bladder wall secure a threatening perforation of a duodenal ulcer.

DR. GEORGE WOOLSEY referred to the color of the bile and its bacterial content. He was inclined to agree with Doctor Meyer that the color of the bile was dark in cases of cholecystitis, and, as the bile was commonly sterile, the bacteriological examination of the duodenal contents did not give any help in diagnosis. Doctor Woolsey asked if he had taken a culture from the wall of the gall-bladder, as it was often possible to get a positive culture from the wall and not from the contents. In regard to these fistulæ connected with the stomach and duodenum, Doctor Woolsey said recently he had removed the gall-bladder, which was very adherent to the stomach a little proximal to the pylorus, and in so doing a small opening was left through the peritoneal coat, the beginning of a perforation of the stomach. Around this opening the peritoneal coat was dissected up, and according to this, there was a ring of yellowish color about the size of a quarter, due to the action of bile. The muscular and mucous coats had not yet been perforated. A large tumor mass, readily seen and felt before operation, proved to be an abscess filling the lesser peritoneal sac with over a litre of pus. The infection was supposed to have come from the commencing perforation of the stomach. It was opened and drained and a good result obtained.

DR. ELLSWORTH ELIOT, JR., said that in one patient in whom he dissected the gall-bladder from the duodenum he found no ulcer in the duodenum, but a small orifice, evidently an ulcer in the gall-bladder, which had perforated through. He closed it with a purse-string suture without further difficulty and no duodenal fistula followed.

DR. DOWNES suggested that, in a case where the gall-bladder was adherent to the liver, it would be a better plan to deliberately open and empty the gall-bladder, then dissect the mucous membrane out, leaving the peritoneal and muscular coats at the adherent point. With proper precautions there was little or no danger from infection. It was worth while to take this chance in order to avoid these severe hemorrhages.

DOCTOR MEYER, in closing the discussion, said one of the points he wanted to bring out was the necessity of making an examination of the duodenal contents previous to operation, and that the facilities for making such an examination should be a laboratory necessity.

In regard to Doctor Woolsey's remarks, the laboratory had reported, not in every case but in quite a number, in fact, in the majority of cases, a sterile bile. He had asked himself whether perhaps some chemical condition might be responsible for the inflammation without presence of micro-organisms. He thought that not much was known about it. It certainly was necessary to let the laboratory make the microscopic examination of the gall-bladder wall, and they had begun doing this at the Lenox Hill Hospital. The pathological report, so far as the gall-bladder itself was concerned, was always chronic cystitis. If surgeons would tap the normal gall-bladder and examine the contents, he thought much more could be learned. This might be done by penetrating the wall obliquely with a very fine needle. Perhaps patients might be willing to consent, if told that it was for the purpose of gathering information.

Regarding the gall-bladder attachment, Doctor Meyer said he was very careful in stripping the gall-bladder from the duodenum. In one of these cases he left a patch of the serous cover of the gall-bladder attached to the duodenum. He felt that asepsis was better safeguarded if one left the gall-bladder closed than by opening it. He always tried to take the gall-bladder out without opening its cavity and to find its point of cleavage between peritoneal and muscular cover of the wall of the viscus. In the case presented, the layers had formed a firm unit.

GANGRENE OF RETROCÆCAL APPENDIX

Dr. WILLY MEYER presented a patient who came under his care with all the signs of acute appendicitis. When he opened the abdomen, he met a gangrenous area representing the base of the appendix, but there seemed no possibility of reaching the tip of the appendix, which was retrocæcal and thoroughly adherent. According to his experience, it was best in many of these cases, particularly of acute appendicitis, to give up working from the anterior incision and add a second one parallel to the crista ilii, commencing at the anterior superior spine; for it was here often of importance not only to feel but also to see. A short retrocæcal appendix could be gotten out best through the intramuscular incision. Sometimes it could also be developed through the para-rectus. But a long and adherent retrocæcal appendix needed an additional cut. In the case presented, the gangrenous organ was fully six inches long and had a peri-appendicular abscess at its tip, near the lower pole of the kidney. The patient made a quick and uninterrupted recovery.

CONICAL STUMP IN THE LEG

Dr. ELLSWORTH ELIOT, JR., presented a lad, aged sixteen years, who was first admitted to the Presbyterian Hospital when he was four or five years old, at which time he was under the care of Doctor Woolsey for gangrene of the leg of embolic origin following diphtheria. Doctor Woolsey amputated the leg at about the middle third. The patient for a time was without material discomfort, walking on an artificial leg. Later he suffered from pain, especially while walking. Eventually a conical stump developed. The divided end of both the tibia and fibula pressed against the scar. These were removed after exposure by incision through and deflection of the cicatrix. Recovery was uneventful.

At the present time, three years after operation for the conical stump, examination of the stump showed it to be in excellent condition. There was ample flap material. At one point there was a slight exostosis on the divided tibia which did not interfere with his wearing an artificial leg. This condition, Doctor Eliot said, was much more common after amputation of the humerus than after amputation of the leg, where not only one, but occasionally several amputations were required for persistent recurrence. The fact that the growth of the upper extremity depended chiefly upon the upper epiphysis of the humerus while that of the lower depended upon the epiphyses about the knee accounted for the occurrence of this condition after amputation through the arm and leg, respectively.

SUBPHRENIC ABSCESS

DOCTOR ELIOT presented a man, thirty-three years of age, who had always been in excellent health until three weeks before admission to the hospital. At that time the invasion was marked by sudden severe pain in the right upper quadrant, which came on while he was working. He had repeated attacks of vomiting and pain, which was severe and sharp in character and was increased by moving the body from side to side. Respiration was somewhat difficult, and his discomfort was somewhat intensified by elevating his head from the pillow. The pain radiated to the right lumbar region and to the scapula. These attacks were repeated at intervals of three or four days for about three weeks. During this time the patient lost twenty-eight pounds. When he was examined, marked tenderness was found over the right costal arch, and an indefinite sense of a mass which prevented palpation of the under segment of the arch. Bimanual examination gave the same sense of resistance, and the right costal arch could not be compressed during respiration. There was no evidence of other peritoneal irritation.

The man was operated upon on September 19, 1919. The peritoneal cavity was opened through an oblique incision parallel to the costal arch. The gall-bladder was found to be covered with adherent omentum extending over the adjacent surface of the liver. On separation of these adhesions, an abscess cavity was found to the outer side of the gall-bladder, occupying the space between the convex surface of the liver and the adjacent costal segment. The pus was not brown in color, and no orifice leading into the gall-bladder or liver was found. The gall-bladder was liberated from adhesions. Nothing abnormal was found about the duodenum or pylorus. There was no evidence of necrosis of costal cartilage. The abscess cavity was so placed that an opening between the overlying costal cartilages for drainage was tempting, but the interval was so narrow that it was thought better to insert the rubber tissue cigarette drain through the abdominal incision, passing first into the peritoneal cavity and then at right angles into the abscess cavity. The remainder of the incision was closed in the usual way. Notwithstanding the irregularity of the drainage tract, the patient was discharged from the hospital four weeks after operation with a superficial sinus which soon completely closed. The fact that it healed promptly and remained healed seemed to indicate the absence of any erosion or lesion in the costal joint. In general, in lesions of this kind, a sinus remained for six months or a year. Doctor Eliot said he recalled one case in which the cavity did not close for eighteen months.

The origin of the abscess cavity was difficult to state. It did not come from the gall-bladder, the liver, or from any part of the intestine. The contents of the abscess consisted in ordinary odorless pus containing streptococcus hæmolyticus aureus. Doctor Eliot said he could account for it only as an abscess of hæmatogenous origin.

CANCER OF THE THYROID

DOCTOR ELIOT presented a woman, thirty-two years of age, who was admitted to the hospital in December, 1916, complaining of a lump in her neck of three years' duration and of gradual growth. This constituted her sole complaint until five months before admission, when she noticed dyspnœa on walking. There was a swelling on the right side of the thyroid the size of a hen's egg. It was firm, smooth, and free from nodules. It showed the normal mobility associated with ordinary goitre. No one would have considered it anything else than some form of simple, benign goitre. A circular incision was made, and there was no difficulty in enucleating and resecting the right half of the thyroid. There were no signs of adhesion nor of infiltration. Ligation at the isthmus was done with chromic gut. The growth seemed to be of the colloid variety. The wound healed promptly without incident. In a few places there were some relatively normal acini, but the major portion of the specimen was a dense mass resembling thyroid acini packed closely. The large mass seemed to be formed of certain lobulations. The stroma was compressed, and in some places the cells were invaded and broken through; necrosis was taking place in some of the masses, and there were several mitotic figures. The diagnosis was carcinoma of the thyroid. Doctor Parsons and Dr. W. C. Clarke made the diagnosis. The symptoms in this case were entirely different from those of malignancy. The fact that one-half of the gland only was sacrificed was contrary to what was taught in the treatment of carcinoma of the thyroid, namely, that the whole thyroid should be removed and myxœdema prevented by the administration of thyroid extract. The thyroid was like most other parts of the body in that it was subject to slowly progressive, as well as rapidly developing, varieties of carcinoma, and in these growths operation was not

NEW YORK SURGICAL SOCIETY

only indicated but gave very satisfactory results. In one case operated on by Doctor Erdmann the presence of glandular metastases on both sides served to make an unfavorable prognosis, yet several years after the removal of the thyroid and glands the patient was still alive and well.

DR. FREDERIC KAMMERER said that Doctor Eliot's case of cancer of the thyroid must have been a very early case. He had had one case of cancer of the thyroid nine years after the first operation, which was done by Kocher. In Doctor Eliot's case the cancer was very slightly developed, and was operated upon sufficiently early to get an apparently permanent cure. All surgeons, he thought, were agreed that only early operation gave a chance of success; in other words, cases in which the clinical diagnosis of cancer was not made, but the malignancy discovered only on microscopical examination. He was unable to account for the good result in the case mentioned this evening, in which metastases were found in the lymph-glands.

DOCTOR ELIOT said that this case was of three years' standing. The carcinoma, however, was of recent formation; it certainly was not of three years' standing. It must have begun, perhaps, six months before operation. The speaker cited a case of extensive carcinoma in a woman of fifty, which developed in a goitre of at least twenty years' standing. In this instance the amount of malignancy was shown both by the development of anæmia and by adhesions to the skin of different parts of the greatly enlarged thyroid gland. In the case reported this evening there was nothing of that kind before or after the operation. If the carcinoma was not of recent growth, it had at least not gone through the capsule nor were there any enlarged glands.

DR. ALEXIS V. MOSCHCOWITZ said that he had had a few cases of carcinoma of the thyroid, and they were of two classes: those in which the diagnosis of carcinoma was made before operation, and those in which carcinoma was accidentally found. In those in which the carcinoma was accidentally found the prognosis was good, while in those diagnosed as carcinoma the prognosis was bad. In other words, early cases only give a good prognosis.

CANCER OF THE RECTUM

DOCTOR ELIOT presented a woman, forty-one years of age, who was admitted to the Presbyterian Hospital three years ago with a history of pain and bleeding from the bowels for three months and constipation for a good many years. Lately the discharge from the rectum had been very foul. The patient had been losing in weight. Examination showed a cauliflower mass of the anterior wall of the rectum at the right side. The finger passing through the lumen of the bowel could not reach the upper limit of the growth. On vaginal examination the growth was found to be movable on the vaginal wall. The case seemed to be favorable for operation, and on October 16, 1916, a colostomy was done, using the intramuscular incision, and the intestine brought out through the incision with a glass rod through the mesocolon. After this had been open several days the rectal mass was removed by the Kraske route. The peritoneum was sewn around the margin of the rectum, which was then unfolded, leaving a smooth surface. Following the operation there was a small sinus, which still persisted, though not connecting with the bowel. The condition of the artificial anus, Doctor Eliot said, was interesting, as both the proximal and distal ends are visible and show no indication of inflammation.

Doctor Eliot said a point to which he wished to call attention was that the prolapsed sigmoid caused no obstruction, and that there was no need of an immediate opening of the bowel. Sometimes, if delayed for a week, the artificial anus would establish itself. Another point was that he thought the intramuscular incision restricted the degree of rupture or hernia. Of still greater interest was the fact that after such an incision the patient might have complete, or if not complete, at least excellent, control of the bowels. The patient with an artificial anus through an intramuscular incision was much better off than with one made through a vertical incision. The woman had three movements during the course of the day and had five or ten minutes' warning. She was capable of doing her household work and was happy and contented. An artificial anus was therefore not incompatible with the comforts of life, and patients should not be allowed to become discouraged by the prospects of such an abnormal opening when the radical removal of the sphincter ani was necessary.

Dr. WILLIAM C. LUSK said that he had previously shown before the Surgical Society two cases of controllable artificial anus. In the construction of this type of artificial anus, the opening for the exit of the bowel through the abdominal wall was made in a transverse line opposite the left anterior superior iliac spine, the incision splitting part way the fibres of the internal oblique and transversalis muscles and cutting through the linea semilunaris well into the rectus sheath to prevent constriction of the gut, avoiding the deep epigastric vessels. A second transverse incision, going through the skin and superficial fascia only, was made one inch above the first, and the bridge of skin and fat between the two incisions raised from the surface of the external oblique. The peritoneum of the lower wound was tacked above and below to the outer surface of the external oblique, and the proximal extremity of the severed, liberated sigmoid, was drawn out of the peritoneal cavity through the opening prepared for its exit, turned upward over the external oblique muscle beneath the bridge of skin and brought out upon the skin surface through the higher incision, the bowel being so disposed, both in the iliac fossa as well as throughout its course of exit, that its mesenteric border always looked inward. Thus the terminal portion of the bowel occupied a position such that, with pressure applied over it externally, it would be compressed against the external oblique muscle. In the first of the cases mentioned, the orifice of the artificial anus accidentally became very small, yet with mucous membrane lining it. In the second case, the bowel end was primarily inverted and sutured tight, and later an opening of small size was made into it, which technic was made possible through the preliminary construction of what the speaker called a "left subcostal colonic vent," which was a tube-sinus entering the descending colon just below the extremity of the left eleventh rib, serving for the prevention of intestinal obstruction and for the introduction of water, following the abdominal portion of the two-stage operation for removal of rectal cancer. In both of these cases, by the use of a flat plate compressing the artificial anus through the agency of a spring truss, continence for both fæces and wind had been attained.

DOCTOR ELIOT said the method Doctor Lusk described had been tried, but was not always attended with success. There were one or two conditions in which it was not available. The first of these was where there was a short cæcum, so that one could not get the cæcum to take a rectangular course, and there might be some objection on account of the possibility of subsequent stricture. He had seen the procedure employed where one, two or three years later they had had to resort to the vertical incision. In these cases, provided one got good control, he thought it desirable to have a good-sized orifice, for if one had a small orifice there was danger of a secondary stricture.

DR. FREDERIC KAMMERER said that for the establishment of artificial ani he had always made the intramuscular incision. He had never known any stricture to follow the use of this incision if primary union was obtained. He always used the glass rod and opened the bowel forty-eight hours after it had been brought out. As to the results obtained, some of his patients seemed to have little trouble, others were very much annoyed by the involuntary passage of fecal matter. A good plan, in his opinion, was to cleanse the large intestine by an irrigation of the bowels through the colostomy opening every evening before retiring. He had seen one of the cases in which Doctor Lusk had followed the procedure he described, and the result was a very good one.

CIRRHOSIS OF THE LIVER

DOCTOR ELIOT presented a man who was first under observation in the Presbyterian Hospital twenty years ago, having come to the dispensary. He had an effusion in both pleural cavities and a moderate effusion of the pericardium and abdomen. He was being tapped at frequent intervals, and his liver was very large.

In 1916 this man was again admitted to the hospital, and the diagnosis of ascites, cirrhosis of the liver, cardiac arrhythmia with auricular fibrillation was made. In 1919 he was admitted to the hospital half a dozen times and was incapacitated. Last October he entered the hospital, after having been tapped repeatedly, for operation with the view of establishing a collateral anastomosis. The abdomen was open above the navel. The liver, which had been very large, had become markedly smaller and smooth; the edge was rounded, and it looked like a "beautifully iced cable," the capsule being one inch in thickness. The omentum was brought through and sutured to bare surfaces of the parietal peritoneum. There was no denudation of the liver or spleen and no drainage, since it had been observed that that procedure markedly increased the operative mortality. In this case the attempt was made simply to establish the collateral circulation between the omentum and the abdominal wall, with the knowledge that the fluid would recur. It was now about four months since the patient had been operated upon, and he had been tapped twice during this time, a large amount of fluid having been obtained each time, but both the interval between the tappings and the amount removed were steadily decreasing. The most striking feature in the case is the improvement in the general condition. The man's appetite has returned, he is stronger, walks better, and is almost ready to go back to work. It is reasonable to expect that in the course of the next six months the recurrence of the fluid will have completely ceased, the collateral venous return having by that time become established.

DOCTOR LYLE said that in 1913 he had performed Routte's operation for cirrhosis of the liver, and there was a temporary improvement. The patient died two or three months later. At the autopsy it was found that the anastomosis between the peritoneal cavity and the right saphenous vein was patent, while the anastomosis on the left was blocked by fibrous tissue.

DOCTOR WHIPPLE asked Doctor Eliot if he had had any difficulty in getting sufficient omentum through for suture to the parietal wall. In some cases the peritoneum and omentum were so altered and atrophied that it was difficult to do this.

DOCTOR ELIOT said that in view of the possibility of an atrophic omentum he always made the incision above the navel and not below. He had fortunately never found the omentum so atrophied that it could not be stitched in the manner described to the abdominal wall. The operation he called a modified talma.

THE OVERHEAD SUSPENSION FRAME

DR. HENRY H. M. LYLE read a paper with the above title, for which see page 760, June, 1920.

DR. JOSEPH A. BLAKE thought there was distinct danger in using a splint that brought the elbow to the body in the treatment of high fractures of the humerus, as there was likely to be a limitation of abduction afterwards. Suspension had given excellent results in all cases. There was no objection to it except that the patient had to stay in bed, and that was not a great objection, considering the rapidity with which repair takes place. Considering the fact that function was absolutely maintained, several weeks were well spent in suspension. Doctor Blake said he had noticed that stiffness took place so rapidly that he never allowed the use of a sling or kept the arm at the side for any length of time. He left the arm free during the day and put it back in the suspension apparatus at night. During the night the man moved his arm and in this way union was often obtained in eighteen or twenty days. The average number of days to obtain complete union, including all cases infected as well as clean, was, he thought, about thirty-two. Of course, in some cases non-union occurred. A certain amount of movement between the fragments did not interfere with union. The old idea of fixation by plaster and other splints in the treatment of all fractures had been exploded, as it had been shown to be not only unnecessary but pernicious.

SEHRT'S METAL TOURNIQUET FOR ARTIFICIAL ANÆMIA IN AMPUTATIONS

Dr. WILLY MEYER stated that in looking through the foreign literature in the summer of 1916 he read an article by Sehrt, of Freiburg, in the *Münch. Med. Wochenschr.* of May 25, 1915, in which he claimed that this method was very superior to every other method known to produce artificial anæmia. It had interested him, and he had followed it up. He had asked the Kny-Scherer Company to import the device for him. As the war came on, it could not be done. But in the fall of last year they asked him if he still wanted it. He said he did, and the apparatus reached him in December, 1919, and he started using it in February, 1920. He had a case of amputation of the thigh in which he made use of this method with the greatest satisfaction, and he had also used it in a secondary operation for recurrent sarcoma of the thigh on the posterior aspect. He thought it would be interesting to the Society to see the apparatus and to learn how it was employed. In looking over recent literature, he found that Doctor Truesdale, of Fall River, had described the same apparatus in the *Journal of the A. M. A.,* of January 31, 1920. Lieut.-Col. J. M. Flint and Lieut. A. Dayton had found this in an advanced surgical hospital which the Germans had evacuated after the battle of Saint Mihiel. Doctor Truesdale said it was sent on to his hospital for trial. He had modified it to a certain extent and found it a great advance over other methods of producing artificial anæmia.

The instrument was made on the principle of a clamp, with two curved arms of steel which in emergency could be covered with cotton or gauze, in times of peace better with rubber tubes. With the screw widely open it could be pushed over the limb, where it was made to compress the large vessels and the screw closed. With a few turns of the screw one obtained complete anæmia. It could be applied high up on the thigh, right in the crotch. They all knew how difficult it was to apply an Esmarch's bandage so high up. Its application was extremely simple, as nothing else was necessary except to tighten the screw, and if, during an amputation or a tumor extirpation, it was not entirely compressing the circulation, all one needed to do was to tighten it a little more. When one began to tie the vessels there was not the annoyance of loosening the elastic bandage. A few twists of the screw to the left, leaving the sterile drapery undisturbed, allowed the return of the circulation.

Doctor Sehrt at first thought this tourniquet should be given to all the soldiers, but said himself that that was incorrect, as it could not be applied for too long a time. But it should be given to advanced posts and stretcher-bearers, as by its use much hemorrhage and many deaths might be avoided.

The instrument described in the *A. M. A. Journal*, Doctor Meyer said, was a slightly modified form of that used by the Germans. The two arms are longer and heavier; an oblong slot is made through the centre of the handle through which passes the screw. This adjustment screw may be pushed either way, releasing compression or renewing control with the greatest ease.

Sehrt's tourniquet represents the greatest advance made in late years for the production of artificial anæmia. It is very simple and efficient and absolutely reliable.

Stated Meeting held March 24, 1920
DR. ALFRED S. TAYLOR in the Chair

SARCOMA OF THE BREAST

DR. BURTON J. LEE presented a specimen of sarcoma of the breast which was removed on December 2, 1919. The patient from whom the tumor was removed had been conscious of its presence for almost a year. She was mentally incompetent and much emaciated, but otherwise physical examination was negative as far as local or general metastases were concerned. The mass occupied the entire breast and was irregular in consistency; the major portion was definitely solid with a few small cystic areas. The circumference of the pedicle was 19½ inches. It measured 27½ inches in the longest and 23½ inches in the shortest diameter. The weight was 10 pounds. There were many superficial dilated veins over the entire skin covering the growth. There was no evidence of involvement of axillary or supraclavicular nodes.

At operation, under local anæsthesia, the tumor was dissected away, the muscle and fascia overlying it being exposed as the breast was removed. The whole area was skin-grafted, but primary union having failed a second skin grafting was done which was successful. Both skin graftings were done under local anæsthesia. The pathologist's report by Dr. James Ewing showed in the gross a tumor with broadly lobulated structure, the lobes being 2 to 6 cm. in diameter. Most of these lobes were necrotic, many infiltrated with blood, and some were soft and opaque. There were no cysts and the tumor was well encapsulated everywhere.

The microscopic examination revealed the general structure of a large spindle-celled sarcoma. The most prominent feature was the large number of huge giant-cells with multi-lobulated nuclei. The tumor probably arose from a fibroma but no remnants of breast tissue could be detected.

The reasons for presenting the specimen were: (1) The relative infrequency of sarcoma of the breast. (2) The unusual size of the growth. (3) That it was possible to remove a tumor of this size under local anæsthesia. (4) That a tumor as advanced as this one emphasized the great need for

establishing a breast examination clinic where presumably normal women
might go at intervals when early tumor of the breast might be discovered.

Dr. Frank S. Mathews related the case of a woman who consulted
him for a number of shot-like masses in the scalp, at first covered by
epithelium but which, if injured by a comb, bled rather furiously. On
questioning the patient, she was found to have had a breast tumor removed six months before. This had been pronounced benign at the time.
No other recurrences were apparent. She died two or three months later.
Histologically, the scalp tumors were pronounced malignant angioma.

OPERATIVE TREATMENT FOLLOWING POTT'S FRACTURE

Dr. Royal Whitman presented a man thirty years of age who was
first seen in January of the present year, having been injured six months
before. He presented a typical equinovarus deformity with almost
complete disability. The internal malleolus was ununited and displaced
toward the interior of the joint. The external malleolus was bent outward and separated from the tibia. The object of operation in such cases
was to replace the foot beneath the centre of the leg and to restore dorsal
flexion and adduction. To accomplish this the external malleolus was
almost completely divided from above downward in an oblique direction,
so that its extremity could be pushed inward by opening a gap between
the fragments, into which a fragment of bone was inserted. The internal
malleolus was replaced, the surfaces of the fragments freshened, and a
thin bone graft was slid downward from the tibia to cover the line of
junction. The tendo achillis was then divided and the foot in an attitude
of adduction and right angular flexion was fixed in plaster.

This patient began to bear weight on the foot as the discomfort lessened, and eight weeks later the plaster was removed; the correction was
satisfactory and the union at the point of grafting well advanced, as
shown in the accompanying picture (Fig. 1).

The shoe was thickened on the inner border, a flat-foot brace was
applied, and the patient instructed in exercises and the proper method of
weight bearing. This was of great importance for functional cure, since
even when the fracture had been properly treated the tendency was toward the passive or flat-foot attitude during the period of reconstruction.
This must be checked by exercises in dorsal flexion and adduction and
by assuring proper balance in weight bearing.

Dr. Nathan W. Green said that these old cases of Pott's fracture in
which there had been bone deformity for a long time were economically
very important. He had had one or two of these disabling cases at the
City Hospital. He had not done a periosteal graft, but had rebroken
them and put them up in inversion, taking care to keep the mortise closed
up, and had been fortunate in getting good results in this way.

Doctor Whitman, in answer to a question as to whether bone grafting was absolutely necessary, said that it was unnecessary except for
ununited fracture of the malleoli.

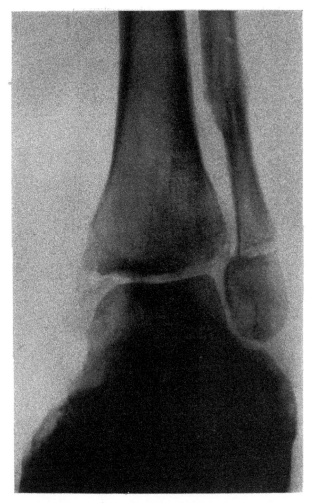

FIG. 1.—Shows the correction of deformity and the bone grafts on either side, also the
original fracture of the fibula.

PEDICLE GRAFT REPLACING ABLATED HEEL

Dr. NATHAN W. GREEN presented a laborer, forty-two years of age, who was admitted to the Surgical Division A of St. Luke's Hospital on April 14, 1917. By the courtesy of Doctor Downes he was turned over to Doctor Green for treatment. His complaint was a painful and tight cicatrix of the right heel with an ulcer on the under surface. This condition was from an injury sustained nine months previous to his admission. The injury was caused by a large paper roll which ran against his heel, removing the skin and cushion of the heel. He was at once taken to a hospital. The wound healed, but whenever he tried to use his foot it would break down and was very painful.

On April 23, 1917, the first stage in the operation for plastic repair was done by Doctor Green. On the sole of the foot a small granulating area was present, the whole right heel being covered with a thin cicatrix. The cicatrix was dissected away from the heel down to the periosteum and ligaments and a large flap, comprising all tissues down to the muscle, was dissected up from the left thigh just above the knee. (This flap was made with its pedicle so placed that it might be elongated and applied to the heel at a subsequent sitting.) The right heel was brought into apposition with the flap which was sutured over the denuded area of the heel. A plaster case was applied from the waist down, holding the heel upon the opposite thigh.

Two weeks later, May 7, 1917, the second stage of the operation was performed. The flap that had been dissected up and applied to the heel was found to be healthy and growing. (Two weeks was thought to be sufficient time for the first part of the flap to have united.) The case around plastic juncture was removed. The flap on left thigh was dissected somewhat further and sutured over the denuded area of right heel with No. 1 chromic gut. The denuded area was now completely covered over except at one place. The plaster case was replaced.

Again, two weeks later, May 21, 1917, the third stage of the operation was performed. The case was removed and the flap found to be viable with practically no slough. The pedicle of the flap was cut loose from the left thigh and sutured to the right heel at the only remaining free point. The wound on the thigh was closed partially and small Thiersch grafts were placed upon the granulating area. The heel was dressed with dry dressing.

The patient was discharged July 6, 1917, with the following note: "Inner side of flap has united perfectly. A small sulcus persists on outer side of heel, which, however, is lined with epithelium" and is "entirely healed." "Motion is somewhat restricted, but improving."

The patient was absent from the hospital for one and three-quarter years and had been working. On account of a small pressure sore on his heel he was readmitted April 14, 1919. On readmission on the plantar surface of graft was an area of induration about 2 cm. in diameter. In the centre of this area there was a small ulceration.

On April 16, 1919 (one and three-quarter years later), a small operation was performed, excising the scar tissue and ulcer, between the os calcis and the heel of the shoe. There was then an ulcerated area of scar tissue about the size of a half dollar. A circular incision was made about the scar tissue. This tissue was dissected free and excised. A small area of the scar tissue deep in the subcutaneous tissue was dissected free and excised. The wound was closed with interrupted sutures of chromic gut. Dry dressing was applied. He was discharged May 9, 1919, improved and is now, March 24, 1920, cured.

The after treatment consisted of directing the patient to follow a suggestion of Dr. P. G. Cornish, Jr., who was then House Surgeon, of wearing within his shoe, under the grafted heel, a rubber bath sponge. This served to distribute the pressure over the entire surface of the graft between the os calcis and the heel.

This case Doctor Green said was shown on account of the general interest which was attached to a large pedicle graft subject to pressure in this anatomical location. It would be seen that the main part of the graft was soft and that hair was growing upon it and that it had now partaken of the nature of the original skin of the heel.

DOCTOR WHITMAN presented a boy fifteen years of age in connection with Doctor Green's case. At the age of five the right foot had been crushed by a street car. He remained in a hospital for two years, for skin grafting and the like, but healing had never been complete. The foot was much atrophied, motion was fairly free in all directions. The heel and the surrounding parts were covered with scar tissue which was firmly adherent to the bone and presented in the sole several ulcers. It was proposed to remove the irregular surface of the os calcis and to apply a flap as in Doctor Green's case.

SARCOMA OF THE ETHMOÏD (THREE AND ONE-HALF YEARS AFTER OPERATION)

DR. A. V. MOSCHCOWITZ presented a woman, twenty-two years of age, whom he had presented before the Society about two and one-half years ago, one year after the operation was performed. She was admitted to Mt. Sinai Hospital a little over three and one-half years ago, at which time she complained only of the disfigurement, which was caused by a unilateral exophthalmos. After a very careful examination by various members of the rhinological and ophthalmological staff, it was concluded that the exophthalmos was caused by a sarcoma, originating in the ethmoid bone, which pushed the eyeball forward and outward. Vision was retained. The problem presented was how to remove the growth in a radical manner, retaining vision, and without any disfigurement. Doctor Moschcowitz evolved the idea of making the incision in the eyebrow and down just to one side of the middle of the nose. The sarcoma which originated in the ethmoid was extirpated. Both the primary and late results were excellent.

DR. WINFIELD S. SCHLEY said this case demonstrated that extensive sarcoma and the squamous-celled type of carcinoma were in many cases distinctly operable in the region of the superior maxilla. Doctor Schley had operated on a number of cases considered inoperable by other surgeons, and a number of these cases had gone several years without recurrence. One patient who seemed almost hopeless for surgery had gone seven years and was alive to-day. Both sarcoma and epithelioma remained localized for a longer time in this region than in any other part of the body. The glands were involved *very* late. Hence, if one did a wide resection before the growth was far advanced the cases were not only distinctly operable, but the prognosis very fair indeed. In fact, the results were far better than had been thought, but depended directly upon the thoroughness of the primary operation. Furthermore, recurrences were local and *not metastatic* in the great majority of instances. If metastatic they were in the neck glands. These should be thoroughly dissected at the time of the primary operation or at a period before it, whether palpable or not.

DOCTOR MOSCHCOWITZ said that the operation in this case began with an incision extending from the middle of the eyebrow and over the nose, a little to the left of the centre. In order to gain good exposure and access to the tumor he now made an incision through the periosteum from the root of the nose outward and downward, and a similar incision at the junction of the nasal bone and the cartilage. The underlying bone was sawn through and fractured in such a fashion that it hung externally upon a periosteal pedicle. The nose was then opened into and the structures of the orbit, including the pulley of the superior oblique, were peeled back. The eyeball was protected by a spoon-shaped instrument. This procedure exposed the tumor, about the size of the end of a finger, attached by broad pedicle to the os planum of the ethmoid. It was removed with rongeur and chisel. Just after having had this case he had two other cases of sarcoma of the ethmoid. The condition was exceedingly rare, and he supposed he would never see another case of that kind. In the second case Doctor Moschcowitz did an evisceration of the entire orbit, saving the eyelids, with which to subsequently line the orbital cavity. The third patient was a very far advanced case, having been treated at other hospitals with palliative operations and with radium, and died after evisceration of the orbit, with metastases in the brain.

ANEURISM OF RADIAL ARTERY

DR. A. V. MOSCHCOWITZ presented the excised specimen of an aneurism of the radial artery which occurred upon his service at Mount Sinai Hospital. By way of introduction Doctor Moschcowitz stated that amongst the drawbacks of Dakin's solution it was often asserted that it was the cause of secondary hemorrhages. His experience had been, however, that Dakin's solution had no effect whatsoever upon well vitalized tissues, and therefore he could not see how it could destroy a blood-vessel. It has been the doctor's experience, that whenever an appreciable hemorrhage occurred, it was due to other, usually mechanical, factors. He had seen one rather alarming hemorrhage in a case of empyema, which was ascribed to Dakin's solution, but was proved to have been caused by the pressure of a drainage tube upon the intercostal vessels. As he was on the constant lookout for such occurrences, Doctor Moschcowitz was not at all surprised at the findings of the case under discussion.

This patient was admitted to Mount Sinai Hospital with a very extensive phlegmon of the forearm. The operation consisted of a thorough opening up of the various intermuscular septa, and subsequent treatment with Dakin's solution, instilled through numerous tubes. The wound cleared up very rapidly and the patient was about ready to be discharged with a superficial granulating wound. Routine examination prior to his discharge revealed a pulsating swelling, about the size of a marrowfat pea, upon the radial artery at a point just where it was crossed by a Carrel tube. The case was watched with great interest for twenty-four hours, during which period the aneurism had increased to double its size. On the following day the aneurism was extirpated in local anæsthesia.

The hardened specimen showed an aneurism of the size described, communicating with the radial artery. The specimen and its exact histological examination will be described in a future paper.

Doctor Moschcowitz said this case proved the following two points: First, that secondary hemorrhages were not caused by the chemical action of the Dakin's solution; and second, that great care must be used in placing rubber tubes in the vicinity of vessels.

CALCIFIED EPITROCHANTERIC BURSITIS SIMULATING SARCOMA

DR. N. W. GREEN presented a girl, seventeen years of age, who was admitted to the Surgical Division A of St. Luke's Hospital on July 16, 1919, on account of a tumor on the right hip. About four months previous to admission the patient fell on her right side and bruised her hip. One month later she began to have pain in the side, which was increased by walking. She noticed a distinct tumor growth on her hip since the time of her injury.

Her past history was unimportant. Physical examination showed a well-nourished girl presenting a tumor in the region of the right hip just below the base of the great trochanter. The tumor was hard, fixed, and slightly tender.

Operation was performed on July 17, 1919, under gas and ether anæsthesia (Doctor Green).

Pathological findings: There was a mass 6 inches long and 3½ inches

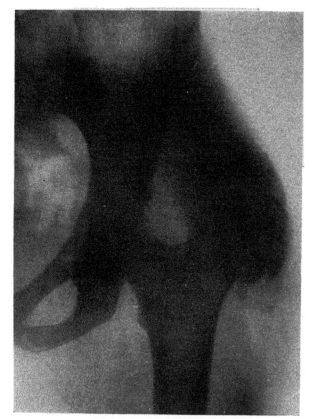

Fig. 2.—Calcified epitrochanteric bursitis simulating sarcoma.

broad, well encapsulated and adherent to the gluteus maximus muscle. The tumor mass was soft, slightly irregular, and contained an area of broken-down material as shown after removal. The mass was situated beneath the fascia of the tensor fascia femoris and the gluteus maximus muscle.

Operative procedure: A long incision was made extending from above the great trochanter down the femur for a distance of 8 inches. The skin, fat, and fascia of the tensor fascia femoris was retracted and separated from the mass on the anterior and lateral side. A portion of the tensor fascia femoris was mutilated in order to get below the tumor mass, which was found adherent to the gluteus maximus muscle. It required the removal of a large part of the gluteus maximus muscle in order not to cut into the mass. (The idea being even at this stage of the operation that it was a fibro-sarcoma.) The mass was removed in its entirety. Bleeding points were ligated and a rubber dam drain inserted. The skin was closed with interrupted sutures of chromic gut and a dry dressing applied. The patient was discharged cured thirteen days after operation. At present she shows no limp and has good motion in every direction.

Pathological Diagnosis.—A calcified bursa situated over the great trochanter.

This case was shown on account of its similarity to a malignant growth and to show the excellent function after a large part of the gluteus maximus muscle had been removed.

X-ray findings: The röntgenogram (Fig. 2) taken by Dr. L. T. LeWald shows a large mass mottled in appearance which shows the presence of lime salts in juxta-proximity to the great trochanter.

This latter, in view of the post-operative findings, proved to be due to a calcification in the bursa. Before operation, and even at the time of the operation, the tumor was thought by several men to be of a malignant nature.

MECHANICAL FACTORS IN THE MANAGEMENT OF RECENT EMPYEMAS

Dr. Frank S. Mathews read a paper with the above title.

Dr. Howard Lilienthal said there were a few points he would like to add to those brought out in Doctor Mathew's paper. First, he would like to add a fourth to the list of the objects of the operation, and that was the prevention of deformity; that was important and should always be borne in mind. Doctor Mathews mentioned that the lungs only con_ tracted by the action of elastic fibres. He thought the lungs contracted because of the intrinsic muscle fibres in the lungs.

In reference to the action of the lungs in cases of traumatic atelectasis, usually this form of atelectasis was confined to one lobe, and that lobe would be so absolutely contracted that it would be like a piece of thick limp leather, and, strange to say, one could not inflate such a lung through the pharynx. This seemed to be due to a spastic condition of the lung itself, and he thought it was a protective effect. He had noticed this behavior of the lung in gunshot wounds where there were spiculæ of fractured rib in contact with the lung, and the lung seemed to have contracted away from the object that was producing the traumatism. Atelectasis usually occurred in the lower lobe but it sometimes occurred in the upper lobe. So he thought there was something more than the elastic fibres concerned in the production of the condition. Doctor Lilienthal said he had suggested in a report to the surgeon general that this would be a good subject to study by animal experimentation to see if it was possible to produce experimental traumatic atelectasis.

As to suction methods, he did not think much of these methods. There had been four or five cycles during which suction methods had been discovered and rediscovered. All had failed. The thing of importance in dealing with empyema was that one was not merely dealing with pyothorax. It was not like a sac of fluid that could be opened at the bottom and drained. It was a condition so multiform that one must have done a large number of operations where there were large exposures to fully appreciate this feature, and one must also have studied the chest with the X-ray.

All these points Doctor Mathews brought out should be considered, but there were other points of equal importance. One of these was the binding down of the lung by dense exudate which rather rapidly became true fibrous tissue and then it took a long time for expansion to occur unless the exudate was removed by the method of Delorme, Fowler, or Ransohof. The patient had to take coughing or blowing exercises in order to keep the lung inflated enough of the time to prevent the exudate from reforming, and retraction again taking place. If much of the lung was bound down healing depended upon two things, either one must get rid of the adhesions and exudate or produce a sterile pneumothorax. In the latter case there would be healing and afterward a gradual expansion of the lung, obliterating the pneumothorax.

Another point that one could not too often emphasize was that multiple pockets were extremely common, so common that one could almost say they were the rule in empyema due to infection through minute and perhaps microscopical openings in the surface of the lung. One could not say that every empyema was caused by minute lung abscesses, but we knew that empyema resulted from large lung abscesses, and it was probable that many empyemas were caused by these tiny abscesses, and there might not be the same organism in each abscess or sacculation. If the sacculations were in different parts of the pleura they had to be done away with either by doing away with all the adhesions, which was a safe and proper method, or else by making a sufficient number of openings to explore and drain every cavity. Only the other day Doctor Lilienthal said he had a woman very ill with empyema. He made a puncture and found the hæmolytic streptococcus. He had demanded an X-ray examination and this showed a general opacity of the chest, but there was one shadow toward the front of the chest, circular in form and more dense than the rest. He predicted that at least two cavities would be found. He opened the posterior cavity and found brown pus which was very thin and contained the hæmolytic streptococcus, as was reported by the medical men who did the puncture some days before operation. A second opening was then made to expose the area in front where the second shadow was located. This opening was made in the fifth interspace near the pericardium. He had been rash enough to predict that he would find green pus, and indeed, this was encountered. The culture showed staphylococcus aureus. These cavities were opened by different incisions and treated separately in the endeavor to keep the hæmolytic streptococcus from getting into the other cavity. This case illustrated what he meant in reference to operation. If this patient had been strong enough to have stood it he would have done a larger operation, using the rib spreader. Doctor Lilienthal said he had seen cases with four different cavities and four different kinds of pus. While one might succeed in clearing up the empyema by draining one abscess at a time, it was better when possible to make a wide exploration, exposing all parts and opening all sacculations at one sitting.

Dr. WALTON MARTIN stated that he was in favor of the views expressed by Doctor Mathews. Doctor Mathews called attention to the fact that the lung expanded at the end of three or four days in many instances. He had recently read an autopsy record of an extensive suppurative pleurisy in which the entire chest was involved. The patient had been drained by a wide intercostal incision and on the sixth day died from heart disease. At autopsy the lung was almost entirely in contact with the chest wall and only a small collection of pus remained.

Dr. A. V. MOSCHCOWITZ would put the mechanics of the cure of the malady in about the following manner: Up to three or four years ago there was only one method of treating an empyema, and therefore the mechanics of the cure consisted in one thing; namely, slow expansion of the lung and its adhesion to the chest wall. During the last four years other methods of healing had been evolved, and the mechanics of the cure were entirely different. It was shown by Tuffier and others at the War Demonstration Hospital of the Rockefeller Institute that an empyema cavity could be sterilized by means of Dakin's solution, and, when sterile, the external incision could be closed by secondary suture. In a certain number of cases permanent healing resulted; and these permanent cases proved an entirely new principle in the healing of empyema. Finally, Doctor Moschcowitz stated that he had a very interesting experience in one of the cases under his care at General Hospital No. 12. In this particular case routine physical examination, subsequently verified by X-ray examination, showed that a case healed for quite some time had a very definite pneumothorax. The case was watched with great care, as it was feared that a recurrence of the empyema would take place.

Much to Doctor Moschcowitz's gratification, the unexpected occurred; namely, instead of a recurrence, there was found a disappearance of the pneumothorax. It was this case that gave the clue for the procedure subsequently adopted. Whereas up to that time operations for the cure of chronic empyema were of almost daily occurrences, all operations ceased. Instead, when definite sterility was obtained in a case of empyema, all treatment was discontinued, and the outer opening was merely allowed to close. The mechanics of the last method were very interesting. The expansion of the lung which occurred could best be explained upon the theory that the air within the pneumothorax became absorbed, thereby creating a vacuum which aided in the expansion of the lung.

DR. ALFRED S. TAYLOR said that a skin flap could be made that acted like a valve. This allowed the pus to come out, and after each expulsion the flap came back against the opening and created a partial vacuum in the pleural cavity. Such a flap had been found to work well in children, and the lung was found down to normal range on the second day.

DOCTOR MATHEWS, in closing, said he removed drainage tubes much earlier than formerly. After their removal he considered air in the cavity a disadvantage. Doctor Moschcowitz had mentioned the sterilization of the cavity by antiseptics, but he considered it safer to have a cavity obliterated by apposition of its walls rather than leave a pneumothorax. Very little was said in the literature about the method of lung expansion. Bronchial communications in empyema seemed commoner with a streptococcus infection. Even with such infections, they would seem to be comparatively infrequent as was shown by our ability to aspirate the fluid without producing a pneumothorax.

Stated Meeting held April 14, 1920

The President, DR. WILLIAM A. DOWNES, in the Chair

SUBPERIOSTEAL RESECTIONS

DR. JAMES I. RUSSELL presented five patients of whom all except one, the subperiosteal resection of the humerus, had been shown to the Society before. In none of these cases had there been secondary foci and none required further operation after the primary operation for removal of the shaft. With this operation the convalescence was slow, but it was rewarded with permanent cure.

CASE I.—The first patient, who had a traumatic separation of the lower epiphysis of the right femur, was shown before the Society October 23, 1912, one year after operation, when he was five years old. Doctor Russell said he presented him now, nine years after operation, to show the final result. There was perfect function and no shortening. He was shown to demonstrate that there had been no arrest in the growth of the bone.

CASE II.—This patient, Doctor Russell said, had had a subperiosteal resection of the fibula, reported and shown before the Society January 28, 1914, at which time the fibula was not completely regenerated. The X-ray, at the present time, still showed the fibula not completely regenerated. The patient's function, however, was excellent, and it might be that in this bone, bearing so little of the body weight, Nature had not found regeneration necessary.

Lantern slides showed the process before operation, at the end of the first, second, third, sixth, and ninth months following operation, and three and seven years after the operation.

CASE III.—Doctor Russell stated that this patient, who had a chronic suppurative osteomyelitis of the shaft of the right humerus, had never been reported. He was admitted to Roosevelt Hospital March 12, 1914, at the age of seventeen years. Five weeks before his admission to the hospital he struck his arm above the elbow and suffered some pain immediately. Five days later he had severe throbbing pain in arm above the elbow, was feverish and very ill. The forearm was swollen. He was in bed for ten days when the pain became somewhat diminished.

When admitted to the hospital the right arm was held in position of mid-flexion. There was one-half inch of atrophy of the upper right arm as compared with the left. The skin was not reddened nor hot. The upper arm had a firm, brawny consistency. There was tenderness over the entire upper arm, except the upper third; it was thickened and there was marked tenderness on the outer side of the humerus. The white blood-cells numbered 16,000, and polymorphonuclears 81 per cent.

At operation, two days after admission, a subperiosteal resection of the greater part of the shaft of the humerus was done. The periosteum was more calcified than any other case on which Doctor Russell had done this operation. It separated in flakes rather than as a thickened membrane. The patient was discharged from the hospital one month later, with the arm in a plaster cast.

X-rays were taken before operation, immediately afterwards, at the end of the second, third, fourth, and sixth months after operation, and the final one six years later. There was no shortening and he had excellent function.

CASE IV.—Doctor Russell said he had presented this patient before this Society January 28, 1914, following subperiosteal resection of left tibia. It was now nearly nine years since her operation, at which time she was eighteen months old. There was about one-half inch shortening of this leg and the child walked with a slight limp.

X-rays showed the condition before operation, one week after, at the end of the first, second, third, fourth, and eighth months, and nine years after operation.

CASE V.—This patient, Doctor Russell said, had had a subperiosteal resection of the right tibia. He was shown before the Society January 28, 1914, five years after operation, which was done at the age of six years. It had now been eleven years since his operation. He had about one-half inch shortening, and a very slight limp. He has been perfectly well since operation.

Slides were shown at the end of the first month and at intervals of two months throughout the first year after operation, and at the end of each successive year for five years, the last slide having been taken eleven years after operation.

Doctor Whitman thought these late results very satisfactory, indicating that the epiphyseal cartilages had not been damaged by the original disease.

The fibula was very useful as a prop during the regeneration of the tibia after such operations, but under normal conditions only the malleolus was indispensable. As was well known, portions of the shaft were sometimes removed to serve as pegs in the operative treatment of ununited fracture of the neck of the femur without functional impairment.

Dr. Robert T. Morris said that in the case with incomplete regeneration bridging of defects in bone might be done. He had had under his care a boy twelve years of age in whom there was very good regeneration of bone after the removal of the diaphysis of the tibia, excepting at one point where two fragments tapered so that there was a hiatus between the two ends of about an inch. He divided the narrowed periosteum longitudinally at this point and put in a piece of rib and obtained a very good growth of bone. The periosteum also replaced the part of the rib from which the segment had been removed. The question had been brought up as to whether osteoblasts developed from bone or from periosteum. In the case just cited there were apparently osteoblasts starting from the graft in the tibia as well as from the periosteum of the rib.

Dr. Howard Lilienthal asked Doctor Russell if he advised the immediate removal of such large pieces of bone or whether he drained first before doing the resection. He said he had always worked the other way, he had not taken out the entire section of bone until it was pretty well proven to be necrotic.

Dr. Wm. B. Coley asked how long extension had been kept up in those cases.

Dr. Seward Erdman asked Doctor Russell just what he meant by primary union in these cases; whether he understood correctly that he removed the osteomyelitis and then closed the wound by primary suture.

Doctor Russell, in answer to Doctor Lilienthal, said that in very acute cases he did not think it desirable to do an immediate subperiosteal resection; thought it better to do a primary drainage, removing the cortex of the bone, and in about three or four weeks, when the periosteum had thickened sufficiently, to do a secondary operation, removing the shaft. In the last case shown, which was an acute case, primary drainage was instituted and a subperiosteal resection of the shaft was done three weeks later.

In reply to Doctor Coley's question about extension, no extension was used except in the case of the humerus; where, as Doctor Whitman had said, there were two long bones the healthy bone acts as a splint to the diseased one and extension was not necessary. The only case in which extension was used was in the subperiosteal resection of the humerus, where extension was continued for about six weeks after the patient left the hospital, making about two and one-half months in all.

In reply to Doctor Erdman's question as to whether primary suture was used; as a rule, these cases were infected and do not heal by primary union. In the fourth case, of nine years' duration, in which there was a chronic process with a sinus in the lower end of the shaft of the tibia, primary union was obtained throughout both the periosteum and the skin with the exception of a small drainage point just above the lower epiphysis. The other cases were all drainage cases.

EPITHELIALIZATION UNDER VOSBURGH'S METHOD OF STRAPPING

DR. SETH M. MILLIKEN presented a man who was admitted to the Lincoln Hospital after a steam burn which burned off the posterior one-half of his scalp, an area on his shoulder, over the scapula and under the arm. Doctor Milliken said he saw the patient for the first time when he came on service at the Lincoln Hospital on February 1st. At that time large areas of sloughing had occurred. The sloughing area on the patient's head was a little larger than his hand. The area over the scapula was about 4 by 7 inches in extent. He had a burn over the olecranon and under the arm. Exuberant granulations were heaped up in these areas.

Doctor Hitzrot, some time ago, had shown a case in which following a burn he had done a skin transplant on the scalp, and it seemed that in this case it would be necessary to follow such a procedure. It was then decided to try Vosburgh's method of strapping. Small grafts were taken off the chest and arm for this purpose, and nothing had been done except to pull the margins of the wounds towards each other. The last graft was put on by the house surgeon one week ago Monday.

The advantage of Vosburgh's method of strapping was that there was less cicatrization than by any other method; the results were much better than by the application of boric ointment or any other form of treatment. The edges of the wound were gently approximated and then adhesive plaster was applied tightly to hold the granulations as flat as possible. This kept the surface in good condition. Nothing else was done in this case except to apply the grafts and strap the granulations absolutely flat.

DR. ROYAL WHITMAN said that the use of adhesive plaster strapping for the purpose of levelling the granulating surface of an ulcer and approximating the margins of the skin was a very old treatment, as was its use in connection with skin grafting of the Reverdin type. Doctor Vosburgh had apparently revived and improved a method that had fallen into disuse.

DR. HOWARD LILIENTHAL said he felt pretty sure that this was not a rediscovery, as Doctor Whitman said, because there was no such thing as F. O. adhesive plaster in those days to which Doctor Whitman referred. He felt quite sure of this, because he had introduced F. O. adhesive plaster himself. It was an improvement on a European plaster. Before that time they used a lead plaster which was used with the idea that it was protective and also to draw the wound edges together. Doctor Lilienthal said that as he understood the Vosburgh method the grafts were glued to the plaster and then the plaster applied, so as to hold the grafts on to the granulations. The plaster did not pull, but was simply a dressing laid on. At the same time, Doctor Lilienthal said he would like to mention another method that was extremely valuable. It was not original with him and he did not know who had originated it. It was a method of grafting infected granulating wounds by first using the Carrel method and getting the granulating surface perfectly germ free and then laying on the graft with a paraffine mosquito-net dressing. Dakin's solution was then applied as a wet gauze dressing once a day. The original paraffine mosquito-net dressing was allowed to remain for ten days. By that method every graft would take if there were no bacteria in the wound. This was better than the Vosburgh method, though he also approved of that.

Dr. H. M. H. Lyle said that in 1915 and 1916 they had used sometimes rubber and sometimes open-mesh material and paraffine as the routine treatment in extensive burns. This method was very satisfactory; with it one might expect almost 100 per cent. of successes.

Doctor Milliken said that zinc oxide plaster was sterile and protective, and if put on firmly kept down granulations and the marginal epithelium formed more rapidly. All he did was to put the graft either on the adhesive plaster or on the granulations and press it down firmly. The new epithelium advanced very rapidly and the zinc oxide kept the surface moist and smooth.

THE METHODS AND RESULTS OF TREATMENT OF CRANIOCEREBRAL WOUNDS

Dr. Harold Neuhof read a paper with the above title, for which see October ANNALS OF SURGERY.

Dr. Burton James Lee said there was one point that should be mentioned in connection with the mortality of head wounds and that was that a large number of those who received head wounds died in the front area, and if one is considering the mortality of head wounds as a whole, these must also be included. The complete records should include all those who died of head wounds in the front hospitals, and also many who died in ambulances on their way to the rear.

Dr. John Douglas spoke of two points in connection with Doctor Neuhof's paper that were applicable to civil surgery. One of these was the implantation of fascial flaps in the dura. He had used such fascial flaps in two operations for traumatic epilepsy and also in a third case, that of a child on whom had dropped a vichy siphon from the fifth story of a tenement, which crushed the skull so that it was like a broken egg shell, with the brain tissue protruding. The dura was impossible to close. By taking a large flap of fascia from the child's thigh, it was possible to close the defect in the dura. For a time the child had hemiplegia, but later the child walked with a comparatively slight limp.

Another point that had been mentioned was the difference in wounds made by war missiles with high velocity and those made by revolvers in civil life. In a case in the prison ward at Bellevue Hospital, that of a man who attempted to commit suicide by shooting himself in the right temporal region, the bullet lodged in the left side of the brain, about one and one-half inches from the surface. The man had hemiplegia and aphasia. He was not operated upon and within one month he was up out of bed and had recovered from his aphasia and later had partly recovered from his hemiplegia. It would seem that in a large number of these head wounds if the victim did not die of immediate hemorrhage or brain injury, and if there were no signs of infection, it was safer to leave the bullet in than to extract it by immediate operation.

DOCTOR NEUHOF, in closing the discussion, said that concerning his statistics he had not obtained them through American official channels with a few exceptions. The chief source was directly from patients by letters, and in this way he had been able to keep track of a large majority of these patients. Doctor Neuhof said he had also had access to the statistics of the British Expeditionary Forces which were collected by the Medical Research Committee. That had been an additional source of information, particularly in regard to reoperated cases. The mortality included all cases up to date. There was no selection of cases for operation in those he had considered; they were taken just as they came under their care. At Mobile Hospital No. 2 Doctor Neuhof said he was in a position to make a certain selection of cases, and he chose the most serious injuries to see what could be done in those cases. No cases were refused operation except those manifestly moribund and those with huge skull defects with the brain extruding that could only live for a few hours or perhaps a day. At his mobile hospital all other cases were subjected to operation.

TRANSACTIONS

OF THE

PHILADELPHIA ACADEMY OF SURGERY

JOINT MEETING HELD WITH

THE NEW YORK SURGICAL SOCIETY

February 2, 1920

DR. GEORGE G. ROSS in the Chair

CASE OF JACKSONIAN EPILEPSY CAUSED BY BRAIN TUMOR. SUCCESSFUL REMOVAL OF THE TUMOR

DR. A. P. C. ASHHURST reported the case of a patient, John T., thirty-one years of age, on whom he had recently operated at the Episcopal Hospital. The man was originally admitted to the hospital November 22, 1919, complaining of "headache and stomach trouble," and was sent to the Medical Ward, then in charge of Dr. M. H. Fussell; and was eventually transferred to the Surgical Service January 3, 1920, by Dr. John B. Carson, who had succeeded Doctor Fussell on duty in the medical service.

Doctor Ashhurst saw the patient first in consultation on January 2, 1920, and learned the essential facts of the history as follows: The patient's family history was negative. He was unmarried. He was born in Poland and came to the United States in 1912. He was a laborer, and his general health always had been good. He smoked and drank very little and had had no serious injuries and no operations. He denied venereal disease.

About a year ago the patient had his first convulsion, losing consciousness. Since then he had had eight other attacks of varying severity at intervals of weeks or months. Three weeks before admission (*i.e.*, about November 1, 1919) his family physician, Dr. Jacob B. Feldman, made a spinal puncture for a Wassermann test.[1] After this the patient developed headache and vomiting. In the three weeks elapsing between this visit to his physician and his admission to the hospital, he had five convulsions. If he tried to leave his bed he vomited. After his admission to the hospital, during the latter part of November and during December, he had five other convulsions, one of which at least was determined to be Jacksonian in type, beginning in the left hand.

The patient, while on the medical service, was seen with Doctor Carson by Dr. Charles W. Burr, Consulting Neurologist to the hospital, who was unable to make a diagnosis. It was learned after operation that

[1] This was reported negative, as was the blood Wassermann after his admission to the hospital.

the patient's physician, Doctor Feldman, had called Dr. Alfred Gordon in consultation, and that Doctor Gordon had suggested an operation on account of a bony lump in the skull in the right parietal region, and after seeing a skiagraph of the patient's head.

Examination (January 2, 1920) showed a young man with rather expressionless face, who felt fairly well when lying quiet in bed, except for a constant terribly severe headache, in the frontal region and on the top of the head. The right eye was kept closed or nearly so, but could be opened. The pupils were equal and reacted (rather sluggishly) to light and accommodation. An examination of the eye-grounds made by Dr. Harold G. Goldberg, Ophthalmologist to the hospital, on November 29, 1919, had shown that the right eye was negative, but that the left eye showed slight paleness of the nerve and disturbance of retinal pigment, and one minute hemorrhage of considerable duration down to the temporal side of the disk. Doctor Goldberg considered it a beginning of neuroretinitis. A subsequent examination by Doctor Goldberg, January 5, 1920, confirmed the above findings, but showed no changes since the previous examination.

There was no paralysis of any of the cranial nerves, and the chest, abdomen and genitalia were negative. The extremities also were negative except for slight accentuation of the knee-jerks. There was no Babinski, no ankle or patellar clonus, and no Kernig's sign.

In the right parietal region of the skull was a sessile exostosis, about 5 cm. in diameter and raised about 5 mm. above the surrounding surface. Pressure on this lump caused some pain. He said he noticed the lump first about five years previously, and that it had been very slowly growing larger. Questioned as to any injury to this region, he said that when he first came to this country (over seven years ago) he attended night school, and there were many fights among those standing in line waiting for admission, but he did not remember any specific injury to his head. Skiagraphs made by Dr. R. S. Bromer, Radiologist to the hospital, showed an area of rarefaction of the inner table of the skull corresponding to the site of the exostosis.

Here was a man, Doctor Ashhurst said, who besides having epilepsy, apparently Jacksonian in type, had intense and persistent headache, had unprovoked attacks of vomiting, had an abnormal bony lump over the right motor region, and who had changes in the left eye-ground suggestive of increased intracranial tension. He considered these facts sufficient to justify an exploratory operation. His opinion was that the exostosis itself might be sufficient explanation for the symptoms.

Operation (January 6, 1920).—Ether (intrapharyngeal). Operator, Doctor Ashhurst; assistants, Doctor Mendel and Doctor McGuire. A bone flap, three of whose sides measured about 8 cm. each, and whose base (in the temporal region) measured 3 cm., was turned down from the right motor region, the exostosis being about in the centre of the flap.

Bleeding from the scalp was controlled by Kocher hæmostats. The bone flap was cut by means of the Hudson trephine, Gigli saw, and De Vilbiss forceps. After raising the bone flap its under surface over the area corresponding to the exostosis was found eroded and hemorrhagic in appearance. The bone flap was therefore removed, together with a portion of the cranial aponeurosis which was adherent to the underlying exostosis (Fig. 1). (Time elapsed at this stage of the operation, fifty minutes.) The exposed dura was granular over an area corresponding to the exostosis, and it was determined to excise it. It felt a little less resistant than the surrounding exposed dura, but the entire surface exposed pulsated normally. After ligation of four or five meningeal vessels with fine silk on a curved needle, the dura was opened and a grooved director slipped inside, and a rectangular incision (5 by 5½ cm.) was made with scalpel upon the director, entirely surrounding the diseased dura. As an attempt was then made to raise the diseased dura by mouse-toothed dissecting forceps, it was found to be continuous with a tumor embedded in the brain. By careful preliminary double ligation (with fine silk on a curved needle) of all pial vessels entering the tumor, and dividing the vessels between the double ligatures, it was possible very slowly and cautiously to outline the tumor. By making gentle traction on the edges of the dura, and wiping away the convolutions of the brain with wisps of cotton (moistened in extremely hot salt solution) held in the fingers, the brain tissue very gradually was peeled off the tumor, millimetre by millimetre, the union between the two being like that of inflammatory lymph adherent to the intestines, and the friability of both brain and tumor being nearly as great as that of the flakes of inflammatory lymph. Only at one point was any apparent damage done to the brain, when the needle passed around one of the pial vessels pricked the cortex, which immediately became suffused with a pink color over an area about 1 cm. in diameter. After the region of pial circulation was passed, the remainder of the stage of enucleation of the tumor was almost bloodless, any very minute ooze being promptly controlled by application of wisps of cotton squeezed out of an almost boiling saline solution. The tumor measured 5.5 cm. by 5 cm. on its surface, and was 4 cm. deep (Fig. 2). The hollow left in the brain pulsated normally, but showed no immediate tendency to fill up (Fig. 3). (Time elapsed at this stage of the operation over two hours, about an hour being consumed in enucleating the tumor from the brain.)[2]

---

[2] The specimen was submitted to Dr. William G. Spiller, at the University of Pennsylvania, who reported, after examining it microscopically, that the tumor could be only one of two things—an endothelioma or a fibroma; and he was inclined to class it as the former. He was further of the opinion that such growths in the brain were frequently the result of irritation from a lesion of the skull, originally traumatic in origin. This had been Doctor Ashhurst's own belief at the time of the operation, and he was glad to have it confirmed by so able an authority as Professor Spiller. Krause [Surgery of the Brain and Spinal Cord; translated

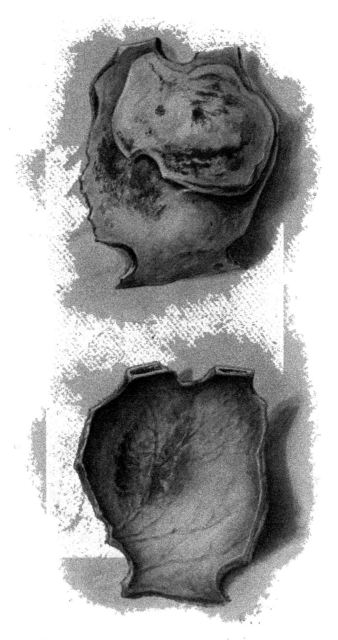

FIG. 1.—J. T., aged thirty-one years. P. E. H. January 6, 1920. Bone flap removed from right parietal region, and containing an exostosis (hyperostosis). Above, the outer surface of the bone, with the portion of the cranial aponeurosis excised because adherent to the exostosis. Below, the inner surface of the bone, grooved by branches of the middle meningeal artery, and showing the rarefied area corresponding to the brain tumor. (Actual size.)

404

FIG. 2.—J. T., thirty-one years, P. E. H. January 6, 1920. Tumor growing from dura in right parietal region. Above, the cerebral surface of the growth, showing some of the ligatures in the region of greatest vascularity. Below, the cranial surface of the growth, showing the adherent dura excised with the tumor. (Actual size.)

During the removal of the tumor, Doctor McGuire cut a free transplant of fascia lata from the patient's right thigh, and this transplant (a rectangle 5 by 5.5 cm.) was sutured to the edges of the defect in the dura by interrupted silk sutures, and was gently pressed down into the hollow left in the brain. The flap of scalp was then replaced and accurately sutured (without drainage) by interrupted sutures of silkworm gut, the sutures being placed about 0.5 cm. apart, and thus effectually controlling all bleeding from the scalp.

The patient's condition was good throughout the operation, which was three hours in duration, and he left the table with a pulse of 128. At no time subsequently were there any unfavorable symptoms. For the first twenty-four hours after operation he said his left forearm and hand felt numb, but at the end of this time normal sensation returned to all but thumb and index finger. By January 18, 1920 (twelve days after operation), the index finger felt nearly normal, but the thumb still felt anæsthetic, though both index finger and thumb distinguished pin contact throughout. At this time the patient was fairly convalescent. He seemed much brighter than before operation, had no headache at all, but still felt giddy on sudden movements or on attempts to sit up in bed.

January 28th: Sitting up in chair.

February 2d: Four weeks after operation. Walking about ward. Has had no convulsions since operation. If symptoms develop later from the skull defect caused by removal of the bone-flap, it is planned to do a second operation and fill the opening by a bone transplant from the outer surface of the neighboring skull.

June 7: Five months since operation. Has gained thirty pounds in weight. Has had no convulsions since the operation. His ears no longer buzz, but he has some consciousness of his brain in stooping (he has returned to his work as automobile mechanic) and in walking fast. On June 10th a bone transplant was cut from the left parietal region. consisting of the outer layer of the skull and overlying pericranium, and was inserted into the defect in the right parietal region which had been previously prepared for its reception. The patient, who was receiving ether by intrapharyngeal insufflation, was in good condition until the head was turned over to the left, for insertion of the transplant in the right. His condition at once became unsatisfactory, and in spite of stimulation he died, apparently of respiratory failure, as the scalp

by H. A. Haubold; New York, 1909, vol. i, p. 71], however, held the opposing view, that tumors of the dura were responsible for the growth of new bone in the skull. The latter view could justify one in replacing the bone flap after removal of the tumor; whereas, if the former is the correct theory, replacement of the same bone might in time cause another tumor to form. In 1899, Spiller reported a case similar to the one now recorded, and in 1907 reported a second case and reviewed the literature (J. A. M. A., 1907, ii, 2059). In advanced cases the thickening of the skull overlying the tumor becomes so widespread as to justify the name of *hæmicraniosis*, applied to it in 1903 by Brissaud and Lereboullet.

was being sutured. The duration of the operation was nearly two hours, but there was no evidence of shock: he ceased breathing some seconds before the heart beat stopped, and artificial respiration and cardiac massage (through the unopened chest and abdomen) were of no avail. No autopsy was permitted.

HÆMATOMYELIA, WITH CROSSED PARALYSIS
(Sensation on Left, Motion on Right)

DOCTOR ASHHURST also presented notes of the following case. He found the patient in the ward at the Episcopal Hospital when he took over Doctor Frazier's service from Doctor Mutschler, August 1, 1914. For the ward notes he was indebted to Drs. J. Walker Moore and J. P. Jones, the surgical internes.

The patient, a young man twenty-five years of age, was admitted July 23, 1914, and discharged October 29, 1914. On the day of admission at 7.30 A.M. he had been knocked backward from the deck of a ship to the deck beneath, landing on his forehead. He was not unconscious at all. He had no pain for the first five minutes, but then felt intense pain all over the body. After the fall he was unable to move a muscle of his body below the chin, but he could talk and move his eyes and eyelids normally.

On admission, at 2 P.M., the patient is paralyzed below the sixth cervical vertebra. He has great difficulty in breathing. He can talk, open his mouth, and protrude his tongue, but is unable to move his head or the rest of his body. There is no bleeding from the ears or nose.

He was placed on a water bed.

Physical Examination.—Fairly well nourished and developed young fellow. Temperature 102° to 101° F.

Head: Eyes react normally to light and accommodation; pupils are equal. Nose and ears are negative. Tongue is moist and clean, no paralysis. There is an abrasion and some slight swelling of the forehead. Complains of intense pain in the neck when the head is moved. There is no displacement of the spinous processes of the cervical vertebræ. He is unable to move his head at all.

Chest: The breathing is shallow and difficult. Lungs and heart are normal.

Abdomen: No respiratory movements of the abdominal muscles. There is a scar of a hernia operation in right inguinal region.

Extremities: All four extremities are paralyzed. The patellar and cremasteric reflexes are absent. The hamstrings and calf muscles contract when the overlying skin is pricked with a pin. The toes move when the sole of the foot is touched. There is loss of sense of pin prick on the entire left side up to the neck, but this sense is retained on the right side.

Six Hours Later.—Slight motion is perceptible in left arm and left leg; sensation remains about the same.

Ten Hours After Admission.—Is able to move the right arm also; can flex but not extend the elbow. Unable to move the right leg. Breathing is better. Pain is less. Knee-jerks still absent.

July 24th: Can move the right arm slightly. Has to be catheterized. No other changes. Temperature 101° to 100° F.

July 25th: Given a purge.

July 26th: Voided urine, and has control of his bowels. Slight increase in power of triceps in left arm. Fibrillary contraction of both lower extremities. Still unable to move right leg. Cannot move the muscles of shoulder girdle.

July 28th: Can move his shoulder muscles, no other change.

July 30th: Temperature has reached normal.

August 1st: Notes by Doctor Ashhurst:

Can rotate, flex and extend the head, but not strongly.

Right upper extremity: Can move the right shoulder. Trapezius, deltoid and axillary fold muscles all act slightly. Subscapularis, good. Biceps, good. Triceps, no power. No power in wrist or fingers.

Left upper extremity: Shoulder muscles are all good. Elbow good, but weak. Slight power in the extensors of the wrist and fingers.

Left lower extremity: Fair power throughout. Increased reflexes. Ankle clonus and Babinski present.

Right lower extremity: No power; spastic. Increased reflexes. Babinski present. Fibrillary contractures.

Sensation: Over the entire left side from the ninth intercostal space down, sharp and dull are called dull. The remainder of the body has normal perception of sharp and dull. Over the left lower extremity cannot distinguish hot from cold. Over the left abdomen and thorax both hot and cold are felt as hot. Elsewhere sensation of heat and cold are normal.

Neck: Third cervical spinous process appears to be more prominent than normally.

Diagnosis: Hemorrhage into substance of cervical cord; hæmatomyelia.

August 3d: Can flex right knee and hip with ease. No other changes.

August 4th: Skiagraphs negative for fracture of cervical spine.

August 13th: Can turn from side to side in bed, and raise entire body from bed. Sensation continues impaired on left side. Is moved from water bed to ordinary mattress.

August 15th: Good movements in arms and legs, but very little power in the hands.

August 18th: Can sit up in bed. Hands still very weak, but arms are becoming stronger. Perfect movement in lower extremities.

August 21st: Gradual improvement in all movements except the right hand.

August 29th: Can flex right index finger, but can move none of the other fingers or wrist on right. Can move all the right toes, but cannot move the ankle-joint. The reflexes on right are greatly increased. The left extremities are normal.

September 2d: Able to move right thumb.

September 10th: Gradually getting more motion in fingers. Has now limited use of all fingers of right hand. Walks all over ward with spastic gait.

September 14th: Except for delayed sensation in left leg and foot, sensation is normal all over body.

September 20th: Goes up and down stairs, but with difficulty. Holds right hand flexed at wrist, and with metacarpo-phalangeal joints extended (Fig. 4).

October 20th: Very little spasticity in gait. Sensation now normal in left leg.

October 29th: Discharged and referred to Orthopædic Dispensary.

July 9, 1917: This date (three years after injury) he paid his first visit to the Orthopædic Dispensary of the Episcopal Hospital, when the following notes were made by Doctor Gill:

Has some atrophy of essential muscles of right hand with a tendency to contracture. Has weakness of triceps of right arm. Active abduction of right shoulder is slightly limited. Has loss of temperature sense on entire left side of body, except left hand and forearm. Has loss of tactile sensation on right side. He is unable to raise toes of right foot from floor. Works as toolmaker.

Proper treatment was advised, but the patient never returned, and cannot now be found; though it is known he was a visitor to a patient in the ward less than a year ago.

END RESULTS OF CERTAIN METHODS OF BRIDGING DEFECTS IN PERIPHERAL NERVES

DOCTOR ASHHURST presented two patients as clinical evidence of nerve regeneration after methods employed to bridge gaps in the peripheral nerves which are condemned by many neurologists and experimental physiologists. Both nerve stretching and nerve flaps are held to be not only useless, but positively harmful; but he believed these cases prove the contrary. No electrical reports of the muscles supplied by the damaged nerves are presented, because he had come to the conclusion after a not inconsiderable experience in such matters, extending over a period of seventeen years at the Orthopædic Hospital and Infirmary for Nervous Diseases, that where the voluntary contraction of a certain muscle is visible, such evidence is much more reliable than is that obtained by electrical reactions.

Nerve stretching to bridge gaps he had employed timidly and without much elongation of the nerves in his earlier cases; it was not until after repeated attempts at feeble stretching had showed no permanent dam-

408

age was done to the nerve, that he had been emboldened to employ such forcible stretching as was adopted in Case III (William B.). And the result in this case is so satisfactory, and the method of operation by lateral anastomosis after stretching the ends until they overlap is so much easier than that by nerve-flaps or free transplants, that he should feel no hesitation in preferring it in future cases. It is no doubt probable that in this case the use of free transplants of fascia lata to surround the anastomosis promoted the return of function; but he believes the chief factor was apposition without tension, of broad areas of denuded nervous tissue. The idea of union by lateral anastomosis followed the recognition of the possibility and desirability of determining the extent of scar tissue in the nerve bulbs not by gradually advancing cross-sections as is usually done, but by a longitudinal splitting of the bulb. During suture the bulbs are still in place and by them the nerve may be easily controlled; and after suture he had not excised them, but merely left them as they were. Cases II and III were presented; Case I was absent.

CASE I.—*Primary neuroplasty of the ulnar nerve.* Fred B., twenty-eight years of age, had his left forearm crushed between freight cars, early on the morning of December 12, 1909. He was brought to the Episcopal Hospital, in the service of Doctor Frazier, and was operated upon by Doctor Ashhurst about eight hours after injury. There was a compound comminuted fracture of the radius and ulna, with extensive laceration of the soft parts below the middle of the forearm. The bone ends protruded, and the laceration of the skin extended entirely around the forearm with the exception of about 3 cm. on the extensor surface.

Operation.—Ether. Esmarch band below shoulder. After débridement the ulnar artery was found crushed and its two ends widely separated; both were ligated. The ulnar nerve was crushed, nothing but a grease stained strand of sheath, 3.25 cm. long, joining its ends. After enlarging the incision to within 7.5 cm. of the internal condyle of the humerus and dissecting the ulnar nerve as high as this, as well as down to the wrist-joint, a gap of 1.25 cm. at least remained between its ends, even when put under considerable tension. After repair and fixation of the fractures, a flap 3 cm. long was turned down from the proximal end of the ulnar nerve and was sutured without tension to the distal end by one through-and-through mattress suture, and three sutures passing through the epineurium only. All these sutures were of fine silk. The severed muscles were repaired as well as possible, after swabbing the entire wound with very hot 5 per cent. solution of carbolic acid. The limb was dressed with alcohol-soaked gauze, was placed on splints, and was kept in vertical suspension for twenty-four hours.

The patient's temperature rose to 103° F. on the third day after operation, and there was some suppuration and a great deal of sloughing of skin and muscle; but the wounds were all healed by the end of February, 1910, about two and one-half months after the injury. Good union was secured in the radius, but the ulna remained ununited. About a year after operation a sequestrum worked itself out from the radius.

The patient was last examined November 17, 1919, ten years after the operation. He continued his work on the railroad, and has no disability from his injured arm. His grip is strong, and he has normal power in forearm, elbow, and wrist. The ulna remains ununited. There is slightly diminished sensation in the ulnar distribution to the fourth and fifth fingers, but normal sensation in the ulnar distribution to the hand. All motions of the thumb and fingers can be performed—there is absolutely no paralysis of any of the thumb muscles, interossei or lumbricals. He cannot make a perfectly tight fist, but this is due to adhesions of the muscles in the forearm to the cicatrix in the skin. It is to be particularly noted that there is no deformity of the fourth and fifth fingers—there is full extension in the phalangeal joints and full flexion in the metacarpal joints, evidencing regeneration of the ulnar nerve.

CASE II.—*End result of primary neuroplasty of the median nerve.* James F., fifty-two years of age, caught his right forearm in a carding machine in the spinning mill where he worked and was at once brought to the Episcopal Hospital. On admission to the Receiving Ward, October 21, 1916, a large gaping wound on the flexor surface was found, and an Esmarch band was at once applied above the elbow to check the free bleeding. The wound was washed with carbolic acid solution (1 : 40), 1500 units of anti-tetanic serum were given, and he was sent to the operating room.

Operation was done by Doctor Ashhurst two or three hours after injury. There was a lacerated wound extending from the styloid process of the ulna to the internal condyle of the humerus, and on the flexor surface from the radial to the ulnar border, except for about 5 cm. at the upper end, where the wound tapered to a point at the internal condyle. In the lower part of the wound the radius was exposed, with some superficial destruction of the bone surface. The median nerve was exposed and torn, the radial artery severed, and the muscle bellies and tendons were exposed throughout, but were so lacerated that their identity could not be determined by inspection.

The wound was cleansed with turpentine, followed by soap and hot water, by alcohol, and finally bichloride of mercury solution. The proximal end of the radial artery was identified about 10 cm. below the bifurcation of the brachial and was ligated. The distal end was ligated at the wrist, the intervening portion having been carried away by the injury. The Esmarch band, applied in the Receiving Ward, was then immediately removed. An area of damaged skin, about 2.5 by 10 cm., was cut away. The ends of the median nerve were next identified, and a defect of 5 cm. discovered; even by gentle stretching both ends of the nerve and flexing the wrist it was impossible to make even the damaged ends meet, much less healthy nerve tissue. Therefore, a flap (about 3 cm. in length) was cut from each end of the nerve, the flaps were inverted, and sutured end

410

to end, without tension, by fine chromic catgut (Fig. 5). The damaged ends of the nerve were not excised, but two ligatures were tied around each to prevent the flaps from splitting all the way to the ends, as indicated in Fig. 5. The lacerated muscles and tendons were repaired as well as possible, and a few silkworm-gut sutures were applied across the wound from one skin edge to the other, but an area about 7.5 by 16 cm. had to be left uncovered. The hand and forearm were wrapped loosely in gauze soaked in alcohol, the limb was placed on a splint, and was suspended vertically for the first twenty-four to thirty-six hours; and for the first week the dressings were kept constantly moist by alcohol douches.

Ward Notes.—October 23, 1916: Patient claims he has perception of touch in hand and fingers, in area of median nerve distribution.

October 28, 1916: Belly of brachio-radialis is beginning to slough. Pain sensation in ulnar distribution. In middle, index and thumb only sensation of touch. Stitches beginning to cut and removed. Temperature 99° to 101°. Wound is 17.5 by 8.5 cm. Still alcohol douches.

October 29, 1916: Tendon of palmaris longus removed for sloughing.

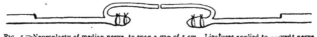

Fig. 5.—Neuroplasty of median nerve, to span a gap of 5 cm. Ligatures applied to prevent nerve ends from splitting beyond the bases of reflected flaps. Case of J. F., 52 years, P. E. H., October 21, 1916.

October 31, 1916: Wound clean except over radial side, where is some exudate. Sensation in thumb, index and middle fingers.

November 1, 1916: Temperature normal and steady.

November 28, 1916: Sixty-two skin grafts applied by Dr. I. M. Boykin.

November 30, 1916: These all disarranged by patient moving, and to-day eighty-two others were applied by Doctor Boykin.

December 10, 1916: All grafts failed to take (infection).

January 6, 1917: Eighteen grafts by Doctor Boykin.

January 8, 1917: Grafts have taken; heliotherapy.

January 31, 1917: Discharged. Slight motion in fingers. Is able to flex and extend elbow somewhat. Wrist extends only to 150° or 160°.

February 5, 1917: Orthopædic Dispensary, Episcopal Hospital. Skin grafts have taken well, wound healed. Wrist flexed to 135°, cannot be extended. Fingers partly flexed. No active motion except slight flexion of fingers. Hand very stiff. To have massage.

May 21, 1917: There is an area of anæsthesia of the thumb, forefinger, and diminished sensation in radial side of middle finger. There is some rotation in the forearm.

October 15, 1917: Can almost touch palm with middle and ring fingers. Forefinger flexes to right angle. No motion in thumb. Sensation present except on inner side and dorsum of thumb.

October 7, 1918: No active motion in thumb except at metacarpal joint.

411

Can barely touch thumb to little finger; slight passive motion in meta-carpo-phalangeal and inter-phalangeal joints. Unable to make a complete fist. Can barely touch the middle and ring fingers to thenar eminence. Little finger about ⅛ inch from palm, forefinger about one-half normal flexion. None of the fingers can be completely extended. At work since January, 1918, in spinning mill; not the same work as before injury, but almost same wages.

November 20, 1919: Examined by Doctor Ashhurst. He was out of work sixty-four weeks in all. He now makes higher wages than before injury, but in a less important position with the same firm. He uses both hands all day long, in hard manual labor, with grasping actions.

No anæsthesia. All the interossei act, all the lumbricals act. Adduction and abduction of thumb normal. Can appose thumb to index finger *strongly*. Can appose thumb to middle finger with fair power. Can appose thumb to ring finger, mere apposition. Can appose thumb to little finger with difficulty. All the voluntary thumb motion is at the carpo-metacarpal and metacarpo-phalangeal joints; but if the proximal phalanx is held by the examiner's fingers, slight active motion in the distal phalanx (flexor longus) becomes possible. Impairment of function of the flexor longus pollicis seems attributable to muscular rather than to nervous injury, as the lesion of the median nerve, and the site of its suture, was below the level at which its branch to the flexor longus pollicis is given off.

He can flex the index finger at the metacarpal joint to an angle of 120°, and at the proximal interphalangeal joint to 90°.

He can flex the third and fourth fingers until they touch the palm, and the fifth finger until it almost touches the palm.

There is slight atrophy on the radial surface of the thumb metacarpal, but no atrophy of the thenar eminence.

He can extend the wrist fully (no hyperextension) and can flex it to about 135°. Elbow motions are normal. Supination of the forearm is slightly limited.

The large scar on the forearm is supple and painless, the identity of many of the skin grafts being preserved; but the underlying muscles are slightly adherent to the skin in the middle third of the forearm, and these adhesions somewhat limit motions of the fingers.

CASE III.—*Successful end-result of secondary suture of median and ulnar nerves (lateral anastomosis) and many tendons in the forearm.*—Wm. B., eighteen years of age, on August 28, 1916, broke his fish aquarium, and the falling glass cut his left forearm on the flexor surface above the wrist. An immediate attempt at repair was made in the Receiving Ward of the Episcopal Hospital, by the interne then on duty; a number of severed tendons were sutured and the ulnar artery, completely divided, was ligated. The wound suppurated for several weeks, but healed about October 1st. In November, eleven weeks after the injury, the boy was admitted to Doctor Ashhurst's service in the Episcopal Hospital with a useless hand. There was a cross-shaped scar on the flexor surface of the left wrist, extending to within 3 cm. of the crease of the wrist. The fingers were in full extension and could not be actively flexed, except for very slight power of flexion in the thumb. The fingers were all supple, and could be passively flexed. The wrist motions were normal actively and passively, and the extensor communis digitorum acted normally. There was no action of any of the interossei or lumbricales. There was anæsthesia in the median and ulnar distributions below the cicatrices. There was marked atrophy of the thenar eminence and more marked atrophy of the hypothenar. The thumb, as already mentioned, could be flexed very slightly, but could not be adducted, abducted, nor opposed. The skin above the wrist was adherent to a dense mass of scar tissue, in which all the flexor tendons were caught.

Evidently this was a case of complete block of the median and ulnar nerves, probably from complete division; also of loss of function of all the flexors of all the fingers and thumb, either from complete division or from inclusion in scar tissue.

Operation was undertaken November 15, 1916, nearly three months after the original injury. Under ether anæsthesia, and with Esmarch anæmia secured by applying the rubber band just below the shoulder, the longitudinal portion of the old scar was excised, and the skin on both sides was reflected. It was densely adherent to the tendinous cicatrix in the middle of the incision, but free proximally and distally.

A. By dissection the following structures were identified: (1) Palmaris longus, its proximal end being lost in the scar; no distal end was found. (2) Flexor carpi radialis; by extending the incision through the annular ligament, the flexor carpi radialis was traced and found to be carefully sutured to the distal end of the median nerve (bulbous). (3) Proximal end of median nerve, ending in the mass of scar tissue, with a bulbous extremity 1.25 cm. in length. (4) Ulnar vessels and nerve, both distal and proximal ends terminating in the mass of scar tissue, and their ends separated by 2 to 2.50 cm. The ulnar nerve evidently was completely divided by the injury and not sutured. (5) Cicatricial mass of superficial flexors, the distal ends of thumb, index and middle tendons not being united to the proximal ends. (6) Cicatricial mass of deep flexors, nowhere completely divided but adherent to the underlying bones and to the scar mass of the superficial tendons. All adhesions were dissected free.

B. The proximal end of the ulnar artery was newly ligated, as the dissection had opened its lumen. The following suturing was done: (1) The flexor carpi radialis was detached from its accurate end-to-end union with the median nerve, and was sutured to the flexor pollicis longus. (2) One of the unattached proximal ends of the superficial flexors was sutured to the flexor of the index finger. (3) The palmaris longus was sutured to the flexor of the middle finger. (4) The median nerve ends could not

413

be made to meet even after the dissection, and with the wrist flexed; therefore its proximal end was stretched for 5 cm. by pulling on the bulbous end with hæmostatic forceps. In this way the bulb was pulled down past the distal end. Both ends of the nerve were then denuded laterally on apposing surfaces and united by lateral anastomosis by means of three fine silk mattress sutures passing completely through the nerve (Fig. 1). (5) The ulnar nerve was treated similarly, after stretching its proximal end for about 4 cm. In this way broad surfaces of healthy nerve tissue were brought into apposition without tension. The Esmarch band, in place about one hour, was now removed. It was found no ligatures were required.

C. A portion of fascia lata, about 8 by 10 cm., was next excised from the region of the left great trochanter. This piece was cut in half (4 by 10 cm.), and one of these smaller pieces was again halved, giving two

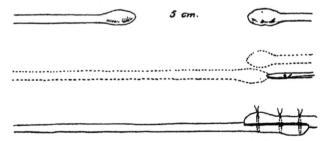

Fig. 6.—The bulbous end of nerve is caught in forceps and the nerve is stretched until the two ends overlap. They are then denuded on apposing surfaces, and united by lateral anastomosis. An actual gap of 5 cm. in the median and 3.25 cm. in the ulnar nerve was thus bridged. Case of W. B., aged eighteen years, P. E. H., November 15, 1916.

pieces about 2 by 10 cm. in dimensions. One of these small pieces of fascia lata was sutured around the median and the other around the ulnar nerve anastomosis, as tubes, being fixed proximally and distally to the nerve sheath by interrupted sutures; the suture for closing the tube in its long axis being continuous. The suture material was No. 000 chromicized catgut, threaded in a fine round needle. The remaining portion of fascia lata, 4 by 10 cm. in dimensions, was arranged so as to form one tube surrounding the bundle of the superficial flexor tendons, including those just sutured; this was to prevent adhesions between the superficial and deep flexors in the depth of the wound, and between the superficial flexors and the skin superficially. This portion of fascia lata was sutured around the tendons and fixed by sutures to the fascia surrounding the tendons as in the case of the nerves. The superficial fascia and the skin were finally closed in separate layers with many interrupted sutures of No. 0 chromic catgut, and the forearm was dressed on a splint.

The duration of the operation was two hours.

Healing occurred uneventfully. The splint was removed at the end

414

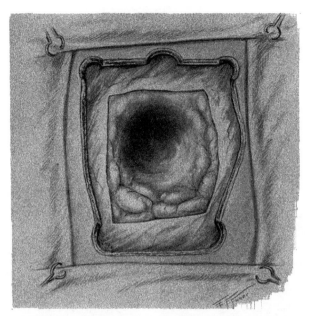

FIG. 3.—J. T., aged thirty-one years. P. E. H., January 6, 1920. Jacksonian epilepsy caused by brain tumor. Depression in brain from which tumor was removed, showing flattened convolutions. Re-drawn from a sketch made at the time by Dr. Mendel.

414

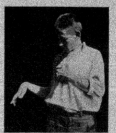

FIG. 4.—Case of hæmatomyelia three months after injury of cervical cord, showing residual paralysis. Episcopal Hospital.

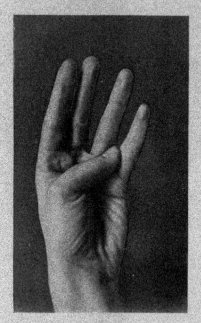
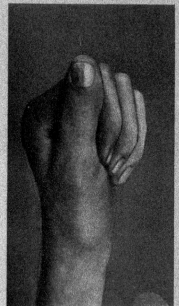

FIGS. 7 AND 8—Three years after secondary suture of median and ulnar nerves, above wrist. Gap of 5 cm. in median and of 3.25 cm. in ulnar; spanned by forcible stretching of proximal ends of nerves, until bulbous ends overlapped. Lateral suture after denudation of opposing surfaces of nerves.

of the second week, and treatment by massage was instituted. This was continued for a year after operation, when approximately normal function had been regained. The patient was able to return to his work in a mill three weeks after the operation.

Examination in November, 1919, three years after operation, shows very little trace of the accident. There is slight fixation of the skin to the underlying tendons at one point. Full regeneration has occurred in both median and ulnar nerves, as evidenced by normal action of all the lumbrical muscles, of the abductor, adductor, short flexor and opponens muscles of the thumb, and by very nearly normal action of all the interossei; the only deficiency in the interossei is slight weakness in spreading the fingers apart (Fig. 7). Each finger can be moved separately in flexion and in full extension, though flexion is possible only until the finger tips touch the base of the palm; they cannot be flexed actively into actual contact with the middle of the palm, but there is normal power in the grip, and no disability in hard manual labor (Fig. 8). The thenar and hypothenar eminences are less well developed than in the normal hand; indeed, the entire left hand is somewhat smaller than the right. The deep and superficial flexors of all the fingers act separately, showing that they are no longer adherent to each other above the wrist. The thumb can be apposed to each finger, but not with much power to the fourth and fifth. There is, however, no power in the long flexor of the thumb, the distal phalanx remaining extended when the flexor brevis acts. As the distal end of this tendon was sutured to the proximal end of the flexor carpi radialis, the fact that it does not act cannot be attributed to failure of regeneration in the median nerve, the nerve lesion having been well below the level where its branches to the flexor longus pollicis and flexor carpi radialis are given off.

The movements of the wrist, active and passive, are normal. The lad works as an electrician, and is conscious of no disability in the use of his hand.

DR CHARLES A. ELSBERG, of New York, regarding the two cases (II and III) showing results of bridging defects in peripheral nerves, said that no matter how good the result one might get in rare instances, all evidence points to the fact that turning down a flap from a nerve from above or turning up a flap from below in order to bridge a defect is inadvisable. If regeneration occurs it has to take place in spite of the procedure and not as a result of it.

The literature of this subject was carefully gone over six months ago by Doctor Stookey, of New York, who published his conclusions in the *Archives of Neurology and Psychiatry* three or four months ago. He showed pretty conclusively that not a single instance, and certainly not in the original case of Letievant, could any regeneration be attributed to the procedure. Throughout the entire literature not a single permanent result was to be found. In one or two cases there was improvement, but

Stookey concluded that the improvement occurred in spite of the procedure and not as the result of it.

Regarding Doctor Ashhurst's third case, he could not agree with him that in sectioning the bulbous ends of divided nerves, it is difficult to determine when normal funiculi are reached. There is an essential difference between the central and peripheral end bulbs. In making successive cross-sections of the central end, one first sees one or two funiculi and the number gradually increases until the whole mass of normal funiculi is seen. In the peripheral end, however, one usually sees nothing but white scar tissue in each successive section until one section suddenly exposes a number of normal looking funiculi. In his experience, the question is largely one of understanding the funicular structure of the peripheral nerves and the appearance of normal funiculi.

The much spoken of case of MacKenzie did not prove anything. In his operation a large flap was turned up from the external popliteal and its branches in order to bridge a large defect of the sciatic. Careful study of MacKenzie's reports do not convince one that there was any real regeneration in his case.

SPECIMEN OF BRAIN TUMOR OF UNUSUAL DIMENSIONS REMOVED FROM A CHILD OF SIX YEARS

DR. CHARLES H. FRAZIER, M.D., presented a specimen to the Academy because of its unusual size, because of its peculiar surface markings, and because of the comparatively short duration of any symptomatic evidence of an intracranial growth. The patient, a child six years of age, was perfectly well until within five months of the operation. At that time the following symptoms were observed in the order mentioned: Vomiting, dulness, apathy, hemiplegia and imperfect vision. Upon examination the following clinical features were observed: (1) Head enlarged, suggesting hydrocephalus with distended superficial veins of scalp; (2) papilloedema of 4 D in each eye; (3) spastic hemiplegia, left; (4) convolutional markings of frontal bone.

Operative Record.—The operation was performed at three sittings. At the first the tumor was uncovered, but the enfeebled condition of the child did not seem to warrant further intervention at that time. One week later the flap was reflected and the tumor removed. It was easily differentiated from the surrounding brain tissue and seemed in size to occupy a space at least half as large as one hemisphere. The surface markings were not unlike that of the brain cortex, and those witnessing the operation thought a portion of the hemisphere was being removed. There was comparatively little bleeding until the tumor was finally separated from the falx. Hemorrhage was then profuse and could not be controlled except by pressure with a large cotton tampon. Any attempt to remove this tampon was always attended with recurrent bleeding.

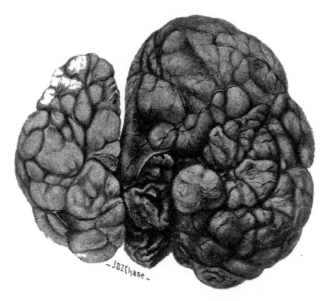

FIG. 1.—An endothelioma of the brain, composed of two sections apparently distinct, the one to the left measuring 7.5 x 4 x 3 cm. and that to the right 10 x 10.5 x 4.5 cm. The surface markings resembled somewhat the cortical convolutions and its capsule a pial membrane.

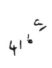

Accordingly the cotton tampon was allowed to remain *in situ* and the wound closed without drainage.

The presence of the large tampon gave rise to no disturbing symptoms until the fourth day, when there was a slight rise in temperature and a convulsive movement of the arm. The patient was taken to the operating room, where under very light ether anæsthesia the flap was again reflected, the dura opened, and the cotton tampon removed. Fortunately there was no recurrence of hemorrhage. The cavity was filled with salt solution and the wound closed for the third time.

Pathological Report.—Endothelioma. Specimen composed of two masses: (1) 10 by 10.5 by 4.5 cm.; (2) 7.5 by 4 by 3 cm. Irregular and nodular, covered with pial-like membrane. Surface convolutional. Interior composed of lobules yellowish gray in color (Fig. 1).

Summary.—Attention is called to the size of the growth; to the fact that despite its size the child was symptom-free until five months before its removal; to the peculiar convolutional markings; to the tolerance of the patient to the three operative sittings, and particularly to the tolerance of the patient to the large tampon of cotton, which replaced the tumor.

CANCER OF BOTH BREASTS

Dr. J. S. Rodman reported a case of sarcoma of the left breast and carcinoma of the right breast in same patient. Double amputation. Subsequent development of mediastinal metastasis. His reasons for reporting the case were: (a) Association of sarcoma and carcinoma in same patient. (b) Unusual length of life considering advanced state of disease. (c) Apparent arrest of mediastinal growth by X-ray.

The patient, a woman forty-six years of age, had known of tumor in left breast for two years. No pain, no trauma, no discharge from nipple, no abscess, but remembers that during first lactation left breast was "sore." Could not nurse second child because she did not have sufficient quantity of milk. Tumor remained about size of English walnut until six months prior to operation. Grew rapidly in this period, during which family physician was treating it with X-rays at first twice weekly and for the last five weeks daily. Was pronounced inoperable by another surgeon six months prior to operation.

Physical Examination.—Large solid tumor mass size of infant's head filling entire left breast. No retraction of nipple. No discharge from nipple. Not tender. Movable on chest wall. Axillary glands palpable.

Operation (October 28, 1910).—Dr. W. L. Rodman. Radical breast amputation, left breast, "Rodman" technic. There was a pathological controversy over the tumor. Two pathologists thought that it was not malignant, but fibro-cyst-adenoma, while the third thought it was unquestionably sarcoma.

In April, 1911, five months after amputation of left breast, she first noticed a small swelling about the size of an English walnut in the lower inner quadrant of the right breast. There has been no increase in size of this tumor mass since first noticed. Breast is painful at times, especially at menses. As was the case with the left breast, there has been no history of trauma, no abscess, or discharge from the nipple. She has noticed a slight retraction of the nipple for the past three months.

Physical examination of right breast shows slight retraction of nipple. There are tender masses throughout the breast tissue, the largest of which is centrally located. Breast freely movable, no discharge from the nipple.

Operation (November 11, 1911).—Amputation of right breast, W. L. Rodman. " Rodman " technic.

Pathological Diagnosis.—Carcinoma of breast. Routine post-operative X-ray treatment following each breast amputation.

About eighteen months after amputation of the left breast and five months after right breast was removed, a bulging of the sternum was first noticed. X-ray showed this to be due to a mediastinal tumor for which she has been under X-ray treatment and observation since. Dr. S. E. Pfaller, who has given the X-ray treatments, states that the mediastinal growth is now calcified. She has gone for one year at a time without X-ray treatment, but is still considered as being under treatment.

Condition at present time, ten years after amputation of the left breast for sarcoma, nine years after amputation of the right breast for carcinoma, and eight and a half years after the mediastinal tumor was first noticed, is reasonably good. Her weight is about normal. The scars of operation show no sign of local recurrence. There is still marked bulging of the sternum, but probably no more marked than when first noticed. For the past six weeks she has had " choking spells " which come on suddenly during which she eructates quantities of gas and from which she gets almost immediate relief after sitting down. Her general physical examination reveals nothing to account for these seizures.

WELCH BACILLUS GANGRENE

Dr. John H. Jopson read a paper with the above title.

Dr. DeForest Willard related a case seen by him in Hospital No. 1 in Paris in which the sera treatment was used in gas gangrene. It was that of a soldier with gunshot wound of the leg in which amputation had already been done in the middle third for gas gangrene. He came in in a distinctly shocked condition, with pulse very high and temperature moderately high. He was perfectly clear mentally. The thigh above the point of amputation was much swollen and very œdematous. The man was in extremis. Previously Professor Vincent, of the French army, whose polyvalent serum was being used exclusively, had given to the hospital staff a talk on his treatment. Professor Vincent was asked to come up and see this case. He gave the man, according to Doctor Willard's recollection, 60 c.c. intravenously. This was at four or five o'clock in the afternoon. The man was then thought to be in extremis. The next morning his pulse was good, below 100; temperature was down, swelling and œdema in his leg had decreased, and he from that time went on to recovery.

ABSCESS OF THE LUNG

Dr. John A. Hartwell read a paper with the above title, for which see page 333.

Doctor Müller said that he had often wondered why abscess has not been more frequently observed after lobar pneumonia. That it is common in cases of pneumonia coming to autopsy was well shown by Lord in 1915. He found abscesses in about one-fifth of the cases of bronchopneumonia and about one-fourth of the cases of lobar pneumonia. He suggests that the clinical infrequency of abscess in lobar pneumonia is more apparent than real and that certain cases of pneumonia are complicated by small losses of pulmonary substance which proceed to full recovery. Doctor Hartwell has shown us how this may occur and quite clearly the etiology of empyema from rupture of the peripheral abscess, a point recently manifested by Doctor Moschcowitz in his several papers. It is necessary to depend to some extent on classification in order to clearly determine in our minds the matter of treatment. Gangrene may be massive from obstruction of its blood supply or minute from the necrotizing action of an acute infection at the point of the abscess. Obstruction by foreign body may result in an abscess with bronchiectasis. Drainage, partial or complete resection, will depend upon the particular type which we encounter.

Dr. Howard Lilienthal said that Doctor Hartwell had shown a magnificent series of lung abscess operated upon by drainage with wonderful success. Other cases he has especially mentioned would probably not be cured by drainage, but only by radical procedures, such as lobectomy. It is my belief that all the abscesses which come from blocking of the bronchi and which are sponge-like are impossible to drain. No patient with a thoroughly established abscess of this kind, which has lasted for more than two months, will be cured by attempted drainage. That patient must be satisfied by such relief as may be afforded by washing out with a bronchoscope, but he has still a progressive disease. To be really cured he must submit to a resection of the lung, which is a dangerous operation. However, when that lung has been resected and the patient has recovered from the operation, he is well. The gangrenous abscesses, as Doctor Hartwell calls them, I have been afraid to operate upon by resection. I have treated them by incision and drainage, with varying results. The chance of curing a case of this kind by drainage is not bad if he withstands the immediate consequences of the operation, but the danger is very, very great in these acute gangrenous abscesses. It had been his custom to watch from day to day with a fluoroscope or with X-ray pictures, and if he saw that they were increasing in size, the patient running septic temperature, he operated, but with a high mortality rate. He did not believe in the indiscriminate aspiration for the purpose of locating an abscess which one wants to operate upon. The X-ray and bronchoscope will locate the abscess without the danger of infecting the chest wall with anaërobes from aspiration puncture. I have recently seen two patients die without operation merely from chest-wall phlegmon following aspiration.

Doctor Hartwell seems to have had very wonderful success by the drainage of these abscesses. In the last six years the speaker had drained twenty-three of these abscesses and had saved 34 per cent. and a fraction. Another 34 per cent. have died and 30 per cent. are alive but not well, not speaking of the bronchiectatic abscesses. Of those he had had eighteen. He had refused none for operation. He had resected the lobe and lost 55 per cent.; the others are well—no cough, no signs of disease. From the therapeutic end of the subject it is important to remember that in the bronchiectatic abscess it is probably wiser even with the big risk to perform resection or removal of a lobe than merely to attempt to drain. I used to drain these cases and lost nearly every one from hemorrhage sooner or later after operation. If an abscess is a very large one and the danger of pneumectomy is too great, an operation has been attempted of ligating the pulmonary artery. There are other procedures which cannot be gone into now. The case which Doctor Hartwell showed in which the lung had apparently disappeared and in which there was a pneumothorax which was not perfectly aseptic but which really closed from the outside, was very illuminating. In a patient of that sort in which he had removed the two lower lobes and part of the upper lobe, and in which the rest of the upper lobe atrophied, the man was perfectly well, but twice has had a reopening with a little discharge from the chest. This closed and the man is now well and at work.

THE MANAGEMENT OF TOXIC GOITRE FROM THE SURGICAL POINT OF VIEW

Dr. CHARLES H. FRAZIER read a paper with the above title, for which see page 155, August, 1920.

Dr. CHARLES N. DOWD remarked that in hearing Doctor Frazier's paper one must be impressed with his method of estimating the patient's strength and then fitting the surgical procedure to it. This is the essence of goitre surgery. The individual surgeon must fit his procedure to the individual patient.

The estimation of the patient's strength depends on clinical observation rather than upon reading. When men write about the grades of toxicity we do not know that their standards are the same. One man's "moderate toxicity" may be another man's "severe toxicity."

Doctor Frazier, in an earlier paper, noted the sparsity of reports from the Atlantic seaboard as compared with the interior of the country. It is possible that different localities differ in type of goitre as well as in its general prevalence, and this difference must be interpreted in planning treatment for the individual patients.

Many observers have adopted a classification which corresponds fairly well with the three main groups of Plummer and Wilson: (1) Non-hyperplastic non-toxic. (2) Non-hyperplastic-toxic. (3) Hyperplastic-toxic.

The groupings on this basis as made by five observers are indicated in the following table:

	I	II	III
Frazier	35.7 per cent.	31.6 per cent.	32.6 per cent.
Wilson and Plummer	43 per cent.	14 per cent.	42 per cent.
Rogers			25 per cent.
The writer (137 hospital cases reported in 1915)	48.1 per cent.	27.5 per cent.	24.4 per cent.
The writer (61 later personal cases)	20 per cent.	55 per cent.	24 per cent.

We thus see that there is considerable variation either in the type of cases or in the interpretation of their toxicity.

Among his later cases the writer has seen many who are either entirely unsuitable for operation or only suitable. For example: (1) A man of forty who had recently come from Ohio with typical symptoms of acute hyperthyroidism, died at his home during the short period which was given to the making of the desirable laboratory tests. (2) A woman of sixty, who had suffered for many years and who had reached the terminal stage of degeneration of the internal organs, was almost moribund when seen and died a few hours later. (3) There were four cases who reacted fairly well to the preliminary ligation of the superior thyroid arteries but who refused, or procrastinated, the secondary operations when the suitable time had arrived, and thus became extremely toxic. (4) There were other cases in whom the diagnosis was not clear. It was doubtful whether the symptoms were really dependent upon the goitre.

It is manifest that the method of dealing with cases must be selected with care and that suitable recourse should be made to X-ray, boiling water injection, rest, medication, anoci procedure, or whatever seems indicated.

Most surgeons must learn some of this by experience. Personally, the writer had developed considerable confidence in the possibility of dealing successfully with the difficult cases by operation, but the procedure was interrupted by three fatalities within two years; one, an extreme case of hyperthyroidism who died under a preliminary ligation, and the other two moderately severe cases who died, one of œdema of the lungs and the other of pneumonia, each two days after operation. These fatalities naturally made a radical revision of standard of operation, and since then it has not been difficult to operate on a continuous series of seventy-six cases without mortality; a series which is not larger when compared with the reports of several other surgeons and which without question embraces a lower average of severe toxicity than does the previous group.

DR. JOHN ROGERS said that he agreed with Doctor Frazier concerning the value of the mechanical tests; that is, they are far from being definite and infallible and to be of any value must be compared with the clinical findings. The calorimeter test which shows the rate of metabolism is the most useful. I was somewhat disappointed in Doctor Frazier's indica_ tions for operation. For it is possible to divide these cases into more or less easily recognizable groups according to the extent and location of the diseased alveoli in the thyroid; and each of these groups can be best treated by its appropriate type of interference. It is now generally accepted that the symptoms of the so-called " toxic " goitres are produced by some abnormal secretion which emanates from certain hyperplastic alveoli. If the diseased tissue is removed the toxic symptoms disappear.

1. When these symptoms occur in the presence of a goitre which is symmetrically enlarged and of even consistency throughout it is presumable that all the hyperplastic tissue cannot be excised unless the entire gland is sacrificed. If one-half or two-thirds of the organ remain this small portion may contain enough hyperplasia to continue the disturbance. In these cases I advise the ligation in two stages of all four of the chief thyroid arteries. My results in several hundreds of such cases show ultimate cures by this operation in the neighborhood of 90 per cent.

2. When one lobe is much larger and denser than the other it is presumable that all or the greater part of the hyperplasia can be removed by excision of the most diseased lobe. In addition, and at the same time, when there is doubt about the remaining lobe, its superior thyroid vessels can be ligated. This limited use of hemithyroidectomy is most satisfactory when one becomes accustomed to examining the gland with a view to the histology of its contents.

3. When the toxic symptoms emanate from the interior or immediate circumference of a toxic adenoma or cystadenoma, the symptoms will disappear almost immediately after enucleation or excision of the adenoma. All the sound tissue possible should be preserved. It is generally immaterial whether at the same time both or one of the superior thyroid vessels are tied. I generally practice this procedure as a precaution against relapse. I wish to protest most emphatically against the present widely accepted advice, to excise in all so-called " toxic " goitres, four-fifths or five-sixths of the gland. In the first place, the symptoms of " toxicity " are by no means well defined nor clearly understood even by the most experienced. In the next, the thyroid gland is far from being a functionally useless or unimportant part of the organism, and experience has abundantly demonstrated that a " toxic " goitre may under indifferent or non-surgical treatment change into a simple or non-

toxic and otherwise symptomless goitre. That is, the hyperplastic alveoli may and can change into the normal type. It is generally understood that these cases will show hypothyroid symptoms at one period and at another, perhaps six months later, show distinct signs of hyperthyroidism. I have observed this so often and in such regular sequence that I have before this called attention to what seems to be the natural history of the disease. It apparently begins with the symptoms and history which are those of fatigue, and it can only be distinguished from simple fatigue by the presence of a perceptible thyroid enlargement. This initial stage may then pass into a true myxœdema or more or less gradually be followed by the signs of so-called hyperthyroidism, to which exophthalmos may or may not be added. If these observations are correct they mean that the patient with hyperthyroidism is suffering not necessarily from too much thyroid but from an abnormal functionation of the thyroid. Such an individual seems to be endowed with, or to have acquired, a thyroid which in attempting to perform its duties "gives out" or "runs amuck." The impulses which thus seem to drive the organ beyond its capacity must in part, at least, reach it through the circulation, and hence it is logical to cut off these impulses and to enforce "rest" upon the gland by ligating its chief afferent vessels. To ruthlessly sacrifice three-fourths or five-sixths of this gland, as is so frequently advised, especially in a patient who gives a history of a longer or shorter period of hypothyroidism preceding that of the hyper stage, is, I am convinced, to inflict in many instances an irreparable calamity. With the prevailing uncertainty in the interpretation of symptoms and the inexperience of the many operators who enter this field, it is far wiser to preach conservation rather than destruction of this important organ. Doctor Frazier failed to discuss, at least at any length, the clinical evidences of "toxicity." In my laboratory studies upon the effects in dogs of the injection of various thyroid extracts and derivatives, the reactions have almost from the outset been recognized as confined to stimulation of the functions believed to be performed by the terminals of the autonomic or vagus system of nerves. The terminals of the opposing or sympathetic system seem never to be affected.

The autonomic system seems to have the general effect, as determined by electrical and chemical experiments, of stimulating vascular and functional activity. The sympathetic terminals, on the other hand, apparently have the opposite effect, or that of inhibition of vascular and functional activity. Adrenalin and all derivatives of the adrenal gland which contain adrenalin are accepted as having a selective and stimulant affinity for this particular group. In general, therefore, the autonomic nerve terminals with their affinity for the thyroid product, may be said to "drive" the viscera, while the sympathetic adrenal combination shows an opposing or "check" influence. Hence, in the presence of an overacting thyroid gland there is evidence in the skin, circulation, and viscera of too much " drive." If the thyroid is underactive there is an apparent insufficiency of " drive "—tachycardia is directly traceable to the influence, not of the vagus, but of the sympathetic nerve, and in my laboratory tests I have never found any normal or pathological thyroid derivatives which would, within the usual period of a few hours necessary for kymograph tracings, excite any appreciable degree of tachycardia. If, however, the thyroid feeding is continued for many days the result corresponds to the accepted dogma. Then there does follow tachycardia and increased metabolism. This does not prove that the thyroid activates the sympathetic. It seems more probable that the tachycardia is due to acceleration of the entire bodily chemistry, and perhaps directly to increased metabolism of the heart muscle itself. Hence, one should at least be cautious in believing that every case of tachycardia with a " goitre " requires the destruction of the greater part of the supposedly offending thyroid gland.

To Contributors and Subscribers :

All contributions for Publication, Books for Review, and Exchanges should be sent to the Editorial Office, 145 Gates Ave., Brooklyn, N. Y.

Remittances for Subscriptions and Advertising and all business communications should be addressed to the

ANNALS *of* SURGERY
227-231 S. 6th Street
Philadelphia. Penna.

ANNALS *of* SURGERY

Vol. LXXII	OCTOBER, 1920	No. 4.

THE INDICATIONS FOR ACTIVE IMMEDIATE MOBILIZATION IN THE TREATMENT OF JOINT INJURIES *

By Ch. Willems, M.D.

of Liége, Belgium

COLONEL IN THE ARMY OF BELGIUM; PROFESSOR OF CLINICAL SURGERY IN THE UNIVERSITY OF LIÉGE

I do not consider it necessary to review in detail the technic and results of this method, all of which I have already published in full in the Transactions of the Interallied Conference on War Surgery, in the *Bulletin of the Societé de Chirurgie de Paris*, the *Bulletin of the Académie de Médecine de Paris*, the *Archives Medicales Belges*, the *Bulletin of the Académie de Médecine de Belgique*, and in *Surgery, Gynæcology and Obstetrics*, the *Medical Record*, etc.

But I learn by a perusal of the published observations of other surgeons, that the method is almost never correctly applied. They content themselves with partial results, because these greatly excel anything obtained by the old classical methods of treatment. But this is not sufficient. In purulent arthritis, for example, it does not suffice to conserve mobility; it is necessary to prevent entirely, or almost entirely, the muscular atrophy. If muscular atrophy is present as a result, it means that the movements have been commenced too late, have been too infrequent or have not been continued long enough.

Frequently the authors indicate that these patients with purulent arthritis have begun active movements, but have been obliged to discontinue them, not having the power to execute them at a given moment. In these cases one ordinarily finds evidences of pus retention, the result of insufficient mobilization. To remedy this it is necessary, instead of stopping the movements, either to enlarge the incisions, which are often too small, or to make the movements more complete. It should be emphasized that a minimum amount of pocketing of pus suffices to arrest voluntary movements.

Further, the patient always attempts at the beginning to escape the obligation of movement, which he regards as a disagreeable task. I am not able to insist sufficiently on the capital importance of having at one's disposal a personal nursing attendant, devoted to duty, and thoroughly familiar with the method, as it is on the nursing of the wounded man that the success in great part depends.

---

* Read by title before the American Surgical Association, May 3, 1920.

What are the indications as to active mobilization in the wounds of joints *complicated by fracture?* In my early publications I have said that the method was not applicable to extensively comminuted fracture of joints when the lines of fracture extended to the diaphysis. Since then the facts have made me admit that we may employ it in all fractures of joints, whatever the extent of the lesions, although, it must be understood, in a modified form. In the elbow, for example, the major fractures admit perfectly of treatment by active limited movements. It is true the movements do not maintain the fragments in perfect reduction, but the fragments are disengaged, pushed back from the interarticular space, and a sufficient regularity of the articular surfaces preserved to insure a certain range of mobility, much better than one could secure by immobilization. In certain cases the result can be improved later by the removal of an osseous spur which constitutes a mechanical obstacle.

Surgical fixation of the fragments which reëstablishes at once the physiological conditions may render great service in these cases, but not when the lesion involves the cartilage, because in war wounds osteosynthesis is often followed by hyperostosis.

If the articular wound is complicated by infection in addition to fracture, mobilization is still more strongly indicated, as it alone can give drainage, which is not perfect by reason of necessary limitation of the movements, but in all cases superior to that accompanying immobilization. Osteosynthesis in the midst of infection may facilitate the movements, but the plates will have to be removed secondarily.

With a fractured knee it is evident that it is not a question of having the patient walk immediately, but mobilization in bed is possible, especially if one adds thereto a continuous extension which furnishes a certain fixation to the fragments, as well as a point of application for muscular action. This mixed method of treatment of articular wounds complicated by major fractures, by extension combined with active movements, gives functional results far superior to those obtained by other methods.

Let us examine now as to whether intra-articular fractures with destruction and removal of a large fragment of the epiphysis admit of treatment by mobilization. I am speaking now of cases where one-third or more of a condyle has been lost. In these cases the danger lies in a lateral bowing of the joint. This danger is especially present at the knee, where lesions of this nature have been considered heretofore as calling for immediate resection. I believe that this is an error. In the elbow in cases treated conservatively after this manner, with active mobilization, I have seen sufficient strength to render good service. I have seen the knee readapt itself rapidly, permitting the patient to walk and use the joint with flexion and without pain. Sometimes it is necessary to protect the limb with a jointed brace, but at the same time the condition in walking is far superior to that accompanying an ankylosis. If unfortunately the result should turn out unsatisfactorily, there is always the opportunity to practice secondary orthopædic resection.

I emphasize then that bony lesions constitute no contraindication to active mobilization, and that in such cases they give unhoped-for success.

I am now at the last class of injuries, comprising extensive destruction of the tissues uniting the joints, especially the ligaments, and particularly the anterior and crucial ligaments of the knee-joints. Whether their destruction is primary or consecutive to joint suppuration does not seem to me to interdict all movement. In cases of this type observed recently, whether accompanied by section of the patellar ligament or by destruction of the crucial ligaments, which have been treated with continuous extension combined with active movements, I have seen a correction of the posterior subluxation of the tibia, and have obtained a cure with partial conservation of movement, even in the presence of a simultaneous purulent arthritis. It must be understood that such treatment demands unremitting attention and perseverance on the part of surgeon and nurses.

In a résumé of the actual state of the question, I estimate that active mobilization knows no contraindications by reason of extent of bony lesions, or extent of destruction of the ligaments. I would urge surgeons not to abandon the method at the first difficulty, but, on the contrary, to pursue it to the end, with the conviction that the functional result will be the more brilliant in the same proportion as the efforts to obtain it have been more energetic and tenacious.

ON FRACTURES OF THE FOREARM IN THE REGION OF THE WRIST

WITH SPECIAL REFERENCE TO THE DIFFERENT TYPES OF RADIUS FRACTURE, THEIR MANNER OF ORIGIN AND MECHANISM *

By Abraham Troell, M.D.

of Stockholm, Sweden

In some papers published within the last few years I have devoted my attention to the question of the treatment of the typical radius fracture—*fractura radii classico loco*. I have therein spoken of my own experiences in consecutive cases during the year 1911, amounting in all to rather more than 200. The essential value of this material was the uniformity with which it was followed, and also the completeness with which it was röntgenologically examined (by Professor G. Forssell and his assistants). That I am now returning to these cases is due chiefly to the fact that they offer no few details of röntgenanatomical interest. For, from an anatomical point of view, they represent, taken altogether, a fairly complete variety of the different types of fractures. And, from a clinical point of view, the röntgenological facts are calculated, if arranged together with certain anamnestic and other data in the records (the kind of trauma, patient's age, stage of development of the respective part of the skeleton, etc.), to facilitate to some degree the understanding of the genesis and mechanism of origin of the radius fracture.

With regard to the question of the different anatomical types of the radius fracture—it is not difficult to prove that our knowledge of the subject has hitherto been unsatisfactory. Up to now the literature obtainable has been lacking among other things in uniform and rational principles of classification for radius fracture, and this, not only when comparing the works of different, yea, even responsible and very experienced authorities, with each other, but also when taking separate cognizance of the statements of individual authors. I will give two examples, both of recent year's date.

Kaufmann divides (the year 1912) radius fractures into the following groups:

I. Radius fracture without dislocation of the place of fracture.

II. Radius fracture with dislocation of the place of fracture.

    1. Transverse and oblique fractures.

        a. Automobilist fractures.

        b. The volar displacement of the peripheral fragments (so-called Smith-Linhartscher type).

    2. Comminute fractures.

---

* From the Surgical and Röntgenological departments of the Serafimer Hospital in Stockholm (Sweden).

428

3. The fracture of the ulnar styloid process.

4. The fracture of the ulnar margin of the radius.

Pilcher, on the contrary, treats (year 1917) the same chapter by dividing it up under the following headings:

a. Perpendicular wedge-like impact of the carpus against the articular cup of the base of the radius.

b. Splitting of the lower fragment by descent into it of the lower end of the upper fragment.

Explosive splitting of lower fragment of radius.

Backward displacement of lower fragment of radius.

Outward displacement of lower fragment.

Anterior displacement of the lower fragment.

Epiphysial separations.

Dorsal untorn periosteum.

Incomplete fractures.

Fracture of the ulnar styloid process.

Associated fracture of the carpal bones.

Associated injuries to the periarticular structures and diastasis of the ulna.

As to the manner of origin and mechanism of radius fracture—it is on the one hand natural that the conception thereof must be built on a due regard not only to the nature of the trauma, but also to the stage of development and solidity of the part of the extremity in question. But, on the other hand, it is remarkable that such regard in the literature on the subject is hitherto either not taken at all, or at most but in incomplete fashion.

The mechanism of the typical radius fracture has been interpreted in various ways. Already at an early period it was established that the fracture arises through a fall on the prone and extended hand, or through other violence having the same effect MacLeod [1] speaks of a case which illustrates the origin of such a fracture with almost the lucidity of an experiment. It concerned a young man who had injured himself whilst boxing with an older and stronger man. The fingers of both of them were entwined in each other's, and the palm of each was pressed hard against the other one's in prone direction. The hand of the younger man was strained to the uttermost and was forced at last to give way, this resulting in violent pains and a typical radius fracture with the usual bayonet deformity. Pilcher relates in connection with the above some characteristic cases of his own. In one of these a woman who was standing on a chair in front of a table slipped, and in falling managed with the fingers only of her one outstretched hand to catch hold of the latter. Her hand was thereby bent violently backwards and a typical radius fracture ensued. Another patient injured himself through letting the weight of a packing-case, which he together with an assistant was to carry down a flight of stairs and which he was nearly about to drop, rest for an instant on his dorsally deflected hand alone. Amongst my own printed matter there occur—which may already be mentioned in this connection—various cases where the details at the moment of fractures are fairly lucidly described. For instance, patient 148 who received a hard blow in the hollow of his hand from a pick-axe, so that the forearm was bent forcibly in dorsal direction (Group IIa). Or amongst other cases 81 (see under Id), cases 54 and 72 (see under IIc), case 27 (see under IId) and the cases 110, 113 (see IIa), case 99 (see IIb), case 76 (see IIc), and case 164 (see IId), the last five being chauffeur fractures.

The theoretical explanation of how the violence thus described may be thought to lead to fracture has, during different periods, given entirely different results.

At first it was more often than not concluded that the radius fracture was a *compression-fracture*, i.e., was caused by the violent pressure of two forces operating in opposite directions to each other (coup et contrecoup). [Dupuytren,[1] Goyrand,[2] Nélaton,[3] and Middeldorph,[4] etc.] The post-mortem experiment by which Nélaton tried to illustrate this theory is well known. The forearm exarticulated in the elbow-joint was placed vertically with the hand extended maximally and resting on a firm support. After sawing off the olecranon a strong blow with a hammer was given on the upper end of the bone of the forearm and the result obtained was, as a rule, radius fracture in the typical area. The clinical analogy to the procedure was thought to be thus, that the forearm when the outstretched hollow of the hand through a fall forwards touched the ground, formed a right angle to the hand, and that the proximal carpal bones ranged themselves as a valve against the support; the weight of the falling body pressed the radius against this valve, with the consequence that either the latter or the radius gave way and broke; if the valve was the stronger, radius fracture set in.

The most usual contrary theory interprets the radius fracture in quite another way as *wrench* (tearing) *fracture*. Already suggested by Bouchet[5] and others, it was completely formulated by Lecomte. Besides the clinical explanation, the latter based his opinions concerning same on the negative result of Nélaton's post-mortem experiment if made after intersection of the ligamentum radiocarpeum volare. [If, however, the radius by this latter experiment is always fixed in the manner described by Brossard, i.e., so that the lower radius epiphysis is not luxated in dorsal direction during the execution of the experiment, then radius fracture ensues (Destot and Gallois).] This opinion has since been accepted in the main by the generality of authors, eventually with certain modifications, such, for instance, as Löbkers, who interprets many of these fractures as pure wrench (tearing) fractures, and with regard to certain of them is of the opinion that "they are caused solely from coup et contrecoup; the typical oblique fracture on the base of the bone ensues through a combined action of both forces mentioned together."

Lastly, Hennequin's theory (resembling that of Nélaton) may be called to mind in this connection, and, on the other hand, those theories which might be called essentially terminological variations to be found in many authors on this subject. I allude here amongst others first, to Helferich's treatise wherein the typical radius fracture is designated as a simultaneous wrenching and snapping (Abknickungs) fracture, caused by drawing on the tightly knit volar radiocarpal ligament, and at the same time violent impact of the proximal carpus against the dorsal margin of the base of the radius. Secondly, I refer to Kuhn's argument, which being interpreted, means that the radius fracture is not a wrench fracture, but a "*Quetschbruch.*" Without going into further details here, I will but express my doubts as to increased perspicuity on the question of the mechanism of radius fracture being gained in this way. The best prospects therefor are obtained by keeping, as far as possible, to the limited, generally prevailing conception of that part of the science of fractures in question—wrench, compression, flexion and torsion fractures—avoiding terms the eventual relation of which to those mentioned is more or less obscure.

A short statement of the purpose of each of the four terms given is to be found amongst others in the author's work on leg fracture. The fact is, however, not therein mentioned that the principal differences between flexion and compression fractures do not need under every circumstance to be so great, that, in other words, in many injuries it is a question of a combination of flexion fracture and (longitudinal) compression fracture. As the drawing to the right in Fig. A shows, a flexion fracture can arise among other things through a strong compression from end to end of a tubular bone with the shape of a crooked staff. The fracturing begins superficially in the cortex on the vertex of the convexity of the bone, whereas the fracture line

FRACTURES OF THE WRIST

afterwards often appears broadest and takes a more or less transverse course. The fracture arises through a disjointing ("Zugspannung") of the different bone particles on the convexity in a longitudinal direction of the bone and towards each of the both ends of the bone, whilst a simultaneous compression ("Druckspannung") coming from the ends of the bone takes place on the bone particles situated on the concavity. In the same degree as the bone in question exposed to violence has from the beginning more the form of a straight than a crooked staff, so is the disjointing component moved from the convex side to the concave, and the compressing component from the concave to the convex. Both components become completely inverted in the event of a flexion fracture arising in the manner shown in the sketch to the left in Fig. A, and this, whether it be a question of a straight or crooked bone. The compression fracture—the character of which is more complicated than flexion fracture—likewise arises under influence of two equally strong forces acting against each other. If the violence concerns a bone which consists mainly of spongiose tissue, e.g., the distal radius epiphysis, then this individual spongiose lamella will be curved, outward bent and eventually fractured, with an intermediary beginning and at first-hand—if it is a question of longitudinal compression—the fracture line longitudinally extended (Fig. B). Has the bone—in this case radius diaphysis—a strong compact, i.e., if it reacts against the trauma in the same manner as a hollow cylinder, then the longitudinal compression ("Stauchung"—Zuppinger), if it continues after the longitudinal fissure has set in, may lead to further fracturing. The latter begins then apparently on the vertex of the already curved convexity of the bone lamellæ (at a and b in Fig. B), thus at the ends of the longitudinal fissure, and continues transversely out towards the surface of the diaphysis, so that a more or less comminute fragment is broken off (according to what is schematically shown in the drawing to the right in Fig. B).

The fractures of flexion, which form the chief part of all fractures, occur in reality most often during simultaneous longitudinal compression, and that more so "because the muscular system extending over the bones violently contracts at the moment of danger" (Zuppinger); that such is the case is shown by the argument just quoted from Zuppinger regarding the effect of the disjointing of the single bone particles on the one side of the bone and the compression on the other. Concerning the nature of the anatomical effect of the violence, even the following circumstance may have some influence—as far as I can understand, in many cases and more especially in the bone of a young person—namely, that the periosteum on account of its considerable relative strength can prevent the fracturing on the vertex of the bone convexity which constitutes the first beginning of the fracture of flexion (see drawing to the right in Fig. A); and thus the continuation of the influence of the trauma is established predominating according to the theories of compression fracture. Finally, with reference to the bone of the young, it must be remembered that it is more elastic, less brittle and therefore offers more resistance to a longitudinal compression than is the case with that of an adult. Thus, before or instead of a longitudinally acting trauma on the bone leading to a longitudinal fracturing, there may be in the case of the young, only that change in the form take place which—according to Zuppinger —"we are accustomed to see as a consequence of stooking (stauchung) in plastic bodies; a circular torus formation which with some amount of reason may be called torus-fracture." (Quervain's and Iselin's stauchung fracture on the epiphysis of the young, the Frenchman's fracture par tassement).

To what has been said here concerning flexion and compression fracture statics may finally, for the sake of completion, be given a definition of wrench-fracture. It is brought about under the influence of two equally strong parallel forces acting in opposite directions to each other. It begins where this disjointing influence first exceeds the elastic power of the bone and passes in the simplest imaginable, fully typical cases rectangularly towards the direction of the pulling (wrenching). It is false to talk about pure wrench fractures in those cases where it is a question of two disjointing

431

ABRAHAM TROELL

but not parallel forces, *i.e.*, in patella fracture or—above all—typical radius fracture (Zuppinger).

I will now return after this deviation to my own material. In the enclosed table I have arranged a concentrated grouping thereof. How the injury in individual cases develops is more completely shown by the following statement (from want of space the records are not given in detail).

I. FOREARM FRACTURES IN THE REGION OF THE WRIST IN INDIVIDUALS WITH INCOMPLETE OSSIFICATION (54 CASES)

A. Transverse Fracture of Radius and Ulna (Figs. 1 and 2, Case 129).— The group embraces 13 cases, the ages of the patients varying from four to thirteen years, with an average age of eight years.[1] In 10 of them both the radius and ulna were with certainty injured (Cases 4, 69, 107, 129, 137, 150, 153, 155, 163, 197), in three was ulna presumably, but according to X-ray plate not with certainty, injured (Cases 109, 169, 199; in the last-mentioned case there was in all probability epiphysial separation in the ulna). The fracture line was transversal (Case 153), somewhat oblique, and lay 2–5 cm. above the radiocarpal joint.[2]

Cases 163, 169 and 199 (respectively, twelve, thirteen, and seven years) have somewhat the appearance of a typical radius fracture with the distal fracture fragment pressed in dorsal and proximal direction and impacted in the diaphysis.

The trauma causing the same was in the case of all the patients a fall (down stairs, from a swing, or such like). One patient (Case 197) had, whilst bob-sleighing, struck his right hand against a tree with such force that the arm thereby came into a rectangular position at the site of fracture. Patient 129 was stated to have been injured by the fall through direct violence to the arm.

B. Torus Fracture of the Radius, Eventually with Simultaneous Ulna Lesion (Figs. 3 and 4, Case 100; Fig. 5, Case 167; Figs. 6 and 7, Case 178).— The group embraces 12 cases with the age of the patients from four to fourteen years and an average age of ten years. In 6 of the patients both bones of the forearm were injured (Cases 20, 57, 100, 167, 186, 194), in 6 only fracture of the radius could be radiologically diagnosed (Cases 19, 101, 147, 178, 181, 187). The radius fracture lay 2½–4¾ cm. above the radiocarpal joint.

The radius lesion appeared—apart from Case 167, where the frontal plate showed a limited transversal thinning in the lateral two-thirds of the bone and which therefore should be placed in group C—as a torus (folding) in the cortex which on the X-ray plate was seen to lie only radially in Case 20; only dorsally in Cases 100 and 101; both radially and dorsally in Cases 147, 167, 181, and 194; in radial, dorsal and ulnar direction in Cases 19 and 57; in radial, volar, and ulnar direction in Cases 178, 186, and 187.

The ulnar lesion was observed as a transverse fissure in Cases 20 and

194; oblique fissure in Cases 57 and 167; epiphysial separation (presumably) in Cases 186 and 187; fracture of the apex itself in Case 100.

The trauma had been caused by a fall in the case of all the patients except one (Case 20, nine years of age), where a play-fellow had wrung him violently by the hand; patient 178 (thirteen years of age) had fallen over whilst cycling, and according to his own statement had, in falling, tried to stop himself with his hand in volar direction. The site of cortex folding (tassement)—also in volar direction—is with regard to anamnestics of interest in this case as in that of patients 186 and 187 (fourteen years of age, right and left arm injured in same individual). The latter had, seven days previous to first visit to hospital, fallen over whilst cycling and driven both hands into the ground. On the day of the visit he had slipped in the street and in falling had his hands extended dorsally.

C. *Transverse or Oblique Fracture with Simultaneous Visible Cortex Torus* (Figs. 8 and 9, Case 111; Figs. 10 and 11, Case 131; Fig. 12, Case 111a; Figs. 13 and 14, Case 131a).—The group embraces 9 patients of an age of from four to eighteen years (average age eleven years). In all of these—possibly with exception of Case 191—were both bones of the forearm injured, the fracture lay 1½–5¼ cm. above the wrist.

Röntgenanatomically the injury was of following character:

Case 23.—Transverse fracture of both bones with suggestion of dorsal cortex torus (folding) on the radius and ulnar (medial) on the ulna.

Case 132.—Transverse fracture of both bones with the ulna fissure broadest on the ulnar and volar side, and radial (lateral) and dorsal cortex torus (folding) of the radius.

Case 111.—Transverse fracture of the radius (which was curved with the concavity in dorsal direction) which began on the volar side (where fissure was broadest) and radially; cortical folding on the dorsal and ulnar side of the ulna which was curved with the concavity on the dorsal side.

Case 111a.—Oblique fracture of the radius with the dorsal concavity and with the fissure broadest on the ulnar side; slight radial and dorsal cortex torus (folding) of the ulna which was curved with radial and dorsal concavity.

Case 191.—Oblique fracture of the radius with the fissure broadest on the ulnar and volar side and folding on the radial side; presumably epiphysial separation of the ulna.

Case 106.—Transverse fracture of the ulna, beginning on the ulnar side (?) and cortex torus (folding) on the radius radially (?) and dorsally.

Case 154.—Oblique fracture of ulna with cortex torus (folding) radially; transverse fracture of radius with cortex torus (folding) dorsally and radially.

Case 131.—Transverse fissure in the radius (broadest on the ulnar side) with cortex torus dorsally and radially; fracture of the apex of the ulnar styloid process.

433

Case 131a.—Transverse fissure in the radius with cortical bone torus (creasing, folding) radially, dorsally, and ulnarally; epiphysial separation—atypical, with small oblique diaphysis crack radially—in the ulna, the fracture line presumably broadest on the ulnar side.

The trauma had been caused in the case of all these patients by a fall (from hammock, tram, and so on), whereby the patient had tried to help himself with his hands.

D. *Epiphysial Separation* (Fig. 15, Case 83; Figs. 16 and 17, Case 156; Figs. 18 and 19, Case 128).—Hereto belong 16 patients of an age from nine to eighteen years (average age fourteen years). In 3 cases only (Cases 25, 128, and 156) was it evident that the ulna was also injured; in the remaining 13 only radius lesion was observable (Cases 63, 81, 83, 88, 95, 119, 120, 142, 143, 146, 162, 166, and 174). In the one (Case 128) of the three first-named patients it was a question of an epiphysial separation even in the ulna, in another (Case 156) no change in the ulna could be discovered on the first plate but a couple of weeks later a distinct callus was found.

In Cases 83, 88, and 120 there was nothing at all abnormal to be discovered on the front-view photograph, whilst the lateral-view photograph showed dorsal displacement on the fracture area. It was identically the same in the case of patient 95, apart from the fact that there, even as in Cases 146 and 162, there occurred an unevenness of the cortex in the vicinity of the epiphysial line. Case 166 showed after replacement nothing röntgenologically abnormal. Case 128 offered, besides the already mentioned character of the ulna lesion, interest with regard to the appearance of the radius injury: close to the epiphysial line a little triangular fragment had been dorsally torn off; similar discoveries were made in Cases 146 and 156.

The trauma causing the fracture was a fall (forwards, backwards, etc.) in all the patients except one (Case 81). The latter's injury was brought about by his hand fastening between a banister and the wall.

E. *Typical Radius Fracture* (Fig. 20, Case 114; Fig. 21, Case 170; Figs. 22 and 23, Cases 151 and 152).—The group embraces four patients of an age from sixteen to eighteen years (average seventeen and one-half years). In the case of patient 114 the ulnar styloid process was also fractured, in the others only radius. The fracture of the radius lay 2¼–3½ cm. above the wrist.

In Cases 114 and 170 the fracture had quite an ordinary appearance. The latter offered a special interest inasmuch as the epiphysial line there appeared broad and distinct (and yet the break in the bone had not occurred there, but in close proximity). In patients 151 and 152—the left respectively right hand of the same individual—there occurred together with the transverse fracture an intra-articular splitting of the distal fracture fragment.

The trauma was caused by a fall in patients 114, 151, and 152. With regard to patient 170, it was a case of direct violence (suggesting the same manner of origin as in fracture of flexion) : the patient had had the dorsum of his forearm trampled on by a horse.

II. FOREARM FRACTURES IN THE REGION OF THE WRIST IN INDIVIDUALS WITH COMPLETE OSSIFICATION (152 CASES[3])

A. Typical Radius Fracture (Figs. 24 and 15, Case 204; Figs. 26 and 27, Case 130; Fig. 28, Case 134; Fig. 29, Case 71; Fig. 30, Case 24; Fig. 31, Case 67; Fig. 32, Case 168; Fig. 33, Case 207; Fig. 34, Case 211; Fig. 35, Case 115; Fig. 36, Case 90; Fig. 37, Case 209; Figs. 38 and 39, Case 52; Figs. 40 and 41, Case 42; Fig. 42, Case 7; Figs. 43 and 44, Case 53; Figs. 45 and 46, Case 113; Fig. 47, Case 10; Figs. 48 and 49, Case 104).—In this group are included 104 patients of an age from twenty-one to seventy-five years of age (average age forty-eight and four-fifths years).

In 64 cases (61.5 per cent.) the ulna was injured as well as the radius; most often in such wise that the ulnar styloid process was fractured, but three times (Cases 10, 104, and 200, Figs. 47 and 49) so that a transverse or oblique fracture was present at the base of the capitulum ulnæ at the same height as the radius fracture, and about 1 cm. above the styloid process. In 4 of the cases with the ulnar styloid process broken off (Cases 74, 77, 78, and 84) this lesion could not be röntgenologically diagnosed until a photograph was taken later on, when a distinct callus or such like betrayed its whereabouts. In 3 of the patients with ulnar styloid process fracture (Cases 58, 70, and 78) there also occurred, judging by röntgen pictures, an abnormally wide diastasis in distal radio-ulnar connection; a positive one of the same kind was, moreover, observed in 4 cases (Cases 61, 62, 68, and 93), a probable one in 2 cases (Cases 90 and 204, in which two the ulnar styloid process was off) (see Figs. 24 and 36).

The radius fracture lay 1½–3½ cm. above the radiocarpal joint in all cases, except one where this distance amounted to 6½ cm. (Case 113, Figs. 45 and 46); in 80 cases, the whole group included in the calculation, the position was 2–2½ cm. above the joint.

Röntgenanatomically the injury appeared when in its simplest and most typical form as a transverse fracture of the radius without dislocation and situated 2 cm. above radiocarpal joint (Case 204, Fig. 24); sometimes with a splitting or smashing of the bone (Cases 130 and 134, Figs. 26 to 28), in some cases even so that small cracks radially (Cases 71 and 24, Figs. 29 and 30) or ulnarally (Case 67, Fig. 31—a triangular fragment broken off) were to be seen. The lateral view shows distinctly the course of the fracture line and the absence (Case 204, Fig. 25—the periosteum appears to be untorn) or the more or less expressed presence of dorsal dislocation (Cases 168, 207, and 211, Figs. 32 to 34), eventually, also, the occurrence of a splitting of the radial dorsal labrum (Case 115, Fig. 35). In other cases (Cases 90, 52, and 209, Figs. 36 to 39) the course of the fracture line is fairly straight, but the distal fracture fragment, without pronounced wedging, markedly displaced in radial and dorsal direction; or there is a considerable typical dislocation together with impaction (Case 42, Figs. 40 and 41), or the fracture line appears in the front-view photograph something like the form of an inverted S, but without dislocation (Cases 7 and 53, Figs. 42 and 43). Already mentioned is Case 113 (Figs. 45 and 46), which concerns a transverse fracture lying considerably higher up on the radius, as well as those cases (Cases 10, 104, and 200, Figs. 47 to 49) where not only the ulnar styloid process is broken off, but where there is a question of a transverse or oblique fracture immediately above capitulum ulnæ. Furthermore, it is interesting to note, firstly, Cases 134 and 113 (Figs. 28 and 46) which show a fold in the cortex reminding one of a cortical torus in the young—which view may possibly have originated partly through reposition measures—secondly, some cases in which a greater breadth of the fissure on the volar side (Cases 11, 207, and 211, Figs. 33 and 34) and on the radial side (Case 113, Fig. 45) is quite obvious.

In all cases but Case 14 the injury has been caused by a fall (from ladder, on smooth ice, backwards, etc.). The patient (Case 171) got a fracture whilst escaping from an encounter with the police; patients 110 and 113—chauffeurs—got a blow when cranking an automobile from the rebound of the winch; Case 148 through bending (see page 434).

Besides the 19 cases reproduced, the following 85 patients have been reckoned to this group: Thirty-two cases of about same appearance as Case 204, namely, 3, 8, 12, 18, 22, 36, 38, 45, 49, 56, 61, 64, 66, 75, 78, 98, 110, 112, 118, 121, 122, 125, 133, 148, 149, 161, 171 to 173, 180, 182, and 184. Four cases with appearance as Case 130 (Cases 124, 139, 140, and 158), and Case 11, most resembling Cases 130 and 42. One case like 134 (192). Six cases like Case 71 (Cases 70, 82, 84, and 93, somewhat impacted in the lateral-view photograph, 188, and 198). One case like Case 24 (51). Two cases like Case 67 (68 and 115 [some splitting]). One case like Case 90 (89). One case like Case 52 (108). Eighteen cases like Case 42 (5, 21, 32, 33, 50, 58, 59, 62, 65, 79, 80, 92, 117, 165, 179, 190, 203, and 208) and Case 13, most closely resembling Cases 42 and 10. Two cases like Case 7 (2 and 136). Nine cases like Case 10 (1, 9, 44, 47, 48, 74, 126, 183, and 196) and Cases 30, 37, 73, and 138, most closely resembling Cases 10 and 204. Two cases like Case 104 (105 and 200).

B. Radius Fracture with Longitudinal Fissures, too, Extending into the Radiocarpal Joint (Fig. 50, Case 159; Fig. 51, Case 29; Fig. 52, Case 210; Fig. 53, Case 15; Fig. 54, Case 99; Fig. 55, Case 97; Figs. 56 and 57, Case 40; Fig. 58, Case 157; Figs. 59 and 60, Case 17; Figs. 61 and 62, Case 17a; Fig. 63, Case 55; Figs. 64 and 65, Case 118a).—The group comprises 28 patients of an age from twenty-four to sixty-nine years of age (average age forty-eight and two-fifth years). In 18 of them (64.3 per cent.) the ulnar styloid process was most certainly injured (this even as in the foregoing group was occasionally only to be verified by an X-ray photograph taken a week or two after the injury). In 4 of the patients with ulnar styloid process fractures (Cases 31, 77, 159, and 210) the X-ray photograph showed a distal radio-ulnar diastasis, which was also observed in some cases with uninjured ulna (Cases 91, 99, 123, and 202) (see Figs. 50 and 54). The position of the radius fracture was 1½–6½ cm. above the radiocarpal joint, one case respectively of 1½, 4¼, 5, and 6½ cm., and 24 cases of from 1¾–3¼ cm.

The picture varied röntgenanatomically, inasmuch as the intra-articular longitudinal fracturing sometimes assumed an ulnar position (Cases 159, 29, 210, 15, and 99, Figs. 50 to 54) and sometimes lay right in between the lateral and medial edges of the radius (Case 97, Fig. 55), or radially (Case 40, Fig. 56), or finally was observed in several places all along the frontal joint surface (Case 157, Fig. 58). Several times longitudinal fissures were verified, even proximally to the transverse fracture (Cases 17, 17a, and 118a, Figs. 59 to 62, and 64 and 65); in a couple of patients a violent splitting in both the dorso-ventral and lateral view (Cases 55 and 118a, Figs. 63 to 65).

The trauma was a fall—through slipping, from a ladder, in lift-cage, etc.—in all cases except Case 55 (Fig. 63), where the patient was run over by a cartload of wood (effect of direct violence), and Case 99 (Fig. 54), a chauffeur who got a blow from the rebound of the winch when cranking an automobile.

Besides the 12 cases reproduced, the following 16 cases belong to this group: Seven with about same appearance as Case 29, namely, 6, 31, 39, 77, 91, 94, and 123. One with about same appearance as Case 15, namely, 189. Three with about same appearance as Case 99, namely, 141, 145, and 202. Three with about the same appearance as Case 40, namely, 43, 102, and 135. One with about same appearance as Case 157, namely, 175. One with about same appearance as Case 17, namely, 41.

C. Fracture of the Radius Styloid Process (Fig. 66, Case 76; Fig. 67, Case 85; Fig. 68, Case 86; Fig. 69, Case 87; Fig. 70, Case 103).—To this group belong 14 patients of an age from twenty to fifty-six years of age (average age 35 and four-tenth years). In 3 of them (21.4 per cent.) even fracture of ulnar styloid process occurred. In one (Case 76, Fig. 66)—without visible ulnar lesion—a distal radio-ulnar diastasis was observed. Röntgenanatomically there was an intra-articular fracturing of a bone fragment, in frontal view of triangular shape and lying towards the lateral edge of the radius. The fracture line went from about the middle of the joint surface, slanting upwards and outwards to 1½–2½ cm. (in 11 patients 1¾–2¼ cm.) above the tip of the radius styloid process. In the lateral view the injury likewise appeared as a triangular fracturing, reaching in volar direction from about 1½ cm. above the joint level, obliquely, dorsally, and distally to the edge of the joint level (Case 87, Fig. 69), or a small bone fragment was seen only dorsally and distally broken off (Case 103, Fig. 70).

The fracture has in the majority of cases arisen through a fall. The exceptions are patient 76 (Fig. 66), a chauffeur, who got a blow from the rebound of a winch when cranking an automobile, and Case 86 (Fig. 68) who was run over by a taxi, and Cases 54 and 72. Case 54 came underneath a wheelbarrow and was severely jammed from beneath by pressure in the thumb grip, whilst the elbow was pressed forcibly upwards and backwards against a plank. Case 72 had been jammed between a plank, against which his elbow was supported, and an iron beam in the flat of the hand, so that a heavy pressure was exercised in the direction of the forearm. A statement regarding the nature of the trauma in Cases 14 and 34 is lacking.

Besides the 5 cases reproduced by X-ray photographs there are the following 9 cases which belong to this group: Four cases closely resembling Case 76 (54, 60, 72, and 176). Five cases closely resembling Case 85 (14, 26, 34, 185, and 195).

D. *Epiphysial Separation* (Fig. 71, Case 27; Figs. 72 and 73, Case 116).— To this group belong six patients of an age from twenty-three to thirty-eight years (average age twenty-six and three-tenths years). In 4 cases even the ulnar styloid process has been injured; amongst these there occurs one patient (Case 116, Fig. 72) with distal radioulnar diastasis.

The fracture line lies 2 cm. above the joint in 4 cases, and 1½ and 1¾ cm. in one case each. According to the röntgen plate, it as good as falls together with the epiphysial line in Case 27 (twenty-four years of age), Fig. 71. Case 116 (twenty-three years of age) constitutes an intra-articular fracture, inasmuch as in ulnar direction a small bone fragment may be seen broken off farthest distally (Fig. 72). In the lateral-view picture the fracture begins in volar direction near the joint (appears broadest here) and proceeds in proximal direction obliquely upwards, dorsally inclined; there is also a fissure extending dorsally into the joint (Fig. 73).

The fracture originated through a fall, except in the case of two patients. The one of these (Case 27) had knocked his left flat hand against a rail whilst hit in the region of his elbow by a heavy cable-bearing falling down from above. The other (Case 164) was a chauffeur and had been injured in the characteristic manner through the rebound of a motor-car winch.

Hereto belong in addition to the two reproduced by X-ray plates Case 16 (fracture immediately above and as good as parallel with the epiphysial line), Case 46 (the fracture as good as in the old epiphysial line), Case 144 (the fracture in and partly contiguous to the epiphysial line), and Case 164 (the fracture almost completely falling together with the epiphysial line).

As will be seen, I have in this representation and as *chief principle* in the classification made use of the *state of development of the skeleton;* the fractures in individuals with incomplete ossification are collected into one group, fractures in those with complete ossification in another. The age limit is nineteen years, that period at which the epiphysial cartilage is customarily completely ossified (Pilcher, etc.; comp. Akerlund [literary notes]).

438

A summary of all the details in my material may here be in its place. I will begin with the 54 fracture cases which *occurred at incomplete ossification* (Division I).

The anatomical appearance of most of these fractures was as the reproduced radiographs (Figs. 1–23) clearly show, on the one hand fairly identical; on the other hand, deviating somewhat from the type of the classical radius fracture.

In the 34 cases which together form the groups *A*, *B*, and *C* is often shown a lesion in both ulna and radius; in practically one-fourth of the cases is, according to röntgen, the ulna intact. The radius lesion lies about 1–5 cm. above the radiocarpal joint and appears, as a rule, as a transverse fracture line (Figs. 1 and 2, 13 cases, Group I*A*, or as an irregularity, or as a folding on the surface of the bone, "torus fracture" (Figs. 3 to 7), 12 cases, Group I*b*, or as a combination of both these variations (Figs. 8 to 14, 9 cases, Group I*c*). The appearance of the ulnar lesion shows the same variations, but in this wise, that in some particular case it sometimes deviates from the picture which the radius fracture in the same patient assumes.

In the remaining 20 cases there occurs either an epiphysial separation of the radius (Figs. 15 to 19, 16 cases, Group I*d*), or a typical radius fracture (Figs. 20 and 23, 4 cases, Group I*e*). There is nothing especially remarkable in the appearance of these injuries, except as to Cases 128, 156, 146, and 170. In the three first named—which are epiphysial separations— it is namely observed that the fracture line, in the same degree as it approaches the radius dorsally, turns off a bit up in the diaphysis, so that a small dorsal triangular bone fragment is broken off (Figs. 17 and 19). And in Case 170—which is a typical radius fracture—the epiphysial line appears broad and distinct, but the lesion of continuity in the bone has not taken place therein, but a little above (Fig. 21). I will return later on to these details (Pilcher calls to mind in his work the occurrence of similar phenomena in certain types of radius fracture).

The greater portion of my fracture material, *i.e.*, the 152 cases which concern individuals with complete ossification (Division II) has an entirely different anatomical character to those forms generally described.

The majority of them, 132 in number, constitute typical radius fractures (104 cases, Group II*A*) or typical radius fractures complicated by longitudinal fissures in the region of the wrist (28 cases, Group II*B*). The radius shows a fracture line going in a transverse or somewhat oblique direction, as a rule, 2–3 cm. above the radiocarpal joint, but with a variation in position of at least $1\frac{1}{2}$ cm., at most $6\frac{1}{2}$ cm., from there. Besides its mildest form, a simple transverse fracture without or with slight dislocation (Fig. 24), the injury appears in several, more or less severe variations. In a great number of cases it may be observed on both front- and side-view plates how the peripheral radial end is displaced, eventually also wedged in in radiodorsal direction in the characteristic manner (Figs. 25 to 27, 29, 35, 37, 39 to 41, etc.). In some there occurs a comparatively slight splitting of the radial dorsal labrum (Fig. 35), or, taking it all round, in the nearest vicinity of the site of fracture (Figs. 26 to 31, 38, and 40). But not infrequently—the already mentioned 28 cases which form the Group II*B*—longitudinal fracturing of the radius right out to the radiocarpal joint has taken place (Figs. 49 to 65), which splitting sometimes even extends proximally to the transverse fracture (Figs. 59 to 62, 64 and 65). With regard to other details of interest, it should be pointed out, firstly, that Case 204, in which the side-view picture would seem to show that the dorsal periosteum was not torn at time of injury, but stood the test (Fig 25); secondly, Cases 134 and 113, where the front respectively side-view picture has a partial similarity to torus fracture (Figs. 28 and 46). The unusual course of the fracture line may be finally mentioned—in the frontal view something like an inverted S—to be observed in some patients (Figs. 42, 43, etc.; compare Fig. 21); likewise, also, the greater breadth in the fracture line volarally (Cases 11, 207, and 211, Figs. 33 and 34) and radially (Case 113, Fig. 145) in some other cases. Simultaneous injury to the ulna occurs in two-thirds of the fracture cases belonging hereto. It constitutes in the great majority of patients fracture at the apex or at the base of the styloid process, but consists in 3 cases (Cases 10, 104, and 200) of a transverse or oblique fracture higher up in the ulna itself at about the same height as the radius injury, about 1 cm. above the ulnar styloid process (Figs. 47 to 49). Besides the ulna lesion, the X-ray plate shows in 7 cases, as far as can be judged, an abnormally wide diastasis in distal radioulnar connection, which complication, moreover, seems to have occurred in 8 cases of radius fracture without accompanying injury to the ulna (see Figs. 24, 36, 50, and 54).[5]

There still remain amongst this category of radius fractures two lesser groups of cases, embracing fracture of the radial styloid process together with epiphysial separation.

Sole fracture of the radial styloid process occurs in 14 patients (Group II*C*). According to X-ray plate, there is an intra-articular fracturing of a bone fragment, of triangular shape in frontal view and lying towards the lateral edge of the radius (Figs. 66 to 68). The fracture line proceeds from the region of the middle of the joint surface obliquely upwards and outwards to about 2 cm. above the apex of the radius styloid process; the lateral-view picture shows a corresponding appearance (Figs. 69 and 70). A slight splitting is observed in a couple of cases (Figs. 67 to 69). Simultaneous fracture in ulnar styloid process occurs in practically one-fifth of the patients. One of these (Case 76, Fig. 66) seems to show an abnormal diastasis in the distal radio-ulnar connection.

A more or less typical epiphysial separation of the radius is verified in 6 patients (Group II*D*, Figs. 71 to 73). Out of them, 4—that is to say, two-thirds—have simultaneous ulna fracture. In one case (Fig. 72) there

I. FRACTURES IN INDIVIDUALS WITH INCOMPLETE OSSIFICATION

A. TRANSVERSE FRACTURE OF RADIUS AND ULNA

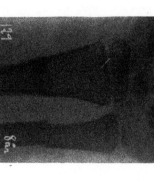

FIG. 1.—Case 129.

B. TORUS FRACTURE OF RADIUS (EVENTUALLY WITH SIMULTANEOUS ULNA LESION)

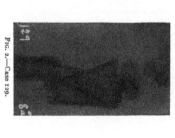

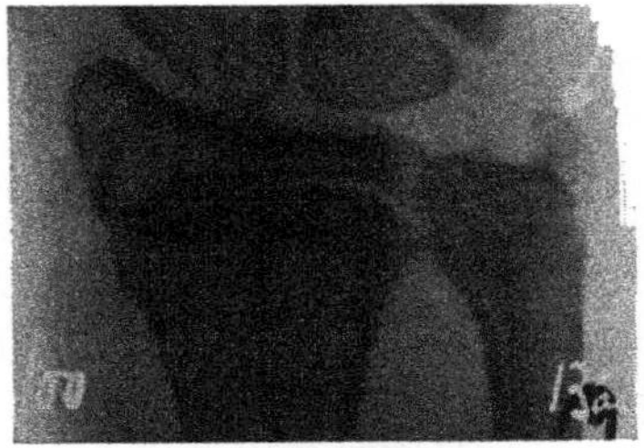

FIG. 2.—Case 129.

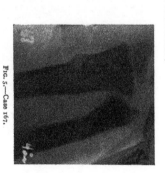

FIG. 3.—Case 100.

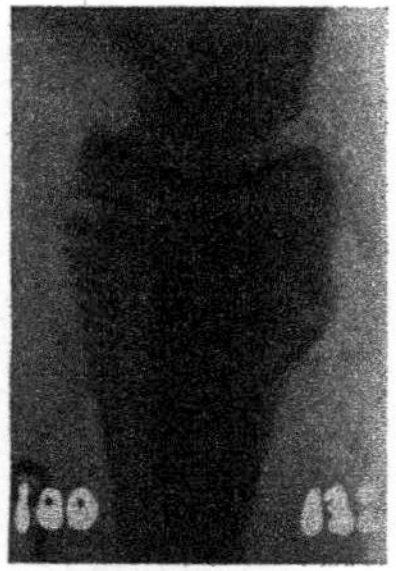

FIG. 4.—Case 100.

FIG. 5.—Case 167.

440

B. TORUS FRACTURE OF RADIUS (EVENTUALLY WITH SIMULTANEOUS ULNA LESION).—Continued

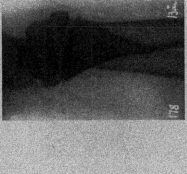

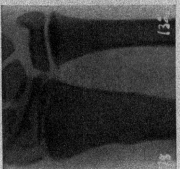

Fig. 6.—Case 178.

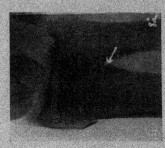

Fig. 7.—Case 178.

C. TRANVERSE FRACTURE WITH SIMULTANEOUS VISIBLE CORTEX TORUS.

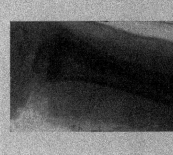

Fig. 9.—Case 111.

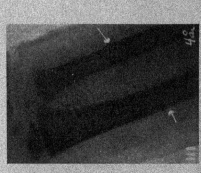

Fig. 8.—Case 111.

Fig. 10.—Case 111.

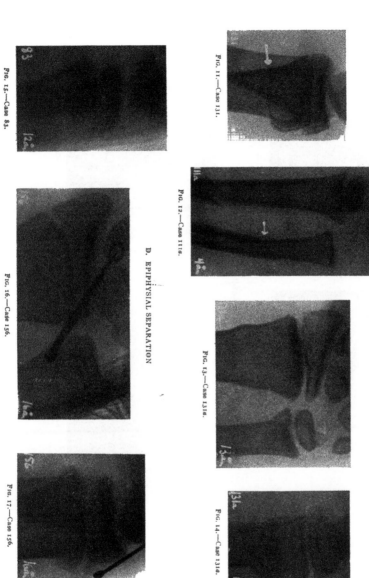

C. TRANSVERSE FRACTURE WITH SIMULTANEOUS VISIBLE CORTEX TORUS.—Continued

FIG. 11.—Case 131.

FIG. 12.—Case 111a.

FIG. 13.—Case 131a.

FIG. 14.—Case 131a.

FIG. 15.—Case 83.

D. EPIPHYSIAL SEPARATION

FIG. 16.—Case 156.

FIG. 17.—Case 156.

D. EPIPHYSIAL SEPARATION.—*Continued*

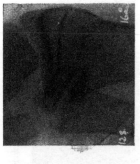

FIG. 18.—Case 128.

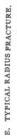

FIG. 19.—Case 128.

E. TYPICAL RADIUS FRACTURE.

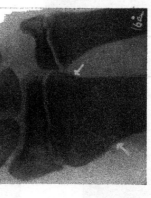

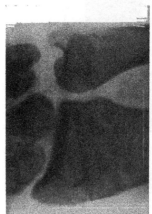

FIG. 20.—Case 114.

FIG. 21.—Case 170.

E. TYPICAL RADIUS FRACTURE.—*Continued*

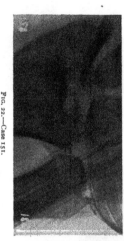

FIG. 22.—Case 151.

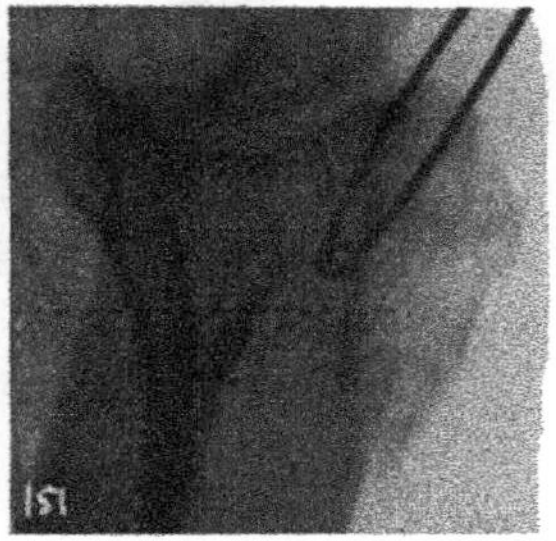

FIG. 23.—Case 151.

II. FRACTURES IN INDIVIDUALS, WITH COMPLETE OSSIFICATION

A. TYPICAL RADIUS FRACTURE

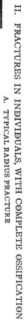

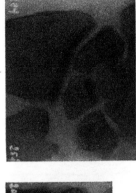

FIG. 24.—Case 204.

FIG. 25.—Case 205.

FIG. 26.—Case 130.

FIG. 27.—Case 130.

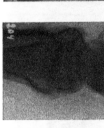

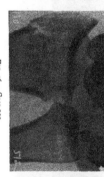

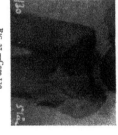

A. TYPICAL RADIUS FRACTURE.—*Continued*

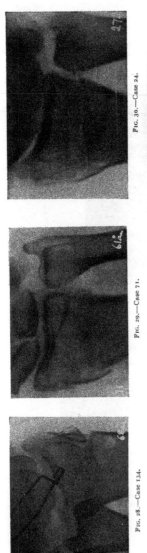

Fig. 28.—Case 134.

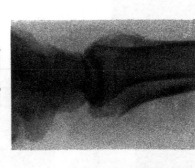

Fig. 30.—Case 24.

Fig. 29.—Case 71.

Fig. 31.—Case 207.

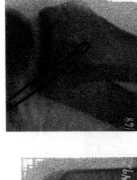

Fig. 32.—Case 168.

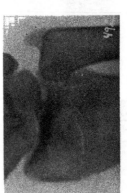

Fig. 31.—Case 67.

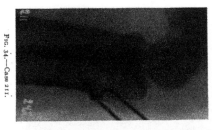

Fig. 34.—Case 211.

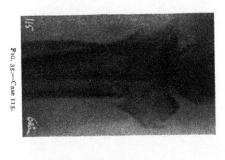

Fig. 35.—Case 115.

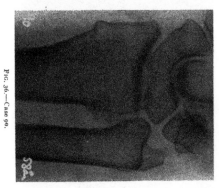

Fig. 36.—Case 90.

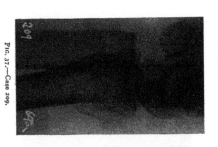

Fig. 37.—Case 209.

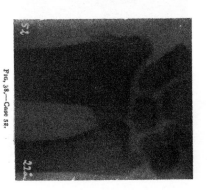

Fig. 38.—Case 52.

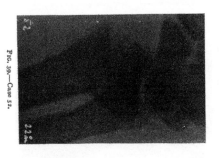

Fig. 39.—Case 52.

440

A. TYPICAL RADIUS FRACTURE.—*Continued*

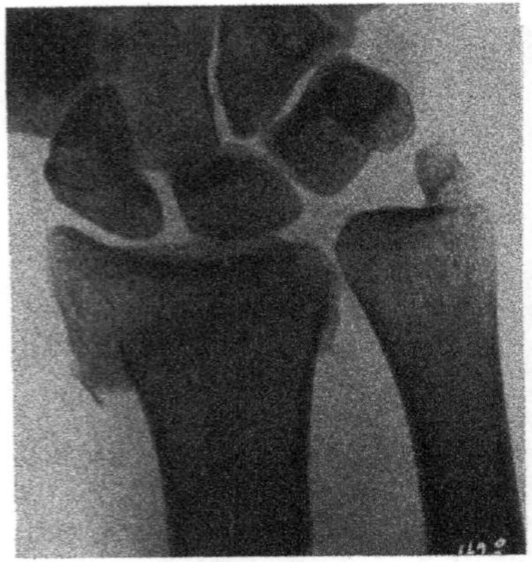

FIG. 40.—Case 42.

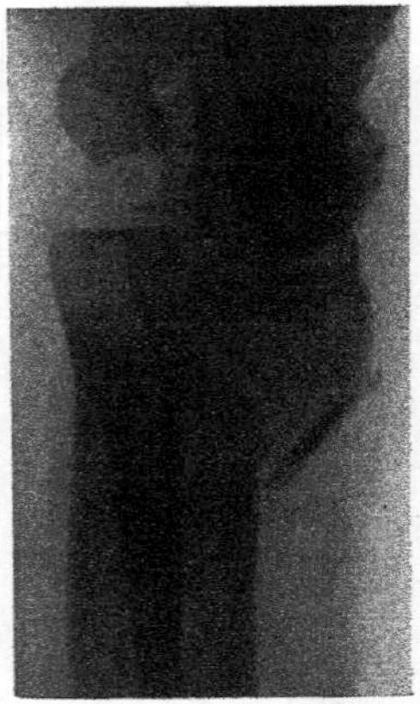

FIG. 41.—Case 42.

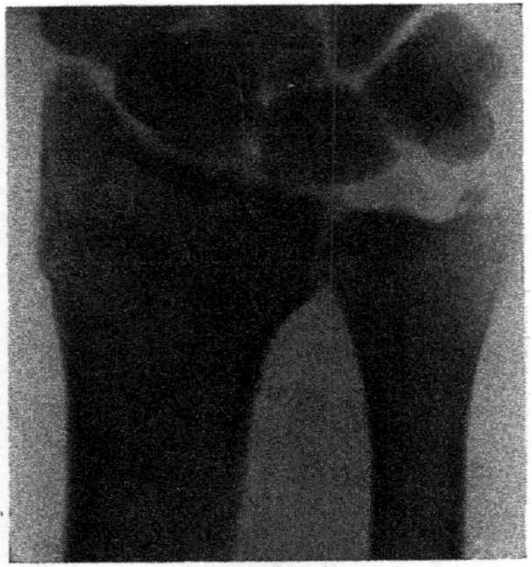

FIG. 42.—Case 7.

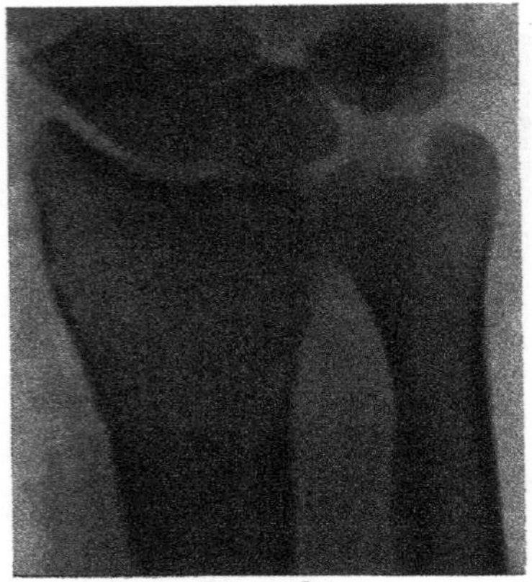

FIG. 43.—Case 53.

FIG. 44.—Case 53.

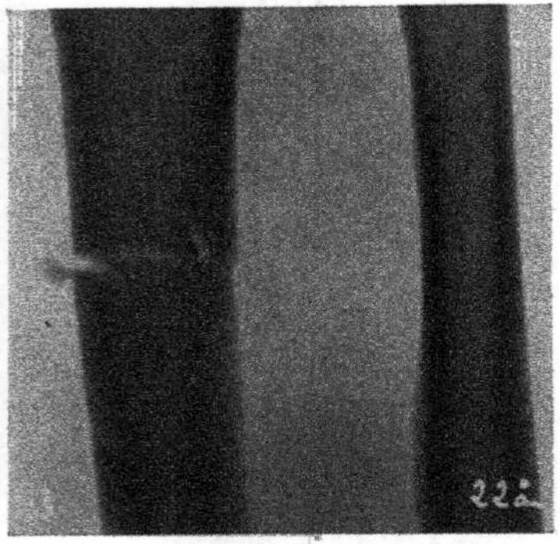

FIG. 45.—Case 113.

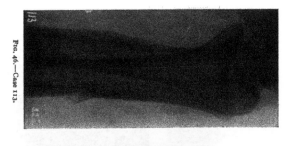

FIG. 46.—Case 113.

A. TYPICAL RADIUS FRACTURE.—*Continued*

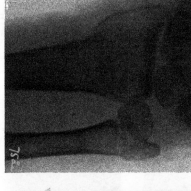

FIG. 47.—Case 10.

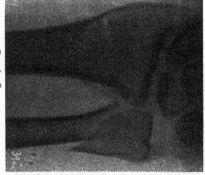

FIG. 48.—Case 104.

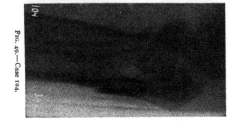

FIG. 49.—Case 104.

B. RADIUS FRACTURE WITH LONGITUDINAL FISSURES TOO, EXTENDING INTO THE RADIOCARPAL JOINT

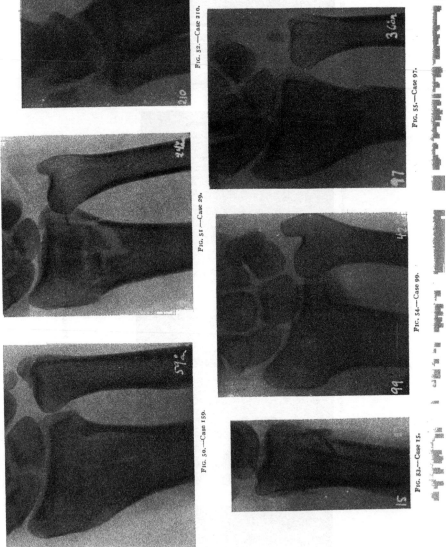

FIG. 50.—Case 159.

FIG. 51.—Case 29.

FIG. 52.—Case 210.

FIG. 53.—Case 15.

FIG. 54.—Case 99.

FIG. 55.—Case 97.

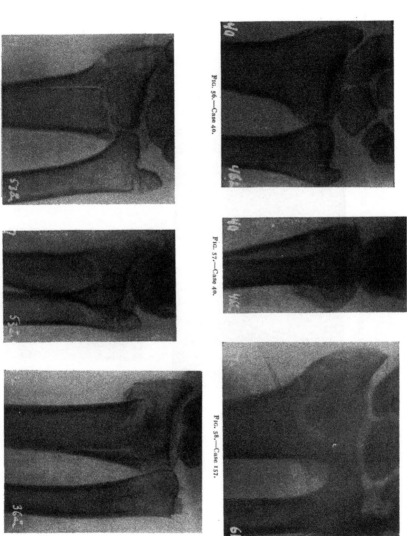

FIG. 56.—Case 40.

FIG. 57.—Case 40.

FIG. 58.—Case 157.

FIG. 59.—Case 17.

FIG. 60.—Case 17.

FIG. 61.—Case 17a.

B. RADIUS FRACTURE; WITH LONGITUDINAL FISSURES TOO, EXTENDING INTO THE RADIOCARPAL JOINT.—*Continued*

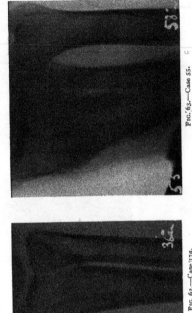

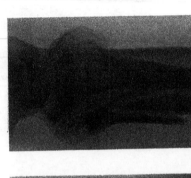

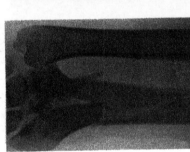

FIG. 62.—Case 17a.

FIG. 63.—Case 55.

C. FRACTURE OF THE RADIUS STYLOID PROCESS

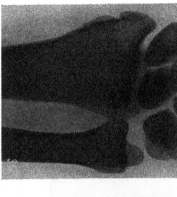

Fig. 66.—Case 76.

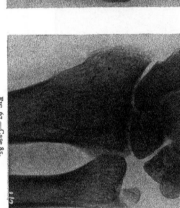

Fig. 67.—Case 85.

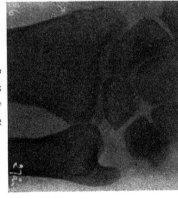

Fig. 68.—Case 86.

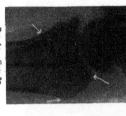

Fig. 69.—Case 87.

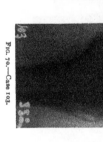

Fig. 70.—Case 103.

D. EPIPHYSIAL SEPARATION

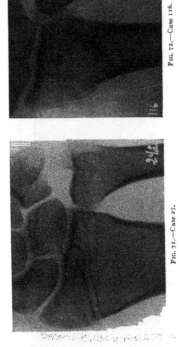

FIG. 71.—Case 27.

FIG. 72.—Case 116.

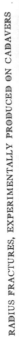

FIG. 73.—Case 116.

RADIUS FRACTURES, EXPERIMENTALLY PRODUCED ON CADAVERS

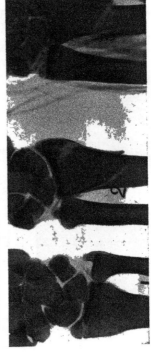

FIG. 74.—Cases 1, 2, 3.

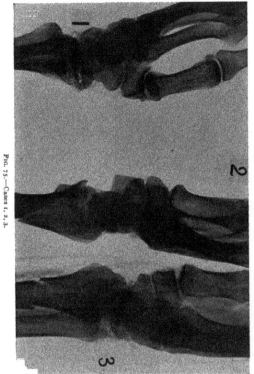

RADIUS FRACTURES, EXPERIMENTALLY PRODUCED ON CADAVERS.—*Continued*

FIG. 75.—Cases 1, 2, 3.

44

SIDE VIEW OF THE RADIOCARPAL REGION FROM A NORMAL HAND

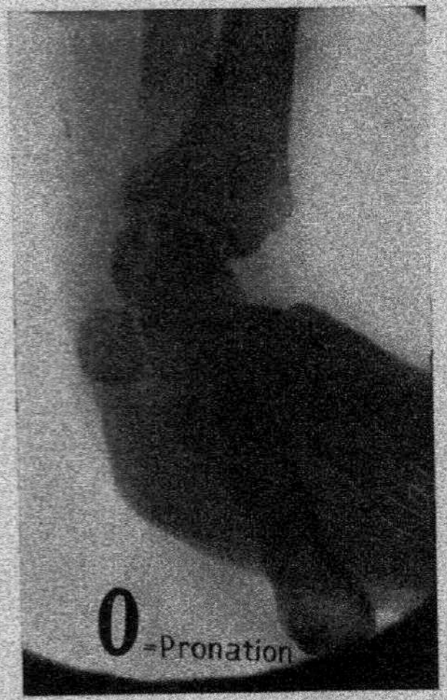

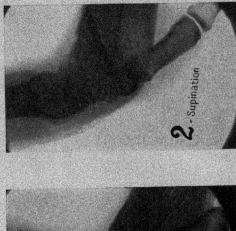

0 - Pronation

2 - Supination

FIG. 76.—Hand pronated.

FIG. 77.—Hand supinated.

occurs, as far as one can judge, an abnormally wide distal radio-ulnar connection. Röntgenologically it may, moreover, be pointed out that the fracture line does not a single time quite join with the epiphysial line. The detail—which should be seen in connection with the already mentioned occurrence of juxtaepiphysial radius fracture in a sixteen-year-old individual in Case 170 (Fig. 21)—is remarkable, but earlier indicated by Ollier and Pilcher. The former, even, is of the opinion that a bone injury of the kind in question seldom, if ever, goes into the cartilage itself, but, on the contrary, into the spongiose bone tissue lying close beside it, whereof thus at least something of it always remains adhering to the epiphysial cartilage.

A closer consideration of the particulars here given should clearly prove that it was both natural and right to divide up my material in the fashion done with reference to forearm fracture in the region of the wrist. It is quite evident that there is a difference in the *anatomical character* of the same, according to if it is a question of individuals under or above the age limit for the completion of ossification. The trauma—in quite the majority of patients a fall on the prone and extended hand—which a child or young person has met with has most often occasioned a more or less transversal fracture in the diaphysis of the forearm, near the wrist, about on the same level of both bones; in scarcely 30 per cent. of the cases has an epiphysial separation set in, and in only about 7 per cent. a so-called typical radius fracture. In individuals above the age of nineteen years, on the contrary, a corresponding violence has with very few exceptions led to a more or less severe typical radius fracture, whilst in only some few cases has it been associated with an equally highly situated transverse or oblique fracture of the ulna, but otherwise has very often been accompanied by fracture of the ulnar styloid process; in a frequency of about 9 per cent. was there a fracture of the radius styloid process at hand, in scarcely 4 per cent. could an epiphysial separation of the radius be recognized.

My division of the fractures in question obtains further authorization inasmuch as it offers the possibility of, as far as one can find, a fairly uniform comprehension of the *manner of origin and mechanism* of these injuries.

I will once again begin with the fractures which have occurred in the case of not yet completed ossification. By way of exception—as, for instance, in Case 170 (Fig. 21, Group IE)—the clinical data already give here a decided suggestion of the nature of the fracture. The patient mentioned had been injured through what for a radius fracture is a very unusual violence, insofar as he was trampled on the dorsum of his forearm by a horse; he had thus been exposed to a trauma whose action is typical for the origin of certain kinds of flexion fracture (compare the sketch to the left in Fig. A).

It is, however, more often the röntgenological details which first convey information of value for the classification of the fracture. Of special interest in this respect are those cases in which radius shows, firstly, a cortex torus (folding) on the surface, and secondly, a fracture line straight through the bone (Group IC, Figs. 8 to 14). Each or both of these details appear, namely, together with an occasionally occurring distinct concavity or angular curving of the fracture area, as characteristic for the majority of fractures belonging to the head group (I). We recognize in the cortex torus (folding) the simplest and mildest effect of a concentrating violence, acting essentially in the longitudinal direction of the extremity —stauchung (Kohl, Quervain, Iselin, Burnham, etc.)—on the juvenile, fairly elastic bone. In the transversal or oblique fracture fissure at hand a similar and previous trauma may be traced. For, in the first place, the fracture is in several cases broader, i.e., there is a larger diastasis, at the edge of one bone than at the other (Figs. 8 and 12, Cases 111, 111a, and 191), and, in the second place, there is sometimes a curving of the bone (dislocatio ad axin) with convexity in that direction where the fracture line is broadest (Figs. 9 and 12, Cases 111, and 111a). The radiograph has, in other words, that appearance which is to be expected after a trauma, the effect of which is shown in the sketch to the right in Fig. A. The bone has evidently been compressed from end to end, momentarily bent, and began to break on the very spot of the vertex of the temporary strain—i.e., the convexity. Röntgenologically the effect is that of a combination of compression (stauchung) and flexion fracture. The closely connected genetic relationship of the cortex stauchung with the transverse or oblique fracture in question is already evinced by those cases where radius shows the former injury and ulna the latter (Figs. 3 and 5, Cases 20, 100, 167,[6] 194, 186, and 187). But it is most clearly visible in those cases where both kinds of bone lesions are simultaneously traced on the same bone. There it is unmistakably to be seen on the plate how a transversal breakage in the bone has begun on the ulnar (medial) and volar side in the ulna and radius whilst a cortex stauchung has arisen radially (Case 132). Or—Case 111 (Figs. 8 and 9)—how a transversal fracture of the radius has begun on the volar and radial side, whilst the ulna was forcibly bent so that a dorsal concavity and a dorsal and ulnar cortex stauchung have taken place. Analogous conditions are demonstrated by the Cases 131, 111a, and 131a (Figs. 10 to 14). In all of them the folding (the torus) lies in the cortex on that side of the bone which is turned away from that where the fracture line begins, or is widest.

In the light of this argument, the cases in Group IB (Figs. 3 to 7) are fully comprehensible. The longitudinal compression, at the age in question, of the fairly elastic bone of the forearm has caused a temporary flexion. But this has not gone so far that a transverse fissure going through the whole continuity of the bone and clearly visible on the X-ray plate has arisen—or, at most, only arisen in the ulna (compare Fig. 5, Cases 20, 194, 57, 167, etc.)—but only occasioned a remaining unevenness.

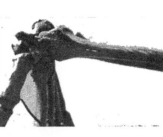

Fig. 78.—Clear lateral view (with hand in dorsal flexion).

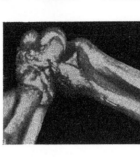

Fig. 79.—Lateral view with the dorsal-flected hand somewhat supinated.

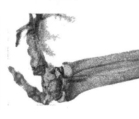

Fig. 80.—Photograph of the volar surface (hand in dorsal flexion.)

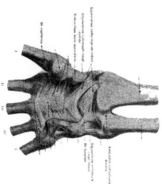

Fig. 81 (from Spalteholz).—The volar ligaments of the carpal joint.

in the cortex of the radius on the spot during the trauma of the momentarily deepest part of the concavity. The seat of the cortex stauchung will consequently be, since the trauma is often brought about by a fall on vola manus, as a rule, on the dorsal or dorsal-radial side (see Figs. 3 to 5, Cases 100, 101, 147, 167, 181, 194, etc.), If, as in Cases 178, 186, and 187, where the patient has been upset whilst cycling, the injury has been brought about in this wise, that whilst trying to save himself with his hand outstretched in volar direction, i.e., with dorsum manus—which patient 178 himself states as having done—then the cortex stauchung will be on the volar, radial, and ulnar side (Figs. 6 and 7). It is less easy to find out röntgenologically the mechanism of origin in the cases in Group I*a*, the pure transverse fractures without visible cortex torus (folding). All the clinical statements at hand should, however, through their agreement in point of principle with the cases in Group I*b* and *c*, be entitled to be compared with these. That there can at least in part have been circumstances—in technical or other respects—which have had some influence with regard to the appearance of the X-ray plate is evinced by Case 197, for instance. The injury was in this case occasioned by a powerful blow in the longitudinal direction of the forearm; it is quite evident, according to the anamnestics, that the patient whilst sledging drove his right hand so hard against a tree that his arm came into a rectangular position. But the radiograph shows—after replacement—that in spite of this, only a transverse fracture ensued, without either special cortex change or dislocatio ad axin.

My material consequently seems to entitle to the belief that *the forearm fractures in the region of the wrist, which are the usual ones for individuals with incomplete bone development* (Group I*a* to *c*), *are, as a rule, with regard to manner of origin, compression fractures, or, a combination of compression and flexion fractures.* The minority of cases of epiphysial separations and typical radius fractures (Groups I*d* and *e*) which in my classification with regard to age have been placed in this category might, in my opinion, in a discussion on the theory of the genesis of the fracture, be suitably placed together with the epiphysial separations and typical radius fractures which occur in and are characteristic for persons with complete ossification. The reason that the trauma, which, on the whole, has been identical in nature, in the former (Groups I*d* and *e*) has shown in point of principle similar anatomical variations to the injuries in the latter (Group II), probably lies in the fact that the solidity of the skeleton has been about the same—in spite of the differences in age.

And it is in reality interesting to notice in this connection how the age of the patients is divided up within the different groups in the fracture category I. As the table demonstrates, the average value shows a steady rise for them in the order that the fractures are spoken of. Transverse and torus fractures in Groups I*a* to *c* occur in persons at an average age of scarcely ten years, epiphysial separations in those at fourteen years, and the typical radius fracture at seventeen and five-tenth years. The occurrence of the first-named fractures, which are diaphysis injuries, in the youngest of all originates, no doubt, in the fact that the distal ossification centre at this stage of bone development, before the age of twelve, is so small—Case 131 (Fig. 10) constitutes an example of an exception—that it scarcely offers even mechanical possibilities for the genesis of an epiphysial separation or a typical radius fracture (see Figs. 5, 8, and 12; compare Pilcher, p. 12) ; the strain of the trauma will therefore essentially assert itself in the diaphysis. But in the same degree as the bone growth approaches completion and the skeleton of the forearm assumes a greater likeness to that of the adult, so will the risk of the lower radius epiphysis reacting in the same manner as is the case with the latter against the trauma, become greater; and, at the same time, when a strong cortex, etc., is developed in the diaphysis, i.e., its strength improved, so will the latter's possibility of sustaining the trauma without fracturing ensuing be increased.

There remain radius fractures in persons with complete ossification (Group II). In their case—on an attempt to make an analysis of the kind here in question—it shows even as in the case of fractures before the completion of ossification what a faulty guidance the clinical analysis gives, as a rule, with relation to a reliable exposition of fracture mechanism.

A brilliant example of this circumstance is offered by the so-called chauffeur fractures, numbering five in all. The trauma has here—from what one has reason to suppose—been of much about the same nature ; the rebound of the winch on the chauffeur's attempting to start the motor car, i.e., a heavy blow operating in the dorsal and proximal direction of the forearm. But the effect thereof has in different cases been very different. Two of the patients received a typical, transversal radius fracture (Cases 110 and 113, Figs. 45 and 46), one, in addition, contracted an intra-articular longitudinal splitting of the radius (Case 99, Fig. 54), another got a radius styloid process fracture (Case 76, Fig. 66), and one finally epiphysial separation (Case 164). All types of fractures occurring within Group II have consequently been represented as a resulting condition of one and the same trauma. The X-ray picture makes it probable that one of the fractures (Case 113, Figs. 45 and 46), by reason of a greater breadth on the radial than on the ulnar side of the fracture line, together with a suggestion of dorsal concavity (dislocatio ad axin), is a case of compression fracture—perhaps more correctly a combination of compression and flexion fracture—according to the drawing to the right in Fig. A ; but for the remaining four cases can the X-ray pictures scarcely be said to give any similar or obvious guidance.

A priori it lies undeniably nearer to hand to suppose that if the trauma causing the injury be somewhat about the same, the mechanism of the forearm fracture in the region of the wrist should most often be in point of principle similar at the period of complete ossification of the skeleton and at incomplete; that, in other words, even in the adult, the injury here concerned would, as a rule, be a compression fracture or a compression-flexion fracture, and in point of fact, much would seem to prove that such is the case.

In Group II several cases occur where the radiograph illustrates that the fracture has been brought about by a powerful compression from end to end in the longitudinal direction of the forearm, according to the sketch to the right in Fig. A. Sometimes the side-view picture shows— absolutely in analogy to what has been demonstrated in several cases in Group I—a greater breadth on the volar (Figs. 33, 34, and 39) or radial (Fig. 45) side of the fracture line than dorsally ulnarally. Sometimes the X-ray pictures show details which best coincide with the presumption that the bone injury has been occasioned by a longitudinal compression, the effect of *coup et contrecoup*. I hereby allude partly to the splitting of the radial dorsal labrum which is observed in solitary cases (*e.g.*, Case 115, Fig. 35), and partly to the longitudinal fissures extending into the radio-carpal joint in a whole group of injuries (Group IIb, at least 28 cases). The reproduced röntgen pictures (Figs. 50 to 65) should fully illustrate that the fracture mechanism of these cases may easily be brought into agree-ment with the description of the effect of longitudinal compression on the long tubular bone in adults, which I have above cited from Zuppinger and which is schematically demonstrated in Fig. B. A further consideration will also give one to understand how difficult—in certain cases (*e.g.*, Cases 55 and 118a, Figs. 63 to 65) impossible—it is to imagine their origin in accordance with the theories on wrench fracture or, in fact, any other kind of fracture than compression fracture.

If we, on the contrary, furthermore take into consideration the fact that in none of my radius fractures is there a case to be met with wherein the effect of the trauma is entirely confined to a fracturing of the radial volar labrum beginning in volar, and proceeding in oblique distal dorsal direction towards the radiocarpal joint, so is even that fact rather re-markable. Such a type of fracture would seem to have been at least a somewhat usual recurring phenomenon if the injury were as regards genesis to be interpreted essentially as a wrench fracture.

In general, the most important anatomical conditions for the genesis of wrench fracture of the radius are described as lying partly in the radial volar labrum projecting markedly in volar direction (see Figs. 34, 46, and first and foremost 76), and partly the strong ligament apparatus, essentially ligamentum radiocarpeum volare (Fig. 81), which emanates from os capitatum and other carpal bones and inserts volarally in the radius. Pilcher, among others, has schematic, very demonstrative drawings of the same. If one, however, carefully inspects an upper skeletted ex-tremity, it will be seen that the volar distal radius area, which in certain lateral-view pictures is so well portrayed as a projecting volar labrum, constitutes the ulnar (medial) radius part (see Figs. 79 and 80) which in comparison with the radial (lateral) part of the radius epiphysis con-

445

stitute but in a very subordinate degree a hold for the ligament in question (Fig. 81). The existence of strong ligaments which are said to insert on the labrum mentioned (on the ulnar side of radius) would therefore seem in point of fact to be more of a schematic construction on the part of the majority of authors rather than a reality. The strongest part of the volar radiocarpal ligament inserts radially (laterally) in the radius, and a strain on the distal volar end of the radius, such as might be thought to occasion a wrench fracture, should consequently, from a theoretical point of view, lead more especially to a wrenching off of the radial styloid process.

The question then arises voluntarily: Is there no visible means or probability of such a fracture arising clinically? The answer must be in the affirmative. A reference to Group IIC, radial styloid process fracture (Figs. 66 to 70; 14 cases), in my material constitutes hereby sufficient grounds. The nature of the trauma is in the case of two of these patients rather remarkable; the one (Case 54) had had a wheelbarrow pass over him and thereby became severely jammed by pressure in the grip of the thumb, whilst his elbow was pressed hard against a plank; the other (Case 72) had been jammed between a plank against which his elbow was resting and an iron beam right in the flat of his hand. The conditions for a simple wrench appear here to be fairly discernible.

Although conscious of the fact that bone and ligament tissue after death (post-mortem) cannot be considered without more ado to react against violence in the same way as during life (intra vitam), I have yet endeavored to ascertain what type of radius fracture one can produce on a corpse which is arranged for by different methods. Only once—in the course of twelve experiments—did I succeed in producing a lesion of similar type to Group IIc. It was a question of a skeleton of an elderly individual from which the muscles had been dissected, and only the ligaments were left. The flat hand of the skeleton was placed on a table and pressed heavily against the support by dorsal breaking of the forearm (hyperextension of the hand). The consequence was that already with but very moderate violence a perceptible cracking and transverse fracturing of the radial styloid process scarcely one cm. above the apex of this apophysis was noticeable (Figs. 74 and 75). Röntgenologically the fracture very much resembles the clinical fractures in Group IIC. In all the rest of the corpse experiments it was, however, impossible for me, with the assistance of either the one or the other methods of violence, to produce a similar fracture type. The result was either a tearing of the ligaments or tension, or there ensued one of the two other types of fracture which are found reproduced in Figs. 74 and 75. The fracture in Figs. 74 and 75 was produced on a forearm on which only the ligaments were left. The flat hand of the skeleton was placed on a stone floor with the forearm supported against a wall at an angle of 45° to the floor. A heavy blow with a broad hammer was exercised on the back side of the forearm immediately above the wrist (also the same mechanism for the trauma as in the drawing to the left in Fig. A). The fracture line takes its course in an oblique, proximal, dorsal, and somewhat radial direction, its uppermost part lies 5½ cm. above the apex of the radial styloid process (Fig. 74). The lateral-view picture seems to show that the diastasis between the fractured ends is broader in volar than in dorsal direction—as the case should be with a flexion fracture. Something akin to this fracture type in the röntgenanatomical sense of the word is Case 53 (Figs. 43 and 44, a fifty-nine-year-old man, who had fallen down sideways and tried to save himself with his hands as he was endeavoring to avoid an automobile) and, although in lesser degree, Case 7 (Fig. 42, a twenty-five-year-old man, wound unknown). The fracture in Figs. 74 and 75 concerns a forearm where,

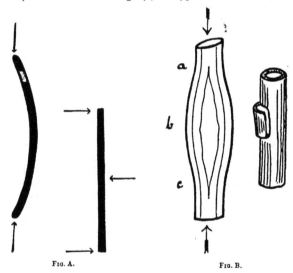

FIG. A.   FIG. B.

besides ligaments, even muscles and tendons—dissected up—were found remaining. The trauma was produced thereby that the hand with vola manus upturned was squeezed in the drawer of a table which was all but shut, the distal end of the navicular bone was hitched up at the top of the edge of the table, the forearm was grasped in the region of the elbow and was broken forcibly downwards. The effect was a somewhat oblique, transversal fracture 5 cm. above the radiocarpal joint. The lateral-view picture with its greater breadth on the volar than on the dorsal side of the fracture line reminds one most of a flexion fracture. The type resembles somewhat the fracture in Figs. 45 and 46 (Case 113, chauffeur fracture). I did not a single time succeed in producing a fracture on a corpse by a direct imitation of Nélaton's postmortem experiment. A powerful blow of the hammer on the upper end of the vertically placed

447

skeleton of the forearm, with the hand of the same dorsally extended and vola manus resting on a hard support, only led to a breaking (tearing) of the radiocarpal ligaments. The reason of this was probably the fact that the dead bodies at my disposal for this particular experiment were not of sufficiently recent date.[7]

A summary of what has been stated concerning the genesis-mechanism of forearm fracture in the region of the wrist, *i.e.*, of the usual radius fracture in its various forms, based upon my own material, amounts to the following:

I. A group—II*B*—comprising 28 or certainly more cases, should undeniably constitute compression fractures. These injuries can scarcely have originated otherwise than by a powerful blow in the longitudinal direction of the extremity (coup et contrecoup). A comminute fracture with long, longitudinal fissures extending out in the joint cannot very well have occurred through wrenching. The latter necessarily appear to have originated primarily—that they really do so is demonstrated by such cases as, for instance, Case 159 and 118*a* (Figs. 50, 64, and 65), where there is an absence of transverse fracturing or where the same retires into the background. The indications of Wolkowitsch and others concerning this latter moment seem to me to be well founded; likewise his suggestion that the area for the radius fracture—that part of the bone where the strong compact of the diaphysis changes into a thin putamen on the extremely spongiose epiphysis which is much broader in extent (Figs. 50, 51, etc.)—on acceptance of this theory is best understood.

II. A group—II*C*—comprising 14 cases, may in consideration of the expansion of the ligament apparatus and the position of the fracture line be interpreted as wrench fracture. The anamnestic statement of the nature of the trauma gives here just as little uniform guidance of any real value as is the case, as a rule, for the rest of the groups, and this so much the less, as amongst the 14 injuries mentioned cases are also met with (chauffeur fractures) where the violence must rather be thought to have been a longitudinal compression and which in consequence with regard thereto are analogous with injuries which röntgenanatomically show themselves to be compression fractures or compression-flexion fractures.

III. For the large groups of fractures—Group II*A*, 104 cases—which have the most usual simple character of the so-called typical radius fracture, there is nothing of either clinical or anatomical moment which conclusively argues in favor of either compression or wrench mechanism. Such an injury (Case 170) belonging to Group I*e* has, however, obviously arisen through a violence, the effect of which is generally a typical flexion fracture, thus an injury closely related to a compression fracture (compare Fig. A); fractures effected on a corpse by similar means of violence have besides in a couple of cases practically obtained the appearance of typical radius fracture.

IV. *Ex analogiam* it lies near to hand to presume that the majority of radius fractures in adults originate as compression fractures, since that fracture form which obviously arises after a similar trauma in children and the young most often has the character of a compression (so-called stooking) fracture or compression-flexion fracture.

The classification now under consideration of fractures of the forearm in the region of the wrist has established the following:

I. The *anatomical nature* of these injuries is to a very great extent dependent upon the stage of development in that part of the skeleton which has sustained the trauma in question. In the case of an individual with incomplete ossification, the fracture most often assumes the character of transverse or torus fracture of the diaphysis of both bones of the forearm. In an individual with complete ossification—*i.e.*, above nineteen or twenty years of age—the injury assumes, on the contrary, the appearance of a so-called typical fracture of the lower radius epiphysis, with, or sometimes without, simultaneous lesion of the ulnar styloid process.

II. With regard to the *genesis mechanism,* the majority of these fractures, judging by the radiographs, would seem in the case of individuals with incomplete ossification to be compression fractures (or compression-flexion fractures). And even for other reasons, there is all authority for interpreting the typical radius fracture also—which is the equivalent at a later age to the transverse and torus fractures in children—as being, generally speaking, a compression fracture, although the X-ray anatomical details do not lend conclusive support to such an interpretation in the same degree for the former as for the latter.

REFERENCES

Reference to notes given at foot of page in the proof, and page number of notes in the translation:

	Page No.	Ref. No.
British Medical Journal, 1879, July 12th, p. 39 (cit. Pilcher)	I	I
Oral lessons, 1839, T I, p. 143 (cit. Wolkowitsch. See also Hennequin)..	I	I
Cit. Lecomte: New researches concerning indirect fractures of the base of radius. General principles of medicine, 1860, p. 654 (cit. Wolkowitsch)	I	2
Cit. Malgaigne: Treatise on bone fractures. Russian translation, 1850, p. 616 (cit. Wolkowitsch and Kranz)	I	3
Supplement to the treatise on bone fractures, 1853, p. 93 (cit. Wolkowitsch)	I	4
Cit. Kranz	I	5
The cases here even as in the material at large have first been collected in the different groups, with the guidance of the appearance of the radiographs; not until afterwards have the statements regarding patients' age, etc., been set up	2	I
Measured up—here as regarding all radius fractures in the material—on the Röntgen plates—in reality lying somewhat nearer the joint.....	2	2
Two cases observed by me from that period which the material embraces are here excluded; the one a 25-year-old man; the other a 22-year-old woman. The injury consisted solely of ulnar styloid process fracture	3	I
Compare note on table	4	I
It is undeniably difficult occasionally to verify with certainty as to whether the interval between the distal ends of radius and ulna, sometimes		

ABRAHAM TROELL

seen on Röntgen pictures, is pathological or not, especially as the
plate put in during the process of photographing may have some
influence. And unfortunately, the uncertainty is by no means always
to be overcome by relying on purely clinical statements, since so
many—eight in all—of the cases in question have not been examined
afterwards. In six of those belonging to group II and afterwards
examined, it was, however, ascertained three-quarters to one year after
the injury, that slight or severe trouble was still experienced in the
hand, whilst three felt nothing more whatsoever of their old injury... 5 1
It must be acknowledged that case 167 could just as well have been classed
with Group IC as with group IB. Since the stauchung on the radius
is the most prominent on the Röntgen plate and no transverse lesion
is distinctly seen going right through the whole bone, it has, however,
been relegated to the latter group 6 1
Regarding material for post-mortem experiments, I owe a debt of gratitude to Professor E. Müller, in whose department the experiments
were carried out 8 1

LITERATURE

Burnham: Fractures about the wrist in childhood and adolescence. ANNALS OF
SURGERY, 64, 1916, p. 318.
Destot et Gallois: Recherches physiologiques et expérimentales sur les fractures de
l'extrémité inférieur du radius. Rev. de Chir., 18, 1898, p. 886.
Helferich. Fracturen und Luxationen, 1903, p. 205.
Hennequin: Considérations sur le mécanisme, les symptomes et le traitément des
fractures de l'extrémité inférieure du radius consécutives aux chutes sur le poignet.
Rev. de Chir, 1894, No. 7 et 9.
Iselin: Stauchungsbrüche der kindl. u. jugendl. Knochen, Beitr. z. kl. Chir., 79, 1912,
p. 440; Korrespondenzbl. f. schweiz. Ärte, 42, 1912, p. 690.
Kahleyss: Beiträge z. Kenntnis der Fracturen am unteren Ende des Radius. Deutsche
Zeitschr. f. Chir., 45, 1897, p. 531.
Kaufmann, C.: Diagn. u. Behandl. der subcut. Radiusfraktur am Handgelenke. Deutsche
Zeitschr. f. Chir., 116, 1912, p. 140.
Krantz: Üb. d. Behandl. des typ. Radiusbruches. Deutsche Zeitschr. f. Chir., 106, 1910,
p. 270.
Kuhn: Der Mechanisms der Fract. radii typ. Deutsche Zeitschr. f. Chir., 63, 1902,
p. 596.
Löbker: Über d. Entstehungsmechanismus der typ. Radiusfraktur. Deutsche med.
Wochenschr., 1885, Nr. 27.
Müller, Ernst: Über subperiostale irreponible Fracturen des Vorderarmes, Beitr.
z. kl. Chir., Bd. 76, H 1, Ref. Zentralbl. f. Chir., 1912, p. 760.
Pilcher: Fractures of the lower extremity or base of the radius. ANNALS OF SURGERY,
65, 1917, p. 1.
Troell: Über die Behandlung der Radiusfraktur. Arch. f. kl. Chir., 101, 1913, p. 511.
Nord. med. ark., 1914, i, Nr. 24, p. 1.
Troell: Über Knochenbrüche am Unterschenkel. Arch. f. kl. Chir., 111, 1919, p. 915.
Wolkowitsch: Einige Daten üb. d. Mechanismus der Entstehung der Radiusfrakturen,
etc., Arch. f. kl. Chir., 76, 1905, p. 917.
Vulliet: Les fractures de l'extrémitié inférieure du radius chez l'enfant. Semaine
médicale, 34, 1914, p. 277.
Zuppinger und Christen: Allgemeine Lehre von den Knochenbüchen. Kurzgefasste
Lehre v. d. Knochenbüchen, von Quervain, u. a., 1913, p. 1.
Åkerlund: Entwicklungsreihen in Röntgenbildern von Hand, etc., im Mädchen-und
Knabenalter, Fortschr. a. d. Gebiete der Röntgenstrahlen, Erg. bd. 33, 1918.

TABLE OF CASES OF RADIUS FRACTURES IN THE REGION OF THE WRIST

Fracture type	With incomplete ossification			With complete ossification			Remarks
	Number of cases	Average age, years	Number of cases with simultaneous fracture of ulna	Number of cases	Average age, years	Number of cases with simultaneous fracture of ulna	
Transverse fra of radius and ulna (see rem.)......	13	8	10(= 77%)[1]				[1] In three cases besides probable ulna fracture
Torus fra of radius (ev. with ulna lesion)......	34 {12	9.5, 10	24(= 70.6%) {6(= 50%)				
Transverse or oblique fracture with simultaneous visible torus......	9	{11	8(= 90%)	6	26.3	4(= 66%)	
torus......							
Epiphysial separation of radius......	16	14	3(= 18.7%)	132 {104	48.8	82(= {64(= 61.5%) 62.1%) {18(= 64.3%)	[2] The figure is in reality surely too low: in, for instance, cases 5 and 204, which are classed with the immediate preceding group, it is pr... tha the radiograph shows a longitudinal fissure ending in the joint, proceeding from the fracture.
Typical radius fra r......	4	17.5	1(= 25%)	28	48.4		
Radius fra with longitudinal fissures out in joint......				152		89(= 58.5%)	
Fracture of radial styl. process......	54		28(= 51%)	14	35.4	3(= 21.4%)	

= 206 cases (whereof simultaneous fracture of ulna in 56.8%)

451

THE RÔLE OF CANCELLOUS TISSUE IN HEALING BONE

By T. Wingate Todd, F.R.C.S. (Eng.)

of Cleveland, Ohio

PROFESSOR OF ANATOMY IN THE WESTERN RESERVE UNIVERSITY

I. Introduction—Studies on the Skeleton.—Ten years ago I began an intensive study of bone growth and metamorphosis. From time to time I have published more or less fragmentary, apparently dissociated, and preliminary reports dealing with various phases of this study. The inter-relationship of bone and nerves as illustrated by cases of so-called cervical rib in their morphological and clinical relationships, the behavior of bone under pathological conditions and under normal conditions at different ages have been touched upon early in the investigation. It soon appeared, however, that an enormous experience would be necessary if this field were to be properly opened up, and this experience must cover every phase of the subject and leave no line of attack unutilized. During recent years I have therefore refrained from further publication temporarily while necessary collections were being made and data gathered. The war with its abundance of bone cases provided for study, in what one might term the experimental phase, an unlimited material of the greatest value. For it is possible to make observations upon growth processes in long bones of human beings whose interest and coöperation can readily be secured, which are difficult or impossible in laboratory animals.

The present paper, therefore, summarizes the result of an inquiry into the regeneration processes of the cancellous tissue of human long bones as revealed by the cases of chronic osteomyelitis which came under my care in 1918, while I was in charge of surgery at the Base Hospital of Wolseley Barracks, London, Ont. I would first of all express my appreciation of the coöperation and encouragement of my many colleagues, and above all to Major G. C. Hale, officer in charge, and to Major David Smith, my predecessor on the service.

The study of the rôle of cancellous tissue in regeneration of bone is urgent because it has received such scanty notice hitherto as almost to be left out of consideration. Periosteum, cambium layer and compact tissue have all had their share of attention, but cancellous tissue has been largely neglected, and this is probably due to the fact that it does not lend itself to study in laboratory animals so well as the other portions of the bone just mentioned.

The cases to which the present paper has reference were all chronic osteomyelitis resulting from compound, more or less comminuted, fractures of bones of the limbs. The cases were of various duration, and in almost every instance the patient was eagerly longing for freedom after many months of confinement to bed. This attitude of the patient, which was fully justifiable under the circumstances, demanded ambulatory treatment whenever and as soon as possible. Nevertheless, my predecessor, Major David Smith, had shown that no treatment other than that of permitting the bone cavity, when cleaned out, to heal from the bottom, held out any hope of a satisfactory and permanent cure. The error of permitting the soft tissues to close in, and the unreliability of the bacteriological examination as an indication of when this procedure might be adopted, were already sufficiently obvious.

The practical problems which faced me therefore were, first, the effects of ambulatory treatment of chronic osteomyelitis and the time when the patient's condition would permit of this; second, the methods to be adopted for encouraging and not retarding the rapid and satisfactory healing of the bone cavity; and thirdly, the prognosis for Headquarters regarding the probable duration of the patient's stay in hospital.

It is apparent that the only solution of these problems lies in an adequate knowledge of the rôle of the cancellous tissue.

II. *Methods of Study.*—In each case a careful summary was made of the previous treatment with its results and tracings of all radiograms taken during the treatment were filed with the case records to check up the progress.

After operation, in which the affected area was thoroughly opened up and adequately drained, the operative wounds were kept open by means to be described later, and the abscess cavity permitted to heal from the bottom. From time to time radiograms were taken and in some cases portions removed under local anæsthetic from the healing walls for histological examination in order that the regeneration process and rate might be adequately checked up. By the courtesy of Professor P. S. McKibben pieces after fixation in 10 per cent. formalin were decalcified, cut and stained in the Laboratory of Anatomy of Western University. The methods of staining adopted were the following: Hæmatoxylin and eosin, Toluidin blue and eosin, Mallory, Wright. I shall therefore describe, in the first place, the histological features of a typical healing bone cavity and then proceed to consider the effect of various factors in retarding or accelerating healing.

III. *Typical Healing of a Bone Cavity.*—In the typical healing of a bone cavity the regeneration occurs from the cancellous tissue in the present series of cases. Some authors have termed this portion of the bone the endosteum, a word which, by the obscurity of its precise significance, is misleading and useless. Instances in which the cancellous tissue had been removed and the wall of the cavity was formed, entirely, or practically, by compact bone, will receive later consideration.

Within a few days of the operation the entire cavity is seen to be lined with vascular granulations, which are of earliest and strongest growth where the remaining cancellous tissue is thickest, and especially in that part of the cavity nearest the mid-point of the length of the bone. A portion of the new vascular tissue, removed carefully under a local anæsthetic two weeks after the operation, shows active growth of bone; and again it is apparent that the earliest and greatest bone growth occurs where the cancellous tissue is most abundant (Fig. 1).

Invading the connective tissue are trabeculæ of recently formed bone, each trabecula having arranged along its surface numerous osteoblasts. The newly ossified bone shows a fibrillar structure, the fibrillæ being arranged in the main in the long axis of the trabecula. Some of these fibrillæ with the accompanying ossein project in among the connective tissue surrounding the bone and more or less enclose osteoblasts on the surface. Near the growing end the newly ossified bone shows as a somewhat flocculent substance obscuring the fibrillæ or entirely obliterating them. In this substance are many lacunar cells, some of which show recent division, either of the nucleus or of the entire cell. In no instance, however, were mitotic figures visible. The term *lacunar cell* is used to indicate a cell which is beyond the osteoblast stage, unsurrounded or only partially surrounded by ossein, but not yet arrived at the stage of the bone-cell, which is apparently completely adult, never again divided, and is surrounded by fibrillar, non-floccular ossein exhibiting canaliculi. Beyond this most recent bone that not so lately formed is of clearer, more evenly translucent character, shows fibrillæ and encloses typical bone-cells each in its lacuna with radiating canaliculi in the surrounding bone.

Occasionally upon the surface of the growing bone can be seen small multinucleated cells, none however exhibiting more than three or four nuclei. The floccular character of the newly-formed ossein and its prolongations into the surrounding connective tissue are shown exceedingly well in preparations stained with Mallory.

Given satisfactory conditions the regeneration progresses steadily until the bone cavity is filled, the rate varying however with the particular bone, the site in the bone, the size of the cavity, and possibly with the age of the patient. This last factor is by no means certain within the usual army limits and is negligible. It is in the later stages of the filling of a large cavity that the growth processes slacken in speed. The march of ossification cannot be adequately followed by means of radiographic examination. In some of the earlier cases, the contraction of the cavity not being discernible radiographically, pieces of the wall were removed for histological examination. This showed that it is only after there is considerable growth of the new bone in density that the radiogram will confirm the satisfactory progress of the case.

It is noteworthy that the cut edges of the compact tissue limiting the bone opening invariably showed little or no tendency to produce new bone, and there was therefore no hindrance from this source in keeping the large superficial opening approximately the same throughout the healing process.

IV. *Effect of Various Factors in Retarding or Accelerating Healing.*—(*a*) *Essential importance of conserving the source of osteoblasts.* That the cancellous tissue is a generous source of osteoblasts has not in the past been sufficiently recognized. Berg and Thalhimer, in a recent paper, however, make the following striking statement [1]: "The few transplants which included endosteum [i.e., cancellous tissue T. W. T.], though not enough to allow any definite conclusions to be formed, showed an even greater growth from the endosteum than from any other transplants, even including periosteum."

The truth of this statement is abundantly borne out by the cases which form the basis of the present paper. While it is essential thoroughly to open up and expose the entire area of infection, remove all sequestra, and provide effective and ample drainage, the cancellous tissue must be conservatively dealt with and under no circumstances removed entirely. It is the bone abscesses which are "thoroughly" curetted out so that only the compact shell remains which result most disastrously from the point of view of healing. Especially is this the case in those instances in which pure carbolic swabbing is used to finish the destructive work of the curette.

Berg and Thalhimer, following other recent authors (e.g., Mayer and Wehner [2]), emphasize the activity of the osteoblasts lining the Haversian canals in regeneration of bone. Whether these osteoblasts come from Haversian systems in the cancellous tissue or from the lining of the spaces in the tissue is immaterial. Doubtless they come from both places. At any rate, there is no doubt that Haversian systems do occur in cancellous tissue. I drew attention to this in 1912,[3] and recently the fact has been reiterated by Arey.[4]

Regeneration of bone from the compact tissue is slow indeed, and may, for practical purposes, even be non-existent (Fig. 2). A typical case falling within this category is the following:

Reg. No. 400349.—Pte. A. W. Gunshot wound right tibia.
Previous History.—April 2, 1916: Shrapnel wound right tibia. Shrapnel passed through the limb. April 3, 1916: Operation; scraping and removal of fragments of bone. June 24, 1916: Operation; scraping; apparently allowed to close superficially. February, 1917: Sinus ceased discharging. August 3, 1917: Sinus recommenced discharging. August 4, 1917: Radiographed. August 14, 1917: Operation; thoroughly opened; cavity is three inches long; curetted thoroughly; swabbed out with phenol, alcohol and iodine. December 18, 1917: Cavity reopened and thoroughly scraped. April 6, 1918: Radiographed. April 12, 1918: Cavity reopened; apparently no filling up by osseous tissue scraped and three sequestra removed from lower part.
Condition on First Observation.—May 10, 1918: Radiographed. At this stage the case came under my control. "The area to granulate has steadily increased with each operation. The wound is thoroughly open and draining well. It should be kept open and left alone as regards operative measures from now on."

Further events justified this decision, for on September 25, 1918, when I last saw the case, healing was occurring from the sides and the lower end and the cavity reduced to one-half the size it had been on May 10th. Examination of the radiograms (Fig. 3) will show how, instead of accelerating healing, the various operations successively created a larger area to granulate. Further, it emphasizes the effect of traumatic and chemical methods in producing the death of bone. There is little doubt in my mind that the late

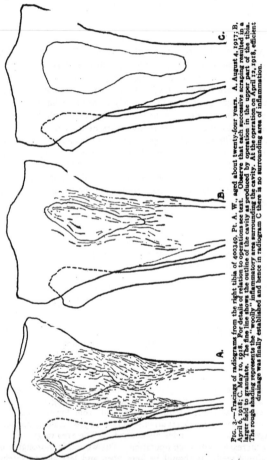

FIG. 3.—Tracings of radiograms from the right tibia of 400349. Pt. A. W., aged about twenty-four years. A. August 4, 1917; B. April 6, 1918; C. May 10, 1918. For details of relation to operations see text. Observe that each successive scraping resulted in a larger field to granulate. The fine line shows the outline of the cavity as produced by operation in the upper part of the tibia. The rough shading represents the "woolly" inflammatory area surrounding the cavity. At the operation on April 12, 1918, efficient drainage was finally established and hence in radiogram C there is no surrounding area of inflammation.

sequestra which were removed on April 12, 1918, were directly due to the vigorous traumatism of the operation of December, 1917. Throughout the healing process it was very evident in this case that little or no regeneration was occurring from those parts of the cavity wall which had been denuded of cancellous tissue.

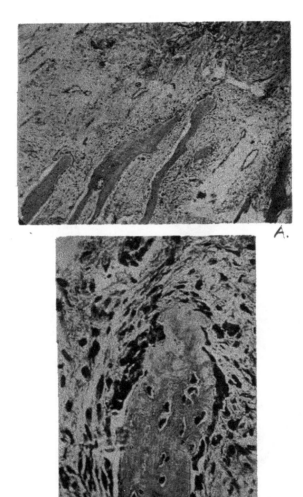

FIG. 1.—Typical regeneration of bone from cancellous tissue of the cavity wall. From No. 400983, Pt. J. R., aged twenty years; gunshot wound left tibia. *A*, Magnification sixty times. Bausch and Lomb Obj. 16 mm.; eye-piece 5.0. Note the bony trabeculæ penetrating the connective tissue of the cavity wall. Hæmatoxylin and eosine. *B*, Magnification 330 times. B and L. Obj. 3 mm.; eye-piece 5.0. Shows the tip of a process of bone from *A*, projecting into the newly formed connective tissue. For description see text.

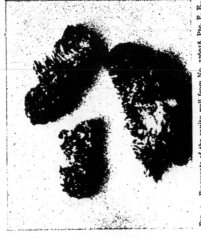

FIG. 4.—Fragments of the cavity wall from No. 226018, Pte. F. E., aged thirty-seven years. Upper left tibia. Twice natural size (No. E. 380, W. R. U.). Note the forest of bony spicules which were imbedded in the pyogenic lining membrane. The upper right-hand piece is shown in profile, the others are shown full-face.

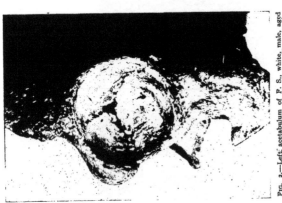

FIG. 2.—Left acetabulum of P. S., white, male, aged thirty-eight years (No. 167, W. R. U.); to illustrate the insignificant role played by compact tissue in regeneration. Healed, stellate fracture, apparently but not actually following the lines of fusion of ilium, ischium and pubis. The femur was uninjured. The floor of the acetabulum contains exceedingly little cancellous tissue and the fracture heals largely by fibrous union. Near the acetabular rim there is considerable cancellous tissue and here firm bony union takes place.

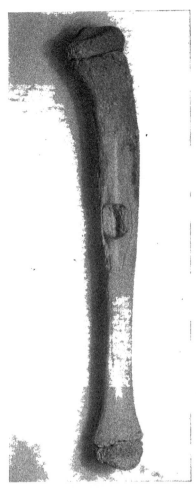

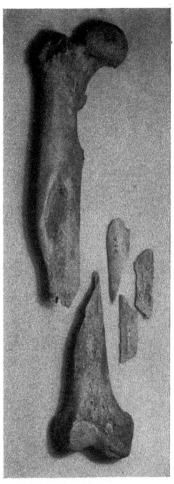

FIG. 5.—Acute osteomyelitis of subperiosteal type. From E. L., male, white, aged nine years, left tibia (No. E. 16, W. R. U.). Note 3 mm. depth of cancellous bone surrounding original incision through the periosteum. This had been deposited under inflammatory conditions in the three weeks elapsing between incision and final amputation. Trephine opening into tibia. The wholly inefficient surgical treatment resulted in infection of the knee-joint and ultimate amputation.

FIG. 6.—Comminuted fracture right femur from J. W., male, white, aged forty-five years (No. 156, W. R. U.), at the stage of commencing callus formation. The callus has been left on the two lower small fragments to show the extent to which it has developed. Callus had formed equally on both sides but not on the edges of these fragments. Such callus as there was has been cleaned off both main fragments and the uppermost small fragment to show the reaction of compact bone to regeneration. Note the generally pitted character of the bone adjacent to the fracture. This is due to the newly developed vascularity of the bone. There is a distinct difference between the upper and lower parts of the fragment which bears the number 156. The upper part shows no pitting: the periosteum was stripped off this and it is dying. The lower part is pitted in consequence of the rarefying action of vascularization. The small amount of callus developed has been removed from this to show the pitted character. *B*

456

Another case which illustrates the fact that the compact tissue is inadequate to supply osteoblasts is the following, but this time it is the superficial or external face of the compact tissue which comes under observation.

Reg. No. 189528.—Pte. E. R. P., aged twenty years. Gunshot wound left thigh.

· *Previous History.*—May 3, 1917: Shrapnel wound left thigh and leg. Compound fracture upper third of femur. Also small wound middle of calf. Incision: drainage; Thomas' knee-splint; removal of sequestra; repeated drainage. November 13, 1917: Large cavity in femur; further drainage; general thickening of femur to knee. February 2, 1918: Knee immobile with wasting of muscles of leg. April 17, 1918: Fibrosis and atrophy of thigh muscles. Six sinuses on front and inner and outer sides of thigh. Knee is swollen but can be flexed slightly by passive movement. Calf muscles wasted. Movements of ankle normal in range but weak. Movements at hip weak.

Condition on First Observation.—May 19, 1918: Multiple sinuses; periostitis palpable as far as knee, which shows fibrous ankylosis not quite complete. Massage. Patient's general condition poor.

July 8, 1918: Operation. Five-inch incision through outer front of upper thigh. Four-inch counter-incision for drainage outer thigh. One large Y-shaped (4½ inches long) and many small sequestra removed from pulpy granulation tissue within an involucrum of sound bone. Much bleeding as Esmarch could not be properly applied to thigh. As patient's condition would not stand further prolongation of the operation, the three lower sinuses of the thigh were not explored, but left for later treatment, since they did not connect with the present operation area.

August 8, 1918: Second operation. Incision to femur through three lower sinuses. No sinuses found leading into bone, and no dead bone, but multilocular abscesses between the bared compact tissue and the raised and much thickened periosteum. The pus and pulpy granulation tissue were removed and the loculi broken down and thoroughly drained, the wounds as in all cases being kept widely open. During the eight weeks following the second operation, while the patient was under my care, the cavity in the upper femur continued to fill up satisfactorily, but there was no marked growth of bone from the outer surface of the compact tissue of the lower femur forming the base of the superficial abscesses, and there was naturally no bony growth from the thickened and fibrosed raised periosteum. The cambium layer had been completely destroyed and the dense walled cavities between periosteum and bone showed the greatest reluctance to fill up. This lack of bony growth is the more remarkable in this case since the periosteal bony growth everywhere, except in the wall of the abscesses, was extraordinarily vigorous.

In addition to examples like the foregoing, it is well at this stage to stress once more the fact that the cut edges of the wound in compact tissue in cases of chronic osteomyelitis invariably exhibit very slow and unsatisfactory throwing out of new bone.

b. Effect of Pressure on Bone Healing.—Pressure may be applied to healing bone in one of two ways: It may be from without, either as a result of the method of treatment or from encroachment of, and confinement by, the soft tissue. Again, the pressure may be intrinsic as a result of contraction, with scar formation in the granulation tissue of the healing bone which precedes the actual ossification.

Owing to the fact that soft tissues granulate and heal much more quickly than bone, the retention of the wounds properly open becomes a most difficult undertaking. When I came on the service I found that the utilization of glass tubes for this purpose, as adopted by Major Smith, served admirably up to a certain point. At the time of operation the dimensions of the wound in the compact tissue were taken, and a large glass tube, long enough to extend from the surface of the limb into the bone cavity, was moulded to fit the aperture in the compacta. On removal of the packing twenty-four hours after operation, the glass tube was slipped into place and retained there either simply by the dressings or by a narrow strip of adhesive, which was arranged so as not to interfere at all with drainage. The glass tube was also arranged so as not to obstruct the drainage, and if necessary, had holes blown in its sides to this end. In this way the wound in the superficial soft tissues was prevented from contracting and was indeed kept of the same dimensions as the opening in the compact bone. Thus the bone cavity could always be adequately studied throughout its healing, and satisfactorily irrigated and treated in whatever way might seem necessary. The only drawback to the glass tube method was that its base eventually rested upon the healing bone, and this pressure effectually put a stop to progress. It was necessary to devise some method whereby all the advantages of the glass tube method might be retained and its disadvantages overcome. Hence I employed a collar of dental impression wax fitted around the glass tube to prevent it sinking in too far. Dental impression wax, being easily moulded when softened in hot water and readily adhering to a clean glass tube, I was able from time to time to make the adjustment necessary in the length of the tube, so that it always cleared the granulating base of the cavity while penetrating the aperture in the compact tissue. Only when the cavity had satisfactorily healed to the level of the compacta was the tube finally removed and the soft tissues permitted slowly to close in. This closing in was regulated indeed by replacing the old glass tube by new ones of successively smaller calibre. Thus the final stages of healing could be adequately observed and controlled.

The effect of slight pressure in retarding and frequently and eventually in inhibiting bone growth cannot be too strongly emphasized. Ossifying granulations will penetrate into the glass tube if it rests upon the healing base of the cavity, but between these and the ossifying granulations around the tube an annular depression remains where the tube was pitted and prevented the formation of bone regeneration.

If some efficient method be not adopted to keep the wound in the soft tissues widely open, it contracts within a few hours, and in two or three days has closed so greatly that further examination and effective treatment of the healing cavity are no longer possible. When our patients reached the ambulatory stage their wounds were always examined immediately upon return to the hospital and the tube replaced if by any chance it had become displaced. This procedure was imperative, for if the tube were withdrawn for even a few hours, the dilation necessary to replace it gave great pain, if, indeed, it were possible. Especially must the soft tissues be prevented from falling in for the first six weeks after operation, for even if the operation has been satisfactory, surgically, in every way. the traumatism necessarily incidental to every bone operation will probably cause the death of some part of the cavity wall, either compact or cancellous tissue. As a result, small superficial flakes will be shed as sequestra, and it is frequently these which keep up the long-continued post-operative suppuration and prevent a satisfactory healing. Such small sequestra begin to be shed about three weeks after the operation and the time they take to separate naturally varies with their size. Not until six weeks after operation can one be reasonably sure that flaking has ceased. It is useless to pretend that such sequestrum formation can be prevented by gentle methods. Chisels, hammers. saws and curettes cannot be gently used, for the term gentle must necessarily have reference to the bone tissue which is exceedingly delicate and sensitive to mechanical or chemical interference. This post-operative flaking constitutes a further reason for keeping the wound open and directly contra-indicates the employment of so-called rapid methods of encouraging healing, such as permitting the soft tissues to fall in or closing the wound after or without the use of antiseptics like pure phenol, tincture of iodine or B. I. P. Again the healing cavity must be kept under close observation, for in some cases the granulations which normally are red become fibrous. When this occurs their color changes to gray. Once fibrosis has occurred in the recent granulations, ossification will not penetrate them and healing comes to a stand-still. In such a case nothing will serve but removal of the fibrosed granulations. For this purpose, a further operation under a general anæsthetic is not necessary. It is only needful to remove the fibrosis, and this can readily be done with a curette if the cavity first be anæsthetized with a weak β-eucaine or other local anæsthetic solution to which some adrenalin has been added. The cause of fibrosis in the granulations is often inadequate drainage or cleansing, in which case this must be corrected. but sometimes it occurs apparently from simple indolence of the healing process. Removal of the fibrosis in such cases is usually sufficient to result in restoration of the normal healing process.

    c. Effect of Inefficient Drainage upon Healing of Bone Cavities.— The effect of inefficient drainage may be localized to the healing walls of the cavity, but is usually more widely distributed in the bone. A radiogram of such a bone usually shows a varying depth of inflammation around the cavity. This is indicated by a " woolly " appearance of the cancellous tissue

in the plate. In all cases in which this appearance was noted we radiographed the area again about three weeks after operation. By this time the
woolly appearance has disappeared if drainage has been effective and the
architecture of the bone again becomes apparent and clearly defined.

Local results of ineffective drainage are unhealthy, pale, and exuberant
granulations, later becoming fibrosed, and sometimes sequestrum formation.
If left uncorrected, these granulations fibrosing, form a veritable pyogenic
membrane. Usually, as in the case No. 189528, Pte. E. R. P., previously
referred to, masses of such unhealthy granulations fill the cavity and surround and imbed the sequestra when the cavity is opened at operation.

Sometimes cases are met with in which there is a small intermittently
discharging sinus leading to a cavity somewhat resembling a Brodie's abscess
and lined by a typical pyogenic membrane. Such a case was the following:

Reg. No. 226018.—Pte. F. E., aged thirty-seven years. Gunshot
wound upper leg.

Previous History.—December 28, 1916: Shrapnel wound upper
left leg. This was a through-and-through wound, the shrapnel passing
between the tibia and fibula. The previous records were lost.

Condition on Admission.—August 18, 1918: Healed scar popliteal
space. Small discharging sinus on front of leg leading into upper tibia,
which was very tender locally. Much thickening upper tibia. No
paralysis. No loss of sensation. Radiographic examination showed
much periostitis upper half of tibia with large area of osteomyelitis
occupying upper third or more, and a small perforation in the bone.

August 29, 1918: Vertical incision over subcutaneous surface of tibia.
Area of compact bone four and a half inches long by three-quarters
of an inch broad around sinus opening removed. The entire cavity was
thus laid bare; it was found to be lined by a pyogenic membrane in which
were imbedded innumerable tiny osseous spicules from the surrounding
compact bone (Fig. 4). Practically the entire cancellous tissue of the
upper tibia had been destroyed by the abscess in which were several
small sequestra rendered unrecognizable in the radiogram by the
opacity caused by the abscess with its surrounding inflammatory
zone. The pyogenic membrane was completely removed and careful examination then showed that no further curetting was necessary. In order to provide an adequate exposure of the cavity the
insertions of the sartorius and gracilis had to be raised from the bone
and the subjacent bursæ opened. The bursæ were left widely open.

September 3, 1918: Healthy red granulations springing from entire
cavity wall. The bursæ are also granulating satisfactorily.

September 21: None of the cavity wall is now visible since it is
entirely covered by healthy granulations. Tendons of sartorius and
gracilis have united afresh to the periosteum at the inner margin
of the wound.

At this stage the case passed out of my hands. It will be referred to
again later in the paper, but for the moment, apart from the occurrence of a

pyogenic membrane, the case presents two instructive features. First, a minimum of mechanical interference and abstention from the use of chemicals, like pure phenol violently destructive of bone, preserve the small activity of the compact tissue in regeneration. Probably the osteoblasts in this case appeared from the Haversian systems. Secondly, it is not necessary to remove all the compact tissue covering the cavity; enough must be, however, to provide for the fullest possible observation and the most effective drainage. In other words, all procedures in the operation must be as conservative as surgical efficiency permits. As an example of the effect of conservative treatment and very free drainage in encouraging healing, the following case is worthy of record:

Reg. No. 727638.—Pte. C. M., aged twenty years. Gunshot wound thigh.

Previous History.—April 11, 1917: Rifle bullet wound right femur. Compound comminuted fracture middle third. Five operations in France and England. No bone removed so far as could be ascertained. In the early stage of treatment, to obtain reunion of the femoral fragments in good position, extension from calipers on the upper extremity of the tibia had been employed.

Condition on Admission.—June 10, 1918: Discharging sinus front of thigh just above middle. Pocketing of pus in back of thigh. Sequestrum palpable under skin immediately lateral to sinus. Knee contains fluid and is laterally movable: it cannot be hyperextended. Radiograph adds nothing materially to the foregoing.

June 20, 1918: Operation. Six-inch vertical incision front of thigh, excising an old operative scar. The entire middle third of the femur was removed as nine sequestra. In order to do this it was necessary to cut a long and broad channel through the involucrum to which the upper and lower thirds of the femur were firmly united. The sequestra were found imbedded as usual in soft, pulpy, unhealthy granulation tissue which was entirely removed, but no unnecessary curetting done. So far as could be ascertained no sinus tracks were left at the bottom of which sequestra might be lying. It was apparent in this case that sequestrum formation had come to an end. A large opening was made through the involucrum on the lateral and posterior side of the cavity, including the old sinus through which pocketing of pus had occurred and this opening connected with the surface by an equally large incision in the soft tissues. A smaller drainage opening was also made in the lowest lateral part of the cavity wall through to the outer surface of the thigh. The cavity was packed as usual with iodoform gauze.

June 22, 1918: First dressing: Gauze removed under self-administered chloroform by Sollmann's method. Glass tubes with wax collars inserted through anterior and upper lateral wounds. Rubber tube inserted into lower lateral wound.

July 15, 1918: The cavity has discharged profusely, but there have been no set-backs. Rubber tube removed from lower lateral wound which is now permitted to close.

August 15, 1918: Glass tubes have been shortened from time to time. There is now relatively little discharge, the cavity having largely filled up.

September 21, 1918: A very small cavity remains which should heal completely in a few weeks. Discharge very small in amount.

At this time the patient was lost sight of. As this was one of the largest cavities dealt with, it is particularly unfortunate that the treatment could not have been followed to the very end, for the terminal phase and the final results would have proved most valuable.

d. *Influence of the Site of the Lesion upon Healing.*—One of the most instructive suggestions which this study has brought out is that the rate and facility of healing vary with the site of the cavity in the bone and perhaps also with the particular bone itself. The bones included in this survey are the humerus, femur, and tibia, these being the large pipe bones in which considerable cavity formation is possible. Without much more extended observation it is impossible to assert categorically that the cancellous tissue in one part of the bone has greater regenerating power than in another. In all three bones mentioned cavitation of the middle third is easier to deal with than it is at either extremity, and this is true even of the femur, in the case of which the wound necessarily kept open in the soft tissues is much deeper than in the case of tibia or humerus. That efficient drainage has much to do with the rate of healing is, of course, obvious, but in looking over the records it is noteworthy that in every case where the cavitation lay toward one or other extremity of the shaft it was always that end of the cavity nearest the midlength of the bone which showed regeneration earliest and was the first to fill completely.

Regeneration travelled more slowly as it approached the extremity of the bone, and frequently that end of the cavity nearest the articulation proved almost intractable, so slow was the process of its filling up. Months after the great majority of the cavity was completely healed there would remain a small area near the joint which persistently refused to heal.

As typical of the general rate of healing of a bone cavity in a site where efficient drainage is a simple matter, the following case is instructive.

Reg. No. 400983.—Pte. J. R., aged twenty years, gunshot wound left tibia. October 1, 1916: Shrapnel wound left leg, compound fracture middle left tibia. Three operations in France and England. Discharging sinus: fracture healed.

January 16, 1918: Operation. Opening 1½ inches long made through compact tissue of subcutaneous aspect. Several sequestra, one 1¼ inches in length, removed. Cavity curetted and disinfected.

April 4, 1918: Area again scraped to original size. No sequestra.

June 26, 1918: Glass tube finally removed from wound.

July 23, 1918: Wound healed, skin having dipped slightly into cavity.

Note that the result of the disinfection at the operation of January 16th was to delay greatly the healing so that by April 4th, when a fresh start was given to the cavity and more effective drainage instituted, very little healing had taken place. Until this date the patient was kept in bed. After this the ambulatory method was adopted, yet twelve weeks after April 4th (*i.e.*, on June 26th), the tube could be removed and sixteen weeks after this operation the patient was discharged healed firmly.

This and other similar cases suggest that there may be more rapid growth of bone from cancellous tissue than from the cambium layer of the periosteum. The cavity which filled in sixteen weeks was about 35 mm. long and 8 mm. deep. In a badly treated case of osteomyelitis of the subperiosteal variety in which amputation was resorted to three weeks after the initial incision, obtained in civil practice from a boy of nine years, not quite 3 mm. depth of cancellous tissue had formed upon the surface of the compacta of the subcutaneous aspect of the tibia (Fig. 5).

e. Effect of Inflammatory Reaction upon Healing.—One case in which surgical erysipelas occurred after curetting a cavity under local anæsthetic suggests that inflammation may have a marked stimulating effect on regeneration. .

Reg. No. 405020.—L/C W. D., aged twenty-three years. Gunshot wound left femur.

Previous History.—September 15, 1916: Shrapnel wound left thigh. Compound comminuted fracture femur involving upper third of shaft and both trochanters. Six operations in France, England, and Canada.

March 12, 1918: Operation. Incision 6 inches long outer side thigh. Removal of many small sequestra from region of great trochanter and of one large sequestrum 3¼ by 2 by ½ inches. Until July, 1918, this large cavity very slowly healed, but by then many œdematous granulations had obscured the deeper cavity. These were curetted away under local anæsthetic. Immediately there supervened surgical erysipelas which was treated with antistreptococcic serum and with saturated solution of magnesium sulphate and alcohol locally. After this the area healed much more rapidly and by September 25th only a small cavity was left in the bone, as usual at the end involving the great trochanter.

f. Effect of the Ambulatory Method of Treatment.—As explained earlier in the report there were sufficient reasons for permitting the patient as soon as possible to be out in the open air. Comparing the results with those previously obtained by keeping the patient at rest in bed, this method proved advantageous. There was no retardation of healing, but on the contrary, regeneration occurred much more rapidly than before, probably on account of more effective drainage and improvement in the general health of the patient.

g. Peculiarities of the Lower Tibia.—In several cases where the tibia was involved near the ankle-joint we were tempted to be too conservative, especially when the sinus lay on the back of the bone, owing to a natural desire to leave undamaged the subcutaneous aspect of the bone. These cases are very difficult to drain, for from the anatomical relations the wound is kept open with difficulty. It was found necessary in every case to open through the subcutaneous surface and make through-and-through drainage, after which no set-backs occurred in healing.

h. The Relation of Compact Tissue to Healing.—It has already been stated that regeneration from compact tissue occurs very slowly or not at all. This was found to be invariably the case and there was never any difficulty experienced through the wound filling up before the cavity had become completely filled. This is of course borne out by the usual course of healing of trephine openings in the skull.

The relation of compact tissue to healing of a bone is well shown by the specimen illustrated in Fig. 6. This is from a comminuted fracture of the femur obtained in civil life. Note that the compact tissue in the neighborhood of the healing fracture is filled with small holes, rarefied, in other words, as though the blood-vessels had enlarged. It seems in accord with the views expressed regarding compact tissue by Berg and Thalhimer.[1] In the fragment from which the periosteum was partially stripped off, only the area to which the periosteum was still adherent is rarefied. No change has occurred in the periosteum-free portion.

V. When to Permit the Cavity to Fill Up.—Filling up of the cavity can only be allowed to occur after one is reasonably sure that sequestra resulting from the mechanical damage of operation have separated. Small flake-like sequestra, according to the present experience, take from three to six weeks to separate, those forming from compact tissue naturally taking longer to separate than if they have formed from cancellous bone. Sometimes after the cavity itself had filled and the tube was removed, complete healing was delayed owing to the late separation of sequestra from the edges and surface of the compacta. Once these had been withdrawn healing rapidly took place.

VI. Management of First Dressing and Other Features.—Certain technical features connected with the work upon which the paper is based, though having no relation to the subject matter proper, seem worthy of a simple statement. The first dressing, usually twenty-four hours, but in some of the more extensive cases forty-eight hours after the operation, when the gauze packing is removed, is naturally extremely painful and to men whose nervous systems are already far from normal because of long hospital experience if from nothing else, a source of great mental anxiety in anticipation. I therefore introduced Sollmann's method of chloroform analgesia by self-inhalation[5] and found it entirely satisfactory and without objectionable result in any of the many scores of times it was used.

As regards management of skin and soft tissues there is little to add. The skin was never permitted to creep into a cavity before it had closed solidly to the level of the compact tissue so that the depression in the skin surface should be quite shallow. As regards periosteum it was found best to remove it entirely to the limits of the opening through the compacta. Any redundant periosteum becomes inflamed, acutely tender, and is much in the way of the necessary glass tube. In those early cases in which redundant periosteum was left by way of experiment, it had always to be removed later under local anæsthetic.

SUMMARY

1. Cancellous tissue is one of the chief agents in regeneration of bone, and like the cambium layer of periosteum, should be treated at operation in the most conservative manner, consistent with thorough exploration and drainage.

2. In regeneration the cancellous tissue nearest the mid-length of the bone grows most rapidly, whereas that in or near the articular extremities shows less readiness to proliferate and fill the cavity.

3. Septic bone cavities should be permitted to heal from the bottom, the wound in the soft tissues being kept widely open until this has occurred. The least possible mechanical disturbance of the cancellous tissue should be employed and no " disinfection " of the cavity attempted, for this simply kills the remaining tissue from which regeneration is expected.

4. Regenerating bone is very sensitive to and easily affected by pressure, even of soft tissues, and by inefficient drainage. It is not adversely affected by the ambulatory method of treatment.

5. Compact bone plays a very minor part in regeneration.

REFERENCES

[1] Berg, A. A., and Thalhimer, W.: Regeneration of Bone. ANNALS OF SURGERY, 1918, vol. lxvii, pp. 331-347.

[2] Mayer, L., and Wehner, E.: An Experimental Study of Osteogenesis. Amer. Journ. Orthop. Surg., 1914, vol. xii, pp. 213-244.

[3] Todd, T. W.: A Preliminary Note on the Development and Growth of Bone. Journ. Anat. and Physiol., 1912, vol. xlvii, pp. 177-188.

[4] Arey, L. B.: On the Presence of Haversian Systems in Membrane Bone. Anat. Rec., 1919, vol. xvii, pp. 59-61.

[5] Sollmann, T.: Chloroform Analgesia by Self-Inhalation. Journ. Amer. Med. Assoc., 1918, vol. lxxi, pp. 657-8.

THE RECOGNITION OF DEAD BONE BASED ON PATHOLOGICAL AND X-RAY STUDIES *

By Dallas B. Phemister, M.D.

OF CHICAGO, ILL.

WHEN bone dies rapidly and in appreciable quantity from infection in osteomyelitis, compound fractures, tuberculosis and rarely in lues, it is at first indistinguishable either by gross or röntgenologic appearance from the adjacent living portions. Only after the occurrence of further changes in the living and the dead bone can its extent be determined. A detailed knowledge of these changes is essential for arriving at a diagnosis, especially by means of the X-rays, and for planning suitable and properly timed operations.

The changes in the dead bone are of great importance in establishing its identity. There are changes in color which are of assistance at operation. Dead compact bone turns white from the loss of circulation and of soft parts, but usually it requires some time for their absorption and the difference in appearance early between it and the pinkish living bone is insufficient to make it a reliable guide for removing the dead bone before the line of separation has begun to form. Necrotic spongy bone is frequently dark brown or red, due to the presence of old blood and necrotic marrow in the cancellous spaces where it is sheltered from attack. Granulations may grow into and be removed with a spongy sequestrum, giving it a reddish color which is sometimes difficult to distinguish from living spongy bone. By holding the sequestrum under the tap, blood and granulations are readily washed out, leaving the white cancellous bone.

Granulation tissue soon attacks the dead bone, but its activity becomes most marked after the acute inflammatory stage subsides. The tasks for the granulations are to separate the dead bone from the living, to reduce its volume or break it up by absorption and to extrude it from the field through the discharging sinuses.

Separation of dead from living bone is accomplished more rapidly than the other changes. The granulations attack both living and dead cortex along the line of junction, from both periosteal and endosteal sides, forming two irregular tortuous grooves which are gradually deepened until they meet. This results in the formation of a jagged irregular zone of demarcation two to five mm. in width, depending on the thickness of the sequestrum. These grooves are frequently seen at early operation, or in the X-ray picture as a nick or uneven dotted line in the cortex, before separation is complete. In the separation of dead

---

* Read before the American Surgical Association, May 5, 1920.

466

spongy bone, because of its loose structure, a zone of granulation tissue forms simultaneously along the entire line of junction which results in early sequestration. The time required for separation is extremely variable according to the density and thickness of the bone involved. It ranges all the way from five or six days with very thin cortex or spongiosa of the small bones to five or six months with the thickest portions of the shaft of an adult tibia or femur.

Reduction in volume of the dead portion occurs from lacunar absorption by the granulations along its surfaces. There is no diffuse internal loss of lime salts from dead bone, so that any remaining portions retain

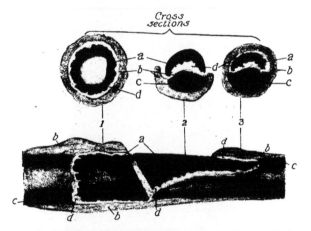

FIG. 1.—Sketch of X-ray of old infected fracture showing atrophy of surviving cortex, involucrum formation and two sequestra with well-preserved fracture lines and external surfaces that are eroded where adjacent to and little or uneroded where remote from living bone; *a*, dead bone; *b*, new bone; *c*, atrophied old bone; *d*, zone of demarcation. Cross sections show sequestra with erosion along 1, external surface; 2, internal surface; and 3, both internal and external surfaces. Differences in density well shown.

their original density. The rate of surface destruction varies greatly in different portions and is dependent largely upon the relation of the surfaces to surrounding living bone and to the channels of purulent discharge. Where living bone is in close contact with dead portions granulations springing from and supported by it attack the dead bone, producing an uneven worm-eaten surface in a comparatively short time. But those surfaces that lie at a considerable distance from living bone may show little or no signs of erosion even after long periods of time. Granulations arising from a soft part's covering attack dead bone slowly, and where they spring from the walls of a bone cavity will not bridge a wide gap and vigorously attack a relatively small enclosed sequestrum. Thus the periosteal surface of dead cortex will become extensively eroded in those portions surrounded by involucrum, but will remain smooth or little eroded where involucrum fails to form. Similarly the condition of the endosteal surface will vary with the degree of involvement of the shaft at any level. If less than half of its circumference dies, endosteal

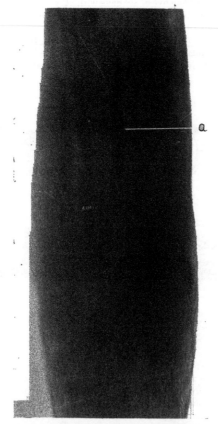

FIG. 2.—Almost stationary sequestrum in osteomyelitis of seven years' standing. *a*, Broad space between sequestrum and involucrum.

new bone will form from the surviving portion and maintain granulations in contact with the dead bone, destroying it from the endosteal surface. But if more than half the circumference is destroyed there will be frequently little or no erosion of the deeper portion of the endosteal surface. When the entire circumference is dead, the endosteal surface will remain unchanged for months or even years, except at the ends of the dead tube where granulations will invade the canal for a short distance. Where an involucrum is present destruction from the periosteal side may

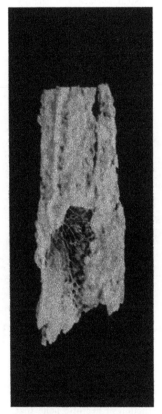

FIG. 3.—Photograph of part of sequestrum from Fig. 2. Periosteal surface markedly eroded, but endosteal surface undisturbed. as shown by presence of cancellous bone seen through window.

finally lead to perforations of the dead cortex, after which endosteal erosion from invading granulations may occur. These features are illustrated in Fig. 1, which is a composite sketch of the X-ray picture in the later stage of infected compound fracture showing different conditions of surfaces in sequestra according to their relation to living bone. Fig. 2 shows an X-ray and Fig. 3 is a photograph of a seven-year-old sequestrum of the entire circumference of the shaft of the femur resulting from osteomyelitis at the age of ten. While markedly eroded externally, it shows through a window endosteal surface and spongy bone that had not been touched by granulations.

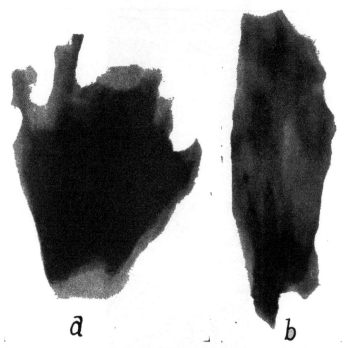

FIG. 4.—Cortical sequestra from gunshot fracture six months old. *a*, possesses original density because uneroded along periosteal or endosteal surface; *b*, eroded by granulations and density unevenly reduced.

There is little destruction of necrotic bone that occupies or borders on discharging channels, as the discharging pus in which it is bathed keeps the surrounding granulation tissue unhealthy. This is frequently seen in infected fractures where the fracture surfaces of the dead ends remain sharp and uneroded for months partly because of the restraining action of pus escaping from the deeper portions (Figs. 1 and 12–4).

Because of this unequal action of granulations upon its surface there may be marked variations in outline of different portions of a sequestrum.

Where unattacked the surface will be unchanged and the volume and density of the sequestrum will be what it was at the time death occurred (Figs. 4 *a* and 12–3). But where extensively eroded with deep pockets and sharp, irregular projections, the density will be unevenly reduced (Figs. 4 *b* and 5 *b*). Any portion that remains will have its original internal structure. These are all points of the greatest value in the X-ray diagnosis of dead bone.

The rate of destruction is greater while the dead piece is still at-

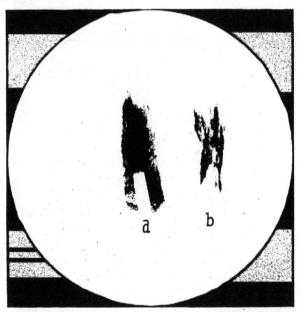

FIG. 5.—X-rays of *a*, involucrum from Fig. 13, No. 5, showing even, spongy character. *b*, sequestrum eroded, showing reduced uneven density but compact character.

tached to or incarcerated by living bone. Once it is loosened and the sequestrum moves into a freer position, especially if into a large bone pocket, destruction proceeds at a much slower rate. Splinters killed at the onset in infected fractures may be found little eroded at operation months afterward. In case of death of the entire circumference with complete encirclement of involucrum, the periosteal surface of the shaft is rapidly attacked at first, and where cortex is thin, especially in young children, it may be eaten through and fragmented, after which the pieces may be destroyed or extruded through the sinuses. But where cortex is thick, continued concentric erosion gradually leads to the development of

a wide space between sequestrum and involucrum as the latter becomes
dense and does not fill in about the dwindling dead piece. This retards
the action of the granulations, and such loosely enclosed sequestra may
then stand for years with only slight reduction in size. This is illustrated by Fig. 2, showing a practically stationary sequestrum with a wide
space between it and sclerotic involucrum.

Destruction of dead cancellous bone occurs more readily than of cor-

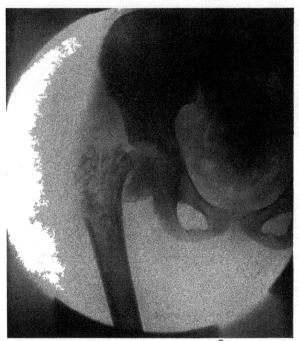

FIG. 6.—Scattered destruction in osteomyelitis of spongy portion of bone; an indirect
sign of the presence of sequestra.

tex which usually gives rise to the first changes shown in the X-ray. In
acute osteomyelitis of the end of the shaft the entire cancellous portion
may become necrotic, but that is not the rule. Usually the dead bone
is irregularly distributed and granulations developing from the adjacent
surviving portions produce signs of scattered destruction. Fig. 6 shows
such a condition in an eight-year-old child with osteomyelitis of the upper
end of the femoral shaft of five weeks' standing and a pathological fracture of the neck. More sequestra than could be identified in the X-ray

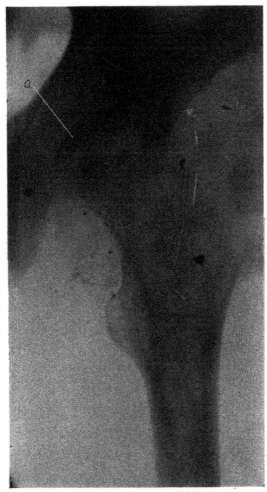

FIG. 7.—Gunshot wound of hip four months old with sequestrum (a) in head casting an evener and heavier shadow than atrophied surrounding bone. Articular surface on sequestrum preserved.

were found at operation throughout the region presenting signs of destruction. Smaller areas are usually completely broken down and it is rare to see large sequestra persist in this location. But in infected comminuted fractures of the ends of the bones, especially from gunshot wounds, large sequestra may form and persist with little more destruction than comes from formation of a wide zone of demarcation. When bordering on the joint cartilage in the presence of a complicating arthritis, the sequestrum stands out prominently because of the preservation of its original density and of the rim of bone supporting the articular cartilage, which on account of its inaccessibility to granulations, is not destroyed;

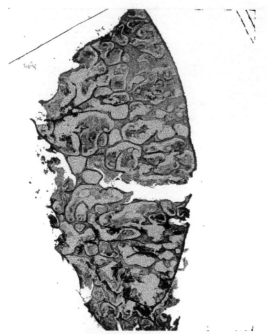

FIG. 8.—Section of sequestrum shown in Fig. 7. Interior trabeculæ intact and articular surface unbroken except in one place.

whereas that over the remaining living cartilaginous surface is irregularly broken down (Figs. 7 and 8).

A cone-shaped area of necrosis of considerable size is not infrequent in tuberculosis of the metaphysis or epiphysis and is usually broken down, leaving a cavity. When bordering on the articular surface of the joint, such a sequestrum is more apt to persist and maintain its original density. Occasionally calcification will occur in its cancellous spaces and thereby further increase its density so that it may cast a heavier shadow than the corresponding normal area on the other side.

Fig. 9.—X-ray of excised wall of tunnel (a), sequestra and shell fragment in gunshot fracture of femur six and one-half months old. Atrophied cortex of most of wall is longitudinally streaked by dilated canals: sequestra compact.

Changes in the Living Bone.—Changes in the living bone consist in local absorption and regional atrophy and transformation of preëxisting bone, and in new bone formation.

Local absorption of living bone bordering immediately on the dead

475

was observed by John Hunter to be of greater importance in the process of sequestration than absorption of the dead bone itself.

Regional atrophy results from disuse and is dependent on the degree and duration of loss of function. A limited osteomyelitis producing partial loss of function for a comparatively short time, may produce little atrophy. Extensive osteomyelitis causing marked and prolonged loss of function, produces much atrophy. Infected fractures, because of prolonged and complete loss of function produced by the fracture, infection, and immobilization, frequently show, after five or six months, the highest degree of atrophy. In the case of cortex, it occurs by diffuse absorption of lime salts, mainly along the course of the haversian canals, and is slightly more marked on the endosteal than on the periosteal side. This produces an even loss in density which, when marked, may be striated longitudinally by the lines of dilated canals (Fig. 9). In cancellous bone there is reduction in numbers and size of trabeculæ in a way that frequently gives a spotted appearance in the X-ray. Atrophy of the living bone usually occurs faster than destruction of the dead bone, hence after a length of time varying with the size of the bone, the dead portion casts a heavier shadow in the X-ray than the living (Figs. 1 and 12). This relation obtains until there is resumption of function and increase in density of the atrophied portion, or until there is further destruction of the dead bone. Then the two portions may be of equal density, but in the living bone it will be evenly and in the dead bone unevenly distributed.

In case of cancellous sequestra bordering on joints this process may be reversed, as the texture of the dead bone is even, while the surrounding living bone shows areas of spotted atrophy and absorption from osteomyelitis. This is illustrated in Fig. 7, of a gunshot wound of the right hip of four months' standing with sequestrum formation in the head of the femur. Fig. 8 is of a section showing the even texture of the sequestrum.

Transformation of preëxisting bone is of less importance in the recognition of dead bone. In osteomyelitis with sequestrum and involucrum formation, the old cortex at the limits of the sequestrum may develop a greater degree of porosity than does the remaining living bone from the atrophy alone. It also gradually shifts to align itself with the involucrum, leaving the dead cortex in its original position. This shifting occurs fairly early, especially in the thin bones of children, but so late, where thick cortex of large bone is concerned, that it is of little diagnostic value. Transformation occurs late in infected fractures healed in malposition, but other signs make it possible to recognize the dead bone much earlier.

New Bone Formation.—New bone formation occurs along the course of the dead bone from the periosteum, unless there is also death of its osteogenetic elements, which is frequently extensive in infected fractures, but limited in osteomyelitis. It also occurs from the endosteum of the affected level unless the entire circumference has been killed. It extends back on the

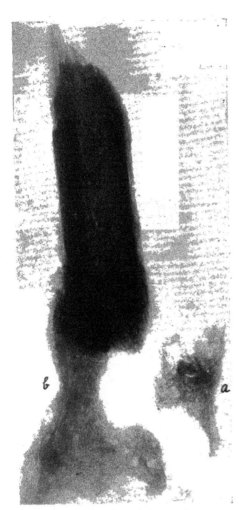

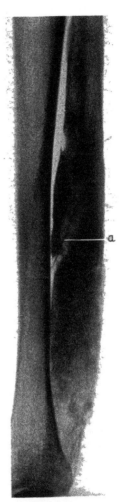

FIG. 10.—Secondary sequestrum (a) from wall of tunnel (b) in gunshot fracture of femur seven months old. Sequestrum resulted from denudation at operation five weeks before it and tunnel wall were recovered. Both have same density.

FIG. 11.—Old hypertrophic osteomyelitis of fibula, cancellous except about sequestrum. Acute recurrent osteomyelitis three and one-half weeks old in lower half producing extensive irregular absorption. At operation extensive irregular areas of necrosis and absorption found.

living shaft at the limits of the dead bone and gradually tapers off at a distance, depending on the cause of the infection. The newly formed bone is spongy early, but gradually increases in density (Fig. 5 *a*). With the resumption of function it slowly assumes a lamellated character. But if there is protracted disuse, as in ununited gunshot fractures, it may in turn undergo atrophy, vacuolation, and absorption.

There is a definite line of demarcation between the newly formed bone and dead bone, but none between it and old living bone. However, peripheral callus on the ends of living cortex may be laminated with an inner spongy and an outer compact layer, which occasionally may simulate involucrum and dead space about a sequestrum. Careful inspection of good X-ray plates will show the presence of a spongy shadow forming a narrower inner layer than is represented by the dead space about a sequestrum.

Irregular osteophytes and islands of new bone develop, especially as a result of gunshot fracture and secondary to operation with displacement of osteogenetic elements. The islands are frequently hard to distinguish from displaced sequestra, but, as a rule, have a more even density with dull fading margins, and their spongy nature can be made out in the X-ray. Displaced sequestra are usually derived from cortex and have a compact texture with sharp irregular outlines.

Secondary Bone Necrosis.—Secondary necrosis is not uncommon from a flare-up in the course of chronic osteomyelitis or from the spread of infection following operation in which extensive fresh-cut or denuded bony surfaces have been created. It differs from primary necrosis in that it usually occurs in atrophied old bone, spongy new bone, or a combination of the two. As a rule, large sequestra do not form since the infection is limited. Also further atrophy does not ordinarily occur in the surrounding living bone as is the case after primary bone necrosis. Consequently, the shadow cast by the new sequestrum is not heavier than that of the surrounding living bone and may be even fainter, as increase in density of the latter can occur from resumption of function during the time required for sequestration. Very small secondary sequestra frequently form from the cut or denuded surfaces produced at operation in chronic osteomyelitis or infected fractures. Because of their reduced density it may be difficult to distinguish them from islands of new bone formed from stripped-off osteogenetic elements or from small chips. The zone of separation forms faster in secondary than in primary bone necrosis because of the more porous character of the necrotic portion. Fig. 10 shows a secondary sequestrum *a,* which separated four weeks following operation, from one wall *b* of a tunnel, in a seven-months-old gunshot fracture of the femur. The wall was removed two weeks later and the sequestrum, placed alongside its defect, casts the same density as the portion from which it was separated.

Shaft that has first hypertrophied from old osteomyelitis and then become porous from years of quiescence of the infection may become reinvolved from lighting up of a neighboring focus. In this case the infection will spread in the spongy hypertrophied portion and produce irregular areas of necrosis similar to that in cancellous bone of the ends of the shaft and epiphysis. The X-ray appearance is quite similar in the two conditions. This is well illustrated in Fig. 11. There had been an old osteomyelitis of the lower four-fifths of the fibula beginning nineteen years before, at the age of twelve. It discharged intermittently from the middle and lower portions for four years at which time dead bone was removed at operation and the lower portion healed. But a discharging sinus leading to the middle portion persisted. There had not been an acute exacerbation of the infection and no interference with function until three and one-half weeks before, when an acute osteomyelitis developed in the lower half leading to extensive abscess and fistula formation. X-ray shows a markedly enlarged lower four-fifths of the fibula with three distinct types of change. The upper one-fourth is enlarged and fairly evenly porous with a smooth surface. The second fourth is hypertrophied and contains an irregular canal with dense walls casting a heavy shadow in which lies a sequestrum, *a*, the lower end of which protrudes through a cloaca. The old fistula leads down to this. The surface in this region is also smooth. The lower half is enlarged and spongy, but throughout there are numerous small irregular areas of reduced density and marked irregularity of the surface, indicative of bone destruction. The entire hypertrophied portion except the external malleolus was excised subperiosteally, and the lower one-half found to be the seat of diffuse acute osteomyelitis with irregularly distributed areas of necrotic bone and bone absorption. The upper one-fourth was cancellous, but free from acute disease. No doubt the lower one-half possessed a similar but more marked cancellous structure, which permitted the acute infection, starting from the neighboring chronic focus, to spread throughout its entire extent.

Diagnostic Points in Septic Necrosis.—To sum up, the points by which we distinguish between dead and living bone are density, demarcation, and contour. These are best determined from a practical standpoint by means of the X-rays, and, after advent of the period when they may be of assistance in the management of the condition, can be expressed as follows:

The density of dead bone is greater than that of an equal volume of surrounding living bone. It retains its original compact texture. Living old bone has its density evenly reduced by atrophy and is occasionally streaked from dilated longitudinal cannular markings. Newly formed bone is of low density and spongy in texture. These are well illustrated in Fig. 12, showing a gunshot fracture of the femur seven months old. Differences in density are striking. Eight sequestra were removed. Fig. 13 is a photograph of the four large ones that could easily be identified in the X-ray and of a piece of involucrum (5) that encased sequestrum No. 2. the surface of which is markedly eroded. while that of Nos. 1 and 3.

DALLAS B. PHEMISTER

which were not covered by involucrum, are smooth. No. 4, presenting a flat surface, was identified by its sharp fracture lines.

There are numerous variations from these general statements. Dead

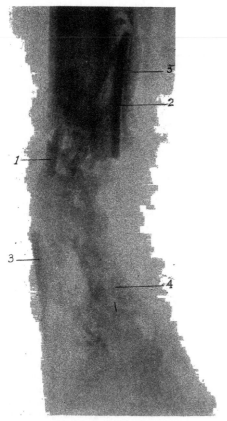

Fig. 12.—Gunshot racture of l. femur seven and one-half months old, showing extreme variations in density of dead bone, new.bone and old living bone. Dense uneroded sequestra, 1 and 3, uncovered by involucrum; eroded sequestrum, 2, covered by involucrum; 5, thin sequestrum; 4, seen on flat and identified by its fracture line. Photograph in Fig. 13.

bone when extensively eroded has its shadow density reduced, which may be equal to or below that of the living-bone, but is distinguished from the latter by its blotchy uneven character. Secondary sequestra usually show no variation in density from the adjacent living bone. The line of demarcation between dead and living portions is usually sufficiently wide and clean cut to be of great value in diagnosis, but any oblique or tortuous portions, especially when overlapped by heavy living bone, may be indistinguishable or very imperfectly made out. Notches

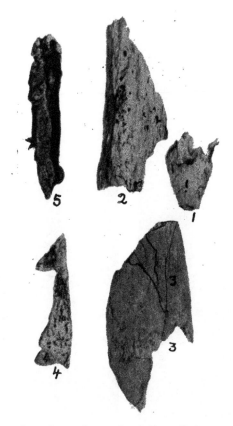

FIG. 13.–Sequestra from case shown in Fig. 12. Numbers same, but pieces reversed.

or unevenly streaked or dotted lines may indicate incomplete separation of the dead piece.

The outline of the sequestrum is of great diagnostic value. Its surface is smooth, sharp, and straight where unattacked, but irregular and jagged where erosion has occurred. Sharp spicules, especially about the ends, are frequently to be made out. Preservation of the smooth curved cortical rim in sequestra bordering on an articular surface and of clean-cut fracture lines late in infected fractures are points of value. The compact texture of dead bone gives its outlines a sharpness that the less

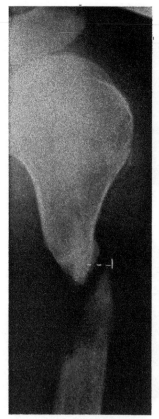
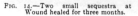
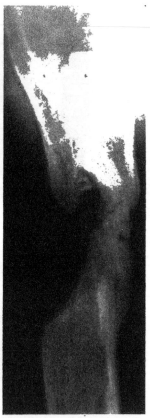

FIG. 14.—Two small sequestra at 1. Wound healed for three months.   FIG. 15.—View at a right angle to Fig. 14. Sequestra in fork of upper fragment.

dense and frequently growing living surfaces do not possess. Evidence of irregular destruction of spongy bone at the ends of the shaft in osteomyelitis is indirectly a pretty safe sign that dead portions are present even though their outlines cannot be determined.

There are many difficulties in distinguishing dead bone in the X-ray, the greatest of which results from overlapping of shadows of necrotic and living portions which obscures the details of each. This can usually be obviated by obtaining views from different angles. Thus a line of de-

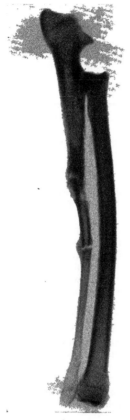

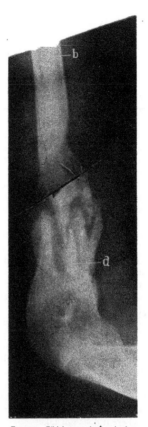

FIG. 16.—Transplant of ulna ten weeks old in adult dog. Casts heavier shadow than atrophied cortex above and below.

FIG. 17.—Tibial transplant *a–b* three months old in non-union of humerus. Lower 2 cm. (*a*) infected and separated as sequestrum casts a heavier shadow than the rest of the transplant which took and has been transformed.

marcation, a sharp point, or worm-eaten surface, may show plainly at one angle and faintly or not at all at another, and a flat piece of sequestrum seen from the side may show a low density and be unrecognizable, but seen on edge is easily recognized by its greater density. Thick overlying soft parts frequently obscure the finer details of internal structure of different types of bone.

The presence of dead bone can nearly always be diagnosed, but frequently the exact number of pieces can not be determined, especially when they are small. It is a not uncommon experience to find, at operation in osteomyelitis and infected fractures, twice as many sequestra as were suspected from the X-rays.

Fistulæ usually persist as long as dead bone is present, because bacteria invade its canals and cancellous spaces, rendering sterilization impossible and keeping up a discharge. In marked contrast, projectiles in gunshot wounds usually heal in after subsidence of the acute infection, as their interior contains no bacteria and surface sterilization takes place. In old gunshot fractures it is common to see several pieces each of dead bone *with* sinuses at the seat of fracture, and missile fragments *without* sinuses in the adjacent soft parts. Wounds containing small sequestra may heal and remain closed indefinitely, but eventual lighting up of the infection usually occurs. Ununited fractures and defects requiring bone transplantation should be scrutinized, especially for the presence of tiny healed-in sequestra, and if such be found they should be removed and the transplantation postponed until the wound has been sufficiently long healed.

Fig. 14 shows the X-ray of an ununited gunshot fracture of the humerus healed for three months. The two small, sharp, dense spots (1) in the shadow of upper fragment suggested dead bone, consequently, a view at right angles was obtained (Fig. 15). It shows two small shadows in the fork of the upper fragment which at operation were found to be produced by two wheat-grain sized sequestra that were surrounded by moist granulations.

Density of Transplants.—The difference in density between dead and living bone in septic necrosis suggested the possibility of a similar occurrence in aseptic necrosis, such as takes place in uninfected bone transplants. Histological studies have shown that nearly all of the transplanted compact bone undergoes aseptic necrosis which, after reëstablishment of the circulation, is gradually replaced, through a process of creeping substitution, by new bone formed from the surviving unossified osteogenetic elements of the transplant in case the latter takes, or growing in from the surrounding bone where it does not take.

Atrophy would be expected to occur more rapidly in the adjacent living bone than in the transplant, because time would be required for the reëstablishment of circulation and the beginning of absorption in it with replacement of the dead cortex by new and less dense bone. Experiments on dogs, details of which will be published later, show this to be the case. A section of ulnar shaft two-thirds to one and one-half inches long, excised and reimplanted, is denser and casts a heavier shadow from the fourth to the tenth week than the adjacent atrophied fragments. This is well shown in

Fig. 16 of a ten-weeks' experiment. After this time the density of the transplant gradually approaches that of the fragments.

That a difference in density gradually develops between the infected and uninfected portions of a human transplant is illustrated by the following case: A tibial inlay graft was inserted for ununited gunshot fracture of the lower end of the humerus. Mild infection occurred with fistula formation at the seat of the fracture. Fig. 17 shows the X-ray at the end of three months. Two centimetres of the lower end of the graft underwent septic necrosis and separated as a sequestrum. It casts a heavier shadow than the rest of the graft which took and has undergone considerable transformation.

ON THE DIAGNOSIS AND THERAPY OF
BONE TYPHOID

By G. Bohmansson, M.D.

of Orebro, Sweden

First assistant surgeon at the orebro hospital

In the March number, 1919, of the Annals of Surgery I have published a case of multiple typhoidal bone-foci in an eighteen-year-old girl, where the diagnosis could not be made until after the chiselling up and cultivation of bacteria from one of the closed bone-foci, where Widal's reaction was negative in the blood and the pathological-anatomical examination did not give any fixed points for an etiological diagnosis, and where finally the patient had not previously gone through any fever-sickness which could have been interpreted as typhoid.

In the case in question an experiment was even made with autogenous vaccine therapy, which turned out well and encouraged me to continue in the same direction. I therefore beg to give a short account of yet another similar case which seems to me to support in every respect the conclusions which I had drawn from the first case.

Case II.—The patient, a woman, aged fifty-three years, sickened in August, 1918, with headache, pains in stomach and back, accompanied by diarrhœa, which continued for two weeks. No cough and no catarrhal symptoms from the upper bronchial tubes. Afterwards lay another five weeks languid and weak and with pains all over her body. Was taken into the internal department of the hospital here, October 13, 1918. The *status* was then: The spleen palpable, somewhat enlarged. On the apex of the right lung a good deal of rustling. Heart without remark. The abdomen considerably distended. Temperature, 39°–40° C. Pulse 100–110.

On the ensuing few days a slight further enlargement of the spleen was observed. Blood. Red blood-corpuscles, 3,200,000; white blood-corpuscles, 3900. Ficker for paratyphoid negative. The patient afterwards lay in an almost unchanged condition with a febris continua which subsided lytically in the middle of November, but afterwards lay subfebrile with nearly 38° C.

On December 27, 1918, a slightly painful swelling over the fourth right rib. Sound of friction in the neighborhood of auscultation. The white blood-corpuscles now 6900. The following day the patient was moved over to the surgical department.

Under the right breast, corresponding to the fourth or fifth rib, was a non-fluctuating, slightly painful swelling as big as a plum, adhering fast to the bone.

On December 27th operation (Lange). Resectio costæ, ribs III and IV. Scraping out of granulations. On an incision being made a granuloma was discovered, partly infiltrating in the pectoralis major. The seat of granulation may be traced under the costal cartilage into the pleura, from which latter it seems to have emanated. Iodoform tamponade. Microscopical examination: Granulation tissue (Westberg).

On February 1, 1919, I saw the patient for the first time. The fistula after the operation is still discharging. On the right tibia shaft and in centre of same a lightly-rounded, slightly-painful swelling. Temperature still subfebrile. Röntgen shows on the corresponding place a thin periosteal layer. Wassermann negative. Widal negative for typhoid and paratyphoid.

The anamnesis with the prolonged high fever, enlargement of spleen and leucopænia seemed to me to favor the belief of its being typhoid, in spite of the negative result of Widal. Further localization of the multiple bone-foci; rib and tibia diaphysis, as tuberculosis with the last-mentioned localization were exceedingly unusual. I therefore decided to make a bacteriological examination from the tibia focus as being the only sure method of obtaining an etiological diagnosis. The focus was laid bare and the limited hyperplastic periostitis cut away (writer). Under the periosteum a shallow concavity in the corticalis. The histological examination now answered to tuberculosis (Professor Westberg).

The sterilized preparation was sent in for the purpose of bacilli-culture to the bacteriological laboratory of the public institute of medicine (Professor Pettersson). It was here found that stave-like bacilli in cultivation were growing from the same which were agglutinated by typhoid serum in strong dilution, less strong by paratyphoid A and B. Vaccine was subsequently prepared from the cultivation received in the same way as in the case previously referred to.

On February 23, 1919, a vaccine therapy was introduced with doses increasing from 5,000,000 up to 5,000,000,000 in subcutaneous injections every other day. Moderate rise in temperature and slightly increased pain in the bone-foci on the days ensuing the first injections. After four injections afebrile. *Widal positive typhoid,* afterwards quick healing. The patient remained for control of the result until March 24, 1920, and was then discharged as cured. Subsequent examination on April 12, 1920: Perfectly healthy. Widal negative.

What appears to me to be of special interest even in this case is the state of reaction in accordance with the Widal method before and during vaccine therapy. In conformity with a previously expressed opinion, I consider that this argues in favor of a low virulence of the bacteria and would further emphasize the already well-known fact that the intensity of the primary disease does not appear to be of any importance with regard to an eventual appearance of pyæmic bone typhoid.

SURGICAL ASPECTS OF THE CHARCOT JOINT AND OTHER SYPHILITIC BONE AND JOINT LESIONS *

By Frederic J. Cotton, M.D.
of Boston, Mass.

BECAUSE of disasters, everyone is afraid of the Charcot joint. Because of poor results no one is interested—clinically. I suspect we have done very badly by them.

This paper can be only the expression of a lately awakened interest on my part, and can cover only the clinical aspects of a small group of cases in which treatment seems to have helped. Already colleagues have volunteered notes of isolated like cases, and perhaps a few months of further painstaking may teach what I think we have not known—the whole " natural history " of these joints: The clinical picture; in whom they occur and why; how they progress; what speeds or stays this progress; why certain cases reach a limit of damage while others go from bad to worse; how far general or local antisyphilitic treatment or treatment of the cord lesion can help; whether they are, or can be made, reasonably safe for operative interference, etc.

We have all seen Charcot joints that had reached a certain stage of tolerance or quiescence: it was a couple of cases that showed, under salvarsan (given on general principles), a real reparative process that aroused my interest. An astonishing proportion of the Charcot joints, as we all know, occur in cases of tabes so early as not to have been diagnosed or even suspected—so early that motor function is intact—the working problem is only that of the joint, and of the preservation of its function.

CASE I.—A man, seen in 1915, who had " dislocated " a hip in bowling, while in supposedly perfect health. The hip had been " reduced; " the X-ray showed a supposed fracture, really a plaque of *new* bone. Examination showed some limitation of motion, no pain; also no knee-jerks, and a suggestion of the Argyll-Robertson pupillary reaction.

Careful questioning elicited the story of a half-forgotten infection, of twenty years before—a history of severe " neuralgia " in the legs, two years before, and in some measure to date—at irregular intervals, resistant to treatment given by his physician. There was not a trace of ataxia discoverable. Patient lean but healthy, exceptionally vigorous and active.

Rest in bed, fixation in abduction for three weeks, then a leather pelvic spica belt, steadying the trochanter, and crutches. A course of 606 treatments by Dr. Otto Hermann.

* Read before the American Surgical Association, May 5, 1920.

488

Very enterprising, he discarded crutches for a cane earlier than I wished, and after about four months even the belt went into the discard. The process was followed with X-rays (many of them unavailable now, with other plates of the late Dr. Walter Dodd) and destruction went on apace for a number of weeks, then after completion of the 606 course, it checked, and the joint, now obviously subluxated, grew firmer.

To-day he is as active as ever, does an unusual amount of walking, is known as a very successful and progressive man in his business, and considers himself well, though he has a limp and carries a cane, though more from habit than from apparent necessity.

CASE II.—A widow, aged fifty-two years, was sent to me for results of a fracture of eight weeks' duration.

The skiagraph showed an obvious Charcot joint, and I was able to get from her doctor the first X-ray taken at the time of the fracture. There was a fracture of the radial styloid, but even then obvious preceding pathological changes were evident in the plate. There was no history, then or since, of any kind of infection, but reflexes and pupils confirmed the story, and the Wassermann reaction was positive. She, too, had a course of salvarsan treatment by Doctor Hermann.

Then I tackled the wrist—useless, swollen, shapeless and grating—opened it, cleaned out the loose original fragment, detached plaques of new bone, loose capsular tissue, etc., closed it, and got first intention, and presently, with the aid of a steel reinforced leather brace, a return of fair function in the hand. She then developed a mental condition which the neurologist, Dr. J. W. Courtney, called general paralysis; this yielded only slowly to the after course of mercurials.

Now, after three years, on reëxamination, she is mentally normal or thereabouts, conducting her business—a lodging house—without obvious non-success, and the wrist, weak, of course, from lack of the removed section of the radial base, is at worst no worse, is without reaction of any sort, and the hand is useful.

CASE III.—A fireman of forty years, was seen by me while I was still in military service. He had a Charcot joint of the left ankle, a sufficient history of infection of many (20 plus or minus) years ago, with some treatment and no later signs of trouble noticed until the ankle began to give a bit of trouble after a slight wrench. Out of practice at the time, I referred him to the City Hospital, where Doctor Nichols did a thigh amputation, precipitated by sepsis at or about the ankle. I understand that the amputated specimen showed an extraordinary degree of syphilitic endarteritis throughout.

What is of interest in this case is the great toe of the *other* foot, which "went bad" shortly after the amputation.

The X-rays shown give the before and after of a treatment with salvarsan and a reasonable protection of this joint by proper, heavy-soled shoeing (in a policeman's boot).

This patient is, or was at last report, an active citizen of these

United States now sojourning in Canada, with one artificial leg and one police shoe, and I think the X-rays confirm the fact of real repair in this once sad-looking joint.

CASE IV.—Next comes the case of a man of forty, supposedly in good health, who began to have trouble—pain and some weakness, in his knee after some unusually heavy lifting. This grew worse and he went to one of the hospitals where a diagnosis was made on the basis of the X-ray of an early hypertrophic arthritis. The X-ray is here shown and corresponds pretty closely with that of the other knee taken at the same time. I have examined the plates. He grew less able to use the knee, though in no great pain, and when I saw him, about two months later the condition clinically was obvious—a thickened knee with some fluid, nearly painless, with marked abnormal lateral mobility, no muscle spasm. The patellar reflexes were gone, the pupils characteristic. There was not and is not now any ataxia. Nearly twenty years ago there was an infection about which he remembers little. There was no systemic treatment.

In the unfortunate shuffle of hospital responsibilities he dropped into other hands, was told the case was hopeless, and no treatment recommended. About three weeks later I saw him with his own doctor in consultation, told him of my more recent views that I am trying to express here, and had him fitted to an apparatus of the convalescent Thomas knee-splint type with a slide lock at the knee and with special plates and pads to correct the bow-leg deformity which had increased in the three weeks to a marked extent. Otherwise there was no essential change in his condition. He was then put through the usual 606 treatment. The Wassermann reaction was positive.

The knee was kept quiet for a time, but after a month put into active moderate use—with the support of the apparatus which was modified at intervals to keep pace with the correction of the bow-leg deformity. Now the leg is practically straight—the abnormal lateral motion decreased from about 25 degrees to less than 10 degrees and he gets about comfortably and pretty solidly. At present he is looking for a job. His general condition is excellent. The X-rays in this case show, what is suspected we are going to find regularly in these cases properly treated, a stage of disintegration before repair starts. In the last plates there is certainly an increase in density of bone, and no destruction since the last plate of a month previous. This joint will never be cured, of course. Whether it will ever be good enough to go without apparatus I do not know as yet. But at least the destruction has been checked and a derelict has been transformed into a reasonably useful citizen.

CASE V.—The next case is a tabetic, not an early case, a real advanced tabetic, diagnosed a dozen years ago, known to me for four years or more, but never a patient of mine until this winter when I was called in to treat the results of one of his many falls. He had fallen five weeks before, striking his right shoulder from behind, injuring his left thumb at the same time.

The thumb showed thickening and subluxation of the first phalanx forward on the metacarpal with abnormal mobility and loss of power. The shoulder was a loose joint subluxating forward to the coracoid and back to its socket. There was much swelling—fluid—in front. Pain was little, but loss of ability to help himself about very distressing to him as his legs and hips are not very useful, and there is a good deal of ataxia of the arms. The X-ray taken at this time showed almost nothing in the shoulder and only the subluxation in the thumb.

Fixation in this case was very difficult, but with a shoulder cap and adhesive something was done with the shoulder and the luxation of the thumb was reduced and held by firm adhesive strapping. The collection of fluid in front of the shoulder persisted. It was tapped twice and permanently reduced. The first tap produced about ʒii of serous fluid. Examination showed sterile culture and no spirochætæ to be found by dark field illumination. He was turned over to Doctor Hermann and put through a course of salvarsan treatment.

To-day his thumb is still strapped and shows thickening, but the mobility is less, the usefulness greatly better. The shoulder still shows abnormal mobility and thickening and a collection of fluid and the subluxation has become permanent, but at much less than its maximum range. Consequently there is some loss of forward motion of the arm, but the usefulness of the joint is much increased. He still wears a shoulder cap held down by straps.

CASE VI.—In this man there was a practically spontaneous fracture of the thigh a year before I saw him. He was treated in the City Hospital; X-rays taken at that time show, first, no pathology in the plate taken directly after the fracture; secondly, union, prompt and with enormous callus as one sees at times in tabetics. This was a tabetic fracture not the result of gumma. A year later he came to my service in January with a spontaneous fracture of the other hip, intracapsular without impaction. I was suspicious and found an early tabes present, never suspected before. Also I found a definite *severe* Charcot joint in the great toe-joint of the other foot, which had been opened up in another hospital six months before and had promptly healed without essential improvement.

The usual systemic treatment with protection of the hip, first in plaster, later in a Taylor splint, has at least slowed up any progress. The fracture ends show only a little erosion—increased density of bone is beginning to be evident. The characteristic shadows of bone plaques about the capsule have become obvious, and clinically the abnormal mobility is less; he is not yet bearing weight on the leg.

The tabetic process in this case was so little advanced that the neurologist hung in doubt for a time before confirming my diagnosis.

CASE VII.—Seen in February in consultation with Dr. McIver Woody, was sent to him with regard to the results of a Pott's fracture sustained last July. The lateral deformity was extreme, the mechanical defect disabling through clumsiness and fatigue, though there was no pain. A rather too short antisyphilitic treatment cut

491

short by his business followed the diagnosis and the confirmation of
a positive Wassermann test; an outside upright and strap reduced
the deformity a little, relieved strain, and gave fixation. He is now
in Canada active in business and with at least great relief from
his disability.

CASE VIII.—Shown by this X-ray is of a transition class. This
man, an Italian of fifty years of age, otherwise vigorous, sustained
an ankle injury over a year ago. He came to the hospital for dis-
ᴵⁱility, without much pain in walking. The picture is suggestive
particularly in relation to the extent of the process without pain.
Aside from this he shows only a local thickening of periosteal bone
in one humerus. Wassermann positive, weakly. Tabes doubtful,
but J. J. Thomas, the neurologist, finally decided for very early
tabes, and the patient is under anti-specific treatment and presently to have brace support. The absence of history is of little use,
he being no speaker of English and not very alert mentally aside
from that.

This seems to me a borderline case—syphilitic beyond a doubt—
and to be classed as a Charcot joint clinically, but showing much
likeness to the non-tabetic specific bone lesions, particularly in the
massive overgrowth of the bone ends themselves.

I have lately been following two cases interesting from this angle.

CASE IX.—A boy of ten years of age, three years under treatment for congenital specific changes in the tibia, hyperplastic and
ulcerative, now cured as to the destructive process and the symptoms,
but with no retrogression in the overgrowth of bone.

CASE X.—A knee in a woman twenty-four years of age, syphilitic,
but not tabetic. The knee lesion, of a year's duration before I saw
her, variously treated in that time under mistaken diagnoses, gave
trouble because of weakness and of muscle atrophy with pain present, but in no proportion to the destructive lesion present. There
was thickening, grating, and considerable free fluid. After treatment for the syphilis and proper fixation for the knee the case is
clinically cured. But the X-rays before and after show no change
save for return of normal bone density about the local erosion on the
joint surface and the last was taken after considerable use of the
joint without recurrence of trouble. Further than this the case can
hardly be distinguished from the early stages of the other knee
shown, Case III, clinically or by the X-ray.

In these two cases as in the ankle just shown, we have retrogression
of symptoms, retrogression of the process in the soft parts, but no definite retrogression of bone overgrowth. The same is true of the thigh in
Case VI, the colossal callus of the tabetic fracture of a year ago
remains unchanged.

This is true of all these few joint cases and perhaps the general similarity of the X-ray picture has misled us in these cases as it has misled
some into thinking syphilitic bone changes in the shaft unaffected by
treatment. In both instances may we not say that proper treatment first

sets a limit to the bone changes; that under proper treatment bone repair does occur and that symptoms, save those from mechanical damage already done, are done away with?

There is nothing new about this you will say, and there is not. We have all seen the remarkable tolerance of some horrid looking Charcot joints under prolonged use; some cases have been helped with supports, and many have been given routine treatment as syphilitics. All that is new is the point of view, I think.

We have thought of Charcot joints as one loss not recoverable in the losing game of the patient with locomotor ataxia. Please think of the lesion as I have come to think of it, as a joint disease that occurs in syphilitics, not always or even usually crippled by ataxia, a lesion not completely curable, but not without power of repair or destined to inevitable progress, but capable under proper handling of restoration to safe use.

Probably such cord changes as exist are permanent—whether antisyphilitic treatment will safely check such changes where they are is doubtful. But as to the joints, let us handle them as syphilitic joints. They may be dependent on cord changes; they are certainly aggravated, as they are said to be caused by the trauma of use of an insensitive joint, but that they are traumatic has no support in any other traumatic process. Personally, apart from any spirochætæ in the joint which others have found, though I did not, I cannot believe the condition other than syphilitic.

Properly handled, they certainly show a checking of the destructive process even if this is not prompt, and certainly a regenerative capacity in the bone, a tightening and shrinking of the capsular tissues, and absorption of waste fluid and soft tissues are uniformly evident. Two cases in this series besides the one I operated had been cut into without disaster or notable slow repair of soft parts.

The many operative disasters I know of in these cases all antedate proper syphilitic treatment, and it is not unlikely that many cases may by proper treatment be brought within the safe operative field for ankylosing operations. At all events, here is a class of joint lesions mainly in cases of a tabes so early as to have given no other symptoms, hitherto almost uniformly "given up" and neglected, in which it appears that useful work can easily be done, with some prospect of better developments to come.

FORWARD DISLOCATION OF THE ASTRAGALUS AND WITH IT THE FOOT*

By Robert Henry Fales Dinegar, M.D.

of New York, N. Y.

Stimson in his work on fractures and dislocations divides the possible tibiotarsal dislocations into five groups, namely: Forward, backward, inward, outward, and upward. Of these there are but relatively few collected cases, of the backward variety about 26; forward, 10; inward, 26; outward, 27; and upward but 4.[1] No doubt at the present time other cases have been added, but it is fair to assume that the relative proportion of these must all be the same.

If we leave out of consideration the very rare upward dislocation, of which Stimson found but two records (though some have seen four cases[2]), there remain but the four commoner varieties. From the figures given above we see that, of these the forward dislocation of the astragalus and with it the foot, is by far the rarest. It is a case of this variety that I wish to report.

Case Report.—A young adult male, aged twenty-two years, an iron worker by trade, was carried into the Emergency Department of the hospital, from a building upon which he had been working, twenty minutes after the accident had happened. The following was the history given by the patient. While engaged in working on the construction of a building, the patient's position was such that his right leg and foot were advanced about 2½ feet in front of the left extremity. The patient's weight was borne on the forward (right) leg, while his left extremity was used to balance with. This leg was tense from the contraction of the muscles, and was extended at the knee, the foot dorsi-flexed at the ankle. The right leg was slightly flexed at the knee and the foot was at right angles with the line of the tibia.

While in this position the patient was suddenly hit on the left heel by a rapidly moving iron beam of great weight. This naturally exerted considerable force. The astragalus, and with it the foot, was dislocated forward; at the same time the patient lost his balance and fell to the side, inverting his left foot. The mechanism of dislocating the foot forward is in part the causative factor in fracturing the tips of the malleoli and displacing the internal fragment forward (by avulsion through the ligaments). But more especially the inversion and lateral displacement of the astragalus is the chief factor and, it would appear, the means of displacing the fragment of the tibia laterally outward.

* From the Surgical Service of Dr. Charles N. Dowd, at the Roosevelt Hospital, New York City.

494

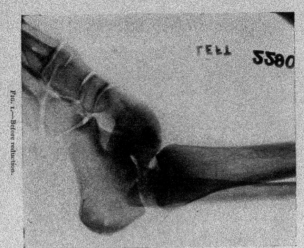

Fig. 2.—Before reduction.

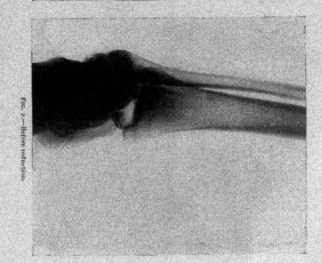

Fig. 3.—Before reduction.

494

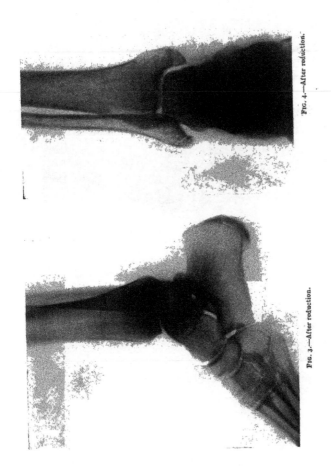

FIG. 3.—After reduction.

FIG. 4.—After reduction.

The man was a relatively normal white male; the left foot was swollen about each malleolus and across the dorsum. The skin here is very tense. An abnormal bony prominence is easily palpable in the upper dorsum of the foot. The foot appears lengthened, feels cold, is cyanosed, and the discoloration reaches the tips of the toes. The heel appears to be shortened and it is impossible to grasp the os calcis in the usual manner. The normal sulcus on each side of the tendo achillis is obliterated. Motion is impossible. There is tenderness over both malleoli with crepitus at the external. The foot appears to be more plantar-flexed than the opposite, and the hollow of the instep is increased. The malleoli appear to be nearer the sole and heel than normal. The patient is unable to bear any weight on the foot.

From the physical signs and symptoms a dislocation of the astragalus was apparent. The X-ray being immediately at hand, skiagraphs were taken before reduction was attempted (Figs. 1 and 2). In these pictures the following points are noted: Before reduction, Fig. 1: (a) The astragalus is dislocated forward. (b) The posterior portion of the os calcis is further forward and nearer the malleoli than normal. (c) The foot is more plantar-flexed than normal. (d) The hollow of the instep is increased. (e) Malleoli are nearer the sole of the foot than normal. (f) The tip of the internal malleolus is fractured and is displaced forward. (g) The tip of the external malleolus is fractured but not displaced. (h) The relation of the astragalus to os calcis and navicular is normal. Fig. 2: (a) Tarsus slightly inverted. (b) Astragalus displaced laterally outward and inverted. (c) Fractured tip of the internal malleolus is displaced inward. (d) Fractured tip of the external malleolus is in good position.

While the pictures were being developed the dislocation was reduced. The method consisted in traction on the os calcis and dorsum of the foot, while with the fingers of the hand, making traction on the dorsum, the astragalus was pushed downward and backward. The surgeon was assisted by counter-traction at the knee. The patient was in the recumbent position. The astragalus slipped into place easily, with the usual feeling of crunching snow. Almost at once the cyanosis began to clear and the foot to feel warmer. Great relief from pain was experienced. The reduction required no anæsthetic. The foot tended to keep the normal position when at rest.

X-ray plates were again taken and when seen the position was as is indicated in " after reduction," Figs. 3 and 4. The corrections of the points enumerated above are noted.

A padded plaster case extending from just below the knee to the base of the toes was applied. The foot was put at right angles with the line of the tibia. The patient experienced such relief from the reduction and the support of the case that he was able to leave the hospital on crutches. The next day he was seen in the Out-Patients' Department; his foot felt very comfortable in its plaster encasement, and very little pain was experienced at the site of the

trauma. The patient reported at frequent intervals and the case
was removed on the twenty-first day. No deformity and only a
moderate amount of stiffness and limitation of motion was noted.
These soon disappeared under active and passive motion, baking,
and massage. When the patient last reported, six weeks from the
date of the accident, he had an excellent result and practically
perfect function.

Discussion.—There are two classical modes of producing this dislocation, according to Stimson,[2] namely: (1) When the foot is in dorsi-
flexion and pressure is exerted through the long axis of the tibia downward and backward; (2) when direct pressure is made forward on the
foot, at the same time the leg is pushed backward while making an angle
of 90°. In the case reported above I believe the mode of production to be
slightly different from either of the two accepted methods. The position
is quite characteristic of the first, except that pressure was not made
down through the long axis of the tibia (as even the body weight
was on the opposite leg), but by a force pushing the foot forward. In this
respect it resembles the second method, only the angle between the foot
and leg was considerably less than 90°, about 55° in fact, and no pressure
was made backward on the tibia.

This manner of dislocation, when the upper fragment is not fixed,
except by muscle spasticity, could only be accomplished under certain
conditions. First, although the leg and dorsum of the foot made an angle
of 55°, the muscles were so taut that they, while not exerting pressure,
rendered the leg so stiff as to splint it. Secondly, the object exerting the
force on the foot was one of great weight. Thirdly, that this object
moved quite rapidly. (Just as a sufficiently quick flick of the finger will
displace a card from beneath a penny on the finger without carrying away
the penny.) All these I believe to be potent factors, because if the blow
was of less force and slower, it would have tended to push the extremity
out from under the individual rather than to quickly dislocate the
foot forward.

REFERENCES

[1] Stimson, L. A.: A Practical Treatise on Fractures and Dislocations, 6th ed.,
pp. 837–842.
[2] Wendel: Beitrage zur klin. Chir., vol. xxi, p. 123 *et seq.*
[3] Stimson, L. A.: A Practical Treatise on Fractures and Dislocations, 6th ed.,
pp. 837–842.

ADVENTITIOUS LIGAMENTS SIMULATING
CERVICAL RIBS *

By ARTHUR AYER LAW, M.D.
OF MINNEAPOLIS, MINN.

THOROUGH study, by many observers, of the clinical entity known as cervical ribs, has crystallized into a definite symptom complex, the reaction which follows when the eighth cervical and first dorsal nerves of the brachial plexus are lifted up, stretched taut and angulated over an adventitious rib, and, in addition, are pinched in the angle formed by the scalenus anticus muscle and the first rib and there subjected to the constant hammering trauma from respiratory movements during the excursion of the lungs.

With the pressure neuralgia of the brachial plexus cords, there is a coincident angulation and pinching of the subclavian artery as it arches over the extra rib and is crowded forward into the angle formed by the muscle and the rib; this insult occasionally results in the symmetrical dilatation of the artery distal to the rib which simulated a fusiform aneurism and which has been so thoroughly studied by Keen and Halstead.

That only about 10 per cent. of the cervical ribs give local and peripheral symptoms is conceded. When these local and peripheral symptoms do occur, they are manifested in the root of the neck and in the forearm and hand, and are an expression of nerve irritation, with motor and sensory changes, with loss of trophic control and with ischæmia of the extremities from vasomotor changes; these symptoms are now thoroughly well established and recognized.

Minor points of discussion as to the physiological mechanics which produce these symptoms in cervical ribs still give zest to study, notably Todd's and Kieth's assertion that the circulatory changes in the forearm and hand are the result of pressure upon sympathetic fibres in the lower cords of the brachial plexus—these fibres from the rami communicantes entering the plexus with the eighth cervical and first dorsal nerves. They affirm that pressure of the cervical ribs upon the lower cord of the plexus causes irritation or even obstruction of these sympathetic fibres which produces trophic changes in the intima and media of the arteries, followed by secondary proliferation and hypertrophy of these coats which results in a coincident pallor and coldness of the hand and upon occasion in gangrene of the finger tips. Other observers assert that the anæmia of the extremity results from a mechanical obstruction and angulation of the subclavian artery in the neck at the site of the offending rib. The British have reported this same symptom complex following pressure from a high first rib.

In 1914 and 1915, while clinically studying a series of cervical ribs, the

* Read before the American Surgical Association May 5, 1920.

writer noted what he finds other observers have reported, that in the cases of some of the shorter and more rudimentary ribs, the forward projecting tips of these ribs were occasionally attached by a definite ligament to the first rib or to the sternum.

When, then, a case presented itself for relief from symptoms which were typically those of cervical ribs, yet in which the radiographic evidence revealed no hypertrophy or elongation of the transverse process of the seventh cervical vertebra, we remembered the ligaments attached to the rudimentary ribs and venturing to explore the neck found a definite adventitious ligament arising from a normal seventh cervical transverse process and being inserted into the first rib at the scalene tubercle with the scalenus anticus muscle. This ligament was about four millimetres wide and two in thickness, it looked like any ligament and had definite longitudinal fibrous bands; it was as taut as a bowstring and tightly stretched over it and sharply angulated were the two lower cords of the brachial plexus and the subclavian artery. Mobilizing the phrenic nerve and pulling it aside, the scalenus anticus muscle was sectioned and then the adventitious ligament; when the ligament was cut, the marked tension upon the nerves and artery was immediately relaxed.

Since the first case noted in 1916 we have operated upon three others, differing only in minor details from the first one, while each of them gave typical cervical rib symptoms, yet in no instance were cervical ribs present. Radiographic study, although it showed no adventitious ribs, did show what seemed to be a tendency on the affected side to a pulling down of the last cervical transverse process closer to the transverse process of the first dorsal vertebra than was shown on the normal side. Three cases showed no hypertrophy of the transverse processes of the last cervical vertebra, while the fourth was of the "cow-horn" type with the process slightly longer than on the other side.

There was in all four of the cases the invariable angling over the ligament and the pinching of the nerves and artery between the ligament and the scalenus anticus muscle, just as these structures are pinched between the muscle and rib in the cervical rib cases. The ligaments were all tightly stretched, and while they all had their origin from the tip of the seventh cervical transverse process, they varied markedly in their point of insertion, for one was inserted with the scalenus anticus muscle into the scalene tubercle of the first rib, another into the costo-clavicular ligament, the next into the sterno-clavicular ligament, while the last was inserted well towards the mid-line into the interclavicular ligament close to the head of the clavicle. In none of the cases studied was there a tendency to dilatation of the subclavian arteries distal to the ligament, and only in one was the pulse appreciably weaker on the obstructed side. Röntgen rays in one of the cases showed a marked osteoporosis of the phalanges of the ring and little fingers of the affected side; this was undoubtedly trophic in origin.

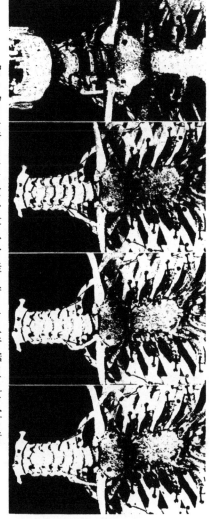

FIG. 1. Demonstrating constant point of origin of adventitious ligaments and the different points of insertion.

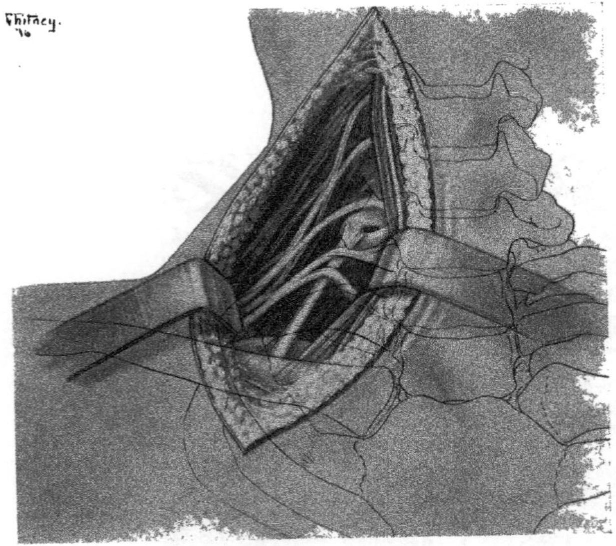

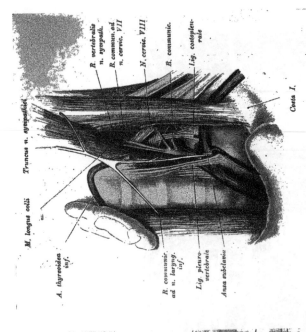

M. longus colli

Truncus n. sympathici

R. vertebralis n. sympath.

R. commun. ad n. cervic. VII

N. cervic. VIII

R. communic.

Lig. costopleu- rale

A. thyreoidea inf.

R. communic. ad n. laryng. inf.

Lig. pleuro- vertebrale

Ansa subclavia

Costa I.

Fig. 206. Linke Pleurakuppel und deren Nachbarschaft.

Fig. 3.—Taken from Zuckerkandl showing Sibson's fascia and abnormal and inconstant ligaments inserted into dome of the pleura.

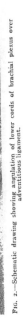

Fig. 2.—Schematic drawing showing angulation of lower cords of brachial plexus over adventitious ligament.

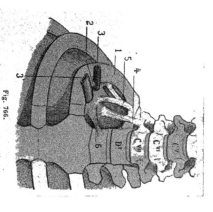

Fig. 766.

Appareil ligamenteux sus-pleural (d'après les dissections de Sebileau).

1, première côte. — 2, tubercule de Lisfranc. — 3, 3, arcs et veine sous-clavière. — 4, ligament pleuro-transversaire. — 5, ligament costo-pleural. — 6, ligament vertébro-pleural. — Cᵥ, CᵥI, CᵥII, cinquième, sixième et septième vertèbres cervicales. — Dᴵ, première vertèbre dorsale.

Fig. 4.—Taken from Poirier and Charpy, showing abnormal bands inserted into the dome of the pleura.

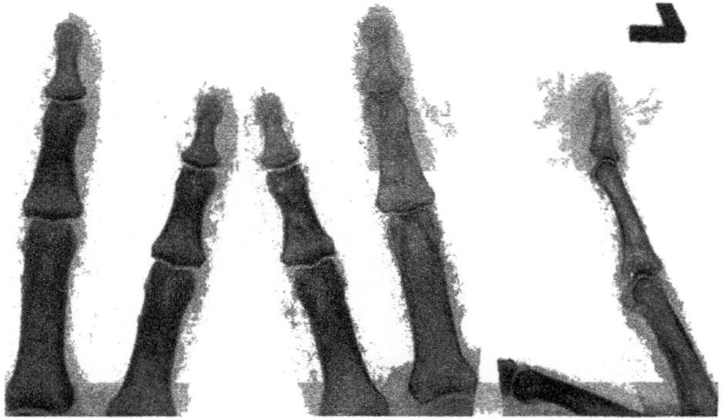

Fig. 5.—Osteoporosis of phalanges of third and fourth fingers compared with normal and showing trophic changes due to pressure on brachial plexus.

The cases were equally divided between the sexes and the ages were forty-seven and forty-eight years in the males and nineteen and forty-four in the females. In each instance after operative interference, while the neuralgia persisted for a while, it promptly became less severe and ultimate and complete relief was obtained.

Searching the literature in an attempt to find an etiological explanation for these bands, we found that those springing from short cervical ribs were reported; the nearest description of anything resembling the complete ligaments is described by Zuckerkandel who, in his dissections, discovered that there were certain inconstant and extremely variable bands which have been associated with Sibson's fascia and which are occasionally found reënforcing and helping that fascia to fix the dome of the pleura. This fascia and associated fasciculi, according to Zuckerkandel and to the French observers, Poirier and Charpy, is derived in man from a tiny rudimentary, inconstant muscle, which itself is extremely variable in its origin, distribution, and insertion, the so-called scalenus minimus; this little muscle, unusual in the human, is normal to a number of the Simian species. These bands of Sibson's fascia as well have been designated according to their distribution as the pleuro-transverse, the costo-pleural, and the vertebro-pleural ligaments.

Whether the adventitious bands we have described are a remnant of supernumerary ribs, are a variation of the Sibson's fascia, or are in themselves a distinct entity has not been determined. We believe, however, that they should take their place and be recognized as structures which are actually as definite and give as plain a symptomatology as do cervical ribs themselves. A knowledge of their occasional presence may help to explain some of the circulatory and trophic conditions of the hand and arm of obscure etiology which heretofore from want of exact knowledge we may have designated as Raynaud's disease, intermittent claudication, spontaneous gangrene, or thrombosis.

The writer hesitates to report so meagre and so inconclusive a series of cases, but hopes that by so doing attention may be directed to a condition which, judging from the barrenness of the literature, must be relatively rare or rather generally overlooked.

SPERMATOCELE

By Edward T. Crossan, M.D.
of Philadelphia, Pa.

Spermatocele is accepted to-day as meaning a retention cyst of the scrotum, containing spermatozoa, and arising either from the vas efferentia, the canal of the epididymis, or from the embryonic remnants around and about the testicle and lower end of the cord. Like many other medical terms, it is not quite exact, for it is claimed that spermatocele can exist without spermatozoa, and furthermore there are a few cases on record in which the cyst extended beyond the external inguinal ring. In view of the varied opinions as to the genesis and etiology it would be better to define it as a cyst originating in the scrotum and which is, or has been, in communication with the semen-carrying system.

The term spermatocele appears to have been primarily employed by Guerin in 1785 in reporting an obscure inflammatory condition of the testicle, which in no way bore any resemblance to what is now recognized as spermatocele. In the literature of that period these cysts were doubtless diagnosed as encysted hydroceles.

In April, 1843, Liston wrote an article, the title of which was " Some Observations on Encysted Hydrocele." In this article he mentioned two cases in which the fluid withdrawn from these sacs contained spermatozoa. Two months later Lloyd reported three similar cases, the first of which was revealed when he was using some fluid from an " encysted hydrocele " to dilute blood for microscopical examination. These findings were confirmed by Paget, Curling, Sedillot, Gosselin and others, and though these proofs seemed to point toward a pathological entity, the term encysted hydrocele survived until 1860, when Cavasse used the term spermatocele as applying to cysts containing spermatozoa. The subsequent studies of this condition were conducted chiefly by the French and Germans, and to Dolbeau, Hanusa, Kocher, Luschka, Hochenegg, and von Hoffman we owe much of the information which we possess.

The American literature is very scanty on the subject. Ellis, in 1858, reported the finding of spermatozoa in hydrocele fluid. From that date until 1876 we find no further reports; in the latter year, Dr. William Hunt and Dr. John B. Roberts reported a case which had been diagnosed as hydrocele, but on aspiration they found the fluid was of a milky color, and the microscopical examination showed spermatozoa. Following the above records only an occasional report is found until 1907, at which time Whitney published a thorough review of the literature, and then comes a hiatus which extends to the present year.

To understand the origin and etiology of spermatocele, a review of the relation of the epididymis and testicle, and of the embryonic remnants to the epididymis and testicle is quite essential.

The testicle hangs suspended in a space, the cavum vaginale, from which it is separated by the visceral layer of the tunica vaginalis. The latter is continued on to the epididymis, at the lateral margins of which it is reflected forward as the parietal layer, and as this is more extensive than the visceral layer, the above-named cavity results. The testicle is enclosed in a thick capsule of fibrous tissue, the tunica albuginea. The tunica albuginea sends prolongations inwards, dividing the testicle into lobules. Each lobule contains the seminiferous tubules, extending from the base where they end blindly, towards the apex, at which point they unite

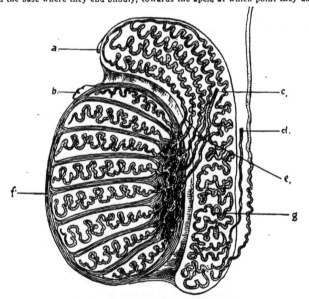

Fig. 1.—Diagrammatic sketch of relations of testicle, epididymis and embryonic remnants. *a*, pedunculated hydatid; *b*, hydatid of Morgagni; *c*, vas aberrans superioris; *d*, vas aberrans inferioris; *e*, vasa efferentia; *f*, testicle; *g*, epididymis.

to form the tubuli recti. The rete testis is formed in the mediastinum testis by the tubuli recti, and from it spring 12 to 15 vasa efferentia, which pierce the tunica albuginea and pass backwards in the ligamentum epididymis superioris, to form the coni vasculosi in the globus major. The canal of the epididymis arises from the coni vasculosi and at the cauda becomes the duct of the vas deferens.

The epididymis is attached to the testicle at three points by two-leafed folds of serous membrane, which are nothing more or less than the extension of the visceral layer of the tunica vaginalis on to the epididymis. The fold of the globus major is called the ligamentum epididymis superioris, and between its leaves pass the vasa efferentia. The double fold at the body encloses a space, the saccus epididymis. The ligamentum epididymis inferioris is the fold at the cauda.

There now remain to be considered the embryonic remnants, viz.: the hydatid of Morgagni, the pedunculated hydatid, the vasa aberrantia and the organ of Giraldes.

The origin of the hydatids is still in dispute. Luschka claimed that the sessile hydatid arises from the upper Wolffian tubules and the pedunculated hydatid from the Mullerian ducts. Virchow and Kocher claim that the sessile is a remnant of the Mullerian ducts. Stohr believed that the pedunculated is a representative of the Wolffian body.

The sessile hydatid is found at the upper pole of the testicle close to the globus major, and it has been stated by Kocher, Hochenegg, Lewin, and Luschka that there is a communication between the canal of the epididymis and hydatid. The pedunculated is attached to the globus major by a stalk; the stalk and head are usually solid. The vasa aberrantia are two in number, the superior and the inferior. The superior rises from the rete testis and ends blindly in the globus major; the inferior springs from the canal of the epididymis or from the duct of the vas deferens and ends blindly after extending up the cord about two inches. Kobelt proved that the inferior one was a remnant of the Wolffian body. Concerning the origin of the superior, there is some doubt; Langer-Toldt looked on it as a vas deferens that had lost its connection with the epididymis.

The organ of Giraldes is a group of vesicles and tubules situated in front of the vessels of the cord at the height of the globus major.

Origin.—Liston regarded the cysts from which he had withdrawn the fluid containing spermatozoa as enlarged seminal tubules.

Curling, Broca, and Paget advanced the theory that these cysts were neoformations. Curling and Broca maintained that the presence of spermatozoa was due to a rupture of seminal tubules into the cyst. Paget thought that the spermatozoa were produced by the epithelium of the cyst.

Following this, Follen and Verneuil produced the idea that this peculiar condition was a remnant of the Wolffian body.

To Virchow is given the credit for the theory held to-day, namely, that spermatoceles are retention cysts; however, he believed that they arose only from the vasa efferentia and the organ of Giraldes.

Kocher contended that the constant site of the spermatocele was at the vasa efferentia; that the latter structures offer a favorable location was confirmed by Hochenegg, who found the width of the seminiferous tubules to be 0.1–0.2 mm., that this diminishes to the size of the capillaries in the rete testis; in the vasa efferentia there is an expansion to 0.6 mm., followed by a contraction of 0.2 mm. in the coni vasculosi. This anatomical arrangement places the vasa efferentia between two obstructions, and as the testicle and globus major are covered with a dense capsule which would impede the formation of retention cysts, while the vasa efferentia are only surrounded by loose connective tissue, it is quite readily seen that dilatation of these ducts could easily occur. As a matter of fact, Dolbeau proved this experimentally by the injection of one hundred testicles with mercury, which caused a dilatation of the vasa efferentia.

The vas aberrans inferior has an origin similar to the vasa efferentia, and since it has similar surroundings, together with the fact that it ends blindly, can be considered as a point predisposed to retention cysts. As far as the vas aberrans inferior, a retention cyst here would mean an obstruction of the duct of the vas.

If the hydatids or the organ of Giraldes are in communication with the semen-carrying system, the origin of spermatocele from these areas is quite possible. However, since the organ of Giraldes and the pedunculated hydatids are usually isolated, not very much credence can be put into any theory including these organs as the points of origin of spermatocele. From the clinical and anatomical data, it seems probable that the sessile hydatid is often involved.

Therefore, in summing up, it can be said that spermatoceles should arise most frequently from the vasa efferentia and vas aberrans superior, often from the sessile hydatid and only occasionally from the vas deferens, pedunculated hydatid and organ of Giraldes.

Causes—1. *Trauma.*—Gosselin was the first to give trauma as a cause, and later Hochenegg described the *modus operandi* of this factor. According to the latter, on violent concussion, the testicle, which is more or less mobile, is able to descend, whereas the epididymis, which is fixed, cannot follow the motion, and as a result there is tension on the folds of the serosa, and as the tension increases the vasa efferentia are torn. This laceration, he states, usually occurs where the vasa efferentia pierce the tunica albuginea; the ends obliterate and blind pouches are formed. Another method is given by the same author, namely, that on account of the very free blood supply, trauma may cause sub-serous bleeding, which becomes organized and converted into connective tissue, and as this shrinks later, the vasa efferentia or the canal of the epididymis are obliterated.

In support of the trauma theory, Hochenegg reported two cases; one in a man fifty-two years of age, in whom after a sudden fall a stinging pain in the groin was felt and followed six months later by spermatocele; the other, a boy of fourteen years, after lifting a heavy load, had a history similar to the above.

Princeteau, Verneuil, Krebs, and Bonneau reported spermatoceles following injury. In Bonneau's case it followed an operation for hydrocele. Krebs found trauma as a factor eight times out of fifteen cases.

2. *Sexual Abstemiousness.*—Cavasse reported the first case that gave rise to this theory, but it has neither strong clinical nor pathological support.

3. *Gonorrhœa.*—It is to be expected, of course, that to venereal disease would be ascribed a rôle in this condition. However, there is very little clinical evidence to support it, and yet why should it not be, particularly when the epididymis is involved?

Of the causes above named, trauma seems to be the most logical one, yet it must be of a peculiar variety, for injury to the scrotum is not rare, while spermatoceles are a curiosity. As before mentioned, it is quite logical to expect that gonorrhœa might be an etiological factor; however, one cannot understand, in that event, why spermatoceles should not be as numerous as cases of hernia. In sexual abstemiousness, the overflow finds its way first to the seminal vesicles and then gains exit through pollutions instead of forming retention cysts.

Evidence has been produced to prove that spermatoceles are more numerous than suspected; Lewin found 8 of these cysts in 100 testicles of cadavers, while Hochenegg found 27 in 362 testicles of cadavers.

In the cases reported, the incidence seems to be equal on the two sides. They may occur at any age after the testicle has commenced to function.

Classification.—Von Hoffman divided them into intra-vaginal and extra-vaginal, though he claims that most of the extra-vaginal cysts commence intra-vaginally.

Extra-vaginal.—This variety arises from the vas aberrans superioris, from the vasa efferentia, and very rarely from the vas deferens and the paradidymis.

Those from the vas deferens and paradidymis are primarily extra-vaginal, whereas those from the other two, according to von Hoffman, become so by first occupying all the space in the ligamentum epididymis superioris, thereby displacing the epididymis backwards, and then they grow upwards in the tissues of the cord, when they become extra-vaginal. In this latter type of cyst the testicle is displaced downward and forward. The position of the testicle is unchanged in the variety arising from the vas deferens and the organ of Giraldes.

The site of insertion of the cysts arising from the vas efferentia and vas aberrans is in the rete testis; from the vas deferens and paradidymis, in the cord. The extra-vaginal cysts are usually unilocular. If multi-locular ones are found, they are probably due to several cysts arising at the same time. The extra-vaginal cysts are larger than the intra-vaginal, and in one case reported by Stanley, 49 ounces were removed at the first tapping and 57 at the second. These cysts are supposed to have a pear shape, which when seen is characteristic, but the larger cysts take most any form. When seen macroscopically, it is noted that the walls of the cysts are thin and that distributed in the sac walls are fibrous cords, which when the sac is greatly distended cause bulgings, giving the balloon shape described by Savariaud.

Intra-vaginal.—These arise from sessile hydatid, or the canal of the epididymis, and project into the cavum vaginale. That these cysts do occur at the hydatid of Morgagni was demonstrated by Hanusa, who found, during an operation for hydrocele, a dilated sessile hydatid, the size of a cherry and containing spermatozoa. As the walls of the hydatid are very thin, rupture into the cavum vaginale can easily occur, giving rise to a hydrocele containing spermatozoa. The intra-vaginal cysts become intimately connected with the tunica albuginea, and as they grow they take on the form of the globus major. It is this latter character-

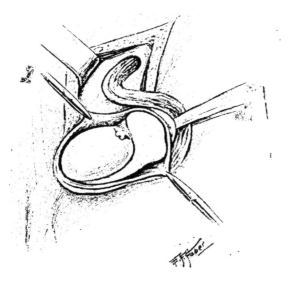

Fig. 2.—Sketch of the operation, showing the cyst at the globus major.

504

istic that gives rise to the impression that there is an accessory testicle superimposed on the normal organ.

Pathology—Structure.—The walls of the cysts are made up of interwoven strands of connective tissue, among which can be found bundles of smooth muscle. These bundles arise from the smooth muscle of the vasa efferentia and the canalis epididymis, and when found, it is claimed, surely point to the presence of spermatocele. The cysts are lined with ciliated or cylindrical epithelium when recent; in the older varieties the lining is of pavement epithelium.

Contents.—The contents are usually milky or soapy in color. On microscopical examination lymphocytes, fat globules, epithelial cells, and spermatozoa are found. The spermatozoa may be rigid or mobile, and in the cysts arising from a testicle which has become senile the spermatozoa may be absent. The fluid is feebly alkaline, has a specific gravity of 1.002–1.006, and contains 0.2 to 0.5 per cent. albumin.

Symptoms—Subjective.—There is a group of symptoms, which though rarely found, is pathognomonic, namely, severe pain in the testicle and swelling on sexual excitation. In the majority of cases there is no pain, only a feeling of distress. The swelling or tumor is what is most complained of, and if this is a slowly progressive affair following trauma, it would cause one to be suspicious of spermatocele. A certain number consult a physician, believing they have a third testicle, and as Liston says, " flatter themselves in thinking they are thus unduly provided."

Objective.—Here, too, the only finding will be a tumor. In the intravaginal variety it is a globular mass sitting on top of the testicle, but as sometimes occurs in this variety, a hydrocele may be coexistent and the tumor will not be recognized.

In the extra-vaginal cysts, the testicle will be found displaced downward and forward.

Diagnosis.—The history of trauma, followed by a slowly progressive tumor in the scrotum, would be circumstantial evidence. If a pear-shaped mass is found with the testicle displaced downward and forward, the diagnosis of extra-vaginal hydrocele is probably correct, as is also the finding of a globular mass on the top of the testicle, indicative of the intra-vaginal cyst. Presence of spermatozoa in the aspirated fluid is not a positive proof, for hydrocele may contain these elements.

Hochenegg resorted to chemical examination for differentiation of hydrocele and spermatocele fluid; spermatocele fluid, as stated above, is feebly alkaline, has a specific gravity of 1.002–1.006, and contains 0.2–0.5 per cent. of albumin, while hydrocele fluid is strongly alkaline, has a specific gravity of 1.020–1.040 and has from 4.4 to 7 per cent. albumin. No dependence can be put on the light test, as spermatoceles transmit light as well as hydroceles.

Treatment.—Aspiration, injection of irritants and incision have all been abandoned, as recurrences were frequent.

EDWARD T. CROSSAN

The radical operation is now performed. In the cysts arising from the sessile hydatid and the vas efferentia, a portion of the tunica albuginea must be removed and the defects covered with serosa. In the other varieties the cyst can be easily enucleated from its bed and the stalk ligated close to its base. If the testicle is atrophied castration is the logical procedure.

CASE REPORT.—L. O., aged eighteen years, male, white, was admitted to the Episcopal Hospital September 12, 1916, and discharged September 30, 1916.

Family History.—Negative.

Past Medical History.—Has not been ill since childhood. Denies venereal infection.

History of Present Illness.—For the past six years the patient has noticed sagging in the left scrotum, and for about the same period has noticed a tumor attached to the testicle. At first was the size of a pea, now has grown to the size of a walnut. On account of the tumor the patient was given the nickname of " Hock Shop." Never any pain in the testicle nor any interference with genito-urinary functions. Comes to the hospital to be operated on, as he wishes to enter the Navy and has been rejected because the Navy doctors said he had a " third testicle."

Physical Examination.—Scrotum: Varicocele left side. Attached to upper pole of left testicle at the site of the globus major, is a mass the size of a walnut. It is firmly attached to the testicle, and pressure over the mass is transmitted to the testicle. A diagnosis of spermatocele was made.

Operation.—September 15, 1916. Operator: Dr. A. P. C. Ashhurst. Assistant: Doctor Crossan. Incision over left inguinal canal three inches long. Fascia of the external oblique is split and the testicle delivered into the wound by traction of the cord. Tunica vaginalis seemed to be slightly distended and did not show any masses on the external surface. Tunica vaginalis is then opened and a few drachms of clear, straw-colored fluid evacuated. Tunica is split throughout its whole length, and it was then ascertained that the globus major showed a cyst the size of a lima bean. This was aspirated and about 4 c.c. of a milky fluid removed. The walls of the cyst were then opened. On opening the wall of the globus major it was found there was another cyst wall inside of it at a depth of 0.5 cm. This was dissected free and removed, having no dense adhesions. Portion of the wall of the globus major is removed for examination. Remainder is closed with No. oo chromic catgut. Before the above procedure a small portion of the tunica vaginalis was removed at the upper angle. The tunica vaginalis is then closed with No. o chromic interrupted gut. It was impossible, however, to make the edges meet at the upper limit of the sac. Testicle and its covering are replaced into the scrotum. Varicose veins separated from the remainder of the cord and divided between ligatures, a length of about 6 cm. being excised, and stumps approximated by tying the corresponding ends of the ligatures. External oblique is then closed by continuous No. 1 chromic catgut. The skin with No. o lock stitch of chromic gut. Dressings are then applied.

October 30, 1916: Discharged. Testicle is still swollen and tender on pressure.

Pathological Examination.—1. Cyst wall: Fibrous tissue wall, lined with columnar cells.

2. Fluid from cyst: 2 c.c. in amount, contained two spermatozoa, specific gravity 1.050.

Further History.—Patient was seen on March 2, 1920, at which time it was found that there was an atrophy of the left testicle. The latter was reduced to a mass 1½ cm. long by 2 cm. wide. The above unfortunate occurrence was probably due to some impediment at the globus major completely obstructing the semen-carrying system. Briaud produced a similar condition in rabbits by ligating the vas deferens.

SUMMARY

Spermatocele is a retention cyst of the scrotum which is or has been in communication with the semen-carrying system. The cysts arise most frequently from the vasa efferentia, the vasa aberrantia superiori, and the sessile hydatids. The main symptom is swelling, with sometimes a history of previous trauma.

I wish to express thanks to Dr. A. P. C. Ashhurst for permission to report the above case.—AUTHOR.

BIBLIOGRAPHY

Liston: Med. Chir. Tr., London, 1843, xxvi, 216–222.
Lloyd: Ibid., 368–373.
Guerin: J. de med. mil., Par., 1785, iv, 66–74.
Cavasse: Gaz. d. hop., Paris, 1860, xxxiii, 378.
Sedillot: Mem. de Sec. de med., Strasb., 1853, xiii, 33–42.
Ellis: Boston M. and S. J., 1858, lviii, 99.
Gosselin: Bull. gen. de therap., etc., Paris, 1852,, xliv, 110–112.
Baker: Edin. M. J., 1876–7, xxii, 1085–1087.
Bennet, E. H.: Irish Hosp. Gaz., Dub., 1873, i, 290.
Curling: Month. J. M. Sc., London and Edinb., 1848–9, ix, 1023–1027.
Hunt, W. B.: Phila. Med. Times, 1875–6, vi, 368.
MacDonnell, R. L.: Brit. Am. J., Montreal, 1860, i, 60–62.
Paget, J.: Med. Chir. Jr., London, 1844, xxvii, 398–404.
Ebert, Walter: Ueber Spermatocele, Leipz., 1902.
Von Hoffman: Ergebn. de Chir. u. Orthop., Berlin, 1914, viii, 698–701.
Whitney, C. M.: Am. J. Urol., N. Y., 1907, III, 175–197.

A CONSIDERATION OF THE VARICOCELE OPERATION AND THE AVOIDANCE OF POST-OPERATIVE INDURATION *

BY PENN G. SKILLERN, JR., M.D.

OF PHILADELPHIA, PA.

AN undesirable sequel of operation for the cure of varicocele is the column of induration that frequently forms and that extends from the testicle upward through the scroto-abdominal passageway to the external inguinal ring. This column of induration may persist for several weeks, and to this extent the cure may be said to be worse than the disease. So disabling was this column of induration considered in recruits that in the first period of the World War official bulletins advised not to operate upon varicoceles unless they were of very large size and productive of symptoms. The writer had occasion to perform the varicocele operation in perhaps several dozen cases during the past three years, and the following observations are based upon the study of this series of cases.

The causes of this column of induration seem to be: (1) Limited resection of veins with end-to-end suture of stumps: this results in stagnation of blood in closed vessels, with a lump at the site of the stumps; (2) failure to obliterate the dead spaces established by dissection of the fascial layers: these dead spaces furnish room for the outpouring of blood and tissue juices after operation; (3) irritation of the vas deferens from rough manipulation: I have found the vas very sensitive to trauma, to which it reacts by swelling to several times its original size.

Many operations have been devised for the cure of varicocele, but to the writer it seems that there need be but one operation—an operation that will remove the disease and yet not be followed by the above undesirable sequelæ. No operation removes the disease which does not remove the entire mass of veins involved. No operation is satisfactory which does not obliterate dead spaces left remaining by mere edge-to-edge apposition of the divided fascial layers, or perhaps no suturing of these layers at all. No operation is satisfactory which brings about irritative reaction of the vas to trauma from rough manipulation.

The writer obtains satisfactory results as regards the above details by performing the operation as follows:

An incision is made over the inguinal canal as for herniorrhaphy, dividing skin, Camper's fascia, Scarpa's fascia, and the aponeurosis of the external oblique muscle, opening into the external ring. The cremaster muscle with its fascia is next divided and retracted, exposing the spermatic-cord enclosed in the thin infundibuliform fascia. The part of

---

* Read before the Philadelphia Academy of Surgery, April 5, 1920.

the spermatic cord first seen is the anterior group of veins which are varicose, and which constitute the bulk of the varicocele. This anterior group of veins is picked up at the internal ring and freed from the infundibuliform fascia as far as the testicle below. During this manœuvre the anterior veins are drawn away from the posterior veins and vas, so that there is no occasion to disturb the vas in any manner whatsoever, nor even to touch it. By keeping away from the vas there will be no misgivings as to the integrity of the circulation of blood to the testicle *via* the deferential artery and veins, nor any as to the post-operative irritational swelling of the vas. While freeing the veins close to the testicle the tunica vaginalis may be opened inadvertently: such an opening, however, is not undesirable, for it prevents post-operative acute hydrocele formation in a closed sack. The opening, when made, should not be closed: it will heal of itself within a few days.

The anterior tortuous veins having been freed are ready for ligation. Removal of the entire pathology requires that these ligatures be applied at the testicle below and at the internal ring above. The thickest part of the varicocele is at the testicle, and the thinnest is at the internal ring, where usually but two veins are present to return the blood from the varicocele to the spermatic vein. In certain cases the varicocele extends into the inguinal canal, where it forms a bulge simulating hernia. The advantages of opening the canal are that such a varicocele extending into the canal may be dealt with, and also that isolation of the veins may be begun where the veins do not contact with the vas, *i.e.*, at the internal ring. The ligatures are applied as follows.

Using No. 1 plain gut carried by an aneurism needle the vein mass is transfixed close to the testicle and the suture is tied on both sides of the mass. A clamp is applied to the vein mass proximal to the ligature in order to prevent soiling of the field with blood escaping from the veins when divided, and the vein mass is divided between the ligature and the clamp. In similar manner the two veins at the internal ring are transfixed and ligated, care being taken not to pinch in the ligature the little pouch of peritoneum which appears anteriorly when the veins are freed close to the internal ring. For safety's sake a second ligature is applied close to the first, for if but one ligature be applied and should slip off, annoying retroperitoneal bleeding from the retracted stump would arise. A clamp is applied to the vein mass distal to the second ligature, and the veins are divided between the clamp and the second ligature. The vein mass between the clamps is now removed from the field: its length varies from four to six inches. The inguinal canal is now occupied by the vas with its vessels and the posterior set of veins, which usually are not varicose. The cremaster muscle with its fascia is now sutured snugly down upon the vas, this being accomplished by passing the sutures at a distance from the cut edges. If it is desired to draw the testicle to a higher position, the cremaster muscle with its fascia is sutured transversely, although I have rarely found this step necessary. I may say in passing that I do not believe in shortening the scrotum by resection, for when an undue weight is removed from the scrotum, the latter contracts soon or late, when the dartos and cremaster muscles recover their physiologic tonus.

The retracted ilio-inguinal nerve is now replaced, and the incision in the external oblique aponeurosis is closed. Scarpa's fascia is closed as a separate layer and tacked down upon the external oblique aponeurosis, thus obliterating the dead space that otherwise would exist between these two layers, and also approximating the cut edges of Camper's fascia and skin. The skin is closed by interrupted sutures of silk-worm gut. After the dressing has been put on a suspensory is applied to the scrotum, and the latter is elevated over the pubes to counteract gravity.

Since employing the above technic I have not seen the column of induration arise. All the palpating fingers find after operation is the ligature stump at the top of the testicle and above this the normal-sized vas pursuing its course up to the inguinal canal. There may be a transitory enlargement of the testicle while the deferential vessels are establishing the compensatory circulation, but atrophy of the testicle is no more frequent than after orchidopexy for ectopia: indeed, it is very rare, and should not be as frequent as in the latter condition.

The patient is allowed out of bed in two days and discharged from hospital on the sixth day, cured of varicocele without undesirable sequelæ.

CUTTING THE BONE FLAP IN CRANIAL SURGERY

By Harvey C. Masland, M.D.

of Philadelphia, Pa.

Cranial surgery is resorted to for the treatment of traumatic conditions and for those the result of disease. In considering the question of
opening the skull it is recognized that many cases, and particularly those
of the traumatic type, must be treated by no set rule, but according to the
indications present.

It is accepted as axiomatic that two motives should dominate one in
performing any surgical operation. First, the objective desired should
be gained with the greatest expedition, safety and facility. Second, with
the first objective attained the tissues left should show the least mutilation
and so promise the best possible physiologic and cosmetic end-results.

The method I wish to present follows the usual basic lines of procedure, but the instruments used are presented with the belief that they
offer certain advantages in the performance of the operation and also
secure better end-results.

The bone cutting is done quickly with safety to the soft tissues and
under perfect control. There is minimum wastage of the bone, so that
in replacement the bone edges are closely apposed and good mechanical
protection is provided. The scalp flap remains adherent to the bone flap,
thus guaranteeing the vitality of the resected bone. It is adapted to
operate upon any portion of the cranial vault.

A brief reference to the advantages and defects of the more commonly
used instruments might be appropriate.

The old trephines served their day and with the ability of the more
modern implements to do better surgery in every way are justifiable in
but a few restricted cases. The cylindrical trephine is more dangerous
than the conical. Either one is very prone to cut the dura and brain at
some thin part in the circumference of the cut. This tendency increases
with the size of the trephine, owing to the greater likelihood of variability
in the thickness of the skull. The button of bone retains no vital connection.

The Hudson linear-biting punch forceps, if properly used, will not
injure the dura. It will make a vitally connected flap of any size or
shape. There is a tendency of the punch to jam in the wall of the incision. It cuts slowly and with increasing tire to the operator, according
to the density and thickness of the bone. It destroys so much bone that
in replacement the bone flap does not touch the surrounding skull wall
for support.

The power-driven spiral osteotome protects the dura, permits a vital
flap of any dimension, and is a useful instrument. Ordinarily, the osteotome is directly attached to the motor and the operator must hold the

motor in his hands. Practice and skill are required with this unwieldy mechanism to give a sufficient degree of sensitive control. Such a spiral osteotome, to be sufficiently strong and yet reasonably slender, must have but a shallow cutting edge. Searing of the bone is inevitable. As with the Hudson punch, too much bone has been removed to secure any coaptation of the bone edges. This can be prevented by leaving the bone partially cut at a few points and by fracturing the inner table, leaving a supporting shelf.

The Gigli saw reduces the width of cut very considerably as compared to the preceding instruments. Considerable skill is required to use this saw without breaking. The preliminary openings should be numerous as the saw occupies the position of the chord of the inside arc of the bone. The greater the curve the more does the saw press upon the dura and brain. Thus the soft tissues are cut before the saw starts to cut the bone in the middle portion of the arc. As the saw is but a square steel wire twisted it loses its slight cutting edge quickly and then chafes rather than cuts.

The thin saw, whether the Doyen hand saw or the power-driven circular saw, gives the least wastage of bone that could be expected. A vital bone flap can be cut with these instruments which on reposition will have bone support from the apposed edge of the skull. When these instruments are used the procedure is to determine the thickness of the skull by making preliminary openings. Gauges for the saw are set to cut through the outer table and partially through the inner table. Herein arises one danger. There is no means of discovering an unexpected thin point, and consequently there is always danger of cutting the underlying tissue. Should the inner table not be severed sufficiently there is the possibility of splitting and separating the two tables of the bone.

The circular saw referred to is of the type where the saw is directly attached to the motor shaft without adequate guards against possible injury to the tissues. All these motors are high speed, and consequently the bone is seared, even markedly carbonized, immediately on contact of the saw and bone. A drip quickly cools but does not prevent burning of the bone. The unwieldy hold on the instrument requires much skill to gain a fair degree of control.

The addition of a new instrument to our armamentarium is justifiable when it facilitates the performance of an operation, when its use lessens the possibility of mishaps, and when the end-results are better.

The enthusiasm of one who claims any or all of the above features is to be weighed in the exacting balance of experience and fact. It is appropriate to state that this equipment has been used clinically in several hospitals in our city as well as experimentally in the performance of different bone reconstructive operations. The equipment is adapted to all general bone plastic work. Each tool has been planned to perform most efficiently the particular work required. The accompanying photographs

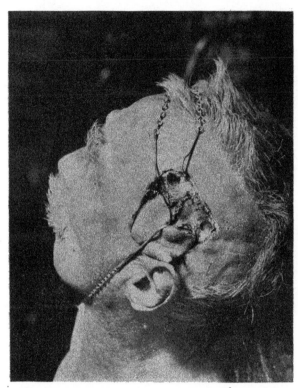

FIG. 1.—Preliminary openings made with Roberts trephine and Masland multi-tool handle.

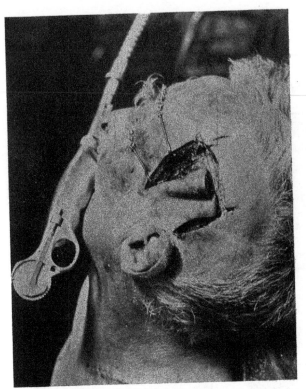

FIG. 2.—Incision through the outer table. Note that the inside guard on the saw is removed and the outside guard adjusted to cut the outer table only.

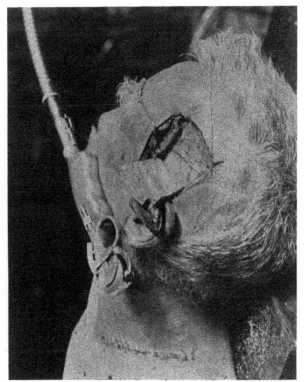

Fɪɢ. 3.—The bone flap with soft tissue attached laid open. The dura is intact.

57 2 β.

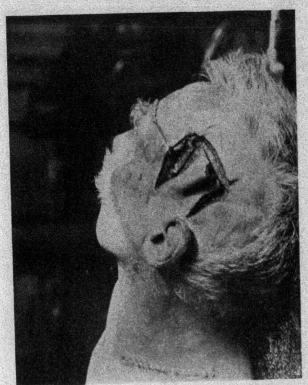

FIG. 4.—The flap replaced, showing the close approximation of the edges.

are of some experimental work done to illustrate the operation, the title of this paper. The instruments for opening the skull comprise the multi-tool handle and a quarter-inch Roberts trephine and a circular saw as illustrated in the photographs.

The Roberts trephine works upon the principle of the Hudson burr. It jams and stops the motor before injuring the dura. The only possible way to prevent this jamming is for the operator to rock his instrument and destroy the tight-fitting bony wall of the opening. These instruments are driven by a low-speed completely enclosed aluminum motor, and a flexible sterilizable cable. Cables formerly used were properly condemned for their irregular delivery of power. This cable is one taken from the industries and especially constructed to sterilize in boiling water. It is sufficiently heavy and strong to deliver steady power without back lash. It is strong enough to stop the motor. The low speed possible with a selective current motor obviates the burning of the bone.

In performing the operation the skin incision is preferably made as illustrated, though, of course, modifications can be made where indicated. The part to be fractured, however, should be reasonably narrow. The preliminary openings are made at the upper angles of the wound. The very small diameter of the trephine practically excludes the likelihood of any great variation in the thickness of the bone. The trephine should be held vertical to the bone surface.

For the next stage of the operation I prefer to use the saw with the inside guard detached. The outside guard is adjusted to cut through the outer table only. This bone incision marks my line of cut. It reduces the final cutting with the inside guard to the inner table. The bone cutting can be done safely using the inside guard alone, but the increased fineness of control has appealed to me as worth while.

The upper incision can be bevelled to insure a stronger support in replacement of the flap. There is no advantage in making a small flap.

After making the cuts through the outer table the outside guard is turned back out of the way, and the inside guard attached. With the thumb this guard is held rigidly wide open and the tip inserted in a trephine opening. The tip is so shaped as to separate the dura from the bone with ease. When the guard arm has advanced its length under the bone the power is turned on and the saw gently brought down upon the bone and through the bone to the guard. Drawing the saw backward and forward and dipping it a bit all the intervening bone is severed. The guard can now follow after the saw through the groove and the cutting can be advanced. Failure to cut any portion of the bone is instantly felt by the pressing forward of the thumb pressing on the finger tip of the guard. The thumb should press backward on the guard so keeping the tip firmly against the inner surface of the bone. The remaining bone is divided quickly.

When one wishes to go across a sinus or large meningeal vessel an absolute assurance of protection is gained by resorting to the method employed in making the primary cut at the trephine opening. The saw is lifted up and the guard tip used to dissect the vessels and all underlying soft tissues the permitted distance of the guard arm. The power is then turned on and the saw cuts this portion. If any lack of confidence or other indication exists this plan can be pursued throughout. The operator quickly gains a tactile sense, however, that assures him that the tip is sliding along the bared bone of the inner wall.

The rotation of the saw is in a direction to throw the débris away from the operator. Any kick that may occur from too hard application of the saw is backward into the region of safety.

The serrated edge of the fractured side does not permit a perfect replacement. This is sufficient to take up the wastage of bone at the opposite side and bring the bone edge in contact with its apposed cranial edge. A slight elevation is usual. In this connection it has occurred that where provision might be desired for a subsequent easement under internal pressure the bone flap might be sectioned longitudinally to give the effect of laths as they are applied on a wall. This would give a bone reinforcement in the flap and also allow for a stretch of the soft tissue.

To summarize the features of this operation and the instruments used. The preliminary openings, usually but two, are small. The relations of the power and of the construction of the trephine to the skull opening are so adjusted that the trephine must jam before penetrating the dura.

If the preliminary saw cut through the outer table is used the guard is immediately adjustable to the depth desired.

The inside guard is of a shape to secure easy separation of the dura, and there is fine tactile sense of its efficiency in this respect.

There is no burning of the bone and so the vitality of the exposed osteoblasts is preserved.

There is bone support for the replaced bone flap.

If a greater provision for internal pressure is desired the bone flap can be variously sectioned in vital fragments to gain the desired end.

514

TRANSACTIONS

OF THE

PHILADELPHIA ACADEMY OF SURGERY

Stated Meeting held April 5, 1920

The President, Dr. George G. Ross, in the Chair

TOTAL CYSTECTOMY—CONDITION OF PATIENT FIVE YEARS AFTER OPERATION

Dr. B. A. Thomas presented a man, forty-six years of age, who was exhibited before the Academy four years ago. The case has been one of particular interest in view of his present state of health, and the nature of the apparatus necessary for deviation of his urinary stream. To the best of the reporter's knowledge this is the only case that has survived, for any length of time, the operation suggested by Watson, of Boston, in 1906; namely, separate nephrostomies, followed by total cystectomy as a third operative procedure.

The patient is employed at present as a mechanic in the Pennsylvania Industrial Home for the Blind. He is able to care for his apparatus routinely. His drainage apparatus is shown in the adjoining cuts (Figs. 1 and 2). It at present consists of two catheters, held in position in the fistulæ with the aid of safety pins and adhesive plaster, and connected by metallic joints to rubber tubing leading to two rubber bag urinals. In this connection it is worthy of note that perhaps no drainage apparatus, in such cases, will be permanently satisfactory. In this case, in the beginning, Watson's apparatus was used, but was soon found to be too bulky and heavy and was strenuously objected to by the patient. Subsequently, one of the urine receptacles of Watson's apparatus was placed over the hypogastric region, suspended by an abdominal belt, to which rubber tubing led from silver-flanged tubes placed in the urinary fistulæ. These at first were bulbous on the inside and fenestrated, but owing to phosphatic incrustations, necessitating their cleansing from time to time, and the difficulty of removal, had to have their bulbous expansions cut off, the tubes then being held in position by adhesive plaster, placed over the external flanges.

This patient had his first cystotomy in January, 1912, for nodular formations at the apex of his trigonum. A few months later these nodular formations recurred, and he was treated in another hospital by fulguration, with little or no improvement in symptomatology. In October, 1913, the patient was admitted to the Polyclinic Hospital and with Young's cystoscopic rongeur two or three of the small intravesical tumors, which at that time completely filled the lower half and neck of the bladder, varying in size from a small pea to a cherry, were removed and submitted to Dr. John A. Kolmer for histopathological examination, who reported them to be inflamed polypi. The bladder was opened and the interior thoroughly cauterized with the electro-cautery, care being taken to destroy all evidence of these multiple polypoid growths. A few weeks later cystoscopy showed recurrence of the growths, and in January, 1914, the left ureter was ligated close to the renal pelvis and nephrostomy under ether anæsthesia performed. Five weeks later the right kidney was treated similarly, under stovain spinal anæsthesia, and on November 6, 1914, total cystectomy under ether anæsthesia was done, together with religation of the left ureter, because the lumen of the ureter had become reëstablished. This ligation was done with silk; the first having been done with catgut.

Three months later the patient complained of pains in his prostatic region and perineum, of a severe character, and on the presumption that the polypi were reforming in the prostatic urethra, where a few had been previously observed, on March 23, 1915, a perineal extracapsular prostatectomy and total posterior urethrectomy were performed under ether anæsthesia, from which the patient convalesced remarkably satisfactorily. In spite of this strenuous surgical treatment, he is still living and in remarkable health.

INTRAPERITONEAL HERNIA OF THE ILEUM THROUGH A RENT IN THE MESENTERY

DR. HENRY P. BROWN, JR., in presenting the patient, said that from a fairly thorough review of the literature of the past twenty-five years it seems that hernia through a rent in the mesentery, while not being rare, is unusual. He had found reference to nineteen cases, to which he wished to add one that was admitted to Doctor Hodge's service at the Presbyterian Hospital, and upon which he allowed the reporter to operate.

The patient, a white boy of five years, was admitted to the hospital June 23, 1916. Chief complaint was pain in the abdomen and vomiting. While playing on June 21st he fell down two steps, striking on the dorsolumbar region. He was apparently uninjured and resumed play. That night he complained of abdominal pain and vomited a few times. He was given a dose of magnesium citrate which he vomited. On the 24th the vomiting and pain became more severe, and on the 25th a physician was called who diagnosed acute appendicitis and advised operation. His bowels moved the morning he fell, but not since. Although not complaining of much pain, the patient had the pinched features and fixed stare of a very sick boy. The abdomen was distended and very rigid. Peristalsis freely heard over upper abdomen. Tympanitic to percussion. Patient points to painful spot just below umbilicus, but no mass can be palpated. His leucocytes were 21,000 on admission; temperature, 101° F.; pulse, 140; respiration, 46.

Operation June 25th, third day after onset of condition. Ether anæs-

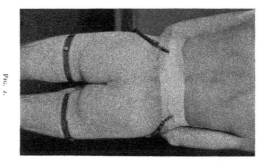

FIG. 1.   FIG. 2.

Drainage apparatus after total cystectomy.

thesia. Incision through outer border of right rectus muscle below umbilicus. On opening the peritoneum about one-half a litre of blood-tinged fluid escaped from the abdomen. A knuckle of twisted gangrenous gut, about 20–30 cm. long, presented in the incision, a coil of lower ileum which had passed through a 3-cm. opening in the mesentery, and had become twisted upon itself two and one-half times. The neck of the volvulus was cord-like in character. The opening in the mesentery, located about 5 cm. above the cæcum, had rough edges, apparently of recent origin. The gangrenous loop of ileum was resected and an end-to-end anastomosis was made with a Murphy button. The hole in the mesentery was closed, and the abdomen closed in layers. Hypodermoclysis was given. The patient died four hours after the operation.

A brief summary of the reported cases as collected from the literature is as follows:

CASE I (Reported by C. G. Franklin).—Man seventy-three years of age. Admitted to the hospital with symptoms of intestinal obstruction. Five days before admission, while in bed, he was seized with sudden abdominal pain and vomiting. Slght action of the bowels. Vomiting daily, it becoming feculent in character two days before admission. Operation day of admission: Coil of small intestine 6 inches long, tightly strangulated in circular aperture in mesentery. Opening enlarged, bowel reduced. It was deep red, port wine in color and deeply indented by the ring. Recovery.

CASE II (Reported by J. G. Smith).—Boy of twelve years. Three weeks before admission had an attack of pain in right abdomen, accompanied by vomiting. Improved. Three days later another attack. Operation: Loops of strangulated intestine, very dark, through hole in mesentery. Easily reduced. Bloody fluid and serum in abdomen. Recovery.

CASE III (Reported by J. S. R. Smith).—Girl of fifteen years. Seized with sudden abdominal pain soon followed by vomiting. Symptoms of intestinal obstruction followed and lasted till operation on the fourth day. Operation: Bowel greatly congested, small loop of bowel in a hole in the mesentery 2½ by 2 inches. Bowel judged capable of recovery—reduced. Hole had smooth thick margins—congenital in type. No history of previous injury. Recovery.

CASE IV (Reported by J. Clark).—Girl nine years old. Four years previously she had been run over by a trap. Went to bed feeling all right. Had sudden attack of abdominal pain and vomiting. When first seen fourteen hours after onset of attack, she was in a state of collapse. Complete intestinal obstruction. Death twenty-four hours after onset of attack. No operation. Autopsy: Thirty ounces of bloody serum in the abdomen. Four feet of lower ileum had passed through an aperture in the mesentery, strangulated. Evidence of old peritonitis in this area of the abdomen.

CASE V (Reported by A. P. C. Ashhurst.—Boy of twelve fell and hurt his hip. Next day, dietetic error. Pains in abdomen, vomiting. Symptoms of intestinal obstruction for three days. Abdomen distended, vomiting fæces, blood and mucus by bowel. Umbilicus suggested presence of Meckel's diverticulum. Operation: Fecal smelling blood fluid—black coil of gut in pelvis resembled volvulus. Resected 14-18 inches of intestine—end-to-end anastomosis—glass tube in pelvis. Death three hours later. Hole in mesentery—ileum passed through till stopped by base of Meckel's diverticulum. Loop of gut was twisted and gangrenous.

CASE VI (Reported by J. B. Deaver).—Sudden severe pain while cranking car—relieved in several days. Six months later while again cranking car had sudden severe abdominal pain which did not subside. Admitted to hospital in dying condition. No operation. Post-operative examination: Strangulated gangrenous coil of intestine through a congenital hole in the mesentery.

CASE VII (Reported by W. A. Lane).—Boy of ten had sudden violent pain in central part of lower abdomen—vomiting. Thoroughly purged by family physician— two days later collapsed.. Complete obstruction of bowels—no previous history of injury or discomfort. Attack came on while asleep. In dying condition when admitted to hospital.

Operation: Second day, after onset. Mass of dark bluish intestine 3½ feet long passed through ⅞-inch hole in mesentery. Lower end was 2 feet above ileocæcal valve. Opening was rough. Foul smelling bloody fluid in the abdomen. Patient died on the table.

CASE VIII (Reported by L. J. Mitchell).—Boy of eight fell down-stairs, landing on abdomen—apparently unhurt. Two days later complained of severe pain in abdomen. Diagnosed peritonitis by outside physician. No operation. Died four days later. Post-mortem examination: Opening in mesentery near ileocæcal junction, smooth margins. Several loops of strangulated bowel, dark cherry red in color, had passed through it.

CASE IX (Reported by A. B. Atherton).—Boy of fourteen years. Subject to attacks of abdominal cramps since six years of age. Present attack started with dietetic indiscretion—was well purged with calomel. Seen two days after onset of symptoms, which were those of obstruction. Died three days later.

Operation: Removed a twisted Meckel's diverticulum, which relieved the obstruction. Died three days later. Post-operative examination: Loop of ileum 1 foot long through hole in mesentery, 6 inches from ileocæcal valve. It was not gangrenous and was easily reduced.

CASE X (Reported by Mauclaire).—Woman twenty-one years. Signs of complete intestinal obstruction for five days. Mass palpated between umbilicus and pubes.

Operation: Strangulation of 30-40 cm. of intestine through hole size of palm of hand in mesentery. Margin of opening denoted that it was of long standing. She fell some days before the appearance of symptoms. Death ten hours after the operation.

CASE XI (Reported by E .C. Staab).—Woman of thirty-eight. Always suffered with constipation. No history of abdominal injury. Eleven days before admission she had severe abdominal pain which lasted five days, and ceased. Complete obstruction since first attack of pain. In state of collapse when admitted to hospital. Abdomen distended, not tense, no pain.

Operation: Large intestine collapsed from cæcum to sigmoid. On exposing small bowel, a portion slipped out of a hole in the mesentery. Circular hole in mesentery, ⅝-inch in diameter, 3 inches from cæcum. Blood supply to intestine was good. Died from collapse eight hours after operation. Post-mortem—nothing further was found.

CASE XII (Reported by F. W. Speidel).—Man shot by companion while out hunting, part of charge entering thigh and arm. While on way to hunt had sudden attack of cramps, and had a bowel movement. At the instant shot was fired, he threw up his hands and pitched forward on the ground. He had severe abdominal cramps which became more severe while on his way home.

Examination showed no evidence of wound to the abdomen. Pain one inch below and to right of umbilicus—vomiting bile. Was given morphine freely, in three hours he having received ten ½-grain doses by mouth and five ⅛-grain doses by hypo. "In short time he was given a dose of opium and in fifteen minutes he was quiet." Next day he was worse—obtained 2 ounces of urine per catheter. No vomiting. Bowels did not move since the accident. Calomel, oil and enemas failed to move him.

Operated on the eleventh day after onset of symptoms. Found a loop of intestine imprisoned in a hole in the mesentery—reduced. Patient died seven days later, eighteen days after the onset, his bowels not having moved in that time. Fecal vomiting from tenth day to end.

CASE XIII (Reported by N. Macphatter).—Woman seventy-three years. No history of trauma. Complained of not feeling well—inability to move the bowels. On the fourth day she showed symptoms of acute intestinal obstruction.

Operation: Loop of intestine through mesentery—twisted—not gangrenous. Enlarged the hole in mesentery—reduced the bowel—closed the hole. Recovery.

CASE XIV (Reported by G. K. Dickinson).—Man forty-five years. Symptoms of acute obstruction.

Operation: General peritonitis. Hole in mesentery in region of cæcum—smooth margins—2 inches in diameter. A 2-inch coil of small intestine through the hole held in place by tip of gangrenous appendix.

Author does not mention duration of condition, condition of bowel, what was done, whether there was history of trauma or result.

CASE XV (Reported by W. D. Hamaker).—Woman seventy-two years. Obstinate constipation for many years. Sudden onset of symptoms of intestinal obstruction.

Operation third day after onset of acute symptoms: Meckel's diverticulum rolled up in one edge of gangrenous omentum. Rent in upper part of mesentery, through which passed all of transverse colon and omentum. Condition evidently of long standing. Opening was size of an egg. Removed Meckel's diverticulum and gangrenous omentum—reduced hernia. Recovery.

CASE XVI (Reported by C. H. Frazier).—Man thirty years. No history of trauma or dietetic indiscretion. Symptoms of acute obstruction.

Operated upon third day after onset. Exposed 18 inches of dilated congested small intestine, protruding through a slit in the mesentery. Easily reduced. Slit probably of long standing. He had an attack somewhat similar to the present one, thirteen years ago—vomiting, pain, constipation and cramps frequently since this first attack. Recovery.

CASE XVII (Reported by J. B. Roberts).—Man nineteen years. No stool for five days. Pain—distended abdomen. Somewhat similar attack one year previous. Symptoms of acute obstruction.

Operation: In ileocæcal region, small intestine entangled in an opening in the mesentry—easily reduced—no gangrene. "There was apparently no actual protrusion of a loop through the mesenteric opening, but the bent intestine was seemingly thrust into the orifice in such a way that the sharp bend closed the lumen." Orifice seemed congenital. Recovery.

CASE XVIII (Glovanoff).—Incarceration of intestines in aperture of mesentery in closure of vitello-intestinal duct. Recovery.

CASE XIX (Herczel).—Intestinal incarceration with double volvulus in mesenteric opening. Operation. Recovery

Of these 20 cases, 3 that showed strangulation recovered. Seven with strangulation died. Two without strangulation died. Six that were not strangulated recovered. In one, the condition of the bowel and the result are not mentioned.

In no case was the condition diagnosed before operation. One condition of bowel not mentioned (gang?) died.

REFERENCES

[1] Franklin, C. G.: Lancet, London, 1894, i, p. 334.
[2] Smith, J. G.: Brit. M. J., 1897, i, p. 1022.
[3] Smith, J. S. R.: Lancet, London, 1897, ii, p. 1111.
[4] Clarke, J.: Brit. M. J., London, 1905, i, 594.

[9] Ashhurst, A. P. C.: ANNALS SURG., Phila., 1910, i, p. 34.
[6] Deaver, J. B.: Surg. Gyn. Obst., 1920, vol. xxx, No. 1, p. 30.
[7] Lane, W. A.: Brit. M. J., London, 1890, i, p. 890.
[8] Mitchell, L. J.: ANNALS SURG., Phila., 1899, xxx, p. 505.
[9] Atherton, A. B.: Brit. M. J., 1897, 2, p. 975.
[10] Mauclaire: Bull. et Mem. Soc. Anat. de Par., 1899, lxxiv, 247.
[11] Staab, E. C.: St. Thomas Hospt. Reports, London, xxi, p. 172.
[12] Speidel, F. W.: Louisville Med. Monthly, 1895-96, ii, p. 479.
[13] Macphatter, N.: Am. J. of Surg., 1904-05, xviii, p. 232.
[14] Dickinson, G. K.: J. A. M. A., 1907, xlviii, No. 15, p. 1267.
[15] Hamaker, W. D.: J. A. M. A., 1914, lxii, p. 204.
[16] Frazier, C. H.: Phila. Med. Jour., 1899, iii, p. 174.
[17] Roberts, J. B.: Therapeut. Gazette, Philadelphia, December, 1915, p. 1964.
[18] Glovanoff: Voyenno Med. J., St. Petersburg, 1901, lxxix, med. spec., p. 1964.
[19] Herczel: Orvosi betil, Budapest, 1897, xli, 42.

LARGE STONE IN THE BLADDER REMOVED BY SUPRAPUBIC CYSTOTOMY

DR. GEORGE ERETY SHOEMAKER presented a calculus and reported the case of a man, aged sixty-nine years, whose history was as follows: A rectal abscess was incised by his physician some four years ago, since which there has been occasional discharge of pus, and soreness in the perineum. Bladder symptoms have been confused by the patient with the rectal disorder, but for two years there has been increasing difficulty in urination with pain in both groins referred to rectum, down the thighs to the perineum and glans. The patient sits down cautiously, sidewise. Urination every one or two hours with much straining; it is accomplished only in the standing position with both knees bent and the right hip lowered. This peculiarity of position evidently gives a mechanical advantage over the obstruction.

X-ray and metallic sound demonstrated a large stone very low down and fixed. Only two ounces of fluid could be introduced, owing to the violent straining developed, and because of the valve-like action of the stone only a portion of the fluid introduced could be withdrawn by either a soft or hard catheter. There was a moderate amount of acidosis present; the heart was slightly irregular; there was some cough. The blood urea nitrogen was 14 and 7/10 mg. per 100 c.c. The phenosulphonephthalein test was 5 per cent. first hour, 8 per cent. second hour; total, 13 per cent. in two hours. The urine showed but little blood. The organisms present were staphylococcus and streptococcus of low virulence.

Because the bladder was contracted upon the stone which extended above the accessible point of drainage, it was felt that preliminary drainage would be unsatisfactory as a means of preparation for the strain of operation. The preliminary treatment was therefore confined to irrigation, somewhat imperfect, and a milk diet.

Conditions having improved, the p. s. p. test being now 30 per cent. in two hours, suprapubic extraction was done under gas ether. The peritoneum was successfully reflected without injury, assisted by the introduction of a finger within the bladder. The surface of the stone was rough and friable, some scales adhering to the pocket behind the prostate where the stone was firmly adherent. The scales were carefully picked off and the wound closed down to a drainage tube. A daily irrigation was followed by one ounce of mercuro-chrome 220 one-per cent. solution which was left in the bladder. The drainage tube was out the fifth day. The bladder sinus was closed and normal function fully established the twenty-fourth day. The patient was discharged entirely comfortable, rising not more than once at night and holding the urine from five to six hours. A letter received a few days ago states that he is free from pain or distress; that the urine is clear and free from sediment, and that he rises once in the night. There is no leakage.

Of possible interest in connection with the origin of this stone is the fact that the patient was engaged in business in the far interior of the Honan Province of China some years ago, a region in which stone in the bladder is common. The weight of the stone was $313\frac{1}{2}$ grams when removed. It has been sawed asunder and apparently contains no nucleus. It is composed of calcium oxalates and phosphates.

It may be mentioned that the use of mercuro-chrome appeared to contribute to the comfort of the patient and the freedom from infection during a smooth convalescence.

DR. ALEXANDER RANDALL presented a calculus which he thought was probably the largest human vesical calculus removed in modern times. The specimen belongs to Dr. Elmer E. Keiser. The patient was a foreman carder in a woollen mill, sixty-one years of age, slightly built, of medium height, and the father of ten children, the youngest of which is but four years old. Twelve years ago he passed by the urethra several small stones, since which time he has complained of frequency of urination, constipation, hemorrhoids, and has noticed hæmaturia on a few occasions. He likewise complained of a large hernia and great difficulty in properly retaining it. He consulted Doctor Keiser on July 17, 1919, having worked up to the first of that month. His complaint was severe constipation and difficulty with his hernia. On examination a hard tumor was found occupying the lower abdomen and extending from the symphysis pubis almost to the umbilicus. A hard catheter on introduction to the bladder grated on a surface that was believed to be a calculus, and withdrew one and a half ounces of clear urine that gave no evidence of blood, albumin, or sugar. An X-ray showed a remarkable shadow that was believed to be an osteoma of the pelvis. Operation was delayed in the hope of building up the patient's condition, but with no improvement operation was decided upon as a life-saving measure, and was performed on August 11, 1919, by Dr. Wm. H. Morrison at the Holmesburg Hospital, Philadelphia. The peritoneal cavity was not opened, the bladder wall was found markedly thickened, the stone firmly fixed in the pelvis. The patient died thirty-six hours after operation. The calculus weighed on removal and in its moist state exactly 64 ounces, or four pounds: in its largest circumference it measures 48 cm. and in its lesser 40 cm., the deep impression with the ebonized surface is the imprint of the symphysis, while on the back can be seen the outline of the sacrum and the course of the rectum. The largest human vesical calculus removed as recorded by Gould and Pyle in " Anomalies and Curiosities " is that of Buffen found in 1739, and weighing over six pounds. In modern surgical literature the largest is that reported by Janeway in the *N. Y. Med. Jour.* in 1877 that weighed 51 ounces. Emerson C. Smith in *Surg., Gyn. and Obst.,* November, 1919, reports the successful removal of a stone weighing 38.5 ounces, probably the largest one removed without death. Sir Henry Thompson's " Catalogue of Collection of Calculi," published in 1893, reports numerous specimens of varying size up to 51 ounces. This stone now presented in its dry state weights to-day 56 ounces, and as far as we have been able to discover, is the largest specimen of authentic record.

THE VARICOCELE OPERATION

Dr. Penn G. Skillern read a paper with the above title, for which see page 508.

GUNSHOT INJURIES TO THE CHEST

Dr. George J. Heuer (by invitation) presented a paper, illustrated by lantern slides, with the above title, for which see page 352, September Annals of Surgery.

Dr. John H. Gibbon said that in probably no field of surgery, except-ing joints, has there been greater advance than in the treatment of gun-shot wounds of the chest. Of the very distinct lessons that surgeons can draw from their own war experience and that of others in regard to gunshot wounds, the most striking thing in the presentation of Doctor Heuer's communication is the results obtained in those patients not operated upon, and they constituted a large majority of the whole series. Another notable thing was the comparatively small percentage of cases of those not operated upon which required operation later and in this lies one of the lessons that we must apply in civil practice. There are very few simple pene-trating wounds of the chest in view of this experience that would require immediate operation. One of the most difficult things one had to do was to get away from the habit of operating on these cases and to prevent others from operating upon them. Although we laid down the rule very often, he saw many cases of penetrating wound operated upon that had none of the indications for operation given by Doctor Heuer. To operate and drain means infection and always will. As to the remarks of Doctor Heuer as to what happens to cases in which the skin was not sutured, in a British base hospital in 1917, the speaker saw many cases of joint, abdom-inal and chest wounds that had been apparently properly treated which healed promptly and in which late infection took place under the skin, and required opening up afterwards; in the chest and joints infection of the underlying cavities occurred. The abdominal cavity was not infected because the adherent omentum protected it. Therefore he concluded it would be a good plan to leave the skin open in these cases and later did so in a number of cases at a British casualty clearing station. He is now convinced that was a mistake. Doctor Heuer shows the cases did badly when the skin was closed. In regard to anæsthesia, he thought that all these infective cases, cases that were not operated upon at once and became infected later, should be operated on under local anæsthesia. Practically all the cases Doctor Heuer reports were drained under local anæsthesia. It is similar to operations in empyema which should be always done with local anæsthesia. One of the types of cases most instructive was combined abdominal and thoracic injury. Doctor Heuer reports a number of cases operated upon, although the abdomen was penetrated, in which there was no perforation of the abdominal viscera. They had a number of these cases in his evacuation hospital in which the abdomen had been penetrated and yet in which no operation was done and in which the patient got well. They established the rule there that if we were fairly certain that a hollow viscus had not been perforated and the chest wound did not require operation, no operation should be done. These cases were a great deal better left alone. Hemorrhage of the liver from gunshot wounds takes better care of itself than the surgeon can. When he starts in to stop it he usually makes it worse. These cases require the exercise of the best surgical judgment to determine those which should be operated upon and those which should not.

Dr. GEORGE J. HEUER in answer to the question regarding the expectant treatment of certain combined chest and abdominal injuries, said that in a series of thirty-nine combined chest and abdominal injuries, six cases were treated expectantly. In five of the cases the foreign body was embedded in the liver. Four of the six cases recovered; two died, one of gas gangrene of the leg, the other of lobar pneumonia of the lung opposite to that injured. Regarding the occurrence of hemorrhage and bronchial fistula during the process of sterilization of infected hæmothorax or empyema in fifteen cases of infected hæmothorax under his care abroad, neither hemorrhage nor bronchial fistula occurred following the use of Dakin solution irrigations. In the empyemata of civil life he recalled four cases in which hemorrhage had followed the irrigations. It has been rather interesting to note that hemorrhage in these cases has occurred late, at a time when sterilization of the cavity has almost been accomplished. Bronchial fistula has developed in the course of the irrigations in two cases.

TRANSACTIONS

OF THE

NEW YORK SURGICAL SOCIETY

Stated Meeting held April 27, 1920

The President, Dr. WILLIAM A. DOWNES, in the Chair

FRACTURE OF THE LOWER END OF THE RADIUS, WITH FORWARD DISPLACEMENT OF THE LOWER FRAGMENT

DR. H. H. M. LYLE presented two cases of fracture of the lower end of the radius with forward displacement. He stated that the first patient, a woman, aged fifty-six years, was admitted to the Out-patient Department of St. Luke's Hospital, in the care of Dr. Julius Arnowich, with the diagnosis of Colles' fracture. She gave a history of having fallen on the back of her hand. The X-ray picture showed that instead of a backward displacement there was a forward displacement of the carpal fragment.

The deformity was reduced under gas and immobilized in moulded plaster splints.

Twelve days after the original injury the splints were removed and the wrist strapped with adhesive, bandaged, and supported in a sling. Gentle massage was also instituted. Four days later an X-ray check showed that the carpal fragment had become displaced forward. The fragment was again reduced and splints reapplied. A series of X-ray checks proved the fragments to be in good position. Eighteen days after the second reduction all the splints were removed. The patient had a good anatomical and functional result.

The interesting points in this case were: (1) The rarity of the fracture. Doctor Hitzroth showed a case before this Society and called attention to the extreme rarity of the condition. (2) Absence of crepitus. (3) Difficult of reduction. (4) Tendency to recurrence. (5) Cause, fall on the back of the hand.

The second patient, Doctor Lyle said, showed non-union after sixty-nine days, and gummatous infiltration thirty-three days after reduction. One week before admission to St. Luke's the patient slipped and fell backward. His hands were behind him and he struck on the dorsal aspect of the right hand. He noticed that his wrist was swollen and painful, but there was no loss of function. The patient had been under treatment in the hospital for spinal lues, and for a dilatation of the arch of the aorta.

On examination there was a well-marked prominence on the back of the wrist and opposite it a depression on the palmar side. The styloid of the ulna was unusually prominent. There was a false point of motion, but no crepitus. The X-ray plate showed a fracture of the lower end of the right radius, with displacement forward of the carpal fragment (Fig. 1).

The deformity was reduced under gas and oxygen, a good result being obtained. Three days later the fragment became displaced. It was again reduced and immobilized, this time for thirty days. Thirty-three days after the reduction the patient appeared at the hospital with a swollen and inflamed wrist. He had a temperature of 103° and a pulse of 110, all the local signs pointing to an inflammatory process. An incision was made over the dorsal aspect of the swelling. No pus was obtained, but a thick, red grumous material was encountered. X-ray examination showed that the lower fragment had again become displaced. Energetic antisyphilitic treatment, both local and general, had greatly reduced the inflammatory mass. There was a certain amount of bony growth in the surrounding tissues, but no union.

CONGENITAL DEFECT OF THE SEVENTH CERVICAL VERTEBRA. FIBROUS ANKYLOSIS OF RIGHT SHOULDER-JOINT

DOCTOR LYLE presented a man who was referred to his service at St. Luke's Hospital by the Neurological Department of the Out-patient Department. He had been uncertain in his gait for seven months. He was unable to walk in a straight line. Last October he fell, striking his right shoulder against the curb. The shoulder did not trouble him until a month later; then he began to notice an aching pain in the shoulder if the arm was kept in one position. The pain often awakened him in the night. The onset of pain was accompanied by an increasing limitation of motion. Abduction was limited to 90° and rotation greatly reduced.

The X-ray examination of the neck showed a failure of closure of the posterior arch of the seventh cervical vertebra, the gap being 2.5 cm. wide. The right shoulder showed an atrophy of tissue. No bony lesion was made out. The blood and spinal Wassermann were negative. The luetin was negative.

At operation under gas and ether the adhesions in the shoulder-joint were broken up and free passive motion established. The patient was then returned to bed and the arm suspended from the author's frame in a position of abduction and external rotation. Active motion was begun as soon as the patient recovered from the anæsthetic. The position and active exercises were maintained for forty-eight hours. At the end of this period the patient was allowed up and the treatment of massage and active motions was maintained for two weeks. The patient at the present time has a perfect motion of the shoulder-joint.

The chief interesting point in the case, other than the congenital defect, Doctor Lyle said, was the immediate after-treatment of the stiff and painful shoulder. Early and persistent supervised active movements of the involved joint would give perfect functional results in the majority of suitable cases. Doctor Lyle emphasized the fact that to insure a good functional result the patient must be under the control of the surgeon for the first forty-eight hours.

OSTEITIS FIBROSA OF FIBULA

DOCTOR LYLE presented a third patient who gave a history of having had a dull pain over the outer upper third of the left fibula for six months before coming under observation. For the first four months this pain was irregular. During the last two months it had been severe and constant. The leg had not been swollen. There was no history of trauma, infection, or lues. The Wassermann and luetin tests were negative. Antispecific treatment had no influence on pain or growth.

At the junction of the upper and middle third of the left fibula there was a smooth, hard swelling the size of an almond. There was a localized swelling in the outer border of the fibula 3 cm. in extent, involving the upper third of the bone, apparently representing a persistent lesion of benign nature. X-ray examination of the skeleton was negative.

Operation March 4, 1920, at St. Luke's Hospital. Under ether the swelling was exposed, the periosteum reflected, and a raised area 1.5 by 2 cm., composed of dead bone, was found. This area was chiselled down to the cortex of the fibula and an exploratory incision carried into the medullary cavity. Nothing suggestive of infection being found, the wound was closed.

Pathological report stated that the section showed a very small fragment of bone, and continuous with it smaller isolated areas in which there was a very active bone production with irregular calcification. The osteoblasts were numerous, but not unusually large, and the fibrous tissue intervening between these fragments was only moderately cellular. There was an occasional giant-cell, which somewhat resembled an osteoblast. The bone was not vascular. There was no necrosis, and it did not suggest an active tumor process, and was probably to be considered as an osteitis fibrosa.

The points of interest were: (1) A local progressive growth of bone, probably an early stage of osteitis fibrosa. (2) Pain was a prominent symptom. This was unusual in osteitis fibrosa. (3) The process seemed to be confined to one bone.

END-BEARING STUMP FORTY YEARS AFTER

DOCTOR LYLE presented a patient who had his leg amputated 2½ inches below the knee forty years ago by Stephen Smith. The X-ray of stump showed what excellent condition the bone was in. There was practically no bone atrophy. Despite the shortness of the tibia the patient practically bore all his weight on the end of the stump. The knee-joint having been retained, the jar of weight bearing is materially lessened (Fig. 2).

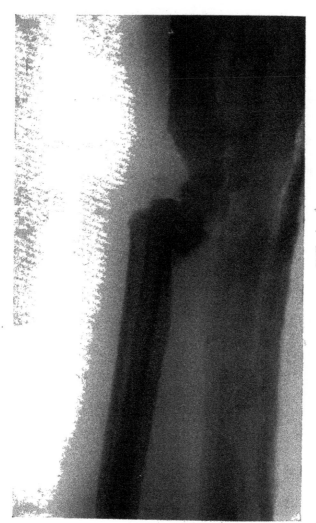

FIG. 1.—Case II.

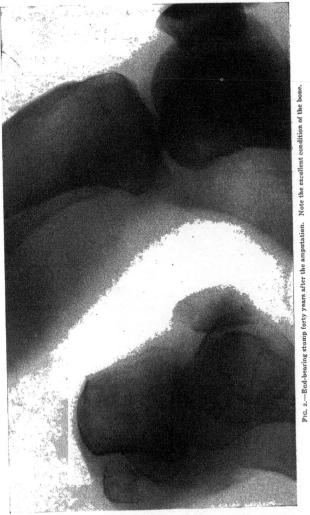

FIG. 2.—End-bearing stump forty years after the amputation. Note the excellent condition of the bone.

Doctor Lyle showed this case for the following reasons: (1) The excellency of the anatomical and functional result. (2) Forty years of use had proven that this end-bearing stump had given a splendid functional result. (3) The value of retaining the knee-joint, even if the stump was short, was clearly shown in this case.

Lately there had been a tendency to decry the end-bearing stump, and also to disregard the great value of maintaining the knee-joint. Hasty conclusions drawn from observing stumps for a short period of time had led to many dogmatic statements which could not be substantiated. The early functional physiologicàl use of a part was the best protection against future trouble. Of all the stumps, an end-bearing one was the best, and no joint yet devised by any artificial maker could take the place of the knee-joint. Lately the author had seen several indirect-bearing stumps that were originally considered perfect; some of these had relapsed into useless painful stumps. As time went on, Doctor Lyle said, more and more of this aftermath of the war would be met.

ACUTE ILEUS

Dr. Ellsworth Eliot, Jr., presented a woman who five years previously had had a hysterectomy. She was well thereafter until three days before admission to the hospital, when she developed the usual symptoms of acute obstruction, namely, severe paroxysmal pain, vomiting, and obstipation. The intestine, however, both by auscultation and palpation, showed signs of peristaltic activity. As a large colonic irrigation failed to produce any result, the peritoneal cavity was opened after excision of the old scar to which the small intestine was found adherent. The acute cause of the obstruction was volvulus of the small intestine, from right to left, the rotation taking place around the adherent intestine as a pivot in such a way as to constrict several feet of intestine beneath the free edge of the mesentery. With the untwisting of the volvulus, after division of adhesions, the obstruction was relieved. Examination then showed a loop three to four feet in length, distended and ecchymotic, but without loss of its glistening appearance or its resiliency. It was returned into the abdominal cavity and the wound closed without drainage. The patient had an interesting post-operative course. For the first five days she had occasional vomiting, especially after fluids by mouth. She received, therefore, fluids chiefly by clysis and the Murphy drip. She also showed a very peculiar mental condition of apathy and slept most of the time, although she could be roused. The urine was much reduced, there being no more than a daily average of 500 c.c. There was a trace of albumin, but no casts. A decided change took place after the sixth day; the patient became clearer in mind and lost her apathy, she retained large amounts of water by mouth, and the appetite improved. The general condition became rapidly normal, and she was discharged on the eighteenth day post-operative.

In this particular instance the degree of constriction, though impairing the circulation of the imprisoned gut, was not sufficient to produce any induration of the intestinal wall, and there was no sharp line of demarcation between the obstructed and non-obstructed intestinal segments. The absence of this more severe form of obstruction accounted for the fact that at no time either before or after operation was there any evidence of shock. It also accounted for the presence of exaggerated peristalsis noted on physical examination prior to operation and demonstrated after operation by the early action of the bowels. It would appear that the occasional vomiting and decided mental apathy in the absence of any post-operative discomfort or distention were due, in part, at least, to the absorption of the toxic contents of the obstructed intestine.

ACUTE ILEUS

Dr. Frederick T. van Beuren presented three patients to emphasize the difference between the severity of ileus with and without interference with the mesenteric circulation, and to illustrate the difference between the effects of immediate drainage and delayed drainage, and the benefit of the former.

The first patient entered the hospital January 1st with a history of vomiting for two weeks and no bowel movement for four days. There was marked distention of the whole abdomen, the colon being clearly outlined. The vomiting was fecal in character. A diagnosis of obstruction of the sigmoid by new growth was made and immediate operation performed. Median incision was made under local novocaine with morphine hypodermically. An annular growth was found in the middle of the sigmoid with enormous distention of the intestines above it. There was no interference of the mesenteric circulation. A puncture was made 1 inch above the constriction and 2000 c.c. of fluid suctioned off. The sigmoid with the new growth was mobilized and brought out through a left colostomy incision near the anterior superior spine. A little nitrous oxide gas was given to secure relaxation and the median wound was closed. A rubber-tube drain was placed in the sigmoid just above the constriction. Fourteen days later the externalized sigmoid with the neoplasm was removed. Later the spur was cut down by clamps and the colostomy wound closed by suture about three weeks ago. The patient made a very smooth recovery, ceased to vomit after the operation, and took water freely by mouth, requiring no hypodermoclysis. She was an excellent example of the beneficial effect of immediate drainage of the obstructed intestinal fluid.

The second case was that of a woman who had had a right inguinal hernia for many years. It began to pain her three days before admission. She had had no bowel movement for two days, and vomiting had commenced twelve hours before admission. It continued frequently and she said the vomitus had a very bad taste. On admission her distention was moderate and her condition fair. The hernia was operated immediately under local anæsthesia, and the intestine found to be in good condition with slight circulatory disturbance, which was relieved by division of a constriction in the sac itself. The intestine was returned and the hernia repaired without removing any intestinal contents. The result was the transformation of a mechanical ileus into a paralytic ileus. The patient's distention was not relieved and she vomited twenty-four hours after her operation. The stomach tube then recovered 60 ounces of foul-smelling fluid. Forty-three ounces were recovered the next day, 22 ounces on the third, 11 ounces on the fourth, and 7 ounces on the fifth day. She retained nothing given by mouth for five days and had no bowel movement until the fifth day after operation, although enemas, colon irrigations, and pituitrin were administered. She required the replacement of water by hypodermoclysis, between 1000 and 2000 c.c. every day, until the vomiting ceased. After one week her recovery was uneventful, but up to that time she illustrated very clearly the bad effects of failing to remove the stagnated intestinal contents.

The third case was that of a man who had had a left inguinal hernia for three or four years. Four days before admission it began to pain him. He had had no bowel movement for twenty-four hours before admission, and he began to vomit twelve hours before admission. Owing to a mistake in believing that the hernia had been reduced, operation was delayed for sixteen hours after his admission. At operation his distension was well marked, and incision under local anæsthesia exposed 4 inches of gangrenous intestine, which showed no signs of recovery after division of the constricting hernial ring. Fourteen inches of intestine was resected, anastomosis being made by Murphy button, and the hernia repaired.

The patient vomited once after operation; otherwise he made an uneventful recovery. His bowels moved on the third day, and the Murphy button was passed on the twelfth. Although he was obstructed a shorter time than the first two patients shown, the mesenteric circulatory obstruction gave him more severe symptoms and caused gangrene.

RELATION BETWEEN INTESTINAL DAMAGE AND DELAYED OPERATION IN ACUTE MECHANICAL ILEUS.

Dr. FREDERICK T. VAN BEUREN read a paper with the above title, which will appear in the November number, ANNALS OF SURGERY.

Dr. ADRIAN V. S. LAMBERT said he had watched this series of experiments with considerable interest. The dogs in which there were few symptoms for a long time were very instructive. The absence of symptoms which were associated with acute ileus was very striking. At the Presbyterian Hospital a series of examinations of the blood and urine of these patients had been carried out. The cases were associated with uræmia, diminution of urine, and lethargic symptoms. There was high blood urea, but the kidneys on microscopic examination showed no particular evidence of kidney insufficiency.

DOCTOR ELIOT said he had no experience with the blood urea content. The paper was most instructive and everybody would emphasize the need of early and prompt exploration in any case of suspected obstruction. Doctor Eliot asked for an opinion as to the time at which aspiration of the contents of the intestine above the point of obstruction should be done. There was a sharp line of demarcation between the cases in which after relief of the obstruction the intestine could be returned intact and those in which either enterostomy or resection was indicated. He was inclined to believe that if either aspiration or enterostomy were indicated enterostomy was the preferable, for it added little to the operative risk and the opening either closed spontaneously (and this usually took place) or it could subsequently be readily closed by operation. In all cases in which the obstructed intestine was unquestionably viable neither aspiration nor enterostomy was necessary, for the amount of toxic absorption would not be sufficient to prevent recovery of the patient, though it might retard it. The experiments on dogs were very instructive, but how close was the relation between symptoms and lesions in dogs and those in human beings, and how advisable it was to draw inferences from experiences in dog surgery to similar conditions in human surgery was debatable. That the peritoneum of the dog was more tolerant than that of the human being could not be gainsaid. Perhaps this increased peritoneal tolerance accounted for the fact that continuity of the intestine after ligation was occasionally, as Dr. van Beuren mentioned, spontaneously restored. In the human being with the same degree of acute constriction at the same distance from the stomach the symptoms would be very much more aggravated and the course much shorter than in dogs, for these are among the worst cases of obstruction. From this standpoint, at least, the clinical subjective and objective symptoms in dogs and in human individuals were unlike.

DR. CHARLES N. DOWD said there were many elements which aided in determining the proper method of dealing with intestinal obstruction. One of these elements was the point of obstruction. The symptoms from obstruction in the upper part of the intestine and those in the lower part of the intestine differed materially. Vomiting and prostration come early in high-lying obstructions, whereas an obstruction might exist for a long time in the sigmoid without giving severe symptoms. Frequently such obstruction might exist for many days. In determining the time of operation and in planning the method of operation this element should be duly considered.

DR. JOHN A. HARTWELL said the lack of water was a most important factor. In some experimental work done by him and Doctor Hoguet one could keep dogs alive no matter where the obstruction occurred, provided they had sufficient water subcutaneously, except in cases where serious damage to the mucosa resulted. With such damage they would die in spite of receiving the water. The degree of this damage seemed to depend upon whether a reverse peristalsis and vomiting was able to prevent overdistention of the bowel, the damage apparently resulting from mechanical stretching. In the case of the man with the strangulated hernia, his stormy convalescence was probably due to the fact that the intestinal mucosa had been damaged, thus producing the toxic elements which result from such damage.

Doctor Hartwell did not believe that the content of the intestine above the obstruction was seriously toxic if absorbed from the normal intestinal mucosa below the site of obstruction, after the latter had been relieved. The continued illness under these circumstances was probably caused more by the toxic absorption from the damaged mucosa than by the intestinal content, which, on the relief of the obstruction, was permitted to pass onward into the normal gut.

DOCTOR VAN BEUREN, in closing the discussion, said that it had been found, in going over a series of ileus cases at the Roosevelt Hospital, that a large number of patients first seen in the later stages of the disease showed marked kidney damage with albumin and hyaline and granular casts in the urine. In response to Doctor Lambert's remark, he said that Dr. G. H. Whipple was the only man he knew of that had done work on the blood nitrogen of these cases.

In reply to Doctor Eliot's remarks on the different reaction of the peritoneum of dogs and of human beings, Doctor van Beuren said that similar results could be observed in both humans and animals but that, in cases of obstruction, perforations were apparently more common in dogs and the intestines on the whole were more easily damaged. He admitted that the difference was very striking between a high and low obstruction, the low obstruction being much less severe; but he said that it was a difference of severity rather than a difference in the quality of the symptoms, and that the replacement of water lost by vomiting sometimes made all the difference between death and recovery in the very sick cases. He repeated that early drainage of intestines was important inasmuch as it was not known how soon the poisonous character of the obstructed contents was absorbed, and he maintained that cases drained early showed a marked improvement.

He explained that there were only three ways of emptying the intestines, by mouth, by anus, or at some point between, and cited his three cases shown that evening as examples of the three types.

BOOK REVIEWS

Urology in Men, Women and Children. By V. C. Pedersen, M.D., Urologist, St. Mark's Hospital, New York City. 8vo, pp. 991. Lea & Febiger, Philadelphia and New York, 1919.

In this work the author has attempted to put before practitioners the clinical and practical side of the subject of urology in its many phases, as is quite evident in the detail of the considerations of the etiology, pathology, symptoms, diagnosis, and treatment of the many subjects. The standard of cure is in each instance briefly stated, so that those not so familiar with the degrees of relief which may be expected from certain forms of treatment may realize that further effort in a given direction will only be a waste of time. This is a phase which we have not noticed in other treatises on this subject.

The general scope of urology is very well covered and in considerations of practice and exact procedure the author is particularly lucid, while the sections dealing with theory are rather more involved and while interesting do not read so easily. However, this is more than offset by the fuller text descriptions of his clinical experiences.

The correlation of the known facts relative to renal functional tests and hæmatological analyses are well expressed and of particular value to those having diagnostic and prognostic opinions to render when there is no specialist to make the interpretations. Not only are normal ranges given, but also pathological proportions and descriptive text of the probable causes of these variations.

The author is inclined to believe that the amplification of physical ' treatment is the next step in the advancement of urological science and practice, and therefore has devoted extended consideration to the subjects of hydrotherapy, heliotherapy, and electrotherapy, and gives much more definite directions regarding the instrument to be used, the type of application, its strength, duration, and frequency, than are usually found when these questions are taken up. A reliable foundation is given the reader upon which he may base such treatment in selected cases.

After-treatment is given careful, thorough, and well-merited prominence, as it is in just such subjects the young practitioner is deficient. If these directions would only be followed there is no doubt that many of the unpleasant sequelæ of urological diseases might be obviated.

Space such as is given to the controversy of the presence of the *micrococcus catarrhalis* in the urethal discharge or to its occasional presence in the normal urethra is useless to devote to this somewhat academic if not impractical question.

Much greater objection must be taken to the inclusion in a tex book of such matter as we find in the second paragraph on page 900, whe in determining the degree of deformity of the renal pelvis the auth counsels the employment of 10 per cent. collargol solution or 50 per cen colloidal silver oxide, or 50 per cent. argyrol, quoting Braasch and Keye as authorities for its use. Both of these men have long since disco tinued the use of these substances as actually dangerous and now u sodium bromide 25 per cent. solution with impunity and obtain equally not more perfectly depicted pelves.

One cannot entirely subscribe to the statement on the same page th a renal pelvis holding 150 c.c. is usually of a non-operative type witho qualifying remarks as to the etiologic factor in each instance—it giv one an entirely wrong impression in so baldly stating the above as a fac

In general, the chapters considering disease of the urethra and bladd are more definite and show greater experience than those on the ureter kidney, and prostate. The impression is that the work is deserving presentation in two volumes, and the matter thus made less crowded an more readable and some chapters markedly amplified.

JAMES T. PILCHER.

THE PRINCIPLES OF ANATOMY AS SEEN IN THE HAND. By FREDERIC WO JONES, D.Sc., M.B., B.S. London. In one 8vo volume of 325 page 2 plates, and 123 text figures. P. Blakiston's Son and Co. Phil delphia, 1920.

In the words of the author, this book owes its inception to two circum stances. " First, it is the result of attempting to teach medical studen such principles of anatomy as may be expected to interest them in the school work and assist them in their after-life as practitioners of med cine. But more immediately its origin is due to the necessity of choosin some circumscribed study in applied anatomy as a subject for a serie of lectures."

The subject matter is well and interestingly presented, and dea with the broad principles of Applied and Morphological Anatomy. N attempt is made to cover nor even consider the surgical anatomy of th hand. There are no suggestions as to the treatment of pathological co ditions, " because we are concerned solely with normal anatomy." Th normal anatomy is in no sense descriptive anatomy such as is found i our anatomical text-books. For instance, in considering the muscle their origin, insertion, nerve and blood supply, and relations are not give It is not the object of the author to describe in detail the course of all th blood-vessels found in the hand. The bones are not considered singl from an anatomical standpoint. The carpal, metacarpal, phalangeal, an digital formulæ, on the other hand, are worked out and presented very tho oughly. The ulnar-carpal articulation is discussed, for instance, as it

533

found in the Macaque monkey. Light is thrown on the puzzling additional toe of the Dorking fowl. Twenty-six pages are devoted to The Flexure Lines, describing the differences found in the various races of man, and comparing them with those found in the different species of the monkeys. Many references to both the older and to the contemporary comparative anatomists abound throughout the text.

The reviewer considers that this book would be a valuable addition to any medical library, not because it would be used daily as a work of reference, but because it presents the subject from a standpoint with which the average medical man is not entirely familiar.

MERRILL N. FOOTE.

REGIONAL ANÆSTHESIA (Victor Pauchet's Technic). By B. SHERWOOD-DUNN, M.D. In one volume, 8vo, 204 pages, with 224 figures in the text. Philadelphia, F. A. Davis Company, 1920.

This work presents a concise and detailed description of regional anæsthesia as practiced by Victor Fauchet, of France, together with a résumé of the writings of Sourdat, Laboure, and Sherwood-Dunn. The text is supplemented by numerous clear-cut, well-drawn plates and figures illustrating its pertinent points.

According to the author, who has worked with Professor Fauchet, any and every conceivable operation, from radical excision of the superior maxilla to partial gastrectomy, may be satisfactorily accomplished under regional anæsthesia. To perfect the nerve blocking in the more difficult operations, it is essential to practice, first, on the skeleton, then on the cadaver, using a hatpin to localize the various foramina in the skull through which the nerves emerge, and to determine the exact positions of the different nerve trunks throughout the body.

For the complicated and more uncommon, as well as for the more common surgical procedures, such as removal of lipomata, sebaceous cysts, hand infections, hernioplasty, appendectomy, etc., explicit directions, full descriptions of the technic, and excellent diagrams are given.

The book is an aid, both to the surgeon and to the practitioner, who may be called upon to use regional anæsthesia. It is a plea to the surgical profession to use, more and more, this method rather than that of general anæsthesia, in all surgical operations.

MERRILL N. FOOTE.

THE AFTER-TREATMENT OF SURGICAL PATIENTS. By WILLARD BARTLETT, A.M., M.D., and Collaborators. In two volumes. St. Louis, C. V. Mosby Company, 1920.

In consideration of the many surgical patients who are made more comfortable by properly directed after-care and the few who are actually lost because of the lack or misuse of it, this work is intended to appeal to those who desire this important subject treated more in detail than is possible in the average system of surgery.

The author truly states in the preface that in the majority of instances the need of surgical after-treatment is in inverse proportion to the accuracy of pre-operative study and the quality of work done in the operating room; a viewpoint with which the reviewer heartily concurs.

Doctor Bartlett and his collaborators have compiled this work in two volumes, the first of which deals with general subjects in surgical after-care and the second with special measures of after-treatment as applied to the various regions and organs of the body. It should be noted in Volume One that thirty-four of the seventy-two chapters have been contributed by Dr. O. F. McKittrick, and these chapters comprise a complete, well-balanced and authoritative review of the more important anæsthetic and operative sequelæ and complications together with their proper management.

This volume begins with a description of the ideal room for the care of patients who have been operated upon and includes chapters on records and charts, the after-effects of anæsthesia, shock, hemorrhage, and the cardiovascular disturbances, acute dilatation of the stomach, post-operative ileus, pulmonary and fat embolism, acidosis, diabetes, nephritis, the various types of bacteriæmia and general infections, the management of operative wounds, the care of the bowels and bladder, dietary measures and artificial feeding, the scope of radium and the X-ray in malignancy, proctolysis, hypodermoclysis, blood transfusion, exercise, massage, hydrotherapy and the reconstruction of the surgical patient.

There is probably no single contribution more important than the chapters which deal with the physical, nutritional, and mental reconstruction of the surgical patient: factors which surgeons have been too prone to disregard, but the necessity and importance of which have been amply proved and exemplified by the experiences of the recent war.

Volume One is concluded with a discussion of post-operative mortality, together with a presentation of some statistical tables representing the combined mortality percentages of a number of operators and hospital clinics in the various types of operations.

In the second volume after-treatment is considered in its relation to the surgical procedures as applied to the various regions of the body. It is here that some phases of operative technic are, of necessity, described and illustrated in order that the reader may have a better understanding of the indications for, and application of, many of the more important post-operative measures.

The volume includes sections on the head and neck, the thorax and abdomen and their contained viscera, urologic and rectal conditions, vaginal and pelvic operations, and the surgery of the extremities, including orthopædics.

The work is complete and compiled with painstaking attention to details; it is well and abundantly illustrated with original drawings and contains many suggestions of value which should prove helpful not only to students, hospital internes, and junior surgeons, but also to the surgeon of experience.

A definite field of usefulness is predicted for this work.

WALTER A. SHERWOOD.

To Contributors and Subscribers:

All contributions for Publication, Books for Review, and Exchanges should be sent to the Editorial Office, 145 Gates Ave., Brooklyn, N. Y.

Remittances for Subscriptions and Advertising and all business communications should be addressed to the

ANNALS of SURGERY
227-231 S. 6th Street
Philadelphia, Penna

ANNALS of SURGERY

VOL. LXXII   NOVEMBER, 1920   No. 5

HYPOPHYSEAL DUCT TUMORS

A REPORT OF THREE CASES AND A FOURTH CASE OF CYST OF RATHKE'S POUCH

By WILLIAM C. DUFFY, M.D.

OF NEW HAVEN, CONN.

ASSISTANT IN SURGICAL PATHOLOGY, DEPARTMENT OF SURGERY, YALE UNIVERSITY

Introduction.—In view of the very small number of squamous epithelial tumors of the hypophyseal region which have been reported in this country and their many points of interest, it seems permissible to call further attention to this group and to report in some detail a pathological study which has been made of three cases occurring in the surgical service of Professor Halsted of the Johns Hopkins Hospital.

The relative rarity of squamous epithelial tumors among hypophyseal neoplasms is suggested by the small number reported in the American literature. Among twenty-six hypophyseal tumors (certified histologically) reported by Cushing (1912), only two belong in this group. Jackson, in 1916, reported a case and referred only to the two of Cushing and another published by Dean Lewis (1910). To these should be added those of Farnell (1911) and Warthin (1916), as well as the three to be presented in the following paper. Erdheim (1904) observed at time of autopsy only two of these tumors, but pathologically resurrected five others which had been salvaged and preserved in the University of Vienna Museum between the years 1828 and 1883. In addition to these he collected about twenty cases from the literature which he decided belonged in the same group. Jackson (1916) tabulated thirty-eight examples, collected from the literature, to which I may add a full dozen, histologically certified tumors, reports of which I have found.

Classification.—Included among the squamous cell tumors of the hypophysis and infundibulum are tumors which range in structure from simple squamous epithelial-lined cysts to tumors which are often reported as teratomas, but which are probably " autochthonous teratoids developed by metaplasia from hypophyseal duct remnants " (Ewing). Case III of the present series and the case of D'Orsay Hecht (1909) appear to be examples of such " teratoids." Tridermal teratomas are rare, but instances have been reported by Wegelin, Rippmann (1865), and Kon. The entire group of squamous epithelial cell derived tumors belong to the general group of *heterogenous* hypophyseal tumors, the so-called *heterotopic* group of Bonin, meaning that such tumors are composed of tissue foreign to the essential structure of the adult gland.

Embryology.—Although the embryology of this region is so well and generally known, it may help the reader to review briefly the salient features that have a bearing in the etiology of this special group of tumors.

Although Rathke first asserted in 1838 that the hypophysis developed from a diverticulum of the pharynx, it was not until 1875 that the essential points in its development were settled and clearly presented. At this time Goette and Mihalkovics demonstrated independently the ectodermal origin of the anterior lobe of the hypophysis. Milhalkovics' work, which was done on canine material, has received most attention and his findings confirmed by the work of subsequent observers.

Meantime, in 1860, Luschka had noted the presence of squamous epithelium in the *normal* hypophysis, but the pathological significance of this finding remained unappreciated for many years. Prior to Luschka squamous epithelial lined cysts had been observed (Zenker in 1857), and subsequently a number of such cases were put on record.

Erdheim (1903) in his studies on the structure of the normal thyroid had been interested in the occurrence of epithelial rests of the thyroglossal duct. Subsequently his observation of numerous squamous epithelial groups in a single "normal" hypophysis stimulated him to undertake a study of *serial sections* of thirteen adult normal hypophyses, in ten of which squamous epithelial cell rests were found (1904). This squamous epithelium occurred as small cell groups (in which intercellular bridges were demonstrable) located usually along the anterior surface of the infundibulum (the *processus lingualis* of the *pars intermedia* of Herring, 190?) or beneath the capsule of the upper surface of the anterior lobe. Turning to Mihalkovics' work, Erdheim found it already demonstrated that the rotation forward and upward of the developing anterior lobe carried the area of attachment of the hypophyseal duct to precisely the location of the *reliquii* (inclusions) of squamous epithelium found in a large majority (about 77 per cent.) of normal hypophyses.

Jackson's (1916) quotation to the effect that Erdheim "on careful examination of thirteen suitable fœtuses discovered that ten of them, or over 80 per cent, showed remains of buccal epithelium in the infundibular region," appears to be somewhat in error, since the thirteen hypophyses examined microscopically were those of adults. Erdheim discarded seven fœtal and new-born hypophyses because of the difficulty of recognizing squamous epithelial cell groups in the presence of incompletely differentiated hypophyseal parenchyma. This detail of Erdheim's work was correctly quoted by Dean Lewis (1910).

An anatomical point of importance in the consideration of the tumor producing potentialities of this region lies in the fact that the hypophyseal vesicle or sac, a later stage of Rathke's pouch, is composed of stratified cylindrical epithelium. Most of this tissue develops into the anterior lobe, but a single layer of cylindrical epithelium persists in the adult gland as the "*cleft*" ("Rathke's" cleft), separating the anterior and posterior lobes. On the contrary, the hypophyseal *duct* is composed of modified squamous epithelium which gradually passes over into the cubical epithelium of the buccal canal (Salzer, 1898). Furthermore, while the vesicle progresses, the duct retrogresses entirely, save for its cellular *reliquii*.

The following extract is of Erdheim's summary of Mihalkovics' illustrated explanation of the development of the hypophysis and the rôle of the hypophyseal duct.

In Fig. 1, " I," we see the *anlage* of the central nervous system, the fore (*v*), mid (*m*), and hind (*h*) brain vesicles, respectively. Between the ectodermal primary buccal cavity (*n*) and the entodermal foregut (*f*), stretches still the oral plate (pharyngeal membrane or "*rachenhaut*"). High above and at the same time behind, one finds a small depression (*h*) in the oral cavity, the "hypophysis angle" ("ch" in this and subsequent stages = chorda dorsalis). In Fig. 1, " II,"

the oral plate is ruptured and the pituitary anlage (*h*) deepened to a small cavity. At (*i*) the infundibulum has already b e g u n to deepen. A further step (Fig. 1, " III,") shows that the small cavity has become the deep pituitary pouch ("*h*" = Rathke's pouch), "*which is lined by stratified cylindrical epithelium.*"

In "IV" the pocket in its upper part has developed into the thick-walled "*pituitary sac*" (*h*), composed of stratified cylindrical epithelium, while the under part has developed the small pituitary or hypophyseal duct (*g*) with a very narrow lumen (not shown in the figure) *lined by low cubical epithelium*. The differentiation of the hypophysis anlage into two totally different (*in both form and cell structure*) parts is an important fact. Whereas the pituitary sac develops into the anterior hypophyseal lobe, the pituitary duct disappears.

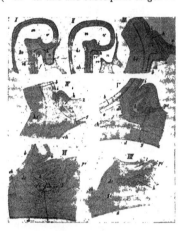

FIG. 1.—Illustrates the developmental cause of the suprasellar and upper sellar location of hypophyseal duct squamous-cell tumors. After the closure of Rathke's pouch (III. *h*) its connection (IV. *g*) with the pharynx is known as the hypophyseal duct. This is lined with modified squamous epithelium continuous with the pharyngeal mucosa. During the further development of the hypophysis the point of insertion of the hypophyseal duct (IV. *g*) is carried forward and upward (VII. *x*) by the rotation of the embryonic anterior lobe. This developmental fact correlates with the frequent occurrence in the mature gland of squamous epithelial inclusions along the infundibulum (in the processus lingualis of the pars intermedia), or near by beneath the capsule of the anterior lobe. The location of these inclusions corresponds with that of many squamous epithelial derived tumors. (After Mihalkovics.)

Already at this stage (Fig. 1, " IV ") one sees that the pituitary sac is slightly curved. The infundibulum (*i*) has grown and lies on the posterior surface of the pituitary vesicle. In a further stage (Fig. 1, " V ") one sees that the angular kinking of the pituitary sac ("*H*") has progressed and that the epithelial wall of the lower part of the sac at the place where it is connected with the canal (*g*) has developed a solid process (*p₁*) anteriorly and above. The lumen of the sac sends forward into the solid process a small cavity. The hypophyseal duct ("*g*") has lost its lumen and remains as a thin solid strand of epithelium which connects

WILLIAM C. DUFFY

the solid process of the primitive anterior lobe ("p_1") with the pharynx and runs between both sphenoidal bone cartilages (Fig. 1, "V").

In the further development of the glandular part of the hypophysis the solid process plays the cardinal rôle. In Fig. 1, "VI," one sees the *process* (p_1) already changed into a large number of solid glandular columns and that the lumen ("h") has come to lie somewhat eccentrically behind. Both sphenoid cartilages are united and the pituitary duct is no longer seen. The infundibulum (i) is still canalized. In the most mature stage (Fig. 1, "VII"), illustrated by Mihalkovics, one sees that the posterior part of the infundibulum ("i") has become the posterior lobe and now lies upon the anterior lobe ("h"). The lumen of the hypophyseal vesicle (about to become the "cleft" between the two lobes) is still present and still sends a small diverticulum into the glandular tissue. The glandular process (p_1) has been pushed forward and upward and lies below and along the anterior surface of the infundibulum. *The region of insertion of the erstwhile hypophyseal duct (Fig. 1, "VII, X") is carried upward, by the further rotation of the developing gland, to the anterior infundibular and upper pars anterior surfaces.*

It is in this locality that squamous epithelial cell groups have been commonly found and where the group of squamous epithelial neoplasms under consideration appear to have taken origin: either from the anterior surface of the infundibulum (Cushing, page 289), or from beneath the capsule of the anterior lobe (*cf.* Case I of the writer, in which the pars anterior was flattened cup-like below by a squamous epithelial cyst situated partly within and partly above the sella).

The Accessory Hypophyses.—A number of interesting researches have been concerned with the questions of patency of the craniopharyngeal canal and the finding of rests of the hypophyseal duct. Among the lower vertebrates it is well known (Jordan, D. S., 1896) that in *cyclostomata* the external pituitary opening remains patent throughout life. In *myxine* the pituitary opening extends into the pharynx and serves as a respiratory tube.

In human cranii Le Double in 1903 (cited by Arai, 1907) found the canal patent in 9 per cent. of newly born (aged one to three months). Arai found with considerable regularity on histological examination of canine and feline cranii three different bodies situated between the sella and the pharynx which, in addition to squamous epithelium, often contained elements similar to those of the anterior hypophyseal lobe. He designated these "*accessory hypophyses*" as: (1) *Hypophysis accessoria cranii* (later, 1911, independently found by Dandy in canine cranii and called the "*parahypophysis*"); (2) *hypophysis accessoria canalis craniopharyngei,* found in the body of the sphenoid bone; and (3) *hypophysis accessoria pharyngei,* the so-called pharyngeal hypophysis or *rachendachhypophyse* of other writers. Haberfeld (1909) found the pharyngeal hypophysis present in all of fifty-one pharynges examined, of all ages from infancy to senility.

540

It was larger in adults than infants, and often differentiated into tissue resembling anterior hypophyseal lobe. Haberfeld concluded that its function must be similar to that of the chief hypophysis. As an example of tumor formation in one of these accessory hypophyses may be mentioned the acidophile adenomatous tumor of Erdheim (1909) which in a case of acromegaly was found within the body of the sphenoid.

E. Christeller (1914), investigating the pharyngeal hypophysis in the human, made serial sections in thirty-one cases, and found the organ present in every case. In three cases in which functional disturbance of the chief hypophysis was diagnosed clinically he looked for possible histological changes in the pharyngeal organ. In one case of typical acromegaly associated with an acidophile adenoma of the chief hypophysis, the pharyngeal hypophysis existed only as groups of squamous epithelium. In the second case, one of *dystrophia adiposo-genitalis* associated with a basophile adenoma, only squamous epithelium was present in the pharyngeal accessory gland, but in the third case, similar to the case just cited, the "*rachendachhypophyse*" was substantially enlarged and composed largely of cells resembling eosinophile anterior lobe hypophyseal elements.

It seems evident that the entire region of the hypophysis from the pharynx to the *processus lingualis* of the *pars intermedia* is peculiarly rich in vestigial reliquii which may be considered as possessing both functional and tumor-producing possibilities. A study of four examples of cystic tumors arising in the region of the upper extremity of this chain of embryonic reliquii will be presented in the following paper.

CASE I.—*Intracystic squamous epithelial papilloma arising from a rest of the hypophyseal duct in the anterior lobe. Enlargement of sella and inclusion of hypophysis in wall of cyst. Headaches and visual disturbances (temporal hemianopsia and amaurosis). Treated for syphilis (positive Wassermann). Operation: evacuation of cyst (lateral intracranial approach); injury to internal carotid, ligation in neck. Exitus twelve days after operation. Autopsy.*

Abstract of J. H. H. Surgical History No. 38232. A white man, thirty-five years old, was transferred October 30, 1915, from the *medical* to the *surgical* service of Johns Hopkins Hospital with the persistent complaint of "blindness and headache." The family history was negative, and aside from typhoid fever at nineteen years of age, measles, mumps, and pertussis as a child, the only fact of importance in his past history was the occurrence of a Neisserian infection several years before. However, he denied all primary and secondary luetic stigmata. Beginning in July, 1914, he suffered with left frontal headaches, not severe enough to interfere with his work. Later the headaches became bi-parietal and more recently general in distribution, and usually started about 10 A.M. each day and ceased toward bedtime.

In November, 1914, visual disturbances began. He noticed distant vision was not as good in the left as in the right eye. The left eye gradually failed. In the spring of 1915 Wassermann tests on the serum and spinal fluid were made at another clinic, and while there he received several injections of salvarsan. Several inunction treatments were given. This therapy is associated by the patient with a progression of visual disability. The right eye began to suffer about two months before admission (August, 1915) and rapidly failed, so that he can barely see to get about. There is only light perception in the left eye. He is practically totally blind.

He has lost forty pounds in the last year, now weighing 152 as compared with 192 a year ago. Thus at the onset of his illness he was fat and is said to have been a red-faced, healthy looking man. There has been no change in the skeletal structures. According to his statement his libido sexualis was perhaps a little below normal before the present illness. Since the latter there has been no *libido sexualis.*

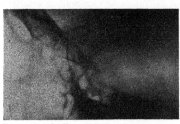

FIG. 2.—Case I. X-ray of base of skull showing destruction of clinoids, enlargement of sella and slight encroachment upon sphenoid space. This tumor, as subsequent pictures will indicate, originated in the upper surface of the anterior lobe below the dural diaphragma sellæ. Hence the enlargement of the sella in contrast to the two other cases in which the origin was suprasellar (cf. Figs. 10 and 13).

No nausea or vomiting. *Examination.* — A well-developed man, rather pale.

Eyes: wide pupils, sluggish pupillary reaction to light on right; no reaction on left.

Fundi: showed marked pallor of temporal margins with swelling of nasal margins and fullness of vessels. Changes more in left fundus.

Visual acuity: left *nil;* right 6/200.

C o u r s e in hospital: While on the medical service a positive Wassermann test was present in the spinal fluid together with a luetic zone reaction in the colloidal gold test. He received salvarsanized serum intraspinously on two occasions.

X-ray report: October 15th (Dr. F. H. Baetjer). " Sella flattened out with destruction of posterior clinoids suggesting tumor " (Fig. 1).

. Visual fields: Temporal hemianopsia on right, no vision in left eye.

Carbohydrate tolerance tests: No sugar in two specimens six and twenty-four hours after taking 100 grams of glucose.

Urine showed slight albumin with occasional granular casts, but repeated examinations were negative.

Operation.—October 30, 1915. Dr. G. J. Heuer. *Evacuation of hypophyseal cyst.* Usual lateral (left) approach as developed by the operator.

Findings: Unusually large collections of fluid in subarachnoid space, possibly related to recent salvarsanized serum injections.

The left optic nerve was stretched and dislocated outward. The tumor bulged forward between the two nerves. It was bluish and apparently cystic. On puncture with a needle probably an ounce of brownish fluid escaped.

On attempting dissection of the cyst wall a hemorrhage occurred which could be controlled only by pressure and with the greatest difficulty. The left internal carotid artery evidently was seriously injured. This vessel was ligated in the neck just above the bifurcation of the common carotid. The cranial wound was then closed after placing rubber tissue drains down to the dura through the decompression opening.

Post-operative Course.—The patient apparently did very well until twelve days after operation, when there was sudden collapse, respirations ceasing. He was kept alive by artificial respiration for several hours, during which time there occurred a series of convulsions involving the left side particularly. Exitus.

The autopsy was made by Dr. A. B. Dayton, to whom I am indebted for the pathological material and use of the protocol.

Autopsy (No. 4508. November 12, 1915.—*Anatomical Diagnosis.*—" Squamous epithelial papillomatous cyst developing from a rest of Rathke's pouch." Operations: (1) lateral craniotomy and evacuation of cyst in hypophyseal region, (2) ligation of left internal carotid artery.

Bronchopneumonia. Pulmonary infarcts. Chronic appendicitis. Phleboliths of spleen and liver.

Body.—Is that of a white man 176 cm. (5 ft. 10 in.) in length. The skin is of smooth texture and the pubic hair is rather scanty, but has the normal masculine arrangement. It is also scanty on the face and in the axillæ. The pupils are regular, the left measuring 4 mm. and the right 5 mm. The scleræ are clear. The nose and ears present nothing of note. The teeth are in good condition. The genitalia are apparently normal. Just below the left angle of the jaw there is a horizontal scar of a recent operation about 4 cm. in length. On the scalp there is the wound of the usual temporal flap operation, which exposes the left frontal and temporal lobes. This, likewise, has healed *per primam.* There is very little, if any, bulging.

Though the patient is not very obese, there is considerable subcutaneous and retroperitoneal fat. There is no excess of peritoneal fluid and the surfaces are everywhere smooth and glistening. The appendix is about 9 cm. in length. Its serous surface is greatly injected, looks swollen and œdematous, is club-shaped, and at its extremity it has a diameter of about 1 cm. There is one delicate, fibrous adhesion. The other abdominal viscera seem normally disposed. The mesenteric lymph glands are not enlarged.

The left pleural cavity is free of fluid and its surfaces are everywhere smooth and glistening. The right pleural cavity is free of fluid. There are a few delicate fibrinous tags binding the edge of the lower lobe down to the diaphragm. There is considerable fat in the anterior mediastinum, and in picking this to pieces it is thought that there is some thymus tissue present. Roughly estimated, the latter amounts to 15-20 grams. The pericardial sac contains 10 c.c. of lemon-yellow fluid. Its surfaces are everywhere smooth and glistening.

Thyroid: Weight 31 grams, soft in consistency and of normal appearance. Parathyroids: Two were dissected out, of normal size and appearance. Adrenals: Together weigh 10 grams. Normal. Testicles: Are of normal size, consistency and gross appearance on section. Heart: Weighs 350 grams,

WILLIAM C. DUFFY

otherwise normal. Spleen: Weighs 150 grams. Acute splenic tumor. Sub-capsular phleboliths. Pancreas: Weighs 110 grams. Normal. Liver Weighs 1900 grams. Phleboliths similar to those of the spleen.

The left internal carotid after dissection showed a double silk ligature just above its point of origin from the common carotid. An antemortem thrombus was present.

Gall-bladder, neck organs and aorta normal.

Examination of Tumor, Brain, and Skull by the Writer.—After the routine injection of the brain *in situ* with 10 per cent. formalin it was removed with the tumor intact. This left the sella (Fig. 4) practically bare. The latter

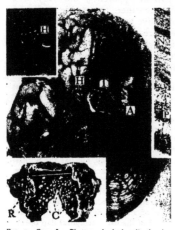

measured 3 x 3 cm. in its antero-posterior and transverse diameters, and was about 1.5 cm. in depth. There was no defect in its floor, which seemed thinned, but the lateral and posterior walls were greatly affected. Poth posterior clinoids were destroyed and the residuum of the dorsum sellæ was only about 1 mm. thick. The left postero-lateral wall showed a gross defect (*A*) corresponding with the prominent pole of the tumor (Fig. 3, *A*) of the same side. The relative uninvolvement of the left anterior clinoid process probably explains why no destruction of the anterior clinoids was apparent in the lateral röntgenogram view of the sella made before operation. The base of the sella showed no defect.

The brain showed only slight flattening of the convolutions over the convexity, but a fairly well-marked compression ring at the base of the cerebellum gave evidence of a moderate degree of herniation through the foramen magnum.

At the time of the autopsy the left hemisphere was quite soft, the ligation of the internal carotid evidently having interfered considerably with its injection with formalin.

Fig. 3.—Case I. Photograph (reduced) showing tumor (*T*) at base of brain (removed after fixation *i i situ* by injection of 10 per cent. formalin). The left lower insert is a retouched print to show the cauliflower-like intracystic papillomatous mass (*C*) on the superior inner surface of the cyst. The lower half of the cyst wall shows a mass (*R*) consisting largely of anterior lobe hypophyseal elements (cf. Figs. 6 and 7). The accessory mass (*H*), enlarged after incision in left upper insert, proved to be a hemorrhage in the right optic nerve. The upper right insert is a low-power photomicrograph of a segment of the nerve bordering the hemorrhage. *P* = large phagocytes laden with blood-derived pigment. *N* = perivascular round-cell infiltration.

The corresponding cerebral vessels on the left, the anterior cerebral, likewise the main cortical vessels and the superior sagittal sinus, were full of postmortem blood clot. The right internal carotid was normal. Both posterior communicating arteries seemed abnormally large, measuring about 1.5 mm. in diameter. The left was considerably stretched by the tumor. The left internal carotid for a short distance was surrounded by tumor and contained a dense clot, which seemed in the gross to be of antemortem character. The optic chiasm was dislocated far to the left and somewhat backward. The right optic nerve appeared rather slender and showed "a small cystic tumor mass" (Fig. 3, *H*) .8 x .7 cm. in diameter at a point about 1.5 cm. from where the nerve left the chiasm this mass seemed to be in the sheath of the nerve. There was no subsequent note concerning this local metastasis

(?) in the protocol. Examination by the writer finds a circumscribed brown to yellow-colored *hemorrhage* in the location of the above-described "tumor mass" (Fig. 3, *H*). The entire small mass in the right optic nerve is excised for microscopic confirmation.

Coronal section of the brain showed some diffuse hemorrhage in the left parietal lobe. Possibly most of this was caused at operation in exposing the hypophyseal region, but ligation of the internal carotid with possible subsequent softening may be a factor in the changes here.

The cranial nerves are normal save for the above referred to optic nerves and slight traumatism to the left olfactory nerve.

The tumor (Fig. 3) was an irregular spherical cystic mass, which measured 3 x 3 x 2.5 cm. in diameter, situated in the hypophyseal region. The hypophysis as a separate organ could not be located. After removal of the brain with cyst attached, the sella (Fig. 4) was left quite bare. Any residuum of the hypophysis must obviously be incorporated in the tumor. Neither was any trace of the infundibulum found at the time of the autopsy. Exami-

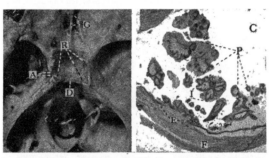

Fig. 4.—Case I. Photograph (reduced) at left of base of skull showing dilated sella. Clinoids (*R*) largely destroyed. Dorsum sellæ (*D*) thinned. Postero-lateral wall shows an erosion (*A*) corresponding with the prominent pole of the tumor (Fig. 3, *A*). *G* = crista galli. The picture at the right is a low power photomicrograph of an upper angle of the collapsed cyst showing the strikingly papillomatous intracystic growth (*P*) composed of squamous epithelium. Lining the fibrous wall (*F*) is a layer of similar epithelium which shows sessile papillomatous masses in places (*E*). The papillomatous mass (*I*) is shown further enlarged in Fig. 5. *C* = cyst cavity.

nation at the present time of the base of the brain discloses no evidence of the infundibulum in the region of the tuber cinereum. Instead this locality appears to have been in close relation with the wall of the tumor mass. The floor of the third ventricle is intact, the ventricle not dilated. The choroid plexus of this and the other ventricles is normal in appearance. The pineal is normal in gross appearance. The region of the tuber cinereum shows some yellow-brown discoloration, apparently hemorrhagic in character.

The tumor then had replaced the infundibulum and largely obliterated the hypophysis, filled the sella and extended above, closely involving the surrounding structures and being in close relation with the floor of the third ventricle.

At the time of removal of the brain the cyst ruptured and "a degenerated portion of the tumor" measuring 2 x 1 x 1 cm. was extruded. It seems probable that this was part of the papillomatous intracystic mass, although it may possibly have been coagulated serum.

Fig. 3 (lower insert) shows the cyst after detachment from the brain. It has been incised and spread open. The wall is seen to vary greatly in thickness, and it seems likely, in view of the microscopic findings, that this is due largely to the presence of hypophyseal tissue in the basal portion (Fig. 3, R) of the tumor wall. On the interior of the wall may be seen numerous small raised papillomatous masses (Fig. 3, C), having a somewhat cauliflower appearance, but the greater part of the cyst contents are lost.

Microscopic Examination.—The Tumor: The cyst wall (Fig. 4, F) varies in thickness from 1 to 6 mm. It is composed largely of fibrous tissue, with considerable hyalinization. Lining the interior of the cyst is a zone of stratified squamous epithelium (Fig. 4, E) with typical intercellular bridges, but no horny layer. In the cyst cavity lie cross sections of papilloma masses (Fig. 4, P) covered with similar epithelium. Of the latter, the more deeply staining layer of basal cells (Fig. 5, B) is sharply differentiated from the connective-tissue framework of the villous-like processes. This central framework (Fig. 5, C) is composed of a fairly loose connective tissue, which carries the nutrient blood-vessels (Fig. 5, S). Where the papillary contents of the cyst have not been lost they loosely fill the cavity (Fig. 4, C) of the cyst. The papillary masses are mostly of a pedunculated character, relatively

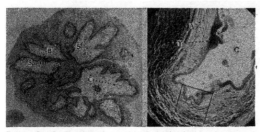

FIG. 5.—Case I. The photomicrograph at the left is a further enlargement of one of the papillomatous processes (Fig. 4, I). The squamous epithelial character of it is distinctly shown. B=basal layer of epithelium. S=blood-vessels which lie in a fibrous stroma (C). At the right is a very low-power photomicrograph of a segment of the cyst wall from which the papillary ingrowth is largely lost. C=cyst cavity. Y=areas of hemorrhage. The squared area is further enlarged in Fig. 6.

few processes of sessile appearance being found (Fig. 4, S). The stalks of the pedunculated processes are rarely to be seen anywhere, so that the absence or presence of these in other parts of the cyst where the contents have disappeared cannot be used as a criterion in determining whether the intracystic papilloma arose equally from all parts of the lining or only in the region where they are still to be seen. It seems probable that the cyst was equally filled throughout with growth similar to that shown in the photographs, and that the mass extruded at autopsy and subsequently lost probably consisted largely of these papillary masses. In the latter the basal layer of cells is everywhere intact. No invasion of the underlying stroma or other malignant criteria are present. The squamous epithelial lining of the cyst in these large sections occasionally sends short processes into the wall, but nowhere do these have a malignant appearance.

The wall of the cyst is well preserved in several microscopic sections. Two blocks for study were taken through nearly the whole circumference of the cyst near the mid-line, and a third, of similar extent but away from the mid-line, consequently of much smaller dimensions. The fibrous tissue of the wall is mostly of a dense type. Extensive areas of hyalinization are present, some of which possess a marked lamellated appearance. This, together with the sinuous outline of the tissue, causes in certain areas a resemblance to an arteriosclerotic *aortic* wall. Numerous areas of hemorrhage (Fig. 5, *Y*; Fig. 6, *H*) are present throughout the wall. Some of these are large and show no attempt at organization. Other smaller ones show fibroblasts extending throughout the clot, while a rich granulation tissue may encompass the periphery of such areas.

Anterior lobe hypophyseal tissue is present in the wall of the cyst (Fig. 6, *A*). In one section strands of anterior-lobe epithelium extend for a distance of about 3.5 cm. Much of this consists of only a few strands of cells in thickness, but over an extent of about 1 cm. there is a thickness of about 12 to 15 strands or cords of anterior-lobe cells, and for a similar extent tissue of about half this thickness is present. These cells are well preserved (Fig. 7, *A*). showing perfectly differentiated eosinophile, basophile and chromophobe cells (the last few in number). In a certain area a recent hemorrhage has widely separated the strands of anterior-lobe tissue, and here the cytoplasm of such cells tends to stain less strongly, although the nuclei still take the stain well and the great majority of cells are apparently still viable. The granules of the eosinophiles are sharply stained (hæmatoxylin and eosin stained celloidin and paraffin preparations). In addition to strands of cells there are fairly large areas, 1 mm. or more in diameter, in which the flattening of the cell groups is not so marked, and they are arranged in characteristic acini. The intimate blood supply of the strands. columns, and acini of anterior-lobe elements is quite well preserved

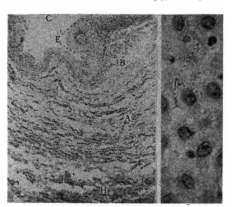

FIG. 6.—Case I. At the left is shown a medium-power enlargement of the squared area in Fig. 5. Strands of anterior lobe hypophyseal cells (*A*) lie in the fibrous wall. *E* - sessile projection from squamous epithelial lining of cyst. *B* =basal layer. *C* =cyst cavity. *H* =zone of hemorrhage. At the right is a photomicrograph (oil immersion magnification) showing the presence of intracellular bridges (*I*) in the squamous epithelium of the tumor.

in spite of the fact that such tissue often lies in a fairly dense fibrous wall. Capillaries in most instances lie adjacent to strands or tubules, and in some cases the anterior-lobe cells delicately line these endothelial spaces. Most of the acinar areas are composed of well-stained cells, but areas are found where such is not the case. One of the latter areas is somewhat detached from the external surface of the cyst wall, and its cells are beginning to undergo necrosis. There is considerable hemorrhage in this area, and the base of it shows a mass of granulation tissue growing into it from the wall of the cyst. None of the cells of this degenerating mass appear to be of the eosinophilic type.

In the large microscopic preparation, which comprises practically the whole median circumference of the cyst wall. is found a large area of necrosis (cf. Fig. 3, *R*). about 3 x 4 mm. in diameter. This is composed of anterior-lobe elements, most of which show a definite acinar arrangement. It occupies almost the whole thickness of the cyst wall at this point, and throughout most of its circumference is surrounded by a vascular granulation tissue. In the latter zone are found isolated anterior-lobe elements, as well as entire acini lined by cells or filled with detached cells, which are in various stages of degeneration (Fig. 7, N, R). Many of these cells show the characteristic granulation of eosinophilic anterior-lobe elements. Indeed such granulation is seen in some cells in the necrotic mass whose nuclei do not take the stain.

Throughout the latter area, but more especially at the periphery, one sees numbers of colloid-like accumulations, some of which are quite homogeneous and refractile, others of which still show a fine granulation. Some of these are several times the size of a large eosinophilic anterior-lobe cell. A few of these hyaline accumulations lie in the meshes of the wall adjacent to the cyst cavity, which at this place has lost (desquamation or trauma?) its epithelial lining. The smaller of these masses resemble the *hyaline*

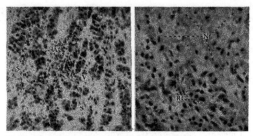

FIG. 7.—Case I. At the left is a photomicrograph showing an area in the wall of the cyst where clumps of anterior lobe hypophyseal elements (A) are thickly scattered through the stroma (S) of the cyst wall. The photomicrograph at the right is of a section taken through the area R of Fig. 3, where a large amount of anterior lobe tissue was present with very little stroma. Much of the area had undergone necrosis and the photomicrograph is taken through the edge of the necrotic tissue. At N are necrotic cells, while at R are cells the cytoplasm of which stains faintly but the nuclei take the stain well

bodies of the pars nervosa described by Herring. (Concerning the latter, it it not clear whether they are the secretion product of epithelial cells of the *pars intermedia*, which may have penetrated the pars nervosa, or whether they may result from the degeneration of single epithelial cells. The occurrence of numbers of similar bodies in close relation to a mass of anterior-lobe tissue undergoing extensive necrosis would seem to favor the view that such material may possibly result from a degeneration of cells in bulk, rather than an accumulated secretion of one or more cells. However, the analogy is not complete, since the hyaline bodies of Herring arise presumably from the intermedia epithelium, whereas the tissue here described is apparently solely anterior lobe.) As to the causation of this necrosis, it would seem most likely due to interference with the blood supply, possibly owing to the operative procedures. It is evidently a comparatively recent affair.

There is evidence also of the presence of *pars intermedia* elements in the wall of the cyst. This consists of a number of epithelial glands lined by cubical or columnar epithelium, and either flattened out, appearing as tubules, or else larger and ovoid in outline. In the latter case they may contain material of a colloid-like appearance, taking the pink stain well. Usually they have been flattened out by the pressure of the cyst, and their long axes lie parallel with the circumference of the cyst wall. There is no apparent evidence of these glands discharging any secretion into the cyst cavity.

No posterior-lobe tissue could be identified, although there was almost similar appearing connective tissue in places.

Polymorphonuclear leucocytes are scattered through the cyst wall, and in fewer numbers occur throughout the structure of the papillomatous processes, both through the stroma and in the epithelial covering.

Numbers of foreign body giant cells lie in the wall of the cyst, usually associated with the absorption of blood pigment, but in places found at the periphery of clear spaces (Fig. 5, A), from which cholesterin crystals have been dissolved out by the process of fixation of the tissue.

Section through the *mass* (Fig. 3, H) in the *right optic nerve* shows a large (1 cm.) recent hæmatoma. This has expanded the nerve to a thin shell. In the wall one sees great numbers of large mononuclear phagocytes (Fig. 3, P), similar to the "compound granular cells," loaded with black hæmatogenous pigment. Occasional small hemorrhages and œdematous areas have further disturbed the remaining nerve substance. A striking feature is the presence of focal areas (Fig. 3, N) of small mononuclears. These areas are usually perivascular in arrangement and are largest in the sheath of the nerve, extending thence inward along the vascular spaces. It is barely possible that these may be unrelated to the hæmatoma, and of a more chronic significance, related to the syphilitic infection (*vide infra*). The blood-cells composing the hemorrhage are well preserved and show no organization. The bright yellow color which was seen in the gross has persisted and appears as a light yellow to brown, finely granular pigment, comparable to bile pigment under similar (fixation and staining) conditions.

Section through the base of the brain and the aqueduct of Sylvius shows two small (¼ to ½ mm.) isolated hemorrhages. Compound granular cells are very numerous. The aqueduct is patent.

The *pineal* shows no microscopic abnormality.

Thyroid.—Acini normal or perhaps below normal in size. Colloid fills practically all of the vesicles, a few of which are distended, with flattened epithelial lining. A small amount of fetal tissue is present here and there between the acini, but no typical adenoma formation is present; no encapsulation of these small areas. The epithelial lining throughout is of low cuboidal, nearly flat, or more rarely low columnar type. The latter, however, is of such small amount in comparison with the flat type as to be practically within normal limits. The gland appears as a whole to be of normal structure.

Parathyroid.—About 2.5 x 1.5 mm. in size, lying near the above described thyroid section in the loose extracapsular fibrous tissue. Essentially of normal appearance; composed of closely packed columns of cells, with here and there a definite acinar arrangement, occasionally with a small lumen. A small bit of colloid-appearing substance was present in one acinus. The cells show what seems to be a neutrophilic staining affinity, with here and there a slight pink variation.

Testicle.—Despite the recorded (protocol) gross normality, the microscopic examination finds a serious alteration of the normal structure (Fig. 8). Spermatogenesis has practically ceased. The seminiferous tubules, for the most part, are lined by one (Fig. 8, S) or two layers of cells, which, in striking contrast to the normal, exhibit no mitotic figures. None of the cells have advanced beyond the stage of secondary spermatocyte. No spermatozoa or spermatids are found. The tunica propria (Fig. 8, T) is hyalinized and considerably thickened. A few tubules are seen, in which the epithelial cells have lost all resemblance to spermatocytes and look like fibroblasts. The *tunica propria* of such tubules show a marked fibrous increase.

The interstitial tissue (Fig. 8, *M*) shows a moderate increase in connective tissue, both diffusely and in strands and patches, the latter of which are 1 mm. or more in diameter. Much of this connective tissue shows well-formed fibrils and elongated flattened nuclei, evidently a connective tissue of not very recent formation. However, most of it is rather loosely meshed, apparently due to œdema. Occasional small areas of round-cell infiltration were found. No miliary gummata were found.

Dr. R. B. Mills, who has recently (1919) made a special study of the testicle, was kind enough to examine sections from this testicle. In his opinion, the cessation of spermatogenesis is complete; practically only Sertoli (supporting) cells remain in the tubules. The interstitial cells of Leydig he found to be present in normal numbers. As to the causation of the changes he gave no opinion.

Thymus.—Isolated, irregular branching clumps and strands of lymphoid

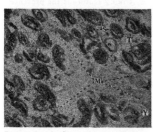

tissue lie scattered through a fatty framework. The Hassell's corpuscles show no proliferative changes, but, on the contrary, a number of them are hyalinized with non-staining nuclei. Some of these corpuscles apparently are being phagocytosed by large foreign-body giant-cells. The capsule of the gland is 1 mm. thick and composed of hyalinized fibrous tissue. Fairly large vessels lie here and there throughout the fatty meshwork, but the vascularization of the lymphoid areas is not striking. Regressive changes in the gland seem predominant.

Fig. 8.—Case I. Photomicrograph (low magnification) of the testicle. Spermatogenesis has ceased. The single layer of cells (*S*) present in most of the tubules is composed of Sertoli cells. The basement membrane (*T*) is thickened and occasional tubules devoid of epithelium (*Y*) are found. At *M* is a patch of loose fibrous tissue. A slight increase in stroma is present elsewhere.

Pancreas.—The islands are numerous and showed no hyalinization. Elsewhere no fibrosis was made out. A special study was not made of the gland, but in the hæmatoxylin and eosin stained preparations nothing abnormal was found.

Appendix.—Shows a marked grade of chronic appendicitis. In places the wall is 4 mm. thick. The mucosa is lost in some places, whereas in others fibrous changes have occurred. The thick fibrous wall is infiltrated with small mononuclears and eosinophilic polymorphonuclears.

Adrenals.—Show no striking changes.

Liver and Spleen.—Normal save for a few uncalcified phleboliths.

Lung.—Purulent bronchitis, section from upper lobe; also a small fibrous-encapsulated calcified area.

The lower lobe—the sections show an infarct, small areas of bronchopneumonia, and large areas of hemorrhagic broncho-pneumonia.

Summary of Case I.—A previously healthy white man, thirty-five years old, began rather abruptly to suffer with severe headaches, progressive diminution of vision, and loss of libido sexualis. In different clinics, although he denied luetic infection, positive Wassermann tests resulted in anti-luetic therapy. Later the diagnosis of tumor in the hypophyseal region was made by means of radiography. The visual fields showed a bitemporal hemianopsia. The exploratory craniotomy was complicated by unusual hemorrhage; however, the cyst presenting above the sella and between the optic nerves was evacuated, and the patient recovered from the immediate effects of the operation, but died twelve days later with symptoms indicating failure of the medullary centres (about one and one-half years after the onset of symptoms).

At the autopsy of this slightly obese man a squamous epithelial intracystic papilloma was found presenting above the enlarged sella with remains of the anterior hypophyseal lobe and traces of pars intermedia preserved in the basal sector of the cyst wall. Death apparently was caused by increased intracranial pressure (cerebral œdema). Testes showed histologically a marked atrophy. Thymus was retrogressive. Other glands of internal secretion showed no definite changes. Changes of subsidiary interest were found in the lung (broncho-pneumonia, pulmonary infarcts) and appendix. *Diagnosis: benign squamous epithelial intracystic papilloma arising from a rest of the hypophyseal duct in the upper surface of the anterior lobe.*

CASE II.—*Cystic suprasellar tumor with adamantinoma characters developing from an infundibular squamous epithelial rest of the hypophyseal duct in a child aged eleven years. Headaches for five years. Excrescence of sex features since age of nine, no marked adiposity. Progressive failure of vision for one year. Projectile vomiting for eight months. Other general pressure symptoms. Operation: Evacuation of cyst and partial removal of cyst wall (lateral operation). Death.*

Abstract of J. H. H. Surgical History No. 42460. A small white girl, eleven years old, was admitted April 20, 1917, to the Surgical Service of the Johns Hopkins Hospital, *complaining* of "headaches," impairment of vision, and difficulty in walking. For at least five or six years, according to the parents, the child has complained of headaches, general in character, but perhaps worse in front than behind. These have gradually increased in frequency until the past three or four weeks, since when they have been almost constant. Within twelve months the vision of both eyes has gradually but progressively failed. This has become so marked that she cannot recognize faces or objects at table. There has been occasional abrupt and forcible vomiting for eight months. During the last six weeks there has been considerable weakness, finally so much that she cannot stand. Gradual impairment of hearing in last year, during which time she has complained of noises in the head. The child was born after a normal labor. The mother is somewhat robust and masculine looking.

Developmental Phenomena.—Following tonsillectomy two years ago for chronic tonsillitis, with "some arthritis," there occurred marked somatic changes. She increased very rapidly in weight. The hair of the head grew much longer and richer. A moderate growth of pubic hair has appeared (see Fig. 9), but the menses are

551

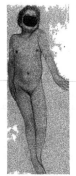

FIG. 9.—Case II. Age eleven years. Growth of pubic hair. Apparent beginning development of breasts. No obesity.

still absent. No distinct increased appetite for sweets, but there is a definite history of polyuria (recent incontinence).

The child was brought in chiefly because of increase in headaches and stupor and visual impairment. Slight increase in size of head.

Examination.—A docile, quiet, rather torpid child. Rich, dark curly hair, well-developed mammary tissue with slight pigmentation of the nipples. The bony pelvis has begun to assume some of the proportions of maturity. Bowing of the femoræ is present.

Hirsuties: Well-developed pubic and axillary hair.

Fingers long and tapering, nails curve and are well kept. No prognathism; teeth normal with no abnormal spacing.

Skin: Somewhat dry and harsh.

General physical aside from above facts is negative.

Visual fields could not be taken.

Grip equal on the two sides. Bilateral optic atrophy with choked disk and proliferative changes. Clonus of legs and equivocal Oppenheim and Gordon signs.

X-ray Report (Dr. F. H. Baetjer).—Marked separation of the sutures, partial destruction of posterior clinoids with calcification just above it, suggesting a suprasellar tumor (Fig 10).

Operation (April 24, 1917, Dr. G. J. Heuer).—*Evacuation of hypophyseal cyst with extirpation of lining of cyst. Lateral approach.*

Findings.—The cyst appeared over the chiasm which was pushed forward. On puncture of the cyst 30 c.c. of thick, peculiar, reddish-brown fluid was obtained. On microscopic examination it showed numerous red blood-cells, a few cholesterin crystals, and some curious rosette-like clusters of small cells, squamous epithelial, apparently. After aspirating this fluid the lining membrane in which were numerous small calcified patches could be stripped away.

NOTE.—Preliminary ven-

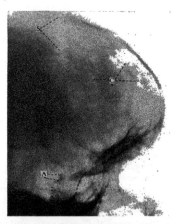

FIG. 10.—Case II. Unretouched print from lateral X-ray plate showing suprasellar calcified mass at *A*. *S*=separation of fronto-parietal sutures. *C*=frontal convolutional atrophy. The latter changes make an internal hydrocephalus probable, due most likely to blocking of the ventricular foramina or the iter by the upward growth of the tumor. The heavy calcified mass above *A* is too far forward to be pineal.

tricular puncture has shown a high grade of internal hydrocephalus; 120 c.c. of fluid which spurted for a height of six or eight inches.

Died on evening of same day apparently of cerebral œdema. Temperature rose to 105°. Autopsy not obtained.

Microscopic Examination.—The tissue removed at operation (part of the lining membrane of the cyst) consisted of a few small bits of tissue too small to photograph. The tissue was hardened in formalin and embedded in celloidin in three separate blocks.

Examination of sections (Fig. 11) from one block shows a predominance of squamous epithelium, present in masses or processes, or strands which line cystic areas, or constitute the periphery of areas of myxomatous connective tissue (Fig. 11, M).

The individual larger mass (Fig. 11, Y) is made up of stratified epithelium with peripheral convoluted processes which are covered by a sharply staining basal layer of columnar epithelium (Fig. 11, E). The nuclei of the latter are oval or slightly flattened, and occupy the greater part of the cell length save for approximately the distal one-third, which is of clear pale pink cytoplasm. The distal periphery of these cells is capped in certain areas by a thin layer of "membrana propria" (Fig. 11, P), which shows an occasional dark flat (shrunken) nucleus.

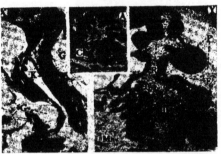

FIG. 11.—Case II. Photomicrographs of tissue removed at operation. The enclosed area in the upper central insert is from the wall of the cyst and presents the adamantinoma picture which is more clearly seen in the enlargement at the right (Y). The mass of stratified epithelium borders a connective tissue area (M). Its peripheral layer of columnar epithelial cells (E) is situated at right angles to the underlying zone of epithelium which shows tendencies to whorl formation (I). The central zone (R) is not strikingly differentiated (cf. Fig. 11, Y and U). Note the delicate elevated membrana propria at P. The insert (X) at the left shows an unusual basal cell epithelioma-like differentiation present in another block of tissue of the same tumor. K = columns of deeply blue staining epithelial cells which lie next to dead masses (G) of keratinized epithelium. This basal cell picture was found in one small area in tissue from this case only.

which lies at right angles to those of the basal layer. Similarly the cells of the latter are at right angles to the subjacent epithelial cells.

The cells beneath the basal layer (the intermediate zone) have larger oval or nearly round, more lightly staining, nuclei, which tend to stain less strongly as the centre of the mass or process is approached. The cell bodies of this intermediate zone are somewhat flattened, with small but varying amounts of cytoplasm. In the central zone intercellular bridges are visible with the high power or else a varying degree of reticulation has taken place. In the latter case the cells consist of almost bare nuclei with thin protoplasmic processes, which stretch out and join similar ones of adjacent cells, often resulting in a "stellate" appearance of such individual cells. In case no reticulation exists, the cytoplasm is larger in amount, giving polygonal outlines to the cells. Such cells show clearly the intercellular spiculæ or bridges.

Concentric-layered epithelial nodules (Fig. 11, I) lie in the convoluted processes of the mass or elsewhere in the intermediate zone below the basal

WILLIAM C. DUFFY

layer of cells. These appear to be the precursors of epithelial pearls, but show no keratinization. Their peripheral layers tend to be flattened, with dark nuclei, the cells centralwards becoming larger, with round, more lightly staining nuclei.

The epithelium which borders the large myxomatous area (Fig. 11, *M*) is a direct continuation of the peripheral basal layer of the above-described processes, but quickly loses its characteristic appearance and comes to consist of a double layer of cells which are flatter and contain much less cytoplasm than the typical basal cells. Also the basal layer of epithelial processes which

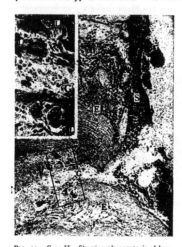

FIG. 12.—Case II. Showing phagocytosis of keratinized epithelium (*E*). *G* = foreign body giant-cells. Those lying within the squared area are shown enlarged in the insert above. Note that the giant cells (*G*) have penetrated the masses of dead epithelium and lie within lacunæ. The phagocyte at the lower right corner of the insert is close applied to the dead tissue, a free space separating it from connective tissue cells whose nuclei take the stain. *S* = viable modified squamous epithelium showing neither typical adamantinoma nor basal cell characters. *n* = clear spaces of dead nuclei.

extend into underlying fibrous or myxomatous tissue tend to lose their typical appearance and become flatter. The myxomatous tissue shows a very loose structure, with fibroblasts and thin-walled capillaries. Besides there is a small amount of adult connective tissue present. Small cystic areas below the main epithelial mass are lined by flat epithelium, which in places extends across open spaces in a single layer of cells.

A single calcified vessel (Fig. 11, *C*) is present in the sections from this block. The wall shows a diffuse infiltration with lime salts. The lumen is filled with a homogeneous material in which the individual elements are fused.

Sections from the other blocks show quite a different variation of the structure above described, with a predominance of degenerative changes. Sections are made up largely of nests and processes of keratinized necrotic stratified epithelium (Fig. 11, *G*, and Fig. 12, *E*), in which a relatively slight but varying amount of calcification has occurred. When present the calcium salts deposit involves alone or more intensely the outer layers of dead epithelium. No ossification is present. A few larger nests or processes composed of viable squamous epithelium, resembling in their essentials those found in the preceding block, are present, but much of the live epithelium is present as attenuated processes (Fig. 11, *K*), which ring the periphery of dead epithelial masses. Only a suggestion is found of the sharply differentiated cylindrical basal cells, and these in no place assume the tall columnar character (Fig. 11, *E*) which is pictured above. Instead, much of the still viable epithelium shows as dense staining solid processes (Fig. 11, *K*) and nests which resemble the familiar picture of a typical basal cell epithelioma of the skin.

Lying in lacunæ' (Fig. 12, *G*) formed in the periphery of the dead tissue, closely rimming the contour of the same, or occasionally lying between the dead masses in the midst of the granulation tissue which fills such spaces, are large, irregularly shaped, foreign-body giant cells (Fig. 12, *G*). In the

554

case of giant cells closely applied to the dead epithelium, either on the surface or lying in lacunæ, a concave surface is usually presented toward the dead tissue, small particles of which may be seen detached from the main mass and about to be enclosed by the encircling cytoplasm of the phagocyte. Other masses of dead epithelium surrounded by giant cells show a disappearance of a dust-like zone of calcification in the immediate vicinity of the phagocytes. This is striking, since calcification in undisturbed necrotic masses is usually more intense at the periphery of the mass. The latter calcified masses are usually surrounded by live epithelium, and no giant cells or fibrous tissue are in proximity to them.

The third and last block contains a small amount of the cyst lining with areas of calcification, large areas of recent hemorrhage, which show, owing to the formalin fixation, much hæmosiderin pigment change. But besides there is a more important small area about 0.4 in diameter composed of obvious hypophyseal anterior lobe element derivatives. These consist of chromophobe and eosinophile cells and a relatively normal amount of connective tissue. Chromophobe cells predominate. In general, traces of the normal structure are to be found in the fairly well-formed acini with delicate fibrous stroma. Marked pressure effects are to be seen in the flattening and convolution of such acini. The latter show no colloid, but in a few a lumen is present. In considerable areas no acini are to be made out, and the picture is of larger masses of cells, such as may be seen in anterior-lobe adenomata.

Summary of Case II.—A female child eleven years old, who had suffered with headaches of increasing frequency for five years, progressive failure of vision for one year, and occasional projectile vomiting for eight months, was brought to the hospital because of increasing disability and the recent appearance of stupor. Instead of retardation of sexual characters, there was perhaps slight exaggeration of same. Radiography showed a suprasellar nodular shadow, due to calcification; partial destruction of posterior clinoids, and separation of the fronto-parietal sutures suggesting a secondary hydrocephalus. At the exploratory craniotomy a suprasellar cyst containing 30 c.c. of fluid was evacuated and partly extirpated. Histological examination of tissue from the wall of the cyst showed definite squamous epithelial cell derivatives presenting the picture of adamantinoma. Death apparently from cerebral œdema. No autopsy.

(*To be continued.*)

THE TREATMENT OF CRANIOCEREBRAL WOUNDS AND ITS RESULTS *

By Harold Neuhof, M.D.

of New York, N. Y.

Craniocerebral wounds in the recent war have differed greatly from those in previous wars. With the close-range firing of trench warfare and the development of more and more powerful explosive missiles, head wounds became not only more common, but also more serious injuries. The use of the steel helmet saved countless lives, reduced the total number of cranial wounds and rendered less mutilating many of those that have been inflicted.[1] Nevertheless, wounds of the head remained very frequent and very grave injuries.

Despite the teeming literature on the subject the evolution in the treatment of head wounds during the war did not, in a general way, parallel that of wounds of the chest, abdomen, and extremities. There developed a certain degree of uniformity of opinion concerning methods of procedure for wounds of these regions, whereas the end of the war saw no such uniformity in the treatment of craniocerebral wounds. The widely held impression that the ultimate results of severe head wounds were at best unsatisfactory discouraged any widespread interest in the subject. Furthermore, there was a general feeling that brain wounds as a class stood apart from wounds of other structures, and hence that their treatment should not be carried out along similar lines. Finally, relatively few of those engaged in military surgery had had sufficient experience in cranial surgery before the war; as a result, head wounds, as compared with abdominal wounds, for example, did not in general receive either the attention or the skill that their importance warranted. These are some of the reasons for the greater divergence of views on the management of craniocerebral wounds even at the close of the war, and, indeed, for the less perceptible advances that were made in their treatment. To the credit of American surgeons it can be stated that under the leadership of Colonel Harvey Cushing they contributed a real share to whatever progress has been made. This was arrived at not through the development of new or original methods, but by adoption and adaptations of the most desirable elements in the methods of Continental

---

* Read before the New York Surgical Society, April 14, 1920. The paper is part of a chapter in a forthcoming volume of Keen's Surgery, and the author is indebted to the Editor and the publishers for their kind permission to use this material.

[1] An appreciable proportion of the head wounds occurred in the temporal and occipital regions below the brim of helmets of the American or British models. Modifications of the brim to protect these regions would certainly have been a valuable added safeguard.

surgeons. In what follows, the evolution of various methods of treatment will be described, procedures that appeal from personal experiences as most desirable will be more fully treated, and the immediate and distant results will be discussed, with a double purpose—to standardize as well as possible the treatment of craniocerebral wounds of modern warfare, and to indicate the applicability of some of the lessons acquired from war wounds to the head injuries and non-traumatic lesions of civil life.

Transportation and Place for Treatment.—The ideal *place* for the operative or other treatment of patients with head wounds is one somewhat further back from the line than the usual situation of evacuation hospitals. This viewpoint is held for the following reasons: Patients suffering from head wounds usually stand transportation well, even over long distances. This is true regardless of the severity of the wound if the pulse-rate is not greatly accelerated. Urgent indications for operation, such as active bleeding, are rarely present. Apparently infection does not spread as rapidly in head wounds as in wounds of the extremities, for example. Quiet is most desirable in the post-operative care of patients with head wounds, so that the place should, if possible, be beyond the zone of loud gunfire. The ideal *hospital* for these patients is one specially planned, equipped, and manned for their care; if that is not obtainable, separate wards for patients with head wounds should certainly be organized. Only in this way can they receive the particular attention they require after operation. Evidence has accumulated to show that patients with head wounds do not stand transportation well *after* operation, for the proportion of complications appears to have been distinctly higher when patients were transferred to base hospitals shortly (within ten days) after operations for severe wounds. Therefore, the ideal hospital plant would be one in which such patients could remain for several weeks or even longer. Unfortunately, very few of these ideal requirements could be attained during the war, especially with the shifting fronts of its later phases. The fact that such arrangements were generally absent in the front area and that patients with head wounds travelled well before operation led (especially in the British lines) to the evacuation of the wounded for their primary operations to base hospitals many miles distant. The unsatisfactory results in the treatment of head wounds under such circumstances was ultimately recognized, for it was found that patients often arrived at base hospitals with wound infections ineradicably established.

Classification of Wounds of the Head.—Many of the classifications that have been advanced were based on pre-war ideas, in which the skull and not the brain injury had been considered the dominant feature of the wound. It may be going too far to say that the classical teaching concerning lines of fracture in gunshot wounds went for naught, but certainly a detailed knowledge of the bending and bursting radiations of the skull injury was no essential requirement for the surgeon. Other classifications pivoted on physical signs and symptoms; these were unsatisfactory, for it was found that patients with wounds involving the brain might walk long distances and appear perfectly fit, whereas others in coma with many signs of serious damage might present trivial lesions at operation. There were also too many other factors affecting the general condition, such as battle exhaustion, starvation, or fear, to have made such a classification tenable.

The greatest single element that determined the seriousness of a head wound was the *condition of the dura, whether penetrated or not.* In other words, the decisive factor was *whether or not the chief portal for the development of intracranial infection had been opened.* The best classification is, therefore, one that hinges on this fact. Using such a classification, wounds of the head can only be placed in various categories at operation, since the external appearances of wounds often give such little information about the extent or situation of deeper lesions. Cushing employed the following grouping of head injuries according to their severity, stressing particularly the condition of the dura. His figures for the operative mortality of the various groups are added[2]:

Grade I. Wounds of the scalp with intact cranium and dura. Mortality, 4.5 per cent.

Grade II. Wounds producing local fractures of variable types, with dura intact. Mortality, 9.2 per cent.
　　　　Type A. Without depression of external table.
　　　　Type B. With depression of external table.

Grade III. Local depressed fractures of various types, with dura punctured. Mortality, 11.8 per cent.

Grade IV. Wounds, usually of gutter type, with detached bone fragments driven into the brain. Mortality, 24 per cent.

Grade V. Wounds of penetrating type with lodgment both of projectile and bone fragments. Mortality, 36.6 per cent.

Grade VI. Wounds with ventricle penetrated or traversed.
　　　　A. By bone fragments. Mortality, 42.8 per cent.
　　　　B. By projectile. Mortality, 100 per cent.

Grade VII. Wounds of craniocerebral type involving
　　　　A. Orbitonasal
　　　　B. Auropetrosal region } Mortality, 73.3 per cent.

Grade VIII. Wounds with craniocerebral perforation. Mortality, 80 per cent.

Grade IX. Craniocerebral injuries with massive fracture of skull. Mortality, 50 per cent.

Unless very complicated no classification of head wounds can be

[2] What is termed "bursting fracture" corresponds to Grade IX in Cushing's classification. Mention of Cushing's Grade VII is omitted, because cases he has placed in that group appear to me to fall more naturally in one of the other grades, depending on their characteristics.

free from a certain amount of overlapping. I have employed a simpler classification, which offers perhaps the added advantage of less overlap, in which each group is arranged in the order of increasing severity:

1. Scalp wounds.
2. Cranial wounds—dura intact:
   (a) Simple fracture.
   (b) Depressed fracture.
   (c) Bursting fracture.
3. Craniocerebral wounds—dura torn:
   (a) Depressed fracture.
   (b) Tangential:
       (1) Ventricle intact.
       (2) Ventricle penetrated by bone fragments.
   (c) Penetrating (metal retained):
       (1) Ventricle intact.
       (2) Ventricle penetrated by missile.
   (d) Perforating.

There are a number of other factors influencing prognosis that enter into either of these classifications, but their inclusion would only serve to complicate the general outlines above given. A few may be mentioned: The degree and nature of contamination or infection of the wound; existence of other serious wounds; physical condition of the patient; terrain of the battle area.

Symptoms and Physical Signs in the Recently Wounded.—A careful local, general, and neurologic examination should be made in every head wound. The reason for the local and general examination is evident. Since it is undoubtedly true that the neurologic manifestations rarely decide the question of operative intervention, its threefold purpose should be stated: (1) To estimate the extent of the cerebral lesion. (2) As a guide for the interpretation of post-operative complications or improvement. (3) For future reference in connection with functional results, late complications, and sequelæ.

Too much emphasis cannot be placed on the fact that the local appearance of the wound is not a guide to the extent of an underlying lesion of the brain or even of the skull. In a considerable proportion of the cases the physical signs and symptoms are very similar whether the wound be superficial or deeply penetrating. A scalp wound, to all appearances superficial, may mask a deeply penetrating wound of the brain. A patient in coma may have nothing more than a chip fracture of the skull, whereas the next patient, mentally alert, may be suffering from a ventricular penetration. To be sure, a man with a deep gash of the head from which brain substance is extruding is severely wounded. But even his lesion may not be as serious as one in which there is a slit-like penetrating wound, where damage of the brain, although invisible, may be much more extensive. Positive evidence of brain injury, such as paralysis or hemianopsia, can be evaluated, but negative evidence is worthless either in the diagnosis, the prognosis, or the indications for treatment. Few or many symptoms and physical signs of cerebral injury may be present in patients suffering from craniocerebral wounds. The following symptoms and signs of those that occur, therefore, should not be understood as manifestations regularly present in the seriously wounded:

Local Signs.—Hemorrhage from a wound of the head is rarely observed except on the battlefield. In the great majority of cases there is little or no oozing of blood by the time the patient arrives at a dressing station or evacuation hospital. This is true even when venous sinuses have been torn across by missiles or fragments of bone. Hemorrhage from injury to the middle meningeal artery is very unusual; indeed, contrary to expectation, extra- or intradural blood-clots of large size are rarely found at operation. The only active hemorrhage I saw from a cranial wound admitted to the front area hospital was one from a divided temporal artery. Of course, bleeding from the ears or nose occurs in head wounds with fractures radiating to the base.

*The Wound.—*Enough has been said concerning the wound itself to indicate clearly the unreliability of drawing any conclusions from it. In many instances the patient enters the hospital with a wound covered by hair matted together by blood-clot and dirt. Only after the head has been shaved will the characteristics of such a wound be apparent. And only then may one or more other wounds of the head that had not been previously suspected be discovered. Finally, at operation the evident wound may turn out to be a simple scalp lesion, whereas the minute, easily overlooked punctured wound may be the entrance of a missile penetrating the brain. Multiple cranial wounds are common or rare, depending on the type of warfare. In the Passchendaele campaign of 1917, when shellfire was employed almost exclusively, I saw multiple wounds very frequently, whereas they were not common with the extensive use of machine guns in the Argonne.

It is futile to make any effort to describe the infinite variations in the appearance of head wounds. Tangential and perforating craniocerebral wounds and " steel helmet " wounds may be selected for special mention. Before the recent war *tangential* (gutter) *wounds* aroused little interest, probably because of their less significance with the lower velocity missiles of those days. Tangential wounds were common and caused serious lesions in the recent war. The wound is generally a characteristic one. The furrow or gutter that is cut through the soft parts is of varying lengths and generally wider in proportion to length than in other types of wounds. A striking feature of tangential wounds is that, if severe enough to involve the dura, brain substance almost invariably presents in, and extrudes from, the gap. Another equally characteristic feature observed at operation is that bone fragments, frequently of large size, are driven into the brain at right angles to the wound. Short through-and-through (perforating) wounds in which the missile has struck the surface of the skull in transit or has tangentially traversed the skull are included in the group of tangential wounds. *Perforating* (bipolar or through-and-through) *wounds* are the most fatal of craniocerebral wounds, owing to the tremendous brain damage that is inflicted. They also form the group for which the least relief can be obtained by operative measures. The fact that the cranial cavity has been perforated by rifle or machine-gun bullets may be readily overlooked and the wound of exit can easily be mistaken for the *only* wound. This is particularly apt to be the case if the minute entry wound is in an unusual situation, such as the nape of the neck or within the auricle. The term *" steel-helmet wounds "* should, I believe, be given to head wounds that are the direct result of wearing this head protector. There are three types that I have noted. In one the helmet has been traversed by the missile and a sharp edge is turned in to be lodged in the skull. The dura may or may not be penetrated. In another the helmet has been driven down on the head, producing a contused or lacerated wound of the scalp, generally in the frontal region. Localized fractures have existed under these lesions in several instances I have seen; in addition, there may be one or more lesions the direct result of missiles. Finally, the skull may be shivered into numerous radiating fractures by the impact of a projectile transmitted by the helmet. A striking feature is that slight, if any, abrasions or lacerations of the scalp are usually found under such circumstances. Such cases belong to the group of bursting fractures. Many of them cannot, of course, be proved to be the result of the force transmitted by the helmet. There are a number of authentic instances, however, and I have seen one in which the deeply dented helmet was brought into the hospital by a companion of the wounded man.

X-ray examination is an absolutely indispensable form of examination of a head wound. Under usual circumstances an operation should never be undertaken without it; in times of stress it has, unfortunately, been necessary to forego the aid derived from röntgenograms. Given, for example, a wound with extruding brain substance, and the difficulties involved in an operation without previous X-ray examination are evident. Not knowing whether the wound is penetrating or tangential, one is forced to grope about for a projectile that may not have entered the brain or may have penetrated in a different direction from the one in which it is being sought. The dangers from such unnecessary trauma need not be dilated upon. Exact localization of foreign bodies is not the only assistance X-ray examination gives. The existence of depressed fractures is established. When skull fragments are driven into the brain, their number, size, and depth of penetration are determined; this is of

great importance to the surgeon at the time of operation.[3] In a consecutive series of 45 cases I checked up carefully the interpretations of stereoscopic pictures that had been made; these exactly described the findings
at operation in regard to size, position, and number of bone fragments
and missiles in 44 of the 45 cases. If X-ray pictures cannot be taken,
fluoroscopic examinations are of great aid in localizing the situations of
fragments of metal, or in determining their absence. During many
months' work in a mobile hospital I had to depend entirely on fluoroscopic examinations, and their reliability is, in my opinion, definitely
established; but the assistance they give the surgeon falls far short of that
derived from X-ray plates.

General Symptoms.—Loss of consciousness is common whether the
wound is slight or severe. It is of very varying duration, from a few
minutes to several days. Stupor or semicoma often alternates with a
peculiar restless irritability, making patients exceedingly difficult to man-
age. Either coma or this irritability is of serious omen if it has lasted a
number of hours. In a series of 100 cases admitted to a front-line hospital
where I was stationed, and in which admissions averaged ten hours after
injury, 37 per cent. entered in one or the other of these conditions. Only 30
per cent. of those in coma or semicoma, and 60 per cent. of those with restless irritability, recovered. Early in the war a slow pulse was interpreted
as indicating cerebral compression. Subsequently, this was found to be
incorrect. A slow pulse is often associated with battle fatigue or with
inanition, and the pulse is not infrequently rapid with cerebral involvement. In fact, a greatly accelerated pulse is of grave significance; upon
examination of my records I find that there was not a single recovery
where the pulse-rate on admission was 130 or more, whether operation was
performed or not. Headache is the most common complaint of patients
entering the hospital; it is generally frontal, regardless of the position of
the wound, and bears no relation to the gravity of the wound. Other
symptoms, such as vomiting, vertigo, vasomotor disturbances, and so
on, occasionally occur.

Neurologic Manifestations.—Detailed descriptions of the many interesting and significant neurologic observations that have been made in
patients suffering from head wounds would take too much space and
must be sought elsewhere. In brief, it may be said that evidence of brain
injury is afforded by disturbances of motor, sensory, reflex, and visual
functions, depending upon the region that has been involved. The important point is that these disturbances are not necessarily due to destruction of brain tissue by the wound, but may be, and often are, in
small or greater part, the result of contusion or œdema of the brain about
the wound. This explains the surprisingly frequent recovery of function

[3] The X-ray picture cannot be entirely depended upon to establish the presence
or absence of slight fractures without much depression, owing to normal irregularities of the shadows.

after head wounds, a recovery that cannot, of course, be ascribed directly to operations that have been performed.

From the foregoing it is evident that neurologic examinations are often difficult and not infrequently impossible of execution in some of the wounded. The presence or absence of gross paralyses and changes in the eye-grounds can, however, almost invariably be determined. The most striking neurologic feature of recent head wounds has been, I think, the relative infrequency of paralyses even when wounds were in the regions in which one would expect them. Thus, in the series of 100 cases, massive hemiplegias with or without aphasia were present in only 7 per cent. and pareses in 9 per cent. An interesting feature, brought out by Dr. L. J. Casamajor in the study of this series of cases, was that the epigastric, abdominal, and cremasteric reflexes were often reduced and sometimes absent on the side opposite to the head wound, even when there were no other evidences of cerebral involvement in the neurologic examination. Cranial injuries having been subsequently found at operation in such cases, the demonstration of reduction or absence of these reflexes, I believe, is of definite value in indicating craniocerebral injury by gunshot wounds. Examination of the eye-grounds is generally of little value. They often show no changes with the severest wounds. Definite choking of the disks is very uncommon. Slighter alterations, consisting in dilatation with occasional tortuosity of the veins and blurring of the disks, are only present (with rare exceptions) in cerebral involvement, and are of value to that extent. Changes in the fundi are most often found in depressed fractures without extrusion of brain substance.

This brief discussion of neurologic signs cannot be left without reference to the so-called "longitudinal sinus syndrome" described by Sargent and Holmes. This striking picture, a rather frequent one accompanying wounds over the midline in the parietal region, consists in a spastic paresis or paralysis of one or both lower extremities, extending to the arms in severe cases. Sargent and Holmes believe the condition to be due to lesions of the longitudinal sinus or of veins entering it. Unquestionably an injury of the vessel frequently coexists, but in the uniform presence of damage to the adjacent paracentral lobes I can see no good reason for attributing the neurologic manifestations to the sinus lesion. I may add that no lesion of the longitudinal sinus or of the vessels entering it was found at autopsy in two patients in whom the syndrome had been present.

Indications and Time for Operation.—These aspects of the subject of craniocerebral wounds were the source of much discussion and wide divergence of views during the war. The question of the indication and the equally important one of the time for operation are intimately linked. It is patent that the indications for operation when the patient is seen two or three days after injury are totally different from those existing shortly after he has been wounded. Yet this basic difference was not generally recognized until the latter part of the war; the result was a confusion of ideas and, unfortunately, the loss of many lives. The purpose of operation in the recently wounded is the elimination of infective material; the chief indication for operation at later stages is the control of infection. In the earlier part of the war operations at front-line hospitals generally consisted in enlargement of the wound, elevation of bone fragments, drainage of brain tracts, etc. Such operations, instead of eliminating infection, established septic wounds and hernia cerebri in many cases. The general impression that resulted was that operations should not be done in the front area, particularly when it was noted that cases arriving not operated on at the base usually ran a more satisfactory course. Only when the correct operation for recent head wounds—one to eliminate contamination—was evolved could opinion logically veer to early operation. Toward the end of the war there was fairly general agreement that the time for operation on craniocerebral wounds was the time for operation on other wounds, and that the main indication for operation on head wounds was the same as in other wounds.

The indications for operation, then, are clear in wounds definitely involving the brain. From what has been said of the ever-open question of deeper involvement in apparently superficial wounds, the indication for operations under such circumstances is exploration. Even though a patient walks without difficulty, does not suffer from any symptoms, has no neurologic signs of injury, is, in short, fit in every way, his scalp wound should be explored as the only means of determining if there is any deeper damage. Cerebral compression from blood-clot is, as has been said, so unusual an occurrence that it need only be mentioned in passing as a rare indication for operation. It has already been noted that neurologic manifestations may be due to destruction of brain substance or œdema and contusion, or to both, and it is impossible to differentiate between these conditions. Therefore neurologic symptoms and signs are not in themselves indications for operation. No matter how severe the cerebral lesion, the patient should be given the chance of operation if there is any likelihood of his withstanding it. The surgeon is not the judge of whether a life is going to be worth while living, so long as there is a chance of the life being spared. Besides, like others, I have had the agreeable surprise of witnessing not only recovery, but also recovery with good function in apparently hopeless cases.

As already stated, the indications for operation on head wounds at later stages, as seen in base hospitals, are totally different; they will be discussed after taking up the operative technic for, and complications following, recent wounds.

Contraindications to Immediate Operation.—An operation for a head wound should not be done at a front area hospital unless it can be adequately performed. This involves a satisfactory armamentarium, arrangements for good asepsis, and the reasonable assurance that patients with severe wounds can remain for at least a week after operation. Operation is contraindicated in manifestly hopeless and moribund cases. It is not indicated, or should at most consist in local toilet of the wounds, in the great majority of perforating craniocerebral lesions. In bursting fractures with insignificant wounds operation is usually not required; if necessary, it consists in a subtemporal decompression. The complete operation to be described is contraindicated in large multiple scalp wounds without evidences of depressed fracture because of the difficulties in closing the scalp under such circumstances. Finally, operation is inadvisable, in the absence of symptoms, in penetrations by very small fragments of metal when the wound of entry is not soiled.

The Operation for Recent Craniocerebral Wounds.—The evolution of the operation for wounds of the head has already been indicated. Wounds were at first freely incised, bone fragments elevated or removed, and brain tracts drained. After the unsatisfactory results of such procedures became recognized the general plan was to defer the treatment of cranial wounds until arrival at base hospitals. Here various methods of flap operations with drainage of brain tracts were evolved; the results were, on the whole, unsatisfactory, but better than the incomplete operations done at the front. A later development, as a consequence of frequent failures by the foregoing methods, was the attempt, both in front-line hospitals and at the base, to secure primary union after excision of the wound. But the principles of *débridement* were not yet established, excision of the wound was accordingly incomplete, and the results were still far from acceptable. The pioneer work of French surgeons (particularly Lemaître) and of Depage and his co-workers in Belgium definitely settled the methods for débridement of wounds in order to insure primary union after suture. There remained the necessity for the application of these principles to cranial wounds. A special adaptation was, of course, necessary, for brain tracts could not be laid open and excised. In fact, the term "débridement" strictly applied to a craniocerebral wound is a misnomer, because brain tracts cannot be so treated. Happily, the deeper portions of craniocerebral wounds generally appear to be less contaminated by bacteria and foreign matter than wounds of other regions because of the combined obstacle offered by the scalp and skull. It was the modified treatment of brain tracts along the lines of débridement, together with the true débridement of the portion of the wound involving soft parts and bone, that led to the best results obtained in operations for craniocerebral wounds.

These are, in a general way, the stages through which operations for head wounds passed. However, there were individual surgeons, mainly French, who practised fairly complete operations with primary closure long before the method was widely accepted. The work of De Martel should be particularly mentioned in this connection, for he persisted along these lines almost from the outset of the war.

Before describing the steps of the operation it may be well to mention the fact that the wound of the head is often only one of many wounds. In an analysis of the first series of 100 cases I treated, the great majority of the patients had wounds other than cranial. These wounds were serious in 11 per cent. of the cases; there were, in addition, 4 cases in which they were the cause of death. The point is that such other wounds cannot be slighted because of concentration on the head lesion at operation; I know that there were at least 2 cases in my experience in which death ensued from infection in these other wounds, most likely the result of the inadequate operations that were performed. The average duration of an operation for a craniocerebral wound is somewhere between an hour and a half and two hours. Therefore, another surgeon with his assistants should operate simultaneously on the other wounds if the latter require prolonged procedures. Furthermore, it sometimes becomes a matter of careful judgment whether or not to defer operation on the head wound in the presence of another serious wound urgently requiring an extensive operation.

Preparation of the Scalp.—The entire scalp should be shaved for a number of reasons. It is impossible to say in advance how extensive an exposure will be needed. Other wounds may be disclosed. Various wide-sweeping plastic incisions may be required for scalp closure. Cushing objects to preparation of the skin with iodine because it is apt to be followed by crusting and scaling, but I believe that that objection is outweighed by the advantages inherent in the penetration of the dried scalp by iodine. He also advocates the application at the field ambulance of a warm soap poultice to the wound, a procedure that is inadvisable, I think, because it would be apt to be a chilling dressing by the time the patient arrived at the hospital. In some French units the scalp was close cropped before the men went into action. This admirable precaution may very well have lessened the infectivity of not a few cranial wounds and certainly rendered less difficult the trying task of shaving the scalp.

Anæsthesia.—The use of local anæsthesia in operations for head wounds was developed chiefly by French surgeons, De Martel in particular. The objections to general anæsthesia are: Increased intracranial tension encountered at operation, with a resulting tendency to herniation of the exposed brain and forcible expulsion of the contents of a brain tract; increased bleeding from the scalp and bone, as well as from cerebral vessels; the tendency to the development of respiratory complications after operation; the necessity for careful observation of the patient until recovery from the anæsthetic, and, of course, the necessity for a skilled anæsthetist. The advantages of general anæsthesia are: Reduction in time consumed in preparation for operation, and the elimination of the difficulties in shaving restless patients. But these are counterbalanced by the many desirable features of local anæsthesia. Besides overcoming these objections, local anæsthesia is apt to encourage gentler and more accurate methods; the patient can be operated upon in a semi-sitting posture (De Martel); he can often coöperate by changing the position of his head when desired, coughing or straining to help express the contents of the brain tract, and so on. Local anæsthesia cannot be satisfactorily employed in some of the patients suffering from the peculiar restless irritability that has been described. Unfortunately, shaving and anæsthetization of the scalp are time consuming, and when many cases have to be operated upon and there is not at hand the assistance required for the preparation of succeeding cases while the surgeon and his team are operating, resort must be had to general anæsthesia.

It is generally advisable to administer some narcotic before operations under local anæsthesia. Omnopon was extensively employed by British, and scopolamine by French surgeons. One per cent. novocaine with adrenalin (added in the proportion of 1 c.c. to 30 c.c. novocaine) is injected about the area of the wound and along the lines of the proposed incision. If sufficient time is given for this to take effect, additional infiltration with the anæsthetic is usually unnecessary during operation.

Excision of Scalp and Bone.—This part of the operation, as practised by De Martèl and other French as well as British surgeons, consisted in turning down a large osteoplastic flap with the wound in its centre, and subsequently excising the wound tract. The objections which I believe to be inherent in flap methods are: Unnecessary difficulties in technic; the need for huge flaps with the larger wounds; the manifest undesirability or impossibility of flaps in certain regions; difficulties in the treatment of post-operative infections, especially hernia cerebri, should they arise; and difficulties in scalp closure after excision. The principle of simple excision of scalp and bone was, therefore, evolved, dependence being placed upon one of a number of methods of plastic incisions if required for closure of the scalp. The method employed by Cushing was an incision about the wound with three radiating (" tripod " or " Isle of Man ") incisions extending from this. By reflecting these flaps adequate exposure of the skull was obtained. In the ordinary type of wound I generally employed a simple long, elliptic incision circumscribing the wound, placed to give the necessary exposure in the desired direction. The ends of this incision were curved one way or another to permit the scalp to be reflected where greatest exposure of the skull was required. The incision employed by Cushing was designed, of course, not only for exposure, but for subsequent plastic closure. I believed that the necessarily extensive reflection and undermining of flaps was undesirable if post-operative infection should supervene, and that the junction of three flaps at one point overlying exposed brain invited infection of the brain and the development of hernia cerebri, should there be any infection in and separation of the scalp wound. As will be subsequently indicated, plastic incisions were not infrequently required for closure after the simple elliptic incision, but I believed that the time for their consideration (as

567

in breast amputations for carcinoma, for example) was at the end of operation. After all, the important point is that, in accordance with the principle of débridement, the wound should be completely circumscribed, not omitting the minutest visibly devitalized or soiled portion of scalp. In the beginning unnecessarily wide areas of scalp were sacrificed, until it was learned that the incision could safely be placed a few millimetres from the margin of the wound. The incision is deepened to bone, all devitalized areas in the soft parts being circumscribed.

The excision of the depressed fracture consists in making a number of small perforations in the skull immediately beyond the bony lesion, and connecting them with linear cuts through the bone. Forceps of the De Vilbiss pattern may be used for the latter, but the Montenovesi forceps is best adapted for the purpose. It makes an excellent linear cut, can be introduced through smaller openings, turns corners more easily, and is less jarring. After the perforations have been joined up, the section of bone is uptilted and scalp and bone are thus removed in one piece. The advantages of this technic are evident. The soiled area is removed in one piece, there is immediate exposure of the underlying lesion, and the mosaic of bone fragments can be examined to see if it is complete. The first point requires no elaboration. The complete exposure that is immediately obtained is particularly advantageous in sinus lacerations, for otherwise removal of a fragment of bone lodged in such a sinus, before the field has been adequately bared, generally leads to hemorrhage that is difficult to control. By possessing the mosaic of bone fragments one can determine if any parts are missing, and accordingly seek them.

This type of block excision was, therefore, strongly urged by Cushing. Although admirable for many varieties of wounds, I found some objections to its routine application. In the first place, it cannot be readily employed in wounds toward the base of the skull, such as those involving the mastoid. In cases in which damage to the skull is merely suspected, or when a superficial bone lesion is anticipated, I believe areas of skull are unnecessarily sacrificed thereby.[4] In such instances I think it better to excise the scalp wound with periosteum and then examine the bone. When extensive depressed fracture exists, block removal of bone can be carried out. If there is a superficial chip fracture, a perforation of the bone can be made to one side, and the involved portion of the skull is then lifted out with a rongeur forceps. The latter is discarded and fresh rongeurs used should the opening require enlargement for the removal of depressed fragments of inner table or for the treatment of a dural tear. Another objection to block removal of skull is that, in that method, the lesion of the outer table is the guide to the amount of bone to be removed. As is well known, fracture of the inner table is often more extensive and the

---

[4] The removal of any more of the skull than is required for the débridement or adequate exposure is no small matter; as will be shown, the question of repair of defects often arises at a later date.

depressed fragments cover a broader area than would be indicated from the fracture of the outer table. In such instances the block removed may well include only parts of the inner table; I recall two instances in which I inflicted unnecessary trauma by depressing fragments of the inner table with the jaw of the bone-cutting forceps under these circumstances. Furthermore, a superficial tear of the dura may be converted into a deeper one upon tilting the block should a pointed fragment of bone be firmly locked in the dura. These objections are not to be understood as outweighing the advantages of block removal, but as indicating what I believe to be its limitations.

A different technic which I have used in many cases may be described as follows: After excision of the scalp with its periosteum, a perforation is made to one side of the bone lesion. With rongeurs and linear cutting forceps the bone is cut away progressively along the margin of the fracture. If more extensive inner table depression is found, the bone is removed widely enough to expose this completely. After the rim of bone about the fracture has been excised, a blunt elevator is used to separate the depressed fragments from the dura. The mosaic is removed in one piece when it appears safe to do so. However, when the lesion is in proximity to a venous sinus, when fragments are firmly attached to the dura, or when a dural tear is suspected, the fragments are lifted out in small sections. In suspected sinus injury removal of fragments is begun away from the sinus region, so that the exposure is adequate and preparations complete to treat a sinus tear upon removing the last fragments. The instruments used for the removal of the mosaic are soiled and therefore discarded. With large defects in the skull, as in tangential wounds, this technic is also very satisfactory for débridement of the bone. Although not as neat as block removal, I consider the method safer under the circumstances that have been indicated; it is always simple of application and attains the same ends as removal *en bloc*.

Whatever technic of débridement is employed, the resultant exposure should be sufficient for the treatment of the underlying lesion. With large dural tears enough bone must be removed to completely expose normal dura all around, except in those regions (tears going down toward the base) in which this is not feasible. Linear fractures radiating from the cranial penetration are not followed except when bone removal along them is required for the exposure of a lesion underneath.

Treatment of the Intact and Torn Dura.—Any blood-clot adherent to the dura may be contaminated and is therefore gently curetted away. The question of incising an intact dura not infrequently arises when its surface is discolored, tense, and not pulsating, especially if paralysis or other functional loss exists. It is always a difficult question to settle in the presence of a soiled wound. Some hold that an intact dura should never be incised; others, that it should be invariably opened if indicated for the removal of blood-clot or disorganized brain. Surely the dura should not be incised under any circumstances unless one is certain of the operating-room asepsis, of the débridement of the wound, and of the uncontaminated condition of the part of the dura it is proposed to open. The possible or even probable advantages of incising the dura must always be weighed against the ever-present possibility of a fatal infection that may result. It is impossible to draw any definite conclusions in favor of or against incision of an intact dura from the literature on the subject, because most writers fail to give facts to support their assertions. In my own experience the dura was not opened in any of the cases in which it was intact, although in a number there were definite evidences of underlying damage. *There were no deaths.* Recovery from paralysis or other loss of function was perhaps slower than it might have been with incision of the dura, but the follow-up notes show a satisfactory outcome in all the cases.

A dural tear is generally large enough for the exploration and treatment of an underlying brain tract; if not, it must be opened to the required extent. Most surgeons contend that the margins of the torn dura should be left undisturbed, the argument being that otherwise adhesions are separated and an infection of the meninges invited. I hold that an adequate débridement includes removal of the devitalized margin of the dura (1 or 2 millimetres) as a necessary step, and I have seen no meningeal complications referable to such excision. When the head wound is definitely infected the stage for true débridement is, of course, past, and the sealed-off meninges must be respected. But in the earlier period every effort is bent toward obtaining primary union, and excision of the dural margin is part of the procedure. It is usually attended by fresh bleeding readily controlled by ligating one or two vessels with fine silk. Débridement of the dural margin is best done after the toilet of the brain tract.

Treatment of the Brain Tract.—This is the most important single step in the operation in wounds with cerebral penetration, for the removal of the cerebral débris, blood-clot, bone fragments, and bits of cloth plugging the tract means the elimination of the greatest factor favoring brain infection. Fortunately, a considerable portion of the contents of the tract will frequently extrude spontaneously (or after removal of superficial fragments corking the tract) if the patient can be made to cough or strain, or with the increased tension that usually exists in general anæsthesia. The method generally used for removing deeper bone fragments, until Cushing introduced catheter suction, consisted in the insertion of a finger to dislodge bone fragments, alternating this with irrigation of the tract. These procedures were repeated until the tract was free from bone fragments and débris. Unquestionably digital exploration may inflict damage to the walls of a brain tract, even when done with the greatest gentleness. Therefore, Cushing's technic is a real contribution, since the tract is well and safely cleaned thereby and the use of the finger is eliminated.

It is employed as follows: " Reliance was placed on the use of a flexible, soft-rubber catheter as a means of determining the exact direction taken by the missiles, whether a metallic body or bone fragments, or both. Without the production of additional trauma one may investigate in this way even the narrowest tract, and it will be found that the presence and situation of any in-driven bone fragments can be detected with almost as great delicacy as by direct palpation. By attaching to the end of the catheter a Carrel-Gentile glass syringe with its rubber bulb it is possible to suck up into its lumen the softened brain, which can then be expelled from the catheter as paste is expressed from the orifice of a tube. The process should be repeated until the cavity is rendered as free as possible of all the softened and infiltrated brain. It will be found that the adjoining normal cerebral tissue, unaffected by the original contusion, will not be drawn into the tube by the degree of suction which can be applied by the average rubber bulb. Not infrequently bits of bone come away in the eye of the catheter, and on one or two occasions a small foreign body has thus been withdrawn. Meanwhile, as the track becomes clean and the tension and tendency of the brain to herniate subsides, it is possible with delicate duck-billed forceps to pick out from the track one by one the bone fragments, whose depth and position can be determined by the unmistakable sensation they impart to the catheter, which thus supplements the information given by the X-ray plates. The technic of the performance will quickly be acquired by any one who may wish to put it into practice."

Before this technic was described I had always explored digitally those brain tracts wide enough to admit the finger freely, reserving the instrumental extraction of bone spicules, débris, or foreign bodies for the narrower tracts. Entirely converted to the routine use of catheter suction, I see no objection and one real advantage in additional palpation of such large tracts, *provided it is done carefully*. My usual procedure in these wider tracts has been painstakingly to cleanse the track with alternate flushing and suction through the catheter, using delicate forceps to remove the bone fragments felt with the tip of the catheter. When the tract has been rendered as clear as possible a finger is introduced and the walls are palpated for any embedded bone fragments that may have been missed. Upon a number of occasions I have found and dislodged such fragments in this way. In fact, bone fragments buried in the wall of the tract can be felt with the catheter only by the merest chance. When felt, it has been safer in my hands to dislodge them with the finger rather than to use an instrument that may readily traumatize surrounding brain tissue.

Although single brain tracts are the rule, it should not be forgotten that two or more fragments of metal may enter through one skull opening (or the missile may be split up in transit through the skull) and penetrate the brain in different directions. The X-ray would, of course, indicate the existence of multiple foreign bodies in the brain, but it is not apt to establish penetration through a single skull opening. I recall an instance of double penetration with the parallel tracts not far apart, and again, a single penetration with three forking tracts in a case with multiple scalp wounds. One must, therefore, be on the watch for multiple tracts in order to avoid missing minor ones; larger penetrations could scarcely be overlooked. Minor tracts require the same detailed attention as the wider, more evident penetrations.

There is no essential difference in the treatment of the tract in the more serious cases of *ventricular penetration*. Until catheter suction was employed the existence of this condition was usually only surmised at operation from the path of the missile, or was found after death. With catheter suction the diagnosis is promptly made by drawing cerebro-spinal fluid up into the syringe. Bone fragments should be extracted from the tract even more carefully than ordinarily for fear of dislodging them into the ventricle. The ventricle can be sucked dry. In wide tracts two long, thin-bladed retractors may then be introduced and inspection made of the interior of the ventricle with reflected light to discover bone fragments or a missile in the cavity. There appears to be a definite tendency (because of the resistance of the fluid) for foreign bodies that have penetrated the ventricle to be retained there rather than to become embedded in brain substance beyond. Their retention in the ventricle is almost sure to be fatal, and therefore every justifiable effort should be made toward extracting them. Fortunately, not a few ventricular penetrations are the result of puncture by one or two long slivers of bone that can be easily removed.

Before catheter suction was introduced ventricular penetration was thought to be a hopeless lesion. We now know that the mortality from penetration by bone fragments is not much higher than when the ventricle is intact. The rôle of dural repair in the results that may be obtained will be subsequently noted. Cases in which the missile penetrates the ventricle appear to be quite hopeless; however, I have had one undoubted case that recovered after operation.

Treatment of Devitalized Brain Tissue.—This aspect of the treatment of the cerebral wound is not usually discussed by writers; yet it is a definite step in the technic. Manifestly the devitalized portions of brain around the cerebral tear should be subjected to débridement as a necessary element in the effort to avoid infection. They are apt to slough and are already contaminated. Snipping off dangling fragments does not suffice. Devitalized fragments should be removed freely enough to obtain some oozing from the surface that is left. It is clear that serious functional loss may occur if one cuts widely into healthy brain substance. By closely hugging the devitalized fragments with a sharp scalpel or fine-pointed scissors no harm will be done. Partially detached tags of pia-arachnoid are generally found where there is much cerebral laceration, and they, too, should be ablated.

Extraction of the Missile.—Subsequently it will be shown that the retention of a missile in the brain is not the essential element in the development of late complications after craniocerebral wounds. Yet the extraction of the foreign body is eminently desirable not only for the elimination of an important element favoring sepsis but also because infective material about the missile and in the tract leading to it is thereby removed. The ideal time for extraction of the foreign body is at the primary operation, for there then exists a tract acting as a guide to its situation. In extractions at a later date cicatricial tissues (or normal brain) must often be traversed, and there is greater likelihood of injuring adjacent brain substance. "Latent sepsis" has been lit up, according to some reports, in late foreign body extraction. Therefore, every reasonable effort should be made to extract the foreign body at the primary operation. When superficially situated in the brain, this is a simple matter. There has been considerable difference of opinion concerning the advisability of the removal of deeply implanted missiles, some urging that they should be left alone. I believe a middle ground between these extreme views is the justifiable position to hold, namely, that every reasonable attempt should be made to extract the missile, always provided that serious damage to the brain be not inflicted by the manœuvres.

Small fragments of metal are not infrequently drawn into the eye of the catheter in the suction method, and removed in this way. After the tract has been freed of débris a foreign body sometimes becomes freely exposed at the apex and can be readily removed. Magnet extraction is usually required for deeply seated missiles. The safest method consists in gently introducing a slender rod (made specially for that purpose) to the bottom of the tract (the length and direction of the tract are determined by the catheter and the position of the foreign body by the X-ray) and then making contact with the portable electro-magnet. The foreign body is withdrawn along the tract. Needless to say, fragments of magnetizable metal are the only ones that will respond. The use of too powerful a magnet, one that will make a piece of metal jump some distance, is most inadvisable. Deeply placed foreign bodies can frequently be extracted either with forceps or with the magnet. In my series they were removed in a little over half the cases. I had one unfortunate experience with magnet extraction. It was an instance of ventricular penetration by a large missile. The fragment was half way out of the tract when (because of its weight, or possibly because of poor contact) it dropped back. It was found in the ventricle only after considerable difficulty, and finally removed with forceps. The patient died about twelve hours after operation. French surgeons have employed extraction by means of the Hirtz localizing compass to which the extractor is attached. They also practised extraction under guidance of the fluoroscopic screen.

Both methods have given satisfactory results, but, unless practised with extreme care (which means that the extractor must remain in the tract), injury to the brain will be inflicted.

Control of Hemorrhage.—Hemorrhage at operation can usually be controlled without any great difficulty except when it arises from a distant region, such as the base of the skull; this, however, is an unusual occurrence. In order to prevent a post-operative collection of blood, that readily can become infected, it is essential that the field shall be dry at the end of the operation. The simplest way to avoid this is to establish hæmostasis step by step. Bleeding from the bone is usually trivial and ceases spontaneously. The application of Horsley's bone-wax ordinarily controls any excessive bleeding, but for large vessels in the bone wooden plugs or small pieces of muscle used as plugs may be required. Laceration of the middle meningeal artery is infrequent. Bleeding from small branches at the torn dural margin is frequently encountered. In either instance hæmostasis is established with fine silk ligatures or by using Cushing's silver clips.

Hemorrhage from torn venous sinuses does not offer great difficulties if the lesion is adequately exposed. The application of a fragment of muscle (or of aponeurosis if muscle is not accessible) is remarkably efficacious. The " postage-stamp " graft is held gently in place with the ' gloved finger for a minute or two, at the end of which time bleeding will have ceased. Large sinus tears may require suture with fine silk, or silver clips may be employed. On several occasions I have seen the longitudinal or lateral sinuses torn completely or almost completely across. In such instances I practised ligation of the divided ends. Muscle grafts might have established hæmostasis, but I felt that secondary hemorrhage might supervene if infection of the blood-clot occurred. Ligatures could not be securely thrown around the ends of the vessels, and I therefore employed the following technic: A short distance beyond the tear small nicks are made in the dura on either side of, and directly adjacent to, the sinus wall. The flat, blunt-pointed end of a probe with the eye carrying a silk ligature is bent to the desired shape (like a small aneurism needle) and gently passed beneath the vessel. Slight pressure on the needle when the membranous fold beneath the vessel is reached suffices to penetrate it. The triangular shape of the sinus in cross-section must be borne in mind, otherwise the vessel wall may be injured. The ligature should be tied only snugly enough to obliterate the lumen.

Bleeding from the lacerated brain requires little discussion. Ordinarily, it is well controlled by the application of moist or dry pledgets of cotton. Sometimes there is persistent oozing from one or two places, and bits of muscle should then be employed for hæmostasis. Bleeding cerebral vessels are ligated with fine silk. Torn cerebral vessels, thrombosed and not bleeding, are occasionally met at operation; if the divided ends are free, the vessels are tied and the excess portions ablated.

Repair of Torn Dura—Suture. Transplantation of Fascia.—This aspect of the craniocerebral wound received scant attention. Surgeons were apparently satisfied with the removal of soiled and infective material and did not devote much consideration to the question of repair. Some sutured the smaller dural lacerations that could be closed, others left them open as a sort of safety-valve in the event of suppuration in the brain tract. The argument against closure of the dura was, of course, the danger of locking in an infection. But the whole plan of treatment as described is based upon the elimination of infective material, and its success is entirely centred thereon. Undoubtedly, suture of the dura would reduce the chances for recovery in some cases by closing off infective foci in brain tracts; however, the prognosis, whether immediate or ultimate, is always bad if such foci are left behind. A detailed consideration of the advantages of dural closure is included in the discussion on fascial transplantation. I believed that dural closure was a required step in the operation, and I therefore employed it as a routine procedure, omitting this step only in a small proportion of the cases under my care. These were wounds in the right temporal regions in which subtemporal decompression was done; wounds with purulent brain tracts; wounds in which the tear in the dura could not be adequately exposed; and finally, wounds in patients in too poor condition to devote the additional time for dural repair. Before dural suture is begun the devitalized margin is excised in the technic I have employed, as previously noted. By passing the interrupted sutures first at one and then at the other end of the tear, and thus working toward the middle, some lacerations apparently too large for suture can be closed.

In many cases, however, the loss of dural substance was too great for closure. For these I employed fascial transplantation. Without entering into details, I may say that fascia lata has been experimentally and clinically proved, by myself and others, to be an eminently satisfactory tissue for the replacement of visceral defects. Implanted into a dural gap, it becomes gradually replaced by a firm fibrous connective tissue almost indistinguishable from the dura, and lined by a layer of cells continuous with the dural endothelium. The reasons for suture of the smaller and fascial transplantations for the larger dural defects may now be enumerated: (1) To obviate infection from without, especially when bone sinuses have been laid open by the injury. (2) To minimize the chances for subdural infection in the event of post-operative infection or separation of the scalp. (3) To prevent leakage of cerebrospinal fluid in wounds with ventricular penetration. (4) To prevent adhesions between the lacerated brain and the scalp. (5) To afford a permanently firm physical protection for the brain surface. (6) To eliminate the possibility of injury to the brain at a subsequent reparative operation.

Before transplanting fascia the devitalized margin of the dura is excised. The technic of fascial transplantation is simple, consisting in removing a portion of the fascia lata of the appropriate shape of, and slightly larger than, the dural gap, and fixing the transplant in place by four silk sutures. Interrupted stitches are placed between these, approximating edge of fascia to edge of dura. The transplants varied in size from 2 by 2 to 4 by 4 cm.

It is evident that fascial transplantation was employed only in serious cases, those in which there was much damage to the brain in keeping with the large dural tear. Of the 19 cases in which I used fascial transplants, 7 died. One of the deaths occurred four months later as the result of sepsis from a compound fracture of the leg. The autopsy showed the transplant well healed in place. The condition of the transplant is known in 4 of the surviving 12 cases, for they were subjected to reparative operations for skull defects. The transplant was described as satisfactory in all; in fact, in two instances operators were not aware that fascial transplantation had been done. Altogether, follow-up reports have been obtained in 9 cases, and in none were there symptoms that could be referable to the transplant acting as a foreign body. The first operation was done more than two years ago, and the last more than a year ago. Sufficient time has thus elapsed to be able to state definitely that the ultimate as well as the immediate results of fascial transplantation in cerebral wounds are satisfactory.

Indications for Drainage.—The sutured scalp incision is drained in one or several places if the head wound was definitely infected. If a brain tract is found to be purulent, or contains manifestly infected bloodclot, its drainage is indicated. Hemorrhage should be a rare indication for drainage. Altogether, drainage should be considered a very unusual feature after a properly conducted operation for a recent wound, for it defeats the purpose of the operation.

Closure of the scalp should and can be complete in the great majority of cases. The exceptional instances are infected wounds or multiple wounds with extensive loss of scalp. In suturing the scalp a separate layer of sutures is devoted to the aponeurosis. Better approximation is thereby obtained, additional support is given, hæmostasis is established, and the external sutures can be removed at an earlier time. With the tripod incisions that have been described closure was generally obtainable by sufficiently extensive mobilization of the flaps. Simple suture of the wound could be carried out in a large proportion (80 per cent.) of the cases in which the long elliptic incision I have described was used. In the remainder some type of plastic closure was required. The one I used most frequently was the S-shaped variety. The scalp is sutured from both ends as far as possible. Then, beginning at one end of the remaining defect, an incision is made through scalp and aponeurosis at right angles to the long axis of the defect. This incision is carried down a varying distance, depending on the required size of the flap, is then curved to run parallel to and for the full length of the defect, and is again turned down to run parallel to the first part of the incision. The resultant flap is now completely freed, slid over the defect, and sutured in place. The plastic incision can be closed completely in most instances by passing the sutures obliquely; a remaining defect at the furthermost part of the incision, however, is of no moment. The success of the S-shaped plastic depends on its accurate placement, and, above all, on its length. The tendency is to make it too small, with an inadequate flap as a consequence. In a large defect over the forehead, for example, I have fashioned the plastic S-shaped incision so that its end reached beyond the occipital protuberance. Some of the defects of the scalp are of triangular or shield shape. Plastic closure of these consisted in prolonging the base of the defect on both sides to lengths sufficient to mobilize the two lateral flaps required for closure. There remained a small proportion of cases in which no typical plastic incision could be employed, and in these various incisions had to be devised to fit the particular case.

Had the war continued the entire question of closure of the scalp might have been put on a very different basis. Following débridement wounds in other parts of the body were either sutured primarily or subjected to delayed primary suture, depending on certain factors, such as the presence of streptococci in the wound. Similarly, delayed primary suture of the scalp in craniocerebral wounds might very well have been developed as a desirable refinement of technic.

Post-operative Course and Treatment.—In the lightly wounded the post-operative course is usually smooth; however, severe headache and dizziness are not unusual. In craniocerebral injuries, on the other hand, the course is often stormy even in those patients who are doing well. Rise of temperature may occur without any evidence of local or general infection. Restlessness is common, and, particularly at night, patients may become very violent, attempting to tear off dressings, get out of bed, and so on. This peculiar " dream state " may last a week or even longer, and yet be followed by complete recovery. It is not in itself of serious omen. Very frequently there is a complete amnesia for the events of the first two weeks after operation even in the lightly wounded. Indeed, many patients have written me that they remembered nothing or almost nothing of occurrences for a month or more after injury. And yet, not a few of these men seemed normal in every way at the time of leaving the hospital one to two weeks after operation. The treatment of some of these patients in the first days after operation, particularly as regards the mental state, the matter of feeding, and so on, is often very trying. The question of nursing is a most important element in the results that are obtained. Loud noises and clumsy handling have very disturbing effects on these patients. The administration of morphine not infrequently results in increased restlessness and violence. Chief reliance should be placed upon the bromides, used as a routine by some.

Aspirin and trional given together are often efficacious for headache. Rectal administration of bromides and of fluids, in patients who cannot or should not take anything by mouth, is very beneficial.

It is usually not difficult to recognize within a day or two after operation the cases that are not doing well. Coma persists, or those who have been alert complain of bursting headache and become stuporous. Signs of meningitis usually make an early appearance. In other instances the first evidence is found in an infection of the wound. Occasionally a series of severe convulsive seizures indicate the change in condition. However, surprises are frequent. One sees recovery in those whose outlook appears hopeless; and, unfortunately, some patients appear to be on the high road to recovery for even a week or more after operation, when a fatal infection supervenes.

In cases that recover the improvement in functional disturbances that often occurs within the first week or two of operation is remarkable. Without entering into details, it may be said that sensory disturbances, aphasias, and defects in visual fields frequently subside completely; the majority of paralyses and pareses (except the type due to brain destruction) begin to improve before patients leave the front area hospital. It is well to reiterate here that paralyses or other losses of function making their first appearance or increasing directly after operation are evidences of damage inflicted by the surgeon. In a considerable operative experience I have not seen such manifestations, and cannot, therefore, accept the theory advanced by some that they are due to cerebral œdema.

Even with rapid improvement in function or in the absence of functional loss patients should not be up and about for five weeks or more after operations for craniocerebral wounds. At best, headaches, blurred vision, pain in the wound, and giddiness on walking are common enough complaints in the earlier stages of convalescence.

In my experience very few complications developed after operation in recovering cases. In view of the grave significance of hernia cerebri I wish to emphasize the fact that I *saw but one instance* of this complication after operation in my series of cases. This was a much soiled penetrating wound in which infection developed at the suture line in the dura. The rarity of hernia cerebri after the complete early operation should be one of the strongest arguments for the adoption of that technic. Epileptic seizures are described as not uncommon after operation, and of lesser and different significance than the epilepsy appearing as a late complication. I have seen only two cases in which epileptic attacks developed shortly after operation; both patients have remained free from recurrence of attacks up to the present time. The great majority of the wounds should heal by primary union. In the small number of scalp infections I saw the majority were slight and readily controlled. Frequently repeated inspections of, and detailed care in, the treatment of the wounds are important elements in successful results after operation. Later infections in the wound are of different significance, being referable to spicules of bone or other foreign matter that had been left behind.

Meningitis or cerebral suppuration after operation are fatal complications for which various therapeutic measures appeared to be of no avail.

Hernia cerebri as an early complication not infrequently recedes under proper treatment. Such procedures as enlargement of the bony opening for supposed strangulation of the brain or ablation of the fungus are mentioned only to be condemned. All the evidence points clearly to infection, and infection alone, as the cause of hernia cerebri. The hernia cerebri is generally the result of an incomplete operation. The hernia varies in appearance and size from a superficially infected, slightly bulging, small area of brain surface, to a large sloughing mass. By the use of the Carrel-Dakin treatment or perhaps, preferably, dichloramine-T in oil, progressive sterilization of the hernial surface can often be attained and, with it, recession of the protrusion. The use of gravity, by propping up the patient's head, is said to be of value. But the most useful therapeutic measure, in addition to attempts at sterilization of the wound, is repeated lumbar puncture. This procedure had many advocates who saw no evidence that infection may spread as the result of evacuating cerebrospinal fluid. The fluid should be withdrawn slowly, and not in large amounts at one sitting, otherwise the hernia may sink back through the cranial defect, and the infection certainly be diffused. The lumbar puncture should always be done with the wound exposed to view, so that changes in the hernia may be observed. In the later stages of hernia cerebri, as encountered in a base hospital, I have seen beneficial effects follow a subtemporal decompression.

Lumbar puncture is of value in the post-operative treatment of cranial wounds not only in hernia cerebri, but also for the relief of intractable headache or other evidences of cerebral œdema. I have, however, seen but few indications for its use in the recently wounded.

The *cause of death* after operations for craniocerebral wounds requires only brief comment. In the patients who die shortly after operation extensive brain destruction, sometimes due to ricochetting of the missile, is usually found. But autopsy shows infection to be the cause in the great majority of those who die at the front area hospital. In my series of cases suppuration was found not only in the brain and meninges, but also invariably in ventricles that had been penetrated by missiles or bone fragments. Not a few of these patients were operated upon twenty-four hours or more after injury, so that there appears to be a definite relationship between fatal infections and the time after wounding at which operation is performed. It is difficult to make a more definite statement because the time at which the wound was sustained could not be determined in many of the serious cases.

HAROLD NEUHOFF

Results of Operation for Recent Craniocerebral Wounds.—Little information can be derived from the voluminous literature on head wounds concerning other than the immediate or intermediate results of operation. Careful studies have been made of results noted after head wounds, but these have not been linked up with various operative measures that were employed, or with the lesions encountered at operation. Since this paper is, after all, an essential commentary on the operative technic of craniocerebral wounds, I will detail the results of operation in my series of cases as based on follow-up reports. The latter have been received from the patients themselves, as well as from those under whose care patients subsequently came.

Before discussing the late functional results and complications the *mortality after operation* in these cases should be taken up. In general, the mortality from head wounds with intact dura is small with any technic that includes removal of the soiled wound and bone fragments. Occasionally, however, infection passes through an intact or bruised dura with fatal issue, so that here, too, the elimination of infective material by a properly conducted débridement is an important element in success. Among my cases death after wounds of the head with intact dura came as a result of other wounds. The usual mortality after operation for head wounds with dural penetration ranged from 50 to 60 per cent. in the different reports. In Cushing's report the significant feature was that his mortality in a first series of cases done in the older way was 54.5 per cent., and in a third series, with the improved operative technic, it was reduced to 28.8 per cent. His publication appeared too soon after the operations were performed to include possible subsequent deaths, so that the figures must be accepted for the mortality in the early weeks after operation. An important point is that deaths from any cause were included, even if unrelated to the head wound. This is the only basis upon which the mortality rates should be given, for there will be no general agreement on conditions that may be justifiably excluded. By paring and pruning, even with the utmost honesty, attractive figures can be produced that will in no way represent the gravity of craniocerebral wounds.

The cases that were under my care fall into two series, the first (95 cases) operated upon in 1917, and the second (80 cases) in 1918. The great majority of deaths occurred in the first weeks, and not a few (certainly 5 per cent.) from other lesions. A number of the later deaths were definitely unrelated to the head wounds, as in a case in which death resulted from sepsis from a compound fracture, and post-mortem examination of the brain showed no evidence of infection. The mortality from every cause is, however, included in the following tabulation. It is based on reports received from time to time until January, 1920, and thus represents the mortality up to the present time. Follow-up reports were obtained in four-fifths of the cases of dural penetration.

580

	Percentage mortality first series, 95 cases.	Percentage mortality second series, 80 cases.
I. Scalp wounds	0	No cases
II. Cranial wounds—dura intact	8.5	6.2
(a) Simple fracture	6.6	No cases
(b) Depressed fracture	0	5
(c) Bursting fracture	100 (1 case)	25
III. Craniocerebral wounds—dura torn	42.5	29.4
(a) Depressed fracture	16.6	0
(b) Tangential wound	33.3	16
1. Ventricle intact	12.5	10
2. Ventricle penetrated by bone fragments ..	75	33.3
(c) Penetrating (metal retained)	30	34.3
1. Ventricle intact	25	20
2. Ventricle penetrated by missile	100	85.7
(d) Perforating	100	66.6

In the first series the technic of operation as described had not as yet been fully developed; the figures are sufficient commentary upon the difference in the results obtained. The results can be better interpreted if I add that a selection of cases was made possible when the second series were operated upon, and that only cases evidently or probably severe were chosen. This is seen in an analysis of the lesions in the 13 patients in the second series who died at the front area hospital: Ventricle penetrated by missile, 6 cases; perforating wound, 2 cases; multiple brain penetrations by missiles, 2 cases; penetration from vertex to base, 1 case; penetration complicated by gas infection of the brain, 2 cases.

The *late results* in the patients who recovered may now be discussed. The most impressive feature of the follow-up in both series of cases is that there is not a single report of late hernia cerebri, meningitis, or brain abscess. Since the great majority of these later complications are known to develop in the first six or nine months, it is reasonable to assume that they will certainly be at least very infrequent at this late date. Next in interest were the changes that occurred in paralyses and pareses. The improvement that took place in the first weeks after operation has already been noted. Reports received from time to time show that this was continuous in a large proportion of the cases. So that at the present time the course of paralyses and pareses can be termed one ranging from progressive improvement to complete disappearance in the majority of cases. Spasticity and persistent paralysis were each reported twice. There was one case of persistent aphasia and two of permanent deficiencies in the visual fields. Epilepsy is considered the most common tardy manifestation after head wounds, yet up to the present there have been only three statements of its appearance. Two of the patients have petit mal and in neither was there a dural penetration; the third, suffering from generalized seizures, had a penetrating wound from which the foreign body was not recovered. The reports in two cases suggest that insanity may have developed; the dura had been penetrated and the foreign body retained in one, and the lesion was a slightly depressed fracture with intact dura in the other. Persistent headaches and dizziness of varying degrees were reported by fully 20 per cent. of the patients. Other subjective symptoms, such as insomnia, hypersusceptibility to sounds, inability to concentrate, and so on, were also frequently mentioned, but these, like headache and dizziness, bear no proportionate relation to the gravity of the wound. Some of the patients have returned to former or other occupations, some are engaged in study, and only a small proportion (6 per cent.) appear to be permanently incapacitated as the result of head wounds. The conclusion that should be drawn from these follow-up reports is that the ultimate prognosis for patients with craniocerebral wounds after radical early operations is far more optimistic and cheering than seems generally thought to be the case.

The Treatment of Infected Craniocerebral Wounds.—The indications for, and the methods of treatment of, this class of cases are totally different from those for recent wounds. As already noted, the attempt to care for infected wounds in a similar manner led to disastrous consequences. Within twenty-four hours of the time of injury the wound may be definitely infected; wounds not operated on are almost certain to be infected by the time patients reach base hospitals. The indications for operation then vary within wide limits and no definite rules can be laid down. The neurologic manifestations and particularly the condition of the eye-grounds are often the decisive factors. Hernia cerebri or other infected lesions can often be successfully treated by the Carrel-Dakin or other non-operative methods for wound sterilization. If operation is decided on, it should be sharply limited to the area of infection, and equally limited to steps for the control of infection. Spreading infection and death may otherwise be the sequel. Loose bone fragments, bits of cloth, or other foreign material may have to be removed, and a purulent brain tract drained.

At best, the results were unsatisfactory in the cases I saw, whether or not secondary operations were performed. Neurologic manifestations and infection showed a tendency to persist and even to progress. The results were, of course, worse with dural penetration. If a hernia cerebri made its appearance the ultimate prognosis became bad, in my experience. Although the hernia may have receded with persistent efforts at wound sterilization, I found, by following the course of these cases, that the hernia often meant either early acute infection of the brain or the focus in the brain for the later development of a brain abscess.

Late Complications and Sequels of Wounds of the Head and Their Treatment.—Final statements upon this very important aspect of the subject of head wounds cannot be made at the present time. Tuffier and Guillain[10] and Sargent and Holmes[9] have made studies of large groups of cases, analyzing the results without direct reference to the types of operative technic that had been employed.

Subjective symptoms, such as those already noted, are without gravity as far as life is concerned, but of great importance from the social viewpoint. I have stated that they bear no relation to the gravity of the wound, yet that does not indicate the significance of subjective symptoms. The size of the cranial defect is not a factor, for they are as common in small as in large breaches in the skull. Possibly a form of malingering in some cases, they appear in others to have a definitely organic origin as established by examination of the eye-grounds and the cerebrospinal fluid. Lumbar punctures often seem to have a favorable effect on subjective manifestations, especially on headache and vertigo. Subjective symptoms in themselves should never be the sole indication for a secondary operation such as cranioplasty or removal of a foreign body.

Organic Manifestations.—Destructive cerebral lesions produce results that, of course, vary widely, depending on their seat and extent. Details cannot here be given. The outcome of lesions of the frontal lobe appears to be favorable, even with large losses of substance; many of the patients suffer no mental disturbance. The improvement that often occurs after lesions in the sensorimotor cortex has already been described. Involvement of the pyramidal tracts usually results in permanent spastic paralyses. The prognosis of persistent aphasia is bad; although some improve, the great majority remain intellectually subnormal. Visual defects from lesions of the occipital lobe have a relatively favorable prognosis, the early symptoms showing a tendency to recede and the residual disturbances often were slight.

Serious mental disturbances are exceptional, and in some cases precise information concerning the antecedent history would have been necessary to establish the causal relationship between the wound and the psychosis. Insanity occurred in 0.64 per cent. of the 6664 cases in the statistics of Tuffier and Guillain.

Epileptic attacks comprise the most common late complication, occurring in over 10 per cent. of the cases in Tuffier and Guillain's series. They may make their first appearance anywhere from a few months to two years after the injury, and even more delayed first appearances ·may be recorded in the future. Generalized seizures are more common than petit mal. Epilepsy has followed wounds in which the dura and even the skull were intact, as well as wounds with proved cerebral injury. Although lesions in the Rolandic area may be followed by epilepsy of the Jacksonian type, injury of the motor cortex as well as of other parts of the brain may result in generalized, non-focal seizures. The latter are, of course, of no aid in localizing the lesion. Occasionally epileptic attacks may be the first manifestation of an acute encephalitis or brain abscess.

Operation is not indicated in generalized epilepsy for the following reasons: There is no indication as to the region of the brain to be explored. The dura should not be opened at the site of the wound merely to divide adhesions that will almost certainly reform; besides, such adhesions are commonly met in old brain wounds in patients who are not suffering from epilepsy. If the purpose of the operation is to reduce tension, other means, such as lumbar puncture or a subtemporal decompression, are more desirable. Repeated lumbar punctures appear to have a favorable effect on the number of attacks. An exploratory operation on the cicatrix is perhaps permissible if the attacks progressively increase in frequency and appear to be leading to permanent mental inferiority.

Jacksonian seizures offer a more favorable indication for operation. A few isolated focal attacks should not, however, lead to operative intervention, for they may be the result of an encephalitis that may clear up, or, in any event, cannot be relieved by operation. The presence of sequestra or a missile in the region of the motor cortex is the chief reason for operation in repeated Jacksonian seizures, and their removal may be followed by prolonged relief.

Late brain abscess occurred in a little over 1 per cent. of the cases, and is thus happily much rarer than would have been supposed. This grave complication is most commonly seen after wounds in which brain substance was exposed and in wounds that have suppurated. A tear in the dura had existed in almost all the reported cases. Too great emphasis cannot be placed on the evidence that the missile itself is not the principal cause of brain abscess; infection from sequestra, bits of cloth or other foreign material swept into the brain is the common etiology. In fact, abscesses about missiles are met in only a small proportion of the cases. The abscess is found at the site of the wound in the majority of cases, either in an existing hernia or in brain substance that has herniated. Abscesses in regions far removed from brain tracts are occasionally found. In 37 cases studied by Sargent and Holmes the overwhelming frequency of brain abscesses in the first three to six months after injury is shown; 28 patients developed abscesses in that period, whereas the complication appeared in the six to nine months' interval in 7 cases. The latest appearance of brain abscess was in the eighteenth month.

In some cases of brain abscess there are no indications of its development, and in others the course is an acute fulminating one, but in the great proportion of instances the usual symptoms and signs of brain abscess are gradually unfolded. An important point is that papilloedema is frequently absent. It is often difficult to make the differentiation between abscess and encephalitis. The value of regularly repeated careful neurologic examinations in patients with old craniocerebral wounds will be appreciated when one realizes that the reappearance of or increase in an old mono- or hemiplegia that was improving, or increase of an aphasia, may be indications of the development of a brain abscess or important localizing signs of the seat of the abscess.

Brain abscess unrelieved by *operation* is fatal; yet the vast majority of patients (97.5 per cent. in Sargent and Holmes' series) die after drainage of pus. The least complicated procedures should be employed. The removal of a projectile or of sequestra in the abscess cavity is indicated, but the extent of dissection should be minimal under any circumstances if spreading infection is to be avoided. Subdural adhesions should not be disturbed. There may be a varying period of improvement following drainage of a brain abscess, but ventricular infection or further spread into the adjacent brain tissue with fatal issue are the common sequels. In my personal experience drainage of the abscess cavity has invariably been followed by death. On the other hand, there was one instance in which the patient has apparently remained free from recurrence for more than a year following *aspiration* of a deep-seated abscess. Such a procedure for brain abscess appears illogic at first sight, but several factors should be considered. The infecting organisms must be of low virulence in many cases. By aspiration of the pus collapse of the walls of the cavity is invited, or in rigid walled cavities a fresh exudation of bactericidal fluids. Drainage of a brain abscess frequently lights up the infection as a result of fresh paths that are laid open, and this appears to be almost inevitably the result, no matter what form of drainage is employed. Theoretically, then, superficially situated brain abscesses might better lend themselves to drainage; deep-seated abscesses, to aspiration. The abscess having been located, aspiration can be repeatedly performed if necessary. If drainage is to be employed, I believe a two-stage operation might be followed by less disastrous results. The first stage would consist in locating the abscess by aspiration, dissecting a tract to its site, and inserting a tube. Several days later the abscess would be entered and the drainage-tube inserted into the cavity.

Hernia cerebri is due to infection and generally masks an abscess or an area of encephalitis. Violent headache, high temperatures, torpor, and occasionally epileptic seizures precede its appearance. *Lumbar puncture should not be employed* in the acute phase, for it may be followed by spread of the infection. In the relatively favorable instances in which an encephalitis is the cause the protrusion may begin to recede in two or three weeks with one of the methods of wound sterilization; lumbar puncture aids in the reduction of the hernia under such circumstances. When an underlying brain abscess is the cause, this must, of course, be cared for. Excision or compression of the hernia or enlargement of the bony opening should be condemned. It may be necessary, however, to remove necrotic brain substance. In some cases of persistent hernia with a low-grade infection contralateral decompression has been done with favorable results; I have seen one case in which striking improvement followed.

Late meningitis is the most fatal of the tardy complications after craniocerebral wounds, but is fortunately rare (0.48 per cent.). As a sequel to brain abscess it has already been noted. Meningitis may also result from fistulæ arising from necrotic bone or infected foreign material. In its localized form the condition exists as an encystic meningitis, and is characterized by cortical irritation and the signs of increased intra-cranial tension. Operation, consisting in drainage of meningeal collections of pus and the elimination of the foreign material, is occasionally successful. The generalized type of meningitis is exceedingly fatal, although occasional cures have been reported following frequent large lumbar punctures.

Encephalitis is a condition difficult to differentiate from brain abscess. It can sometimes be recognized when local cerebral symptoms arise from time to time, to recede spontaneously. In general, the symptoms are not as severe as in brain abscess. They are known to have receded after removal of bone fragments or other foreign material, but have also cleared up after negative exploratory operations. If encephalitis can be diagnosed, operation is not indicated.

Retained missiles in the brain do not in themselves comprise a late complication of head wounds, for a considerable proportion of the patients are free from symptoms. The question arises as to whether foreign bodies should be systematically removed in all cases. This is answered in the affirmative by those who hold that the foreign bodies are only apparently well tolerated, and that the patients are exposed to the possibilities of grave complications, such as brain abscess, or to sudden death. But Pierre Marie, for example, has had under observation more than 80 cases of retained intracerebral projectiles in which there were absolutely no symptoms or signs referable to the foreign bodies. All the evidence at hand at the present time indicates that foreign bodies can be perfectly tolerated. Under such circumstances there should be no routine removal of retained missiles. The operation is not free from danger, and may result in the aggravation of existing disturbances in function, or the development of new neurologic manifestations. A destructive lesion of the brain having been established, removal of the foreign body will not improve it.

Headache, vertigo, and other subjective symptoms are not indications for the removal of the foreign body. It should be removed if it is the probable cause of attacks of encephalitis or of a brain abscess. Lymphocytosis in the cerebrospinal fluid, associated with signs of increased intracranial tension, suggest the desirability of operation. The method of choice for the removal of foreign bodies is an approach through the cicatricial tissue occupying the former tract, and extraction with the electromagnet.

Cranial Defects and Their Repair.—Many papers have been written on the indications for cranioplasty, and more on the technic to be employed. The confusion that exists on this subject will not be cleared up until the sequelæ with and without operation are better known than at the present time. Such symptoms as headache, vertigo, and even epileptic attacks are considered indications for cranioplasty by some, and these very symptoms are contraindications to operation for others. In a study of a number of cases operated on Marie found improvement in subjective

586

symptoms in some, no relief in a larger number, and aggravation of the manifestations in others. Even new symptoms are reported to have developed after operation. Under such circumstances a clear therapeutic indication for cranioplasty cannot be said to exist at the present time.

Cranioplasty may, however, be indicated for protection of the brain and for esthetic reasons; the latter is particularly true for large skull defects in the frontal region. An operation should not be performed until the wound has been healed for several months. Any symptoms that indicate the possibility of a late complication are contraindications; if such manifestations have already appeared, the operation is not justified, even though they are, for the time being, in the background. The cerebrospinal fluid and eye-grounds should show no evidence of increased intracranial tension.

Many types of operation have been performed for the repair of cranial defects, and good results have been reported after all of them. A description of the various operative procedures cannot be here given. They may be classified as follows:

  a. Cranioplasty, which is, strictly speaking, a procedure consisting in plastic flaps fashioned from the skull itself.

  b. Bone grafts, auto-, homo-, or heteroplastic, with or without periosteum.

  c. Grafts of decalcified or macerated bone.

  d. Cartilage grafts.

  e. Osteocartilaginous grafts.

  f. Prostheses of gold, platinum, silver, or ivory.

Cranioplasty, either of the Mueller-Koenig variety or one of its modifications, is only suitable for the smaller defects. It cannot be employed in the frontal region because of the additional scarring that results. Autoplastic bone and cartilage grafts are most widely used; excellent results have been described after both. Villandre, who has had a large experience, reports 100 per cent. success with osteoperiosteal grafts taken from the tibia, and 96.8 per cent. with rib-cartilage transplants. It is as yet too soon to make any definite statements concerning the ultimate fate of such autotransplants.

Application of the Experiences in Craniocerebral War Wounds to Head Injuries and Other Intracranial Lesions in Civil Life.—Cranial injuries with extrusion of brain substance are rarely seen in civil practice, but depressed fractures with or without dural puncture and brain damage are not at all uncommon. A soiled scalp wound is often present in such deeper injuries. It is for these cases that the operative technic as described for gunshot wounds has its main indication in head wounds in civil life. The operation heretofore practised has generally consisted in incision, piecemeal removal of depressed fragments of bone, removal of spicules from the brain, and institution of drainage. The results have, on the whole, been unsatisfactory. I have recently seen two cases in which brain abscess followed such operations. There is every reason to believe that a great stride forward will be made in the treatment of soiled cranio-cerebral wounds of civil life when the technic developed for gunshot wounds shall have been applied with the same meticulous attention to details. On the other hand, it would manifestly be a grave mistake to consider cerebral penetrations by small-calibred, relatively low explosive bullets of civil life in the same category with the injuries caused by war projectiles. In the former case relatively little foreign material is swept into the brain by the missile, the wound of the scalp is generally a non-soiled, punctured lesion, and thus the indications for a débridement of the tract do not exist in the vast majority of instances. Our knowledge as to the surgical treatment of complications encountered at operation has also been enhanced, and this has its direct application not only in traumatic surgery, but also in cranial operations for other conditions. The more logical methods of treatment of late complications of head wounds (epilepsy, hernia cerebri, etc.), evolved during the war, should improve the procedures employed in similar lesions encountered in civil practice. Indications for and methods of repair of dural defects were developed; they will probably have a wider application in cranial operations for other conditions than fractures. The indications for extraction of intra-cerebral projectiles and for repair of cranial defects have been more clearly defined, and the technic of operation greatly developed. Finally, the many advantages in conducting cranial operations under local anæsthesia, demonstrated during the war, will undoubtedly be recognized as existing to a similar extent in cranial operations in civil life, and thus another lasting addition to the technic will have been made.

BIBLIOGRAPHY

The voluminous literature is largely reviewed in the following two volumes:
War Surgery of the Nervous System. A Digest of the Important Medical Journals and Books Published During the European War, 1917. Office of the Surgeon General, Washington, D. C.
Velter: Plaies Pénétrantes du Crâne par Projectiles de Guerre, 1917, A. Maloine et Fils, Paris.
Other references are:
Cushing: Brit. Med. Jour., Feb. 23, 1918.
Cushing: Brit. Jour. Surg., 1918, vol. v.
De Martel: Trait. Opérat. Plaies du Crâne, 2d ed., 1918, Masson and Company, Paris.
Eisendrath: War Injuries of the Skull. A Collective Review, Surg., Gyn., and Obst., 1917, vol. xxv.
Leclere and Walch: Cranial Grafts, Bull. et Mém. Soc. Chir., Paris, 1196, vol. xlii.
Lemaitre: Lyon Chirurg., 1918, vol. xv, p. 65.
Sargent and Holmes: Injuries of Scalp, Longitudinal Sinus, Jour. R. A. M. C., 1918, xxv, p. 56.
Sargent and Holmes: Later Results of Gunshot Wounds of the Head, Jour. R. A. M. C., 1916, xxvii, p. 300.
Tuffier and Guillain: Comp. Rend. Confér. Chir. Interalliée p. l'Étude d. Plaies de Guerre, Paris, 1918, p. 263.

A NEW APPLIANCE TO SECURE PROPER POSITION AND STEADINESS OF THE HEAD DURING BRAIN OPERATIONS

By T. M. JOHNSON, M.D.

OF PHILADELPHIA, PA.

RESIDENT PHYSICIAN, JEFFERSON HOSPITAL

MANY appliances have been designed by surgeons and instrument makers to secure the combination of satisfactory position and firm retention of the head during operations upon the skull and brain. Some of these appliances have decided advantages, each of them has some disadvantages. A combination which will allow satisfactory exposure of the cerebrum may totally fail in permitting satisfactory exposure of the cerebellum.

The purpose of the table described in this article is to permit the placing and holding of the head in a position suitable for operation upon the cerebrum or the cerebellum. The position is attained by easily-effected adjustments.

The table used is the standard operating table with an angle-iron support at the head of the top of the table. On each side are two yokes bolted to the angle iron beneath the glass top. In the centre of the yoke a square rider 12 inches in length and ¾ inch in breadth is placed and holes are bored through it at intervals of ¾ inch. To hold the rider at the level desired, a set-screw is passed through it and into the yoke at the other side where it meets a threaded socket. These side pieces enable us to obtain a desirable height to fit the physique of the patient, and they also allow of the raising or lowering of the shoulders as the surgeon may desire.

The accurate adjustment of the appliance to the breadth of the shoulders of either an adult or a child is accomplished by an expanded portion with a tunnel at the top of the head. This is ¾ inch square. Through it the threaded pieces move laterally or medially as desired. A thumb-screw holds the sliding shoulder pieces. A flared-out shoulder rest 4 inches long and padded with gauze accommodates each shoulder.

By raising or lowering the side pieces and sliding the shoulder supports in and out, the height from the table and the breadth of the shoulders can be adjusted and the instrument can be held in place by two thumb-screws, one through the rider and yoke for elevation, the other in the top of the rider through the sliding shoulder rest. As the pieces are square, composed of ¾-inch steel and held by the threaded thumb-screws, there is no danger of twisting, dropping or unsteadiness of the apparatus when in use.

The head rest is, of course, the more important consideration. The

37   589

standard operating table has a glass plate on either side with a space of 2 inches between the plates. Two rolled-steel rods, each ⅜ of an inch in diameter, threaded at each end and bolted, are fastened to the angle iron beneath the glass plates. On these is placed a saddle bored out to accommodate each rod, the saddle being so designed as to ride back and forth on the rods. On each side of the saddle a thumb-screw is used to fix it in place when the proper position has been ascertained. These screws come flush against the rods.

To obtain the desired height for the head, a hole is made in the centre of the saddle ¾ inch square and through this hole the centre rod of the head support can be raised or lowered and the proper height is set, the thumb-screw beneath the side is tightened. We gauge the distance for long necks and short necks by simply moving the saddle along the rods and setting the screws. The proper distance is quickly found and is certainly maintained.

By means of this simple mechanical device set on a standard table a steady head and shoulder rest is readily obtainable and the surgeon can have a patient upon the face or upon the back as desired. We have found that when a patient is on his back, by simply raising the riders of the shoulder pieces and lowering the head piece an excellent position is obtained for surgical work on the face and on the neck.

The appliances in ordinary use not unusually are out of order when wanted, are hard to adjust, or fail to give exactly the proper position, or lack steadiness.

This instrument can be applied to the operating table in a few minutes. It can be removed by simply loosening the two thumb-screws in the two rods and the three in the saddle and slipping out the pieces, and the table is again the ordinary table for everyday surgical procedures.

The cuts indicate the simplicity and arrangement of the apparatus.

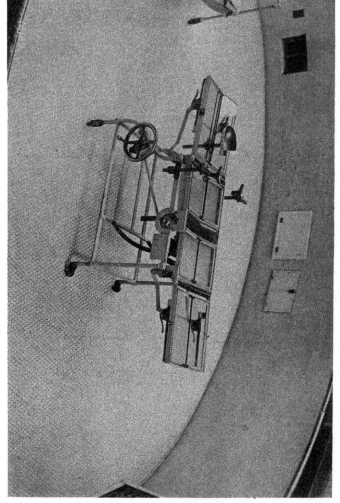

FIG. I.—Apparatus adjusted to standard operating table.

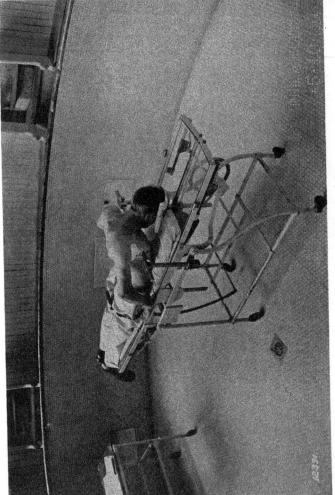

Fig. 2.—Patient posed for exposure of cerebellum.

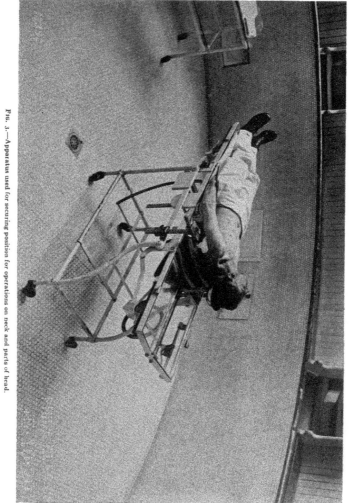

Fig. 3.—**Apparatus** used for securing position for operations on neck and parts of head.

PERFORATING GASTRIC AND DUODENAL ULCER *

By Charles E. Farr, M.D.

of New York, N. Y.

Of the acute abdominal crises perforation of a gastric or duodenal ulcer ranks easily first in its dramatic suddenness of onset, its violence of symptomatology, and its gravity.

During the past six years I have operated upon twenty-four of these acute perforations with three deaths, a mortality of 12½ per cent. Contrary to the usual statistics, a large majority of my cases have been gastric rather than duodenal, but with one exception, all were within 3 inches of the pyloric ring.

The duration of acute symptoms has been within the twenty-four-hour period in all but two cases, both of which died, and many cases were within twelve hours. The peritonitis was localized to the site of perforation in all except the two fatal cases mentioned. The ulcer base varied in size from 2 to 8 cm. and the perforation from 3 to 8 mm. Closure was easily effected in all save two, to be described later in this article. Infolding mattress sutures of fine chromic gut, in two layers, widely placed, were used exclusively. Posterior gastro-enterostomy was done but once, the details of which will be given later.

No " toilet " of the peritoneum was carried out and no drainage used for the uncomplicated cases. The appendix was found markedly involved in all cases and removed except in the three fatal cases and one other very poor risk. One case had a coincident acute cholecystitis and appendicitis. The appendix was removed and the gall-bladder drained. Two cases with coincident cholecystitis and cholelithiasis were treated by partial cholecystectomy and drainage.

Recovery in all but the fatal cases was remarkably smooth and uncomplicated except for a few mild superficial infections.

The end-results in the twenty-one recovered cases are known in about one-half the cases. Two came to gastro-enterostomy for pyloric stenosis. Of these one had had a previous perforation sutured in another clinic. Both were completely relieved. All the remaining cases seemed entirely free from ulcer symptoms and were in excellent general health when last examined.

The diagnosis in all the uncomplicated cases was obvious on the most cursory examination. The exceptions are as follows:

Case I.—A man, aged about forty years, with a history of lues and definite signs of tabes. He had had repeated gastric crises. For

* Read before the Clinical Society of Montclair, June 7, 1920.

about twenty hours he had had severe epigastric pain. Tenderness and rigidity were moderate. There was a slight rise in temperature and in the leucocytes. Operation revealed a small ulcer near the pylorus with perforation a few mm. in diameter. Recovery was uneventful.

CASE II.—Colored female. She was in very poor general health, had signs of tuberculosis of the lungs and rather marked hyperthyroidism. An ulcer of the lesser curvature had been discovered by X-ray and was being treated medically, but she became unmanageable and left the hospital. In a few hours she returned with severe pains and signs of perforation. She was quite hysterical and persisted in sitting upright. Nothing could persuade her to lie down. Operation disclosed an ulcer on the posterior surface of the stomach near the lesser curvature and an acute cholecystitis with cholelithiasis. The ulcer was œdematous and bled freely, but had not completely perforated. It was infolded with great difficulty, the gall-bladder removed nearly entirely, and drainage inserted. Recovery was quite stormy and protracted.

CASE III.—Male, white, aged about forty years. Attack began six hours previously and was typical in all symptoms except that as in Case II the patient persisted in sitting upright and could not be induced to lie down for more than a few seconds. Operation revealed a perforated ulcer near the pylorus and an acute cholecystitis. The gall-bladder was removed, drains were inserted, and recovery was uneventful.

CASE IV.—Male, white, aged about forty years. The history and signs in this case were typical except that the temperature and tenderness were excessive and the leucocytes were high. Operation revealed an acute cholecystitis and cholelithiasis with perforation into the duodenum. Possibly this case should not be included in an ulcer series, but an acute perforation of the duodenum certainly had occurred. A partial cholecystectomy was performed, drainage instituted, and no attempt made to close the perforation. Recovery was delayed and rather troublesome, but finally was complete.

CASE V.—Male, white, aged forty-five years. Had definite ulcer symptoms and had been given a positive diagnosis of duodenal ulcer five years before the acute onset. He was a Christian Scientist, however, and refused treatment. At the end of this time a severe hemorrhage brought him to terms and he began medical treatment. During a month he gained 8 pounds and seemed on the way to recovery when he had a sudden onset of violent pain with slight rise in temperature, pulse, and leucocytes. At operation a very large ulcer involving the pylorus, duodenum, and stomach was found, with perforation into the pancreas from the duodenal side. No safe operative approach was possible and a posterior gastro-enterostomy was done to relieve the stenosis. A drain was inserted. He made a fair rally for twelve hours, but succumbed at the end of thirty-six hours from asthenia. Post-mortem examination showed no extension of the peritonitis and no especial reason for the fatal outcome.

In another similar case I would be tempted to do a simple jejunostomy rather than a gastro-enterostomy. I did not realize his weakened general condition. Of the two other fatal cases, one was in a very stout alcoholic with advanced cirrhosis of the liver and a perforation of several days' standing, with generalized peritonitis. The ulcer was very large and appeared possibly malignant. Death occurred about twenty-four hours after operation. No post-mortem was permitted. The third fatal case was in a feeble subject also, with cirrhosis of the liver. Perforation had occurred two days previously and there was a marked spreading peritonitis. No drainage was used. The wound was opened the following day and drains inserted, but death occurred from exhaustion on the following day. All the cases showed a free perforation except three, two of which have been previously described. The third showed a perforation covered by the liver and partially sealed.

The diagnosis of acute perforation of the stomach or duodenum is remarkably easy except in the complicated cases. On the other hand, acute perforations of the gall-bladder from gangrene, acute pancreatitis, and occasionally high-lying perforated appendices will give symptoms suggestive of stomach perforation. In no case that I have seen, however, has there been any such onset of agonizing pain, nor such board-like rigidity in the first few hours. After twenty-four hours, of course, the symptoms are masked by the spreading peritonitis.

Shock has never appeared to me to be present in any of the cases. Vomiting is not the rule, either.

One case of error in diagnosis caused me great chagrin. A soldier was suddenly taken violently ill at midnight with intense epigastric pain. Examination showed extreme rigidity of the abdomen, and the previous history of loss of weight and vomiting of blood with "dyspepsia" seemed to clinch the diagnosis. The ward surgeon was summoned and, much to my disgust, was able to demonstrate the symptoms were all assumed and that the real diagnosis was a very mild attack of "flu." To the best of my recollection this is the only non-surgical case I have seen at all simulating an acute perforation.

That perforations do occur which become quickly adherent and closed is undoubtedly true. I have seen a few that might possibly have been such, besides one that had gone on to a local abscess formation. Many times adherent scars suggestive of old healed perforations are found at operation or post-mortem. The great majority of acute perforations, however, go on to spreading peritonitis and death if not closed surgically.

The treatment of acute perforations is obvious and, moreover, is easily carried out in nearly all cases. A simple high laparotomy and suture of the opening can be done in a very few minutes. The only question of other procedure is whether a gastro-enterostomy should be added. Deaver urges that this be done in all cases. Conners is just as strongly opposed. Many surgeons, like Peck, take a middle ground, doing the gastro-enterostomy in cases seen early and without peritonitis.

The argument for gastro-enterostomy, of course, is that it tends to aid in the healing of the ulcer and to obviate a later operation for resulting stenosis. On the other hand, it is well known that by far the greater number of all perforating ulcers tend to heal promptly after closure and that reperforation, hemorrhage, and stenosis are exceptional sequelæ. Moreover, it is difficult, if not impossible, to tell at the time of operation whether or not stenosis will occur. The mere fact that it is present after the suturing has been done is not conclusive, as it is very improbable that such stenosis will persist. When one considers how difficult, if not impossible, surgeons have found the operation of pyloric occlusion, surely it can hardly be thought a few fine chromic sutures will bring about this end.

To my mind, however, the strongest arguments against the added operation are twofold. First, the added immediate mortality will be considerable. Even in the hands of such masters of surgical technic as Peck, Deaver, and the Mayos, there is a certain, although low, mortality for gastro-enterostomy, even in non-acute cases. Second, the end-results of gastro-enterostomy, even in the best clinics, are not 100 per cent. good. When one considers that by far the great majority of these acute perforations will always be operated upon by surgeons of much less skill and experience, especially in gastric surgery, it would seem only the part of wisdom to do the simple life-saving operation and await the result, with a later gastro-enterostomy for the small percentage of those requiring it. I feel sure that I voice the feelings of most conservative medical men, including surgeons, in saying that I would not care to have a gastro-enterostomy done on myself if it could be avoided.

The cause of gastric ulcer is yet unknown, but the occurrence of chronic appendicitis in such a large proportion of the cases is suggestive of one etiological factor. Other chronic infections probably have a similar relationship.

In my cases it was usually difficult or impossible to obtain any history of chronic gastric disturbance before operation, but afterward when the severe mental and physical distress were abated, close questioning usually elicited a fairly typical ulcer history.

In conclusion, twenty-four cases of acute perforation resulted in eventual cure in twenty-one patients. One of the fatal cases was hopeless at the time of operation and the other two were in very grave condition.

Early diagnosis and simple closure of the perforation will result in cure in a very large proportion of cases. Gastro-enterostomy should be reserved for the few who may need it later.

I wish to express my most sincere thanks to Doctors Charles L. Gibson, Alfred Taylor, and William Luckett, in whose service these cases, with two exceptions, occurred, and to whom I am deeply indebted for the privilege of publishing them.

NOTE.—Since this paper was read one more case has been operated upon by me in the service of Professor Gibson, the Cornell Division of the New York Hospital. Recovery ensued after a very stormy convalescence.

PERSISTENCE OF PYLORIC AND DUODENAL ULCERS, FOLLOWING SIMPLE SUTURE OF AN ACUTE PERFORATION *

By Richard Lewisohn, M.D.

of New York, N. Y.

ATTENDING SURGEON, BETH ISRAEL HOSPITAL; ASSOCIATE SURGEON, MOUNT SINAI HOSPITAL

There is a prevalent idea that an acute perforation of an ulcer of the stomach or duodenum will result in the spontaneous disappearance of the ulcer. For this reason many surgeons claim that all that is necessary in a case of acute perforation is simple closure of the perforation in order to prevent leakage of gastro-intestinal contents. They consider gastro-enterostomy as an unnecessary, rather dangerous procedure in these cases.

I think we can safely say that operative recoveries are not impaired by an immediate gastro-enterostomy. Reports have been published by advocates of the simple suture method, showing the good operative results of that procedure and warning against the extensive use of gastro-enterostomy in these cases. Shea[1] has reported a series of 9 consecutive cases without death in which he performed simple suture. Gibson[2] has reported 14 cases with one death; thirteen of these cases had simple suture. On the other hand, Deaver,[3] who is a strong advocate of immediate gastro-enterostomy, has reported 25 cases with one death. My personal series comprises 10 consecutive cases without a death. Eight of these ten cases had a gastro-enterostomy performed. Two of the patients were operated upon in 1919, one in 1918, two in 1917, two in 1916, and three date back to 1915. Seven of the patients have been reëxamined during the last few months, whereas I was unable to trace three (one simple closure, two gastro-enterostomies). The seven cases which I reëxamined consisted of one simple suture and six gastro-enterostomies. All the six cases that had gastro-enterostomies performed are entirely well. They are now free from all the symptoms from which some of them had been suffering for years previous to the perforation. The seventh case (simple closure on account of very bad general condition, July, 1919) is still complaining of pains and fullness in the epigastrium and occasional vomiting. The X-ray shows a considerable residue in the stomach after six hours. I have advised him to have a gastro-enterostomy performed.

---

* From the Wimpfheimer Division for Gastro-enterological Surgery (Service of Dr. A. A. Berg), Mount Sinai Hospital.

[1] Shea: A report of nine successive operations for perforated gastric and duodenal ulcers. Annals of Surgery, 1916, 64, 410.

[2] Gibson: End-results of fourteen operations for perforated gastric and duodenal ulcers. Surg., Gyn. and Obst., 1916, 22, 388.

[3] Deaver: Acute perforated duodenal and gastric ulcers. Annals of Surgery, 1913, 57, 703.

Up to the present he has not consented to a secondary operation.[4]

The main points which have been dwelt upon by the opponents of immediate gastro-enterostomy are the spreading of infection and the undue lengthening of the operation. The spreading of infection is a more or less theoretical objection. If the perforation has occurred into the free peritoneal cavity, the whole peritoneum is already infected and the gastro-enterostomy does not spread the infection. If we are dealing with a walled-off perforation and a localized peritonitis, the rest of the peritoneal cavity can be safely protected by packing; the gastro-enterostomy can then be done in a clean field. A gastro-enterostomy can be performed so rapidly that the small loss of time will not play any rôle in the operative end-results. The Murphy button ought to be used in cases of acute perforation, as this method requires less time than a suture gastro-enterostomy.

The great advantage of an immediate gastro-enterostomy, especially if combined with a pyloric exclusion, is based on the fact that the after-treatment (feeding of the patient) is considerably simplified as compared with simple closure. The main advantage, however, of immediate gastro-enterostomy in cases of acute perforated pyloric or duodenal ulcers is the curative effect on the ulcer. The perforation, usually pin-pointed in character, occurs in the centre of the ulcer. In the majority of cases we encounter a rather large indurated area surrounding the perforation. In closing the perforation we approximate the normal serosa and muscularis surrounding the ulcer, and thus push the ulcer-bearing area into the gastro-intestinal lumen. The ulcer, however, is still exposed to the traumatic injuries of the food and to the anomalies of the stomach (hyperacidity).

There can be no doubt that simple closure of the perforation will fail to cure the patient in a large number of cases. I have had occasion to observe four such cases in the short period of two years. These cases had, with the exception of one case (Case II), been previously operated upon in other hospitals for perforated ulcers. In every instance the operative procedure consisted in simple closure of the perforation and drainage of the peritoneal cavity. They were admitted to Mount Sinai Hospital because of the persistence of symptoms after the performance of the operation (simple suture).

CASE I.—S. M., aged forty-one years; admitted March 9, 1917; discharged March 31, 1917.

Diagnosis.—Pyloric stenosis and post-operative ventral hernia.

History.—The patient was operated eight years ago for perfor-

---

[4] I reoperated upon this patient in June, 1920. He had a perforated duodenal ulcer, walled off by the under surface of the liver. The opening admitted a lead pencil. The operation consisted of closure of the perforation, suture gastro-enterostomy and pyloric exclusion. He made an uneventful recovery. The simple closure of the perforation had neither effected a cure of the ulcer nor prevented a recurrence of the perforation.

ated ulcer. He has complained for the last three years of hunger-pain, nausea, and constipation.

X-ray Examination.—The stomach is markedly ptosed; its tone is fair, and the peristalsis normal. The duodenal bulb is complete and somewhat tender. The motility of the stomach is practically normal. A slight residue is present after six hours. The findings are suggestive of duodenal ulcer.

Operation (Doctor Berg).—March 13, 1917. Stomach and duodenum are densely adherent to the anterior abdominal wall. The adhesions are very thick around the pylorus. They were carefully liberated. Typical gastro-enterostomy; ventral hernioplasty.

Post-operative Diagnosis.—Pyloric stenosis due to adhesions.

Reëxamination, February 20, 1920: The patient has felt perfectly well since the second operation. All his previous symptoms have disappeared.

CASE II.—J. B., aged thirty-nine years; admitted January 21, 1917; discharged February 9, 1917.

Diagnosis.—Duodenal ulcer.

History.—Patient was operated upon at Mount Sinai Hospital by Doctor Berg in 1912 for perforated duodenal ulcer, with diffuse purulent peritonitis. The operation at that time consisted in suturing the defect and in extensive drainage. The patient was free from attacks for two years. He has complained since 1914 of abdominal cramps coming on two or three hours after meals and lasting one hour, occasionally accompanied by vomiting. He has frequent gaseous eructations. He suffers from constipation. He has lost about 13 pounds.

X-ray Examination.—The duodenal bulb is complete, the peristalsis very active. There was no tenderness over the stomach nor over the duodenum. The X-ray examination does not warrant the diagnosis of recurrent ulcer.

Operation (January 27, 1917) (Doctor Berg).—A large indurated ulcer with a definite crater was found in the first part of the duodenum just beyond the pylorus. A typical suture gastro-enterostomy, combined with a pyloric exclusion, was performed. Uneventful recovery.

Reëxamination.—July, 1917: Patient feels perfectly well and has been relieved of all previous symptoms.

A reëxamination at the present date is impossible, as the patient is serving a five years' sentence in the State Prison.

CASE III.—S. B., aged forty-two years; admitted February 28, 1918; discharged March 24, 1918.

Diagnosis.—Duodenal ulcer.

History.—The patient was operated upon one year ago for perforated ulcer of the stomach. The symptoms (pains after meals and belching) persisted after the operation. He does not vomit. The symptoms became worse in the last few weeks (frequent belching and sour eructations).

X-ray Examination.—The stomach is markedly ptosed, its tone is poor. The peristalsis is hyperactive with marked incisures around the pylorus. The duodenal bulb was not seen fluoroscopically. Its appearance on plates is rather irregular. The motility of the stomach is delayed, a slight residue being present after six hours.

Operation (March 2, 1919) (Doctor Berg).—A small ulcer is present in the duodenum. The ulcer was excised and the opening closed with chromic gut. Button gastro-enterostomy and pyloric exclusion. The specimen shows a small hard ulcer, with the suture material from the previous operation *in situ.*

Post-operative Course.—The patient developed a hemiplegia and aphasia on the third day post-operative. His post-operative course, as far as the abdomen was concerned, was uneventful. He was discharged from the hospital March 24, 1918.

Reëxamination.—March 1, 1920.—The second operation has resulted in complete relief from all his abdominal symptoms. All the severe symptoms which persisted after the first operation have disappeared entirely. He eats everything. He is still suffering from a slight amount of aphasia.

CASE IV.—A. W., aged thirty years, admitted February 13, 1919; discharged March 15, 1919.

Diagnosis.—Pyloric ulcer.

History.—The patient was operated upon ten months ago for perforated gastric ulcer. The symptoms subsided for three months, then recurred. She complains of burning pains in the epigastrium, which have no definite relation to meals. She has distinct remissions of her symptoms. The pain is often followed by vomiting, which relieves the pain. No hæmatemesis. Bowels are markedly constipated. She is very weak and has lost considerably in weight.

X-ray Examination.—Shows a markedly dilated stomach and increased peristalsis. There was a slight irregularity of the gastric contour in the region of the pylorus. The duodenal bulb could not be visualized properly. No food was seen passing the pylorus during the first twenty minutes. After that period the food started to pass the pylorus, but very slowly. The motility of the stomach was delayed, a marked residue being present after six hours.

The dilated stomach, the irregularity of the pyloric region, the increased peristalsis, the inability to visualize the bulb, and the delayed motility suggest a lesion in the pyloric region.

Operation (March 1, 1919) (Doctor Lewisohn).—The stomach was found to be adherent to the anterior abdominal wall. A large ulcer was found on the anterior wall of the stomach near the lesser curvature, in the region of the pylorus. The ulcer was hard, about the size of a hazelnut. It showed a scar on the serosa, where it had perforated previously. Suture gastro-enterostomy and pyloric exclusion.

Reëxamination (March 1, 1920).—The patient feels perfectly well. The symptoms (pains, vomiting) from which she was suffering after her first operation have disappeared entirely.

These four cases show that the theory that a perforation will automatically cure an ulcer is incorrect. In two of our cases the symptoms persisted for eight and five years, respectively, and the patients were promptly relieved of their symptoms after the performance of a gastro-enterostomy and pyloric exclusion. In one case the ulcer was excised; the other cases did not lend themselves to this procedure.

The findings in the first case did not show an ulcer, though it is very possible that a small ulcer was overlooked on account of the dense adhesions around the pylorus.

It is customary to drain the peritoneal cavity after the closure of the perforation. This drainage (tube or packing) is apt to cause the formation of adhesions between the pylorus and duodenum, the neighboring organs (liver and gall-bladder, etc.), and the anterior abdominal wall. Thus the outlet of the stomach becomes partly obstructed and its motility is delayed. Gastro-enterostomy will safeguard proper drainage in spite of the formation of these adhesions.

CONCLUSIONS

1. Immediate gastro-enterostomy in the treatment of perforated pyloric and duodenal ulcers does not increase the mortality.

2. Gastro-enterostomy and .pyloric exclusion simplifies the postoperative treatment considerably.

3. Simple closure of the perforation will not cause a cure of the ulcer in a considerable number of cases.

4. Gastro-enterostomy will guarantee proper drainage of the stomach contents and overcome partial obstruction of the pylorus caused by postoperative adhesions.

5. Closure of the perforation, gastro-enterostomy, and pyloric exclusion should be the method of choice in the treatment of perforated pyloric and duodenal ulcers. Simple closure of the perforation should be reserved for only those patients whose general condition is so poor that even a rapidly performed gastro-enterostomy would be too much of an operative risk.

CARCINOMA OF THE DUODENUM

By EDGAR R. McGUIRE, M.D.

OF BUFFALO, N. Y.

PROFESSOR OF SURGERY IN THE UNIVERSITY OF BUFFALO

AND

PERCY G. CORNISH, JR., M.D.

OF BUFFALO, N. Y.

CARCINOMA of the intestine is quite rare, forming a very small percentage of all carcinomata. Brill estimates 2.5 per cent. The Mayo Clinic reports 3 per cent. Jefferson reports 3.1 per cent., while Geiser reports 4 per cent. A variety of explanations have been offered for this rarity by various authors, all in accordance with their views on the cause of cancer in general. Some believe that the liquid nature of the contents of the small intestine gives its mucosa a freedom from trauma, as compared with the large intestine. Others hold the abundance of the pancreatic secretion responsible. Those who uphold the parasitic theory believe the comparative sterility of the small intestine has an influence. The imperfect knowledge as to the origin of cancer in general makes such speculations idle.

Inch for inch the site of election for carcinoma of the small intestine seems to be the duodenum, though its total occurrence in the jejuno-ileum is slightly greater than in the duodenum, as shown by the following table:

TABLE I

	Duodenal	Jejuno-ileum
Köhler	9	3
Mayo	5	17
Nothnagel	7	11
M. Müller	6	3
Rüpp	1	1
Barnard	5	10
Lubarsch	2	2
Fr. Müller	6	2
Maydl	2	4
Schlieps	20	16
	63 47.7 per cent.	69 52.3 per cent.

The rarity of carcinoma of the duodenum is well shown in Table I of the hospital autopsies following death from all causes.

This table shows a percentage of 0.033 for duodenal cancer.

In the duodenum the distribution of carcinoma is quite striking. Geiser reports 71.8 per cent. in the second part, while Fenwick reports 57 per cent. and Rolleston 67 per cent. Carcinoma of the second or papillary portion of the duodenum is extremely hard to differentiate from carcinoma of the ampulla—at operation or autopsy—so rapidly do they destroy

600

TABLE II

	Autopsies		Duodenal carcinoma
Maydl	20,480	Wiener Allgemeines Krankenhaus	2
Nothnagel	21,358	Pathologic Institute, Vienna	5
Perry-Shaw	17,652	Guy's Hospital	4
W. S. Fenwick	19,518	London Hospital	18
McGlinn	9,000	Philadelphia General Hospital	1
Achleringer	42,000	Vienna	7
M. Müller	5,621	Berne, 1886–1891	6
Fr. Müller	11,314	Basle, 1874–1904	6
Rüpp	4,248	Zurich	1
	151,201		50

all traces of their origin. Ampullary carcinoma has been thought very uncommon, but the preponderance of the peri-ampullary cancers in the duodenum would lead one to believe that many of them have their origin in the ampulla, and are not true duodenal cancers at all. The first part is affected somewhat more frequently than the third, as shown by the figures of Geiser, 11–9; Forgue and Chauvin, 17–12; Fenwick, 11–7, and Rolleston, 8–3. They are usually cylindrical-celled adeno-carcinoma from the intestinal mucosa. Various theories are advanced as to their origin. Orth believes they arise from Brunner's glands, others consider pancreatic rests found in about 1 per cent. of autopsies to be the points of origin, while some believe aberrant stomach glands to be the primary site. Some emphasis has been laid on old duodenal ulcer as a causative factor in cancer of the first part. Lichty has reported six cases of carcinoma of the first part, none of them at the usual site of duodenal ulcer. He also states that the incidence of carcinoma arising on duodenal ulcer is as 1–80, while that of gastric cancer on old ulcer is as 1–2¼. Jefferson has been able to collect only thirty-one cases—some of them very doubtful, and concludes that the relationship of duodenal ulcer to duodenal carcinoma is extremely difficult to establish.

In reporting the following cases we are conscious of the fact that two of them should not be classed as duodenal carcinomata. The first two cases are primarily carcinoma of the bile-duct with secondary involvement of the duodenum, and really should be definitely distinguished from carcinoma of the duodenum when estimating the frequency of the latter lesion. This is a very frequent error, as many of the reported cases evidently arise from the bile-duct, and we are reporting these two cases to emphasize this point. The two remaining cases are definitely primary in the duodenum, and should be added to the proven cases of the disease.

CASE I.—H. S., aged forty-six years, male. Admitted to the Buffalo General Hospital April 10, 1916, complaining of increasing jaundice, pain and discomfort in the upper abdomen. The jaundice began about six weeks prior to admission, but the pain and discomfort were of long duration, having led to a diagnosis of cholecystitis several years before admission. Had lost weight in the past few

601

weeks. Operation revealed a small mass at entrance of the common duct into the duodenum. Common duct dilated, probe inserted revealed no stone. Cholecystostomy done. Patient died a few days after operation. Autopsy showed a small growth at the papilla of Vater, which on microscopic examination proved to be carcinoma.

CASE II.—A. C., aged sixty-eight years, male. Admitted to the Buffalo General Hospital February 5, 1910, under the care of Dr. Charles G. Stockton. Patient in very poor condition, complaining of nausea, vomiting, jaundice, and loss of weight. Until a few months before admittance he had been in perfect health. He first began to be troubled with nausea and vomiting after meals—not accompanied by pain, but becoming progressively worse. At admission he was unable to retain anything. He became markedly jaundiced shortly after the onset of his symptoms, and had continued so. Had lost a great deal of weight. Stomach showed typical carcinomatous findings. No palpable mass, stomach not dilated. Operation under very light anæsthesia showed a large carcinoma of the duodenum, involving the entrance of the bile-ducts. The condition of the patient was desperate, so that a hurried anterior gastro-enterostomy was done, and the wound closed. The patient rallied after the operation, but died suddenly the following morning. No autopsy allowed.

CASE III.—A. G., aged fifty years, female. Admitted to the Buffalo General Hospital October 16, 1918, with a history of upper abdominal pain, for a period of three or four months—particularly after taking food. This had necessitated a change of diet, until at admission she was taking only semi-solids and fluids. There had been no evidence of pyloric obstruction. She had lost about 30 pounds in weight in the past three months. X-ray examination negative, as was also fluoroscopic examination. There was no palpable mass. Operation showed mass infiltrating around lower border of liver, and connecting with the duodenum. Pylorus entirely free, the connection being about one and one-half inches below it. The mass was considered inflammatory from a perforated ulcer, and was broken into for the purpose of drainage. No pus was found and as the interior of the mass looked malignant, a piece was removed, which on microscopic section proved to be carcinoma of the duodenum. A tube was put into the opening of the duodenum, and the patient given fluids through this for a few days. There was an uneventful recovery. The patient left the hospital and has not been heard from since.

CASE IV.—A. M., aged forty-six years, male. Admitted to the Buffalo General Hospital October 28, 1918, with history of old stomach trouble of mild character. In the last few months this had grown worse, with increasing inability to retain solid food, until at admission, could retain only fluids. Had lost 49 pounds in weight in the last few months. There was no jaundice. X-ray showed an obstruction apparently at the pylorus. Wassermann negative. Operation revealed a hard mass about two inches below the pylorus, about the size of a walnut; further exploration showed a secondary mass in the liver; this was about the size of a marble. Posterior gastro-enterostomy was done, the patient making a good recovery. After leaving the hospital the patient was put on intensive anti-syphilitic treatment, but without benefit. He died about four months later, extremely cachectic.

BIBLIOGRAPHY

Fenwick, W. S.: Cancer and Other Tumors of the Stomach. London, 1902.

Maydl-Nothnagel: Diseases of the Peritoneum. Am. Med. Assn., 1905.

Mayo, W. J.: Carcinoma of the Gastro-intestinal Tract. Collected Papers of the Mayo Clinic.

Brill: Primary Carcinoma of the Duodenum. Am. Jr. Med. Scs., November, 1914, cliv, p. 824.

Rolleston: Carcinomatous Stricture of the Duodenum. Lancet, 1901, i, p. 1121.

Geiser: Ueber Duodenalkrebs. Deutsche Zeits. Chir., 1907, lxxvi, p. 41.

Forgue-Chauvin: Le Cancer Primitif et Intrinsique du Duodenum. Rev. de Chir., December, 1915.

Jefferson: Cancer of Supra-papillary Duodenum. British Journal of Surgery, October, 1916.

Lichty: New York State Journal of Medicine, November, 1918.

Orth: Lehrbuch Spec. Pathology, 1887, l, p. 850.

Kohler: Quoted by Eichorst in Handbuch der Speziellen Pathologie und Therapie. Wien, 1887, Bd. ii.

Müller, M.: Beiträge zur Kenotness der Metast-cisenbild Malig. Tumoren. Berne, 1892.

Müller, Fr.-Rüpp: Quoted by Hinz. Ueber den Primaren Duodenalkrebs. Arch. of Clin. Chir., 1912, xcix, p. 305.

Barnard: Contributions to Abdominal Surgery. London, 1910.

Lubarsch: Ueber den Primaren Krebo des Ileum. Virchow's Arch., 1888, xi, p. 280.

Schlieps: Beiträge z. klin. Chir., 1908, lviii, p. 722 (Lit.).

Perry-Shaw: On Diseases of the Duodenum. Guy's Hosp. Rep., 1893, l, p. 274.

McGlinn, quoted by Outerbridge: Carcinoma of the Ampulla of Vater. ANNALS OF SURGERY, 1913, lvi, p. 402.

Schlerenger, quoted by G. D. Head: Am. Jr. Med. Scs., 1919, No. 2, clvii, p. 182.

PTOSIS OF THE THIRD PORTION OF THE DUODENUM WITH OBSTRUCTION AT THE DUODENO–JEJUNAL JUNCTION *

By Eric P. Quain, M.D., F.A.C.S.

of Bismarck, N. D.

Pathologic descent of the third portion of the duodenum associated with obstruction at the duodeno-jejunal junction has been given almost no attention by the numerous students of visceroptosis. That there are many individuals suffering from chronic digestive disturbances because of this condition is certain. The symptoms may vary in severity from occasional mild attacks of nausea and vomiting to an almost constant invalidism from duodenal obstruction and retention. The symptoms may simulate cholecystitis, gastric or duodenal ulcer or appendicitis, and patients have been operated under such mistaken diagnoses, but, of course, without the expected relief.

The writer has had the opportunity to operate on several patients for this condition and the results have been so satisfactory that a more careful study of the symptoms, causes, methods of diagnosis, and the technic of surgical relief has seemed highly justified.

The usual symptoms are: Epigastric distress or pain beginning and lasting a variable period after meals; periodic attacks of headache; nausea and vomiting of bile—the classic " bilious attack." The pain is usually not severe enough to incapacitate the patient from work, except during the period of vomiting. During these attacks a couple of days may be spent in bed before the duodenum ceases to regurgitate. Fluoroscopic examination of the stomach and duodenum with barium meal will demonstrate the low situation of the dilated loop, as well as the obstruction to the emptying of the duodenum.

At operation the dilated duodenum may protrude into the abdominal cavity like a large pouch below the transverse mesocolon. The jejunum is abnormally small and the obstruction at the duodenal junction is plainly visible. In all the cases operated the superior mesenteric vessels and an abnormal ingrowth of fibrous bands along these vessels have been the apparent immediate cause for the obstruction. More fundamental causes will not be discussed at this time.

In view of the futility of medical treatment in the more aggravated cases and of the impossibility of relieving the obstruction satisfactorily without causing damage to the superior mesenteric artery, a short-circuiting operation was adopted. Duodeno-jejunostomy was made between the bulging duodenum and the descending jejunum. This operation was made in five patients in the years 1916 and 1917. The results have been all that could be desired in the four patients who have been

* Subject presented at the Western Surgical Association, December 19, 1919.

under observation. No report has been obtained from the fifth, but on leaving the hospital this patient was apparently cured from a previous p. c. nausea and distress.

The following clinical history describes one of the two most aggravated of the five cases. A correct diagnosis was not made before incision. With more röntgenologic experience it has been possible later to diagnose the trouble by means of the fluoroscope. It is believed that this pathologic condition of the duodenum is a disease not at all uncommon, and that more careful search with fluoroscope and more diligence in abdominal exploration will prove this belief to be well founded.

E. N., school girl, seventeen years old. With the exception of scarlet fever and measles she was in normal health until about the age of eight, when present trouble began. Chief complaint: " Pain in stomach." During first three or four years the pain would come on immediately after eating and last one-half to one hour. The pain seemed to be worse every second day and was often associated with vomiting of bile. After profuse emesis there would be a certain amount of relief for a day. During the next four or five years the pain and emesis were less constant, but there was vomiting of bile at least once a week. Appendectomy made three years ago did not give relief. The pain has become much worse during the past three months. It is present after each meal and sometimes before breakfast. Quality of food makes no difference. It is worse when riding than when walking. She has a constant, dull headache. Vomiting of bile takes place almost daily and is followed by relief from pain until after the next meal. Bowels are constipated and move only every two to five days. Laxatives increase pain.

Family History.—Father died from accident. Mother well, but thin and looks poorly nourished; has had " poor digestion " always. Brothers and sisters well.

Examination.—Girl rather small in stature, thin and anæmic; narrow chested, thoracic organs normal. Abdomen somewhat prominent, muscles relaxed. Narrow through epigastrium; evident ptosis of stomach and intestines. Very tender to deep palpation in epigastrium and to right of navel. Gall-bladder region not tender. Ptosis of both kidneys. Blood examination showed a simple anæmia and the urine had a trace of albumin. Test meal showed gastric juice practically normal; barium meal and X-ray proved a ptosis of the stomach and to a point near pubes. There was no retention in the stomach and no abnormality found in its walls, but part of meal was found in second portion of duodenum. Most of meal was in ileum (partly confused, no doubt, with the unsuspected descended loop of duodenum), and some in cæcum, both lodged in the pelvis. It was surmised that a chronic ulcer of the duodenum with possible adhesions and traction caused the chief symptoms, and operation advised.

Operation (November 25, 1916).—Median incision. Examination of stomach on both sides negative, except for its abnormal descent. Duodenum showed no evidence of ulcer, but there was a definite membrane attached to the lower part of the descending portion and passing upward and outward to become incorporated with the under surface of the liver to the right of the gall-bladder. Gallbladder and ducts seemed normal and were entirely free from the membrane. There were no palpable lymphatic glands about the duodenum or pylorus. The cæcum rested in the pelvis, and so did the big bulk of the small intestines. A small omental tag was adherent at the old appendiceal scar. When the transverse colon and omentum were lifted up, it was found that the third portion of the duodenum had descended from its usual situation behind the transverse mesocolon and occupied a pocket behind the peritoneum. It was markedly dilated and formed a " U " with its angle reaching to a point near the pelvic brim. The distal end passed upward to the superior mesenteric artery. This ascending part was over two inches in diameter, with a decided thickening of the walls. The dilatation ended abruptly at the superior mesenteric artery in an abnormally narrow jejunum. The dilated duodenum contained fluid and gas and formed a pouch which extended forward into the abdomen, the small jejunum and its mesentery resting against the side of the pouch. It was clear that the bowel was constricted at the point where it passed the superior mesenteric artery and that the constriction had been chronic enough to cause both dilatation and hypertrophy of the duodenum. Moreover, there could be no doubt as to this being the lesion causing the persistent symptoms.

An effort was made to push the duodenum upward, but to retain it in an elevated position so as to insure certain and permanent drainage past the obstruction, seemed impossible. It would have required extensive dissection and preparation of space behind the peritoneum at a higher level together with a permanent closure of the large pocket now chronically occupied by the ptosed organ. Release of the obstruction by dissection of the fibrous ingrowth about the superior mesenteric vessels would have jeopardized their function. It was concluded, therefore, to make an anastomosis between the duodenum and the jejunum, for the purpose of short-circuiting the duodenal contents. An incision one and one-half inches long was made in the peritoneum over the most prominent part of the ascending part of the duodenum. The duodenum was pulled out sufficiently through this incision to permit easy placing of two rows of sutures, an outer linen and an inner chromic catgut—Quain's sewing-machine stitch—around an opening one inch long through the duodenal and jejunal walls. A few plain catgut sutures fastened the margins of the peritoneum to the suture lines and obliterated the small gap between the two loops of bowel above the anastomosis. The wound was closed and the patient made a rapid and uncomplicated recovery.

All abdominal symptoms, with the exception of a continued sluggishness of the bowels, disappeared after the operation. Final results, December, 1919, three years after operation: Had no further stomach trouble; general health excellent; gained 30 pounds in weight; graduated from Normal School.

JEJUNO–COLIC FISTULA *

By MARTIN WARE, M.D.
OF NEW YORK, N. Y.

THE unique characteristics of this case without a parallel in literature, precisely diagnosticated before operation and successfully dealt
with, urge the narrative thereof.

Past History.—J. K., aged fifty-five years, operated thirteen
years ago for hemorrhoids. Five years ago Dr. I. Haynes resected
6 inches of transverse colon and performed a lateral anastomosis for
the removal of an annular carcinoma which manifested itself with
symptoms of intestinal obstruction. Forty-eight hours after operation fecal vomiting and hiccup set in and persisted for two weeks at
intervals. Seven days after operation fecal discharge appeared on
the dressings. At the expiration of the third week patient left the
hospital. The abdominal wound had given way to a large extent,
and because of the continued drainage for two months a long healing of the wound followed. Three months after the operation patient gained thirty pounds. Another three months he began to
complain of pains, unlike the colicky pains before operation, referred
to the left of the umbilicus—digestion and bowels operate regularly. He continued gaining weight up to one year after operation,
and within the next six months he fell off in weight. About this time
(two years after operation) liquid movements day and night, much
flatus, borborygmi, and attacks of pain set in with slight bleeding.

Physical Examination.—Doctor Haynes vouches for the fact that
palpation did not disclose any tumor mass, and Dr. S. Unger, who
conducted X-ray examination, reports colon is normal in outline
with apparently no obstruction in the entire length. In the prone
position the transverse colon is normal, but in the erect posture it is
completely ptosed and encroaches on the sigmoid and rectum.
There are no signs of adhesions at either hepatic or splenic flexure.

Present History.—July, 1919. In 1917, two years after the operation cited above, Mr. J. K. rapidly and progressively lost weight
and flesh, notwithstanding a voracious appetite offset by copious
diarrhœal movements shortly after the ingestion of food throughout
the day and night. These were accompanied by borborygmi and
visible peristalsis and great tympanites and a reduction of weight to
97 pounds. In addition there was a ventral hernia due to a diastasis
of the recti M.M. throughout the length of the abdomen.

Believing at first that the diarrhœal condition was due to some
ulcerative or catarrhal process, I gave large doses of bismuth sub-
nitrate and atropin. The diminution of stool was but temporary.

* Presented before the Surgical Section of the New York Academy of Medicine,
April, 1920.

There was no febrile movement and the patient presented the picture of inanition. This latter impression, together with the pertinent statement of the patient that " what struck him peculiar was that he was possessed of great hunger and that his food seemed to go right through him," led me to the assumption that there was perhaps a communication somewhere between the small intestine and the large gut, due to a perforation from recurrence of the carcinoma. At no time was the stool formed and always accompanied by much flatus, the expulsion of which relieved him. I had recourse to X-ray examination. The report of Dr. C. Gottlieb follows:

Radiographic Examination.—The radiograms obtained either with the barium contrast meal or enema did not disclose any filling defect or stricture characteristic of a recurrence of the carcinoma. On the other hand, the large intestine was conspicuously dilated in its entire continuity. In the screen and in the picture, the barium injected (Fig. 1) or ingested (Fig. 2) was seen to pass from a loop of small intestine high up into the large intestine near the splenic flexure, and *vice versa*. This loop of small intestine shows the striations of the barium-coated valvulæ conniventes by which it was identified. It was dilated, but not so much as the large gut. The outline of the balance of the intestinal tract is wanting. In fact, the ingested barium did not even reach the ileum to sufficiently outline its transition into the cæcum.

The X-ray confirms and locates a communication between a loop of the small intestine, high up, by a small ostium, with the large gut in the vicinity of the splenic flexure.

Operation.—Upon laparotomy by an incision extending the entire length of the abdomen there was no evidence of fluid or scattered miliary deposits of carcinoma. The liver surface and substance were free of any nodules. No enlarged glands encountered in the mesentery or transverse mesocolon. Some adhesions enveloping the omentum, small intestine, and colon were divided. A large extent of small intestine identified as ileum leading down towards the cæcum was found collapsed. A loop of gut identified as jejunum adjacent and intimately fused with the large dilated big gut, proximal to the splenic flexure was divided along the line of adhesion, thereby disclosing the stoma. The defect in both the jejunum and the colon, the size of a lead-pencil, was closed by a purse-string of chromic gut reinforced by a Lembert suture of the same material. Exploration of the site of the lateral anastomosis failed to reveal any evidence thereof other than a larger extent of dilatation in the transverse colon than obtained in the rest of the extent of the colon. Even the transverse mesocolon appeared normal and the haustræ could be traced uninterruptedly over the colon. To overcome the wide diastasis of the recti the abdomen was closed by overlapping side to side of the sheath harboring the atrophied recti.

Post-operative Course.—Within twenty-four hours the diarrhœa so incessant by day and night ceased, never to return. After the fourth day in the face of primary union a light diet was instituted, in turn followed by regular diet. On the fifth day the bowels were first

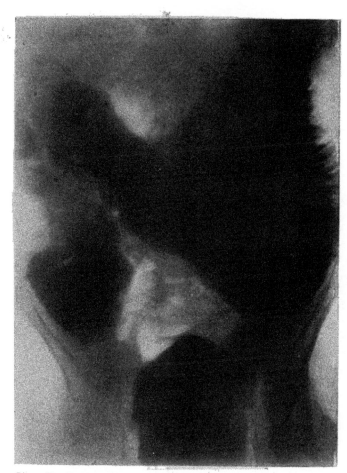

FIG. 1.—Bismuth enema passing from splenic flexure into small intestine outlined by striations of valvulæ conniventes.

608ª

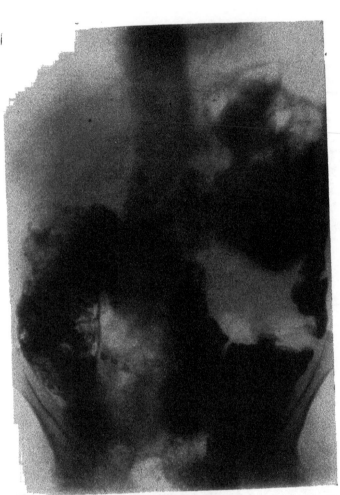

FIG. 2.—Bismuth test meal passing from stomach leaving empty the ileum and being driven into colon by way of jejunal fistula.

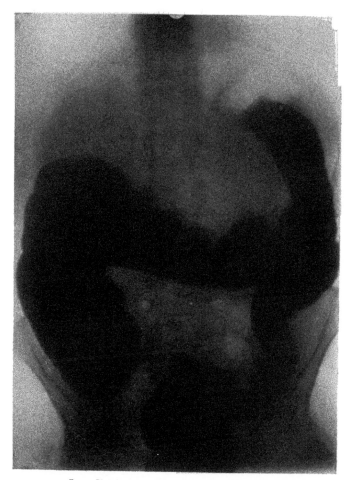

FIG. 3—Bismuth enema recently given showing normal conditions.

moved by pituitrin given intravenously. Thereafter they were made to move by laxatives which were abandoned, owing to the speedy return to spontaneous movements. By the tenth day the patient began to feel stronger. At the time of leaving the hospital on the fourteenth day he was able to walk unaided, having gained 5 pounds above his weight of barely 100 pounds at the time of operation. Up to date he has gained over 40 pounds and enjoys the best of health. The barium X-ray enema of the intestinal tract (Fig. 3) shows restoration of normal conditions.

Comment.—Two and a half years after the otherwise successful operation for removal of the growth, signs of disorder relative to the fistula first became manifest. An X-ray at this time, however, did not disclose the existence of any such process, whereas with the persistence of symptoms X-rays one and one-half years later conclusively demonstrated the fistula. This long interval that lapsed between the operation and the signs of the fistula makes it unlikely that error in suture was responsible for this development. On the other hand, it is more plausible to assume the fistula as incident to the suppuration at the site of the anastomosis. Adherence between the loops of gut was inevitable, harboring a focus of infection which slowly went on to ulceration and perforation. In view of the fact that fistulous communication between the stomach and colon (gastro-colic) arises after a legitimately executed gastro-jejunostomy and which have been assigned to wandering of the non-absorbable sutures, I draw upon the Pagenstecher thread that was used for the anastomosis. Beyond this it is difficult to reconstruct the sequence of events that may have led to this jejuno-colic fistula.

THE RELATION BETWEEN INTESTINAL DAMAGE
AND DELAYED OPERATION IN ACUTE
MECHANICAL ILEUS *

By Frederick T. Van Beuren, Jr., M.D.
of New York, N. Y.

A NUMBER of fascinating theories have been suggested to explain the immediate cause of death in acute mechanical ileus and some of them have given real, practical assistance to the operating surgeon. The "toxæmia" theory has supported the rationality of intestinal drainage, while the "tissue desiccation" theory has affirmed the value of replacing the water lost by vomiting. But there is forced upon the mind of anyone who examines a considerable series of cases of this condition one conclusion which is of the utmost significance. Subject to certain exceptions, it might be stated as a corollary that, if the case is really one of acute mechanical ileus, the longer a patient lives with it before operation, the sooner he dies afterwards! Everyone knows this; and almost everyone acts as if he had forgotten it when he is faced with a case occurring in the convalescence of a patient upon whom he has operated for some other condition.

Acute ileus due to strangulated hernia usually receives fairly prompt attention; but a patient whose intestinal obstruction depends upon adhesion-angulation or peritoneal band-pressure arising in the course of an operative convalescence frequently waits the limit before the attending surgeon makes up his mind to perform an operation that ought to have been an early exploratory, but which often turns out to be a sort of ante-mortem examination. This paper is a thinly disguised brief for early exploration in cases of suspected acute mechanical ileus.

There are several good reasons for urging early exploration, familiar to everyone but frequently forgotten. For example, the longer the ileus exists unrelieved, the greater the patient's fluid loss, the poorer his circulation, the greater his prostration, and the worse his general condition. Moreover, it is probable that the poisonous character of the stagnated gut contents is enhanced during the interval. And it is in most cases unquestionable that the damage to the gut itself increases the longer it is obstructed. This factor was so clearly evidenced in some animal experimentation done in the course of third-year teaching at the College of Physicians and Surgeon last winter—experiments in which the duration of the obstruction was definitely known—that I have thought it worth

---

* From the Laboratories of the Department of Surgery, College of Physicians and Surgeons, Columbia University.
Read before the New York Surgical Society, April 28, 1920.

while to demonstrate the specimens here with the specific intention of urging the plea they make for early operative interference.

Fifteen dogs were operated under ether anæsthesia, and ileus was created by ligating or by dividing the jejunum within 30 cm. of its upper end. The object was to demonstrate the lesions, the course, and the treatment of acute mechanical ileus to third-year students, and care was taken to create a simple obstruction without strangulation of the mesenteric vessels. One dog died within twenty-four hours, and in two there was failure to maintain complete obstruction on account of the cutting through of the ligature; but, in the remaining twelve, complete obstruction was maintained until the intestines had been examined at operation or at autopsy. Four dogs were examined (Nos. 1123, 1169 (Fig. 1), 1173 (Fig. 2), and 1174) at the end of forty-eight hours after the onset of obstruction. Six dogs were examined (Nos. 1130, 1144 (Fig. 3), 1145 (Fig. 4), 1171, 1172, and 1131) at the end of seventy-two hours after the onset of obstruction, and two dogs were examined at later periods, No. 1173 (2) (Fig. 5) at the end of about ninety-six hours, and dog No. 1176 (Fig. 6) at the end of one hundred and eighty hours after onset of obstruction. One of the dogs, who was examined at the end of forty-eight hours and was relieved at that time by resection with lateral entero-enterostomy, showed recurrence of ileus symptoms on his fourth post-operative day, and died four days later on the night of his seventh to eighth post-operative days. Autopsy showed an angulation ileus at the site of the anastomosis, which had presumably existed about ninety-six hours. This made thirteen cases of ileus in twelve animals and accounts for No. 1173 appearing in two places in the series. Of the five intestines examined at the end of forty-eight hours or less, only one showed any gross damage. Of the eight which were examined at the end of seventy-two hours or more, all showed gross damage, excepting two of those in the seventy-two-hour group. In other words, 25 per cent. of the early group showed intestinal damage, and 60 per cent. of the late operative group showed intestinal damage. It would appear from this observation that the third twenty-four hours is a rather critical period in the course of an acute simple obstruction where no element of strangulation of the mesenteric blood supply complicates the condition. In four of these late cases the evidence of damage, aside from distention and thinning of the wall, consisted in the appearance of discolored areas varying in color from purple to green, and in size from ½ to several cm. (Figs. 3 and 6). These areas were taken to be areas of beginning necrosis, areas of beginning gangrene, if you like, because gangrene of the intestine is no more nor less than the persistent interruption of the blood supply, accompanied or followed by the invasion of bacteria and the resultant destruction of that portion of the wall involved in the process. They are apparently dependent upon the intestinal distention, for they were found only in the markedly distended guts, and only one case of marked distention failed to show them (Fig. 4). The distention was in all cases chiefly a gaseous one, and although the cause of the gas formation is not entirely clear, its effects are fairly apparent. The gut becomes distended to three or four times its normal diameter, with a resultant arithmetical increase in its circumference and a geometri-cal increase in its volume. The greater the distention of the intestine the less the residual elasticity of its wall and of the vessels in it. As for the vessels themselves, their elongation results in a narrowing of the lumen and a thinning of the walls. The thinning of the walls results in greater compressibility. These conditions are maximum at the antimesenteric border of the intestine, where the terminal vessels anastomose; and, fail-ing any interference with the mesenteric vessels, tissue damage is earliest and most apparent on the·antimesenteric surface, where these discolored areas were seen. Their shape often corresponds with the distribution of the terminal vessels; and this irregular diamond shape, with its long axis across the intestine, is fairly well seen on the closed end of the oral loop in dog No. 1176 (Fig. 6). A good indication of the same appearance is also observable in the specimen from dog No. 1144 (Fig. 3), although a longitudinal section for microscopic examination has been taken from its middle. If this necrosis extends through the wall, perforation occurs with resultant peritonitis. If the distention is relieved early enough the necrosis may remain superficial, and may heal by scar formation, or by adhesion to omentum or to other viscera. If it is relieved too late, the necrosis may progress to perforation in spite of the relief of the disten-tion. Illustrations of these two possibilities were seen in dog No. 1123, relieved after forty-eight hours' obstruction, and in dog No. 1131, relieved after seventy-two hours' obstruction. In the forty-eight-hour case an area of beginning necrosis was seen about 8 cm. from the pylorus at opera-tion, and after aspirating the intestinal contents by needle through it, it was purse-stringed and the obstruction relieved by resection and anasto-mosis. The dog recovered, and, at autopsy a month later, the duodenum was found firmly adherent to the under surface of the liver throughout the area where the necrotic spot had been seen previously. In the seventy-two-hour case several spots of beginning necrosis were seen at operation, and an effort was made to remove them by resection while the obstruction was relieved by anastomosis. The dog died forty-eight hours after the relief operation, and autopsy disclosed a diffuse peritonitis, due to duode-nal perforation about 15 cm. from the pylorus, and a localized abscess around a leaky anastomosis as well.

Parallel with the increase in intestinal damage went the increase in the mortality of the operated cases in our little experimental series. Dogs Nos. 1123, 1173, 1174, and 1175 were relieved at the end of forty-eight hours. Dogs Nos. 1130, 1131, 1171, and 1172 were relieved at the end of seventy-two hours. Resection of the intestine was done in all but two of the eight cases, and lateral anastomosis was done six times, and end-to-end anastomosis was done twice. Only one of the forty-eight-hour

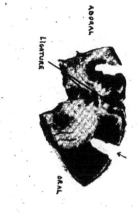

FIG. 1.—Dog No. 1169 (Surg. Path. No. 5035). Intestine examined forty-eight hours after onset of ileus. Longitudinal section showing obliterated lumen at ligated point and little change in thickness of wall. Distention within normal limits. No evidence of gross damage. Arrow points to removal of section for microscopic.

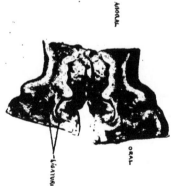

FIG. 2.—Dog No. 1173 (Surg. Path. No. 5922). Intestine examined forty-eight hours after onset of ileus. Longitudinal section showing obliterated lumen at point of ligation and little change in thickness of wall. Distention within normal limits. No evidence of gross damage.

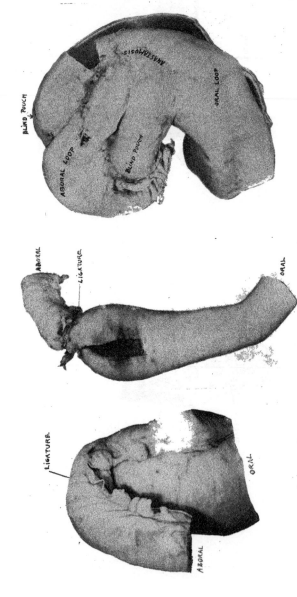

FIG. 3.—Dog No. 1145 (Surg. Path. No. 5883). Intestine examined seventy-two hours after onset of ileus. Showing marked distention of oral segment with thinning of wall above ligature but no evidence of gross damage.

FIG. 4.—Dog No. 1144 (Surg. Path. No. 5882). Intestine examined seventy-two hours after onset of ileus. Showing distention beyond normal limit of oral segment with thinning of wall and area of beginning necrosis (roughly diamond-shaped area with long axis transverse to long axis of intestine—dark colored) through which section has been taken, exposing lumen.

FIG. 5.—Dog No. 1173 (Surg. Path. No. 5944). Intestine examined seventy-two to ninety-six hours after onset of ileus. Showing intestinal anastomosis with distended oral and collapsed aboral segments due to obstruction of stoma from adhesion-angulation of aboral segment. Wall of oral segment markedly thinned and discolored segment. Wall of oral segment markedly thinned and discolored due to distention beyond normal limits.

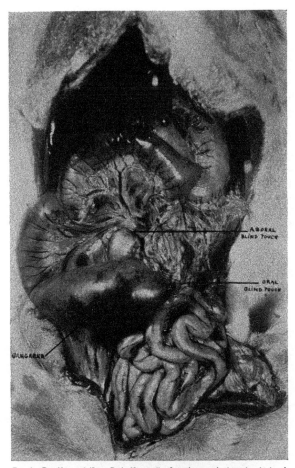

FIG. 6.—Dog No. 1176 (Surg. Path. No. 5946). Intestine examined one hundred and eighty hours after onset of ileus. Showing collapsed gut aboral to section of jejunum and distended discolored gut oral to obstructed point. Note the coalescent areas of diamond shape on the antimesenteric surface of oral segments, near inverted end due to distention beyond normal limits.

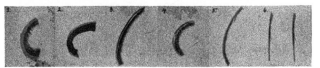

FIG. 7.—Dogs Nos. 1169, 1173, 1145, 1144, 1173, 1176. Showing relative thickness of sections taken from intestinal walls after various periods of obstruction. Nos. 1 and 2, forty-eight hours after onset. Nos. 3 and 4, seventy-two hours after onset. No. 5, seventy-two to ninety-six hours after onset. No. 6 one hundred and eighty hours after onset. The progressive thinning-out is due to the progressive distention.

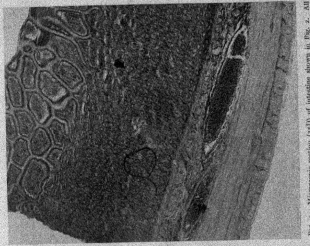

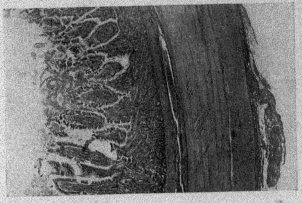

Fig. 8.—Microscopic section (35D) of intestine shown in Fig. 1. All coats of wall intact; layer of mucosa which shows some destruction of villi.

Fig. 9.—Microscopic section (35D) of intestine shown in Fig. 2. All coats intact. Note flattening of surface, due to pressure, and thrombosed vessel in submucosa.

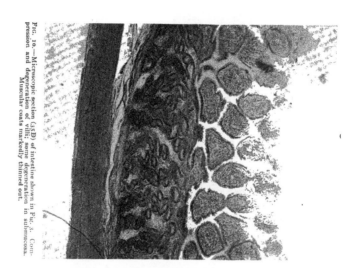

Fig. 10.—Microscopic section (35D) of intestine shown in Fig. 3. Compression and degeneration of villi; some degeneration in submucosa. Muscular coats markedly thinned out.

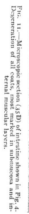

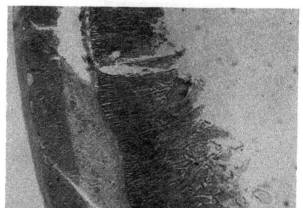

Fig. 11.—Microscopic section (35D) of intestine shown in Fig. 4. Degeneration of all coats, most marked in submucosa and internal muscular layers.

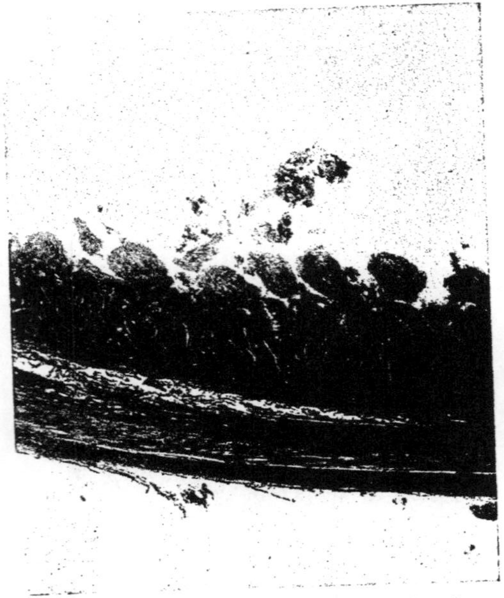

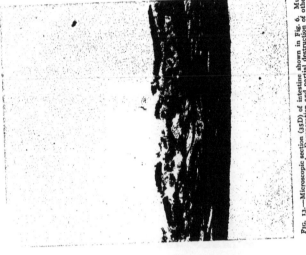

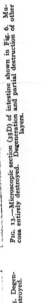

Fig. 12.—Microscopic section (35D) of intestine shown in Fig. 5. Degeneration and thinning out of all coats. Villi practically all destroyed.

Fig. 13.—Microscopic section (35D) of intestine shown in Fig. 6. Mucosa entirely destroyed. Degeneration and partial destruction of other layers.

operation group died—No. 1174—while only one of the seventy-two-hour group recovered—No. 1171. In other words, 75 per cent. of the forty-eight-hour obstructions recovered, and 75 per cent. of the seventy-two-hour obstructions died after operation. On the basis of such evidence as this one feels justified in urging early operation, exploratory, if you like, in cases of suspected acute ileus, without waiting for an absolutely positive diagnosis.

PROTOCOLS OF CASES REFERRED TO IN THE SERIES

Dog No. 1169 (Surgical Pathology No. 5935).
January 17, 1920: 11.00 A.M. Ileus by ligation of jejunum 30 cm. below duodenal-jejunal flexure (upper fixation).
January 19, 1920: 1.00 P.M. Died (fifty hours post onset of ileus) after showing marked symptoms of vomiting, prostration and constipation.

   Autopsy.—About two hours post mortem. Local peritonitis in R. U. Q., with serosanguinolent exudate. Occlusion complete. Duodenum and jejunum oral to ligature moderately distended (2 cm. and superficial vessels congested). No evidence of permanent damage due to circulatory interference. M.M. normal to gross appearance. Intestine below ligature collapsed and pale. Pancreas pale. Apparent hemorrhage into it.

   Microscopic.—Specimen taken 2 cm. oral to ligature. The wall is intact. All coats are relatively normal, although there are small scattered areas of blood extravasation and degeneration in the muscularis and submucosa and some œdema. There is quite marked degeneration of some of the villi of the mucosa.

Dog No. 1173 (Surgical Pathology No. 5922).
January 17, 1920: 11.00 A.M. Ileus by ligation of jejunum 30 cm. below duodenal-jejunal flexure (upper fixation).
January 19, 1920: 11.00 A.M. (Forty-eight hours post onset.) Relief by resection of ligated portion with lateral anastomosis of oral to aboral segments (after showing marked signs of vomiting, moderate prostration and constipation).

   Operative Findings.—No leakage or peritonitis. Ligature is not visible, and smooth glistening peritoneum extends across the furrow which indicates its situation. Obstruction is complete. No signs of permanent damage due to circulatory interference. Intestine is 3 cm. in diameter above ligature and 1 cm. below it. M. M. normal to gross appearance.

   Microscopic.—Specimen taken 1 cm. oral to ligature. The wall is intact. All coats are relatively normal and show no degeneration. The vessels of the submucosa are congested and some are thrombosed, and there are a few extravasations of blood in the submucosa and muscularis.

Dog No. 1144 (Surgical Pathology No. 5882).
January 3, 1920: Ileus by ligation of jejunum about 17 cm. below upper fixation.
January 6, 1920: Chloroformed after showing some vomiting, moderate prostration and constipation.

   Autopsy.—Immediate. No leakage or peritonitis. Obstruction complete. Duodenum is moderately dilated and congested, but shows no marked damage till a few cm. above ligature, where a marked dilation exists (about 3 cm. in diameter) and an area of dark purplish discoloration about 1 cm. in diameter on the anti-mesenteric surface, with a surrounding area of lighter color 2 cm. in diameter. It is believed to be a beginning necrosis of the wall like that seen in other cases, one of which perforated. The wall of the dilated portion is thinned out and the m. m. directly beneath the discolored area appears to be ulcerated.

Microscopic.—Section taken through discolored area. The wall is moderately thinned, and its integrity is threatened by a very marked degeneration of the submucosa and inner muscular coats. The serosa and outer muscular coat are relatively normal and the mucosa shows only a little degeneration of its villi.

Dog No. 1145 (Surgical Pathology No. 5883).

January 3, 1920: Ileus by ligation of jejunum about 17 cm. from upper fixation.

January 6, 1920: Chloroformed after showing very few signs of obstruction (does not eat or drink, but looks well).

Autopsy.—Immediate. No leakage or peritonitis. Obstruction complete. All organs look normal except intestine. Except for marked distention and congestion, duodenum appears fairly normal. No evidence of permanent damage due to circulatory interference.

Microscopic.—Section taken 2 cm. above ligation. The wall is moderately thinned, but its integrity is preserved. The superficial part of the mucosa is markedly degenerated and the stroma of its deeper part infiltrated by round-cells. The submucosa is thinned and partly degenerated, but the muscularis and serosa, although very markedly thinned, are otherwise relatively normal.

Dog No. 1173 (Surgical Pathology No. 5944).

January 17, 1920: Ileus by ligation of jejunum about 30 cm. from upper fixation.

January 19, 1920: Relief by resection of ligated portion and lateral anastomosis of oral and aboral segments. No vomiting for five days. On the fifth day he had a small bowel movement. None after that, and obstruction probably became complete that day.

January 24, 1920: Onset of recurrent ileus due to angulation of gut at anastomosis.

January 27, 1920: Found dead in cage seventy-two to ninety-six hours after onset of recurrent ileus.

Autopsy.—Several hours after death. Local peritonitis in R. U. Q., where loop of duodenum and jejunum are bound by soft adhesions to each other and to liver and omentum. Stomach enormously distended with gas (13 cm. in diameter). Duodenum descending moderately distended and shows purple area at middle, where it is somewhat angulated. Remainder of duodenum and jejunum above anastomosis greatly distended, progressively more so towards anastomosis, where oral segment measures 4 cm. in diameter and shows patches of purplish-green discoloration apparently beginning gangrene. Wall is thin in this area and m. m. is bile-stained and rugæ flattened. Some apparent ulceration in m. m. Aboral segment collapsed and pale, and angulated so as to form obstruction at anastomosis.

Microscopic.—Section taken from oral loop opposite anastomosis. The wall is greatly thinned out, but all coats are present, and the integrity of the wall is preserved. The villi of the mucosa are completely degenerated and the stroma of its deeper part widely infiltrated by round-cells. The submucosa is compressed and the inner muscular coat partially degenerated. The outer muscular coat and serosa are relatively normal.

Dog No. 1176 (Surgical Pathology No. 5946).

January 17, 1920: Ileus by section of jejunum (with inversion of ends) 15 cm. from upper fixation.

No vomiting observed for seventy-two hours post operation, then vomited q. d., but only moderate amount. Had one small constipated stool (one hundred and twenty hours) on fifth day post onset of ileus. Prostration grew progressively more marked and died the night of the seventh day post onset of ileus (one hundred and eighty hours, about).

January 24, 1920, or January 25, 1920: Died during the night. Found dead in A.M., January 25, 1920.

Autopsy.—About thirty-six hours post mortem (in ice-box meantime). No leakage. No free fluid. No peritonitis except locally, where adhesions have bound duodenum to under surface of liver and jejunum; to wound in outer wall and omentum to inverted end of jejunum. Stomach pale and contracted. Duodenum and oral segment of jejunum greatly distended with progressive increase to point of section just above which a large greenish purple area of beginning gangrene appears on antimesenteric surface. This area is irregular in shape, 5 cm. long and 3 cm. in greatest width. It corresponds to the distribution of the terminal branches of the intestinal vessels. The diameter of the gut at this point is about 4 cm. and the wall reduced to approximately ½ mm. thickness. The intestine below section is pale and contracted.

Microscopic.—Section taken through area of discoloration. The wall is extremely thin and the integrity of the wall is lost. The m. m. is absent and the inner muscular coat almost completely degenerated. The outer muscular coat and serosa retain their integrity, but show many blood extravasations.

THE ORTHOPÆDIC TREATMENT OF BURNS.*

By Anthony H. Harrigan, M.D.

of New York, N. Y.

ASSOCIATE VISITING SURGEON FORDHAM HOSPITAL; ASSISTANT VISITING SURGEON ST. FRANCIS HOSPITAL

AND

Samuel W. Boorstein, M.D.

of New York, N. Y.

ADJUNCT ORTHOPÆDIC VISITING SURGEON, MONTEFIORE HOME AND HOSPITAL. ADJUNCT ASSISTANT VISITING SURGEON
FORDHAM HOSPITAL CHIEF ORTHOPÆDIC SURGEON, FORDHAM DISPENSARY

(From the First Surgical Division of Fordham Hospital, the Service of
Dr. Alexander Nicoll)

Since deformities in general can be prevented the orthopædic treatment
of burns should be properly emphasized and detailed. Unfortunately,
however, the leading text-books pass rapidly over this phase of the problem. As a result, medical students receive very little instruction concerning this problem. It is not until they merge into general practitioners
that the treatment of burns becomes of interest and moment, and even
then, occasionally, the incapacitating and crippling deformities may be
overlooked. Of course, the actual deformities following extensive and
deep burns are well known, for these unfortunates with their disabling
scars and contractures are extremely common visitors of the clinic. From
these patients can be elicited, as a rule, the history of numerous and
unavailing operations to correct the deformity and to prevent the recontraction of the scar tissue.

The orthopædic surgeon, by applying the braces or plaster casts commonly used in the treatment of anterior poliomyelitis, peripheral neuritis,
etc., may prevent these contractures. During the war many new devices,
plus the use of fenestrated plaster casts, were employed to use in similar cases. But, it would appear, that some simpler methods are desirable
and applicable for the use of the general practitioner.

We have not only used extremely simple methods in the First Surgical Division of Fordham Hospital, but have gone a step further, in
instructing and interesting the internes and nursing staff, with the ultimate purpose that, every patient admitted with a burn, no matter what
degree, receives immediate attention upon admission. From this co-
operation we have noted, to our great satisfaction, that no contractures
have developed. Indeed, even the nurses in the ward, who have become
acquainted with the technic, and who have learned how to keep the
limbs in proper position, administer the treatment often before the
patients are seen by the house surgeon. Of course, we are not discussing
at present the specific methods of treating burns, such as by paraffine,

---

* Read before Bronx County Medical Society, June 19, 1919.

616

electric light, etc., but are merely pointing out the necessity of prevention of deformities.

MacLeod, in his book on "Burns and Their Treatment," devotes but one paragraph to this topic, though he mentions that the limbs must be kept in a proper position during the process of healing. He describes the best position, but fails to mention the details as to how to place the limbs to maintain their position. Our methods, in short, are as follows: In burns of the front or side of the neck, a collar of felt is applied to maintain the head in the middle line with the chin directed upward. If there exist a tendency toward contraction of one side, the neck is pushed to the other. The collar is made of felt about three-quarters of an inch in thickness. The height of the collar corresponds, generally, to the length of the neck from the chin to the sternum. This collar is surrounded with soft felt or muslin (Fig. 1), though one may use softer material. The collar is sewed following each dressing, although clips may be pro-vided. We have

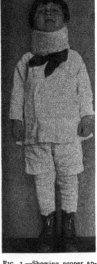

Fig. 1.—Showing proper application of a felt collar in cases of burns of neck.

found that sewing is an extremely simple procedure. As a rule, the nurses after applying paraffine, etc., as a dressing, place oil skin over the wound and then apply the collar instead of bandage. The collar may be made of leather, plaster or celluloid, but since these take time to prepare, felt appears more desirable. Indeed, an ordinary stiff linen collar, with gauze beneath, may be utilized in an emergency.

In burns of the shoulder and axillæ, which are, admittedly, extremely common and which induce severe contractions, the arm must be kept in extreme abduction, in order to prevent its being drawn toward the body to produce the so-called "bat-wing" deformity. In these instances, we tie the hand in slight abduction to the head of the bed, which is elevated, so that the weight of the

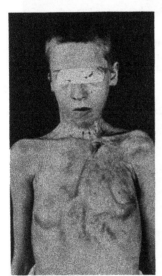

Fig. 2.—A severe case of burn of neck showing the marked deformities that may occur. This patient had no orthopædic treatments. The wounds are healed.

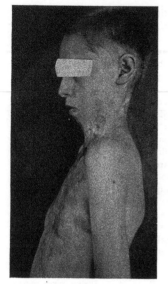 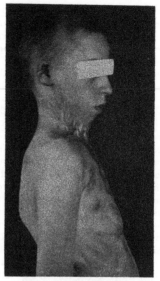

FIG. 3.—Same patient as in Fig. 2.   FIG. 4.—Same patient as in Fig. 2.

trunk tends to drag the patient downward, while the upper extremity remains in marked abduction. In order to avoid constriction of the peripheral circulation, felt may be placed surrounding the wrist before applying the bandage.

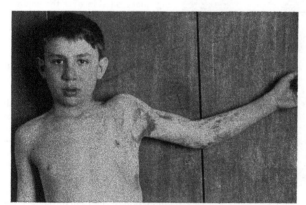

FIG. 5.—Case II. Photograph taken in January, 1920. Note the extensive scar. The limitation of abduction is still present.

618

In case of a burn at the elbow, extension of the arm is maintained by securing the trunk to the opposite edge of the bed, while the affected arm is tied to the corresponding side of the bed, or even perhaps to the ad-

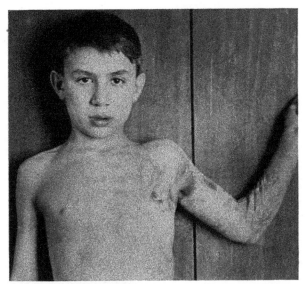

FIG. 6.—Case II. Photograph taken in January, 1920. Note the limitation of flexion.

jacent bed. The body is secured to the side of the bed by passing a sheet round the chest at the level of the nipple. Sandbags are extremely useful in this connection.

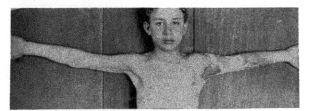

FIG. 7.—Case II. Photograph taken April 11, 1920. Note the good abduction.

In the case of burns of the wrist and fingers, it is extremely important to keep the adjacent raw surfaces separated, in order to prevent adhesions. We have, in some instances, applied oil silk to the wound and then

619

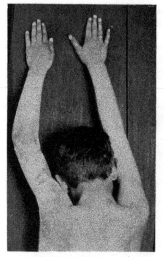

FIG. 8.—Case II. Photograph taken on April 11, 1920. Note the hyperabduction.

made a plaster cast to separate the fingers. This method is somewhat crude, but, as yet, we have not discovered any simpler procedure. We are, at present, experimenting with pestaline, so commonly used by dentists. The pestaline is melted in hot water and then applied with the wrist straight or hyperextended and the fingers separated. A muslin bandage is then applied. For one finger a padded tongue depressor is generally sufficient.

For burns in the region of the hip we usually tie the feet in abduction to the foot of the bed. A sheet is then placed around the chest and brought to the head of the bed. Slight Trendelenburg position is of value. A Cushing knot may be made as follows: After padding with heavy felt the tendo achillis and foot, a heavy webbing strap or flannel is applied to the back of the leg, passed over the tarsus and then crossed under the foot. The position recommended for burns in the region of the hip is also of value in case of burns of the knee.

For burns of the ankle the knee should be tied with a sheet, passing across them to the sides of the bed. A sandbag is placed next the soles of the feet in order to maintain flexion.

Recently we have made use of the Thomas Jones splints, ankle splints and cock-up splints for the knee, ankle, shoulder and elbow. The application of these splints, which has been so markedly stimulated by the war, is well known and needs no explanation. Of course, these appliances are not always at hand, and in their absence the methods we have recommended may be employed. In general, we have found that these simple methods are advantageous, in not only preventing deformities, but save the nursing force a great deal of unnecessary work, which is,

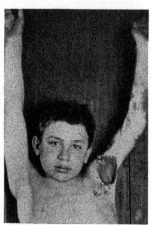

FIG. 9.—Case II. Photograph taken on April 11, 1920. Note the hyperabduction and ability to rotate outwards.

620

of course, a vital point in hospital economy. Moreover, the process of healing and repair has been accelerated. The position of the limbs appear to
be extremely comfortable to the patient; none of the children have complained.

If scar tissue was already present, or even beginning to form, the
proper positions of the limbs were selected and gradual stretching begun.
Though new epithelial layers were necessarily ruptured by this method,
the results obtained have been very encouraging. Many times we have
had to resort to operations under narcosis in order to stretch contractions, but these instances usually have been in neglected or late cases.
Massage and exercises were begun as early as possible, in some instances
even when the wounds were still open. We cite a few illustrative cases:

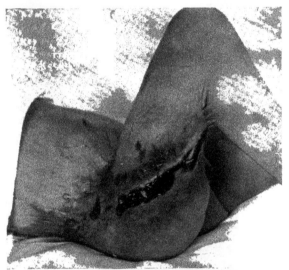

FIG. 10.—Case VI. January 6, 1919. Photograph taken before orthopædic treatments
were started. Note the flexion of the hip and knees.

CASE I.—Becky S., aged four years, second degree burns of both
feet from the perineum down to the knees. Admitted to the hospital June, 1919. Orthopædic treatments begun two weeks after the
accident. Perfect recovery.

CASE II.—Abraham R., aged twelve years, burn affecting the left
upper extremity from shoulder to elbow. Hand tied to the head of
the bed on the second day. Later on a brace used. At present can
abduct arm and rotate it freely. He is still wearing the brace.
Scars are not stiff (see Figs. 5, 6, 7, 8 and 9).

CASE III.—Vera T., aged seven years, both hands and elbows burned.
Second degree burn. Cured in three weeks. .

CASE IV.—Israel W., aged eleven years, burn of left shoulder. Discharged wearing a Jones shoulder brace. Shoulder could be abducted to an angle of 110 degrees. Since discharge from the hospital, has not returned for reëxamination.

CASE V.—Genevieve D., aged nine years, burns of right side of neck, two weeks prior to admission to hospital. Collar applied on November 15, 1919. Cured in three weeks.

CASE VI.—Anthony D., aged eight years. This is not a case of early orthopædic treatments, but of late application of these methods. Patient sustained a burn of right leg and treated for one year. When admitted to Fordham Hospital had contractions of hip on abdomen at an

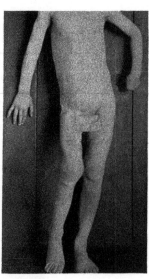

FIG. 11.—Case VI. Photograph taken in February, 1920. Note the good position of the hips and the slightly flexed knee.

acute angle, knee flexed on thigh at an angle of 70 degrees, and leg almost dislocated. Some wounds in the back still open, and not covered with epithelium (see Fig. 10).

Operated on January 21, 1919, when the scar tissue of the popliteal fossa was excised and leg brought down to an angle of 160 degrees. We might have been able to stretch it more, but we feared rupture of the popliteal artery which was probably shorter than normal. The wound healed three months later. Of course, a brace was kept on the knee to prevent recontraction. The hip was operated on May 8, 1919, and the thigh brought down to an angle of 150 degrees, and a brace applied. On June 20, 1919, the brace was changed to a "walking brace," and a raised shoe made and patient encouraged to walk.

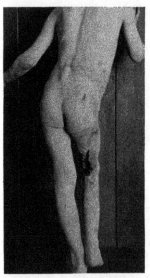

FIG. 12.—Case VI. Photograph taken in February, 1920. Note the shortening of the limb, probably increased by the presence of bone atrophy due to the flexed position in which the limb was kept before orthopædic treatments were instituted.

622

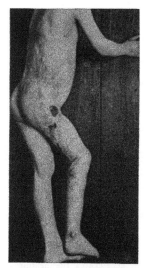 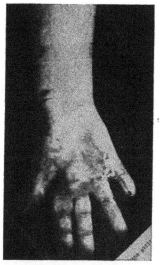

FIG. 13.—Case VI. Lateral view of
Case VI. February, 1920.

FIG. 14.—Case VII. Note the ability to separate the fingers and the good position of the
little finger.

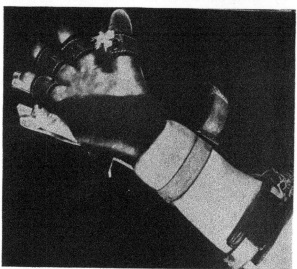

FIG. 15.—Case VII. The brace used to hold the fingers.

623

Examination February, 1920, shows: Thigh flexed at angle of 170 degrees. Knee in good position (Figs. 11, 12 and 13). We intend, however, to operate on him again and gain a better position for the hip.

CASE VII.—Leonard W. Burn of right hand resulted in marked contraction of little and ring fingers and palmar fascia and webbing of the little and ring fingers. Operated on June 7, 1918, the webbing corrected, the palmar fascia excised, and the little finger corrected. There was decided improvement in the palm and in time complete cure. The webbing has been cured, but the contraction of the little finger has recurred. It was very hard to hold it in the brace (Figs. 14 and 15).

These two last cases show the bad consequences of burns and the improvements that can be obtained by orthopædic methods.

CONCLUSIONS

1. Contractures of burns can easily be prevented by early orthopædic treatment.

2. By using simple methods, such as tying the limbs in positions to prevent contractures, no deformities develop and early recovery is obtained.

3. Holding the limbs in proper position accelerates the healing of the wounds.

4. Early massage, exercises, and the wearing of braces aid in obtaining satisfactory positions and proper use of the limbs.

We express our sincere thanks to Dr. Alexander Nicoll, the Director of the Service, for permission to make full use of the material. We wish to thank Mr. Morrison, photographer of the Bellevue and Allied Hospitals, for his coöperation.

TRANSACTIONS

OF THE

PHILADELPHIA ACADEMY OF SURGERY

Stated Meeting held May 10, 1920

The President, Dr. George G. Ross, in the Chair

DISLOCATION OF THE SHOULDER AND FRACTURE OF THE SURGICAL NECK OF THE SCAPULA, CAUSED BY MUSCULAR ACTION DUE TO ELECTRIC SHOCK

Dr. George M. Laws exhibited a man of twenty-eight years, with no history of previous fracture except fractured ribs from adequate trauma, who, in the early days of his experience as an X-ray operator four and a half weeks ago, received a shock in this manner. His hands were outstretched so that they were a few inches from the wires and happened to be cold and wet. The current entered his left hand, passed across his body and out his right hand, holding both of them in contact with the wires. The left upper extremity was fully extended, forward and horizontal, and in order to break the circuit he pulled it downward and backward with all his strength. Suspecting a dislocation of the shoulder from his symptoms he made a film which confirmed it, and then went to his physician who reduced it, whereupon he went back and made another film. A few days later the physician brought him to me to clear up some doubtful features of the case. He then presented the signs of a minor injury at the acromio-clavicular joint and a fracture of the surgical neck of the scapula which was better shown by subsequent radiograms. Union is not yet firm and tenderness persists at the suprascapular notch and at the site of fracture on the axillary border. Incidentally he received a burn on each hand.

Dr. T. Turner Thomas said that he had never recognized a case of fracture of the surgical neck of the scapula. The X-rays in this case are a little bit vague, but show clearly damage done to the glenoid process. He had seen in a number of cases operated on for recurrent dislocation of the shoulder more or less of the anterior part of the glenoid process broken off. He recalled one case where the glenoid process was broken in half; the anterior part being entirely separated from the scapula and the posterior part being continuous with the scapula.

PYOCOLPOS AND PYOMETRA IN A CHILD AGED SIXTEEN MONTHS

Dr. Damon B. Pfeiffer reported the case of a female child aged sixteen months who was admitted on February 4, 1920, to the service of Dr. J. P. Crozer Griffith in the Hospital of the University of Pennsylvania.

The chief complaints were retention of urine and fever. The patient was one of twin girls normally born. Both were bottle-fed, and had been pale and rather delicate, but had had no serious illnesses. This child had always been constipated. The father, mother, and two older sisters were living and well. The child was in her usual health until about ten days before admission, when she became fretful and feverish. The mother noticed that she strained as if in pain and passed no urine. The family physician was called and he removed ten ounces of urine by catheter. Since that time she has required catheterization four times daily. On questioning, however, the mother stated that the child had been "always wet" before the onset of the present illness. On admission the temperature was 103° F., pulse 128, and respirations 28 per minute. The temperature remained high with moderate variations throughout the course of the illness.

The child weighed 19 pounds and was rather fat, but presented an unhealthy, yellowish pallor. She was feverish, fretful, and uneasy. The head, neck, and chest were negative except for slight evidences of rickets. The abdomen was tense and much distended. Above the umbilicus the abdomen was tympanitic. Below the umbilicus there was dulness over an oval area corresponding to the position which would be occupied by an enormously distended bladder. Here a firm, somewhat resilient mass could be felt rising from beneath the symphysis. It was smooth except at the summit, where a definite nodule was palpable. There was no evidence of free fluid within the abdomen. There was tenderness in the right loin posteriorly. Catheterization obtained 12 ounces of urine of specific gravity 1006, acid in reaction, showing a trace of albumin and much pus, otherwise negative. After catheterization the mass previously felt was slightly smaller but otherwise unchanged in character. Rectal examination revealed a mass filling the cul-de-sac anteriorly which was similar in character and evidently continuous with the suprapubic mass. The vaginal outlet was normal in appearance. It seemed to have a lumen, did not bulge, and no attempt was made to examine vaginally. It was the consensus of opinion that the mass was a tumor, probably of embryonic sarcomatous character and inoperable. On the day after admission the blood examination was as follows: Hæmoglobin, 21 per cent.; red blood-cells, 2,930,000; white blood-cells, 23,800; polynuclears, 80 per cent.; lymphocytes, 16 per cent.; mononuclears, 2 per cent.; transitionals, 2 per cent.

The course was down grade. On the ninth marked venous stasis appeared in the left leg. Radiographic examination was inconclusive but suggested to Doctor Pancoast that the mass was cystic. On the following day, thinking that it might be possible to drain a suppurative cystic collection with a minimum of time and trauma, for it was apparent that the child was almost moribund, under light ether anæsthesia the abdomen was opened over the mass, which was at once perceived to be cystic. On the summit the uterus and adnexa were perched, normal in appearance except for distention of the uterus to about 4 cm. in length and 3 cm. in width at the fundus. Recognizing the condition as cystic dilatation of the vagina and uterus, the wound was covered and the vagina dilated. Just within the vestibule was an imperforate septum which was punctured with immediate discharge of about a litre of watery, yellowish pus. Unfortunately, at this stage the child ceased to breathe and died in spite of attempts at resuscitation.

An immediate post-mortem examination showed marked bilateral pyonephrosis and pyoureter. The anatomical conditions and relations suggested that the cavity of the vagina had become infected by direct extension from the lower end of the infected ureters, though it can not be denied that the pyocolpos may have preceded the urinary infection which would then have been favored by pressure and stasis.

RETAINED DRAINAGE TUBE FOLLOWING CHOLECYSTOTOMY

DR. MORRIS BOOTH MILLER reported the following case as worthy of note as an unusual accidental sequel of cholecystotomy. Incidentally it furnishes an additional though rare argument in favor of cholecystectomy in gall-bladder disease. It further carries a lesson to the hospital interne who was probably responsible for the mishap which required reoperation eight years later.

T. F., aged fifty years, a native of Poland, was admitted to the Medico-Chirurgical Hospital on March 18, 1920, with chief complaint of pain in the right epigastrium. As he could only speak Polish a history was obtained through an interpreter and this at its best was inexplicit and unsatisfactory. As nearly as could be learned he had been troubled with pain in the epigastrium since the age of thirteen. He was operated on in Troy, N. Y., eight years ago for this pain and was somewhat improved but not entirely relieved. As to the after-treatment he states that "a large tube was in his side and that when this came out a smaller one was put in." He seemed totally ignorant of the cause which led to the second operation, and naturally and for obvious reasons, he has not been enlightened. Two years ago he commenced to have pains in the upper abdomen resembling sticking of pins; sometimes the pains radiated to the back or right side; no vomiting at any time, but has had occasional periods of nausea; no noticeable loss of weight; has been generally constipated. No history of colic.

Physical examination revealed practically no phenomena of importance. Heart and lungs were normal, no enlargement of spleen or liver. There was a scar over the right rectus commencing at the costal margin running straight downwards for about 10 centimetres. Abdomen soft with no distention, and the only unusual feature which was noticed was slight rigidity over a small area about the upper portion of the scar. Even this was apparently voluntary and thought to be associated with the place where he felt the pain. He breathed freely without increase of pain.

There was no jaundice. The urine reports showed nothing suggestive and gastric analysis gave no material departure from the normal. Blood examination showed a small increase in leucocytes to 8700, dropping in two days to 6500, but otherwise negative. As he was entirely afebrile he was kept under observation as a probable mild case of cholecystitis, possibly due to stone formation. Further investigation, however, with the aid of the X-ray, revealed the cause beyond a question of doubt, as the shadow of a piece of drainage tube was distinctly shown lying transversely below the liver.

Incision through the right rectus revealed many adhesions between the parietes, stomach, duodenum, and liver. Patient dissection exposed the fundus of the gall-bladder lying well under the liver, less than half its normal size, with moderately thickened walls and densely bound down by adhesions. The fundus was probably 8 or 10 centimetres from the surface of the abdomen. Upon opening it a small quantity of foul-smelling bile escaped, and at once a piece of drainage tube 8 centimetres long was picked out. Apparently the gall-bladder had shrunken down until it represented an approximate sheath for the tube. No adventitious stones were found, but one end of the tube was filled with stone formation making a partial cast of the tube. An attempt to do a cholecystectomy was only partially successful as the difficulties of the dissection, as well as the impossibility of identifying relationships, made it necessary to leave a more substantial stump than otherwise would have been done, and even then it was necessary to leave an angled clamp on the stump for seventy-two hours. Recovery was smooth and uneventful.

The probable explanation of this mishap is very simple. When the original drainage tube came away a tube of shorter length and likely lesser calibre was inserted into the drainage track without safety pin or other guard. This shorter tube slipped down the track until it came to rest at the lower end of the gall-bladder, and in course of time the drainage track closed above it. Whether the disappearance of the tube was carelessly explained at the time by being lost in the dressings, or whether the interne or surgeon did have some qualms of misgiving is a matter of interesting speculation.

The reporter had not been able to make a search for similar cases in the literature. For obvious reasons, if they exist in any numbers, they are not apt to be dwelt upon except perchance by the lawyers. He had, however, had his attention called to a case recently reported by Arthur Dean Bevan in the Surgical Clinics of Chicago for February, 1920, in which a gauze sponge was removed from a gall-bladder eleven years after the original operation. In this case operation was performed for supposed malignancy which the physical findings seemed to indicate. It is furthermore interesting in that the meshes of the gauze sponge furnished a nidus for stone formation, so that when removed it had the form of a cast of the entire gall-bladder.

STRANGULATED EPIGASTRIC HERNIA

Dr. Calvin M. Smyth, Jr., said that by epigastric hernia was to be understood any hernia through the linea alba, or sheath of the rectus, between the ensiform and the umbilicus. Epigastric hernia is not common, and strangulation of such herniæ is exceedingly rare. Four types of epigastric hernia are recognized: (1) There is a protrusion of preperitoneal fat through a slit in the linea alba. This is not a true hernia in the stricter sense. (2) In addition to the preperitoneal fat, there is a process of peritoneum protruded, thus forming a sac. The sac, however, is without contents. (3) The sac contains all or a part of the great omentum. (4) Both omentum and gut are protruded.

The last type is the rarest and the one less frequently operated upon. This is due in part to the fact that patients suffering from this variety of hernia do not so frequently present themselves for treatment, because they suffer little or no pain. This is in contradistinction to the other types which give severe pain noted by Moschovitz. In reviewing the literature he had found only about fourteen cases of strangulated epigastric hernia on record, and in only five of these did the hernia contain gut. The most recent of these cases was reported by Gatewood in 1910. In his report he states that only four such cases were on record prior to his. To the best of our knowledge the subject of this report is the sixth one.

The explanation, or at least one explanation of the rarity of this condition, may be found in a consideration of the anatomical factors present. The linea alba is a very strong structure composed of dense fibrous connective tissue, the fibres running in three directions. The transverse fibres are the coarsest and the strongest, therefore, most of the defects are in this direction. Another fact to be borne in mind is the tension of the peritoneum in this region in contrast to the comparative flaccidity of the lower abdominal peritoneum. Then, too, the epigastric viscera are of a size which makes herniation unlikely; for example, a defect which would permit of the protrusion of a loop of small gut would not be large enough to allow a loop of transverse colon to escape from the abdominal cavity. Transverse colon is nearly always the portion of the gut that is encountered in these cases. The rarity of this condition would seem to warrant the report of one more case.

The case reported by Doctor Smyth was as follows: A white woman, aged sixty-eight years, para 6, weighs 268 pounds, was admitted to the service of Dr. G. G. Ross at the Methodist Hospital, December 19, 1919, with the chief complaint pain in the abdomen and vomiting.

For the past eight years she has had a mass in the abdominal wall, above the umbilicus. For the past four years it has been gradually increasing in size, and during this period she has worn a combination truss and abdominal binder. The mass always became prominent at night and it has been her custom to replace it each morning on arising. She has never had any difficulty in accomplishing this until the morning of her admission to the hospital. This morning she was unable to reduce it and sent for her doctor. About half an hour after rising she was seized with a sharp stabbing pain in the epigastrium. The pain was somewhat relieved by vomiting, which she induced. The relief, however, was only temporary, and in the course of the next three or four hours she vomited eight times. The pain became steadily worse. Her physician then ordered her removal to the hospital. No attempt at reduction had been made prior to her admission.

On admission the patient was in a state of exhaustion, although she was not suffering much pain. A mass about the size of a small grapefruit was felt in the epigastric region about four inches above the umbilicus. It projected far out to the right and was hard and immovable. The percussion note was dull. Auscultation of the abdomen disclosed markedly exaggerated peristalsis, and there was a slight distention of the abdomen. An enema which was given proved very slightly effectual.

Operation.—Under ether the abdomen was opened in the midline and the hernial sac was located without difficulty and incised. The opening of the sac was followed immediately by a gush of clear straw-colored fluid amounting to about 250 c.c. The omentum, which had evidently been present in the hernia for some time, was in an advanced state of degeneration. It was adherent to the sac and was freed with considerable difficulty. A loop of transverse colon about five inches long then presented itself, and following this down with the finger, the opening through which the hernia had occurred was located. This opening was found to be a transverse slit in the linea alba which would not admit two fingers. A grooved director was passed into the opening and it was enlarged by cutting upward. The gut was discolored but still retained its resilience, and after the constriction was relieved soon returned to the normal. The gut was then returned to the abdomen and the degenerated omentum excised. The sac was treated in the usual manner. The anterior sheath of the rectus was then dissected up on either side of the opening and for about three inches in the longitudinal direction. The flaps thus made were overlapped and secured by several interrupted mattress sutures. The rest of the wound was closed in the ordinary manner. Uneventful recovery. She was discharged from the hospital on the twenty-first day after operation, and when last heard from was in perfect health. There has been no recurrence of the hernia.

DR. MORRIS BOOTH MILLER said that for many years he had, midway between the umbilicus and the ensiform, a little flat tumor about the size of a 25-cent piece which he could feel through the tissues, but which had never given him any direct trouble. Although for some of these years he had digestive trouble, which some of his friends thought was due to duodenal ulcer, this condition was never definitely diagnosed. During the late winter of 1917–1918 while serving on the United

States ship *President Grant*, they were subjected to severe weather and considerable exposure on the east bound voyage. During the latter part of that trip he caught a bad cold which terminated in cough. The night after Brest was reached he had an attack of coughing which kept him awake. During the night he was taken with an especially severe paroxysm, during which he felt something in his upper abdomen give way, and noticed that the little flat tumor had grown to the size of an egg. He did not vomit, although he had some nausea, but the tumor was so painful that he could not stand erect. The next morning he was sent to Naval Hospital No. 5 where he saw Doctor LeConte and Doctor Ross. The diagnosis was an incarcerated epigastric hernia, and operation was advised. He returned to the United States and was operated upon at the Naval Hospital, Philadelphia. Dr. W. A. Angwin, the operator, stated that on opening the abdomen he found a small sac which had omentum in it which showed evidences of recent inflammation. The opening in the linea alba was the size of a lead pencil. Uneventful recovery.

THE SURGICAL TREATMENT OF BURNS

Dr. W. ESTELL LEE read a paper with the above title.

Dr. HUBLEY R. OWEN said that he had under his care at the present time a child who, three weeks ago, while melting paraffine, set fire to her clothing and she was badly burned. Her burns would undoubtedly have been much more serious had she not had the presence of mind to fall on the floor and wrap herself in a rug. Her burns extended from above her ankles to her groins anteriorly, and from above her ankles to above her buttocks posteriorly. He saw her four or five hours after she had been burned. In the emergency her father had covered the whole burned area with picric acid, and applied it very freely. This picric acid dressing was removed at the first visit and boric acid ointment applied. In spite of the fact that the picric acid had been applied to the burn only a few hours, she developed symptoms of absorption of picric acid the following day.

Amberine was used for a few days until sloughing developed. It was then discontinued and Dakin's solution applied over the burned area. Dakin's solution was somewhat painful, but cleared the burn up wonderfully. Her kidneys were in good condition, and, under light anæsthesia, the sloughs were cut away. Hypertonic salt solution was tried, but this was very painful and had to be discarded.

He believed the whole secret in the treatment of a burn is cleanliness—not only keeping the burned area surgically clean by removing sloughs, but also keeping the surrounding skin clean. This cleansing is best accomplished under an anæsthetic.

One of the worst burns he had ever had occasion to treat was in the person of a child, in the service of Doctor Wharton at the Children's Hospital, many years ago. She was burned around her abdomen, vagina, thighs, and buttocks. In the treatment of that child a cradle was used to hold the bedclothes away from the burned area, and an electric light was placed under this cradle to keep the child warm, and keep the burn surgically clean. Of course, at that time Dakin's solution had not yet been devised, but in that case salt solution was used.

DR. GEORGE P. MULLER said a good many burns are admitted to his service at the St. Agnes and Polyclinic Hospitals. In association with his assistant, Doctor Ryan, he had tried to reduce the mortality and to improve the methods of external dressing. To understand the phenomena of burns one must consider three factors, namely, shock, toxæmia, and infection. Therefore, from the moment of admission to the hospital the patient, usually a child, must be considered as in a state of shock or on the verge of it. Too often they remain in the receiving wards, which are usually cold and draughty and noisy, to have a preliminary dressing applied before admission to the wards. He tried to have a blanket thrown over the patient and an immediate admission made. The patient's clothing should be rapidly cut away, the patient placed on a blanket and covered with some form of frame for holding electric light, over which another blanket can be thrown. When the electric lights are turned on the body is in a warm chamber, the temperature of which can be regulated at will. The foot of the bed should be elevated, moderate doses of morphine given, and a continuous enteroclysis of salt solution started. Hot drinks and the other accessories useful in shock are added.

Many terribly burned cases come out of shock nicely but die a few days later with manifestations of intense toxæmia. Some have lived several weeks and then died, even though the external surface was clean. They had pushed water to the utmost and had used sodium bicarbonate a good deal, intravenously and by the mouth, but it would seem as though the patients became sensitized and then succumbed from further absorptions of the poison.

To control the infection they had in the last year routinely used dichloramine-T, sprayed upon the burned surface every six hours at first and later every twelve hours. He did not find it hurt the patient after the first spraying if the oil is perfectly fresh. If it smells acrid it should be discarded. Some cases crust up too much and wet dressings are useful for a time. In such cases he protected the surface with paraffine mesh, but had stopped entirely the paraffine film method. One gets just as good results from the perforated mesh and a great deal of time is saved. If an occlusive dressing is needed adhesive strapping is as good as the paraffine film. Fortunately, male adults are usually burned on the hands, face, and neck. There is no difficulty keeping women and children extensively burned on the entire body and trunk under the frame and with no covering.

Therefore, he believed that if the shock is controlled and if attention is paid from the very beginning to the nature of infection, practically all burned cases do well except the hyperacute toxic cases who die apparently for no reason at all. Some German writers have advocated removal of the entire burned area by curettage, but it seemed to him that the trauma and the hemorrhage would offset the advantages.

Dr. John H. Jopson said there is one effect of amberine which he had observed and after no other dressing, and that is very rapid epithelialization over the whole surface. He recalled one man who suffered a typical airman's burn over the surface of his face which was unprotected by his helmet. He was dressed with amberine from the start, and the spread of skin over the surface was very different from that observed ordinarily. Each day it was as if one had used a powder shaker over it. These epithelial cells must have been partially undestroyed, but the protection afforded by the amberine had prevented their being washed off. I think Doctor Lee's contribution is a notable one on sterilization. It would be interesting in these cases to plot out the rate of healing by Doctor Macy's method. Fauntleroy in his paper reporting a large series of burns discusses the value of occasional change of character of dressing, which he calls "switching time." In other words, if we treat these cases by any one antiseptic we find that the granulating surface becomes habituated to that type of dressing and healing slows up. We have seen this exemplified in the sterilization of other types of wounds.

Dr. George G. Ross said that he had an unusual opportunity of observing cases treated by dichloramine-T in the service in France. He was impressed by observing what Doctor Jopson noticed, the islands of epithelial cells growing widely over the granulating surface, as if thrown on by a pepper box; healing was much more prompt and the scars better. A great many burn cases came into the hospital at Brest. He remembered on one occasion an ammunition ship was blown up and sixteen men were brought in, four died immediately. On another occasion six or seven were brought in and they had two to sixteen or twenty men real badly burned all the time. They tried out every known method of treatment and finally came to the conclusion that wide mesh paraffine gauze with dichloramine-T was the most comfortable and easiest method by which a burn could be easily sterilized and unquestionably gave the best type of scar.

TRANSACTIONS

OF THE

NEW YORK SURGICAL SOCIETY

Stated Meeting held May 12, 1920

The President, DR. WILLIAM A. DOWNES, in the Chair

USE OF CHINOSOL AND SODIUM CHLORIDE IN THE TREATMENT OF WOUNDS

DR. WILLIAM C. LUSK read a paper with the above title.

DR. ROBERT T. MORRIS stated that the addition of salt to chinosol would offer a great advantage. He had been using chinosol for many years, and it seemed to him that the addition of salt introduced an improvement which should be recognized more often than it was in mixing antiseptic solutions generally, for the reason that ordinary water was distinctly corrosive in its action. This was because of the exosmosis which took the salts out of the protecting tissue-cells and lowered their efficiency. This action could be demonstrated by comparing the action of plain water with that of an isotonic salt solution on the tail of a rat if one was studying the tail tendons. They are dulled at once in plain water, but remained glistening in saline solution. This principle had not been applied enough in eye work. It was important to make up lotions with a salt solution that was isotonic, because a solution that was not isotonic for blood-serum exerted a corrosive influence on account of the laws of osmosis.

RECURRENT FIBROSARCOMA OF SKIN

(Fifteen years after the original operation)

DR. H. H. M. LYLE presented a man who, twenty years ago, first noticed a pedunculated wart in the region of the left shoulder. Five years later this wart began to show evidences of ulceration which led him to consult Doctor Abbe, who made a diagnosis of sarcoma and removed the growth with an extensive area of skin. A small recurrence one year later necessitated a secondary operation. Since this time the man had remained in perfect health, without signs of recurrence for fourteen years. A short time before entrance to St. Luke's Hospital the patient noticed a soft, flat growth in the middle of the old scar. Physical examination showed a cicatrix 6 by 4 inches on the left base of neck and shoulder. This area had been grafted at the previous operation fifteen years ago. The grafted

634

area extended from the border of the trapezius over the shoulder ant_
riorly to the second rib. Just posterior to the middle third of the clavicle
was a round, raised, adherent mass 2 inches in diameter. The mass was red
and was crossed by numerous dilated veins. No axillary or cervical glands
were palpated. X-ray examination of bones and chest was negative.

On July 2, 1919, the area of old skin graft was excised and the tumor
removed *en masse* along with deep fascia covering the upper part of the
deltoid. The superficial portions of the pectoralis major and trapezius
that were in relation to the old skin graft were also removed. The resulting raw surface was covered by skin grafts taken from the thigh.

The pathological diagnosis was fibrosarcoma of skin (recurrent).

ANGIO-KERATOMA OF SCROTUM

Doctor Lyle presented a man who was admitted to St. Luke's Hospital with a diagnosis of a left-side varicocele. Six years before he had
suffered from a swelling of the scrotum which he attributed to a number
of minute blood blisters. These so-called blood blisters had broken at
times and bled profusely. He now came to the hospital to see if a
varicocele operation would help the condition.

There was a moderate varicocele of the left cord. Numerous small,
raised, purplish-red nodules were scattered over the scrotum. These
nodules were firm, and appeared to be in relation to the finer blood-
vessels of the scrotum. There was an extensive port-wine nævus on the
left arm and shoulder. The patient was referred to the Dermatological
Clinic for the condition.

A portion of tissue was removed and a diagnosis of angio-keratoma
made. The patient was then referred back to the surgical service for an
operation on the varicocele, with the idea of lessening the congestion in
the veins of the scrotum. This had improved, but not cured the condition.

Dr. De Witt Stetten said as to this case of angio-keratoma of the
scrotum that he had at present under treatment an almost identical case.
The patient complained that he had multiple bleeding points on the
scrotum, which on examination appeared to be angiomatous warts. The
condition was mainly unilateral, in this instance, right-sided. The
growths, however, were somewhat larger and the slightest irritation
caused profuse hemorrhage. Under local anæsthesia Doctor Stetten excised
these warts individually, removing some twenty odd at one sitting. He
was much gratified to find, when the wounds had healed, that the skin of
the scrotum looked practically normal. There was a large branching
varicose vein at the perineal junction of the scrotum, which was apparently a tributary of the right superficial perineal vein and was probably related
to the angiomatous condition. Doctor Stetten said he intended to excise this
vein before he discharged the patient. He did not believe the spermatic
veins had anything to do with the disease because the lesion was a super-

ficial, cutaneous one and on the side opposite the varicocele. Neither did he think a varicocele operation would affect it at all.

ANKYLOSIS OF THE TEMPORO-MAXILLARY ARTICULATION

Dr. John Douglas presented a boy, five years of age, who was admitted to St. Luke's Hospital June 6, 1919. He began to have difficulty in opening his mouth two years previously, but no previous history of otitis media or of an acute illness could be obtained which would furnish a cause for the temporo-maxillary ankylosis. His trouble progressed until at the time of admission he could only separate his incisor teeth 0.5 of a centimetre. There was no rotary motion. A slight deviation of the chin toward the left side was present.

At operation it was found that there was a complete bony ankylosis of the left temporo-maxillary joint, the production of new bone extending to and fusing with the posterior part of the zygoma. A horizontal incision was made just above the zygoma, its posterior end being extended upward 1.5 centimetres. The articular process and the neck of the mandible was removed with a chisel and the new bone extending to the zygoma and into the articular fossa excised, whereupon the lower jaw opened easily, showing that the other side was not involved; a flap of the temporal fascia with the overlying fat was dissected, its base being along the zygoma. This was turned down and fastened into the articular fossa. There was no injury to the facial nerve and the final result as now shown was excellent, although it was impossible to get the parents of the child to carry out any after-treatment to keep up complete motion in the joint.

Dr. George Woolsey said he had had a somewhat similar case some years ago in a woman physician. She had fallen when a child and had never since that time been able to take anything but liquid food. He found an ankylosis of the left temporo-maxillary articulation upon which he operated by resection and turning in of a flap of temporal fascia, and obtained a very good result. He kept the jaws apart for some time after the operation. He thought it was an advantage to do the operation early in life because the jaw then had an opportunity to develop. This woman had a very poor development of the lower jaw. He thought the development would have been much better had she been operated upon earlier in life.

Dr. A. O. Whipple asked Doctor Douglas why he used the fascial transplant; whether it was to prevent ankylosis occurring again.

Doctor Douglas replied that the condyle of the inferior maxillary was excised and this left a raw surface on this bone and there was also a raw surface on the temporal portion of the articulation. A fascial transplant introduced between these raw surfaces prevented recurrence of the ankylosis due to production of new bone which might occur unless some material was interposed. It was essential to remove enough bone not to cause pressure on the interposed flap.

PLASTIC ON THE FACE BY THE TUBULAR FLAP METHOD

Dr. John Douglas presented a woman, seventy-five years of age, who had a small epithelioma just under the inner portion of the left eye which had been slowly increasing in size for four years. During eight or nine months previous to the time when she was first seen by him, she had been treated with the X-ray and radium. This finally resulted in the skin area healing over, but at the expense of the tissue of the side of the face, so that the contraction of the scar tissue had caused the right nostril to be pulled up and the inner canthus of the eye to be pulled down.

The area had remained healed for only one week when it had broken open again and she was referred to him by the physician from whom she was receiving her radiograph treatment. At this time she had a small ulcer in the area described, through which a probe could be introduced into the antrum of Highmore, a portion of the anterior wall having been destroyed by the growth. In August, 1919, the epithelioma, which was of the basal type, was excised, together with a considerable portion of the anterior wall of the antrum, an opening being made into the nasal cavity to thoroughly drain the antrum. The wound was closed by a sliding flap from the lower part of the face. In performing the plastic operation, it was impossible to lift the inner canthus of the eye without injuring the lachrymal duct, so this was not attempted.

Six months later a small recurrence appeared on the side of the nose. This was evidently deep in its origin as the squamous layer of epithelium was not involved. It was, therefore, necessary to do a deep excision which could not be covered by a skin graft. The loose skin on the side of the face had been utilized for the previous plastic operation. The use of a sliding flap from the forehead would probably have caused considerable deformity, and therefore it was determined to use the tubular flap method of Gillies. The patient had a large goitre with considerable loose skin on the neck. On March 8, 1920, under local anæsthesia, two parallel incisions about four centimetres apart were made in the neck, making a flap about sixteen centimetres long. The flap was dissected up, and the skin edges sutured together, making the tube of skin and subcutaneous tissue which was left attached at both ends.

The skin edges were freed and sutured together underneath the flap, closing the raw area, from which the flap had been removed. Twelve days later, there being a good circulation in the flap, again under local anæsthesia, an area at the left end of the flap was cut out in the skin, which after allowing for shrinkage, would be sufficiently large to fill in the area it was determined to excise from the side of the nose. This was only partly cut away from its deep attachment and left attached to the end of the flap for the further development of collateral circulation from what was to be the base of the tubular flap at the right end. This was loosened a little further each day, and on the third day, under ether anæsthesia, a

deep excision of the carcinomatous area involved was done. It was necessary to excise the periosteum over the right nasal bone and the nasal
process of the superior maxilla, and also a small portion of the nasal
mucous membrane. The flap was then sutured into place to close this
defect. One week later the flap, having become adherent and well healed
to the skin edges of the new area, it was cut off close to the face and
the edge sutured to the cheek and the base end cut off; the wound in the
neck from which it took its origin was closed. Doctor Douglas said the
patient was shown as an example of the use of the tubular-flap method in
plastic surgery of the face.

JEJUNAL ULCER FOLLOWING GASTRO-ENTEROSTOMY

Dr. John Douglas presented a man, thirty-one years of age, who was
admitted to St. Luke's Hospital January 23, 1920. He began to have
severe abdominal pain ten years previously. At this time had repeated
vomiting attacks during which he vomited a large amount of blood and
had blood in the stools. Shortly afterward he had a gastro-enterostomy
done in a Brooklyn hospital for "ulcer of the stomach." He was relieved
of pain for one year after operation while he remained on a diet, and then
as he returned to a regular diet pain returned and has persisted. Pain
had been more severe than at first; it was relieved by food for an hour or
two or by eructation of gas, was worse always at midnight, and was
increased by sweet food.

Two years ago he had a severe attack of vomiting of blood accompanied by syncope. Three years ago and again two years ago he entered
different hospitals where, after radiograph examination of the stomach,
he was discharged without treatment. For the past week has vomited
frequently large amounts without blood or nausea, always after meals.
There had been no blood in the stools. Physical examination showed
the urine and blood-pressure all negative, and a radiographic examination showed nothing diagnostic.

At operation a number of adhesions between the first portion of the
duodenum and liver were found which would suggest an old healed
duodenal ulcer. There was no induration of the duodenum suggestive of
active ulcer, and no narrowing of the pylorus was present. The gastro-
jejunostomy stoma was at the junction of the horizontal and vertical
portions of the stomach and admitted three fingers; there was no thickening about its margin to suggest a gastro-jejunal ulcer. The anastomosis was of the short loop, isoperistaltic type.

On separating the stomach and intestine, a small punched-out ulcer
about .5 cm. in diameter with thickened base and edges was found on the
jejunal wall about .5 cm. proximal to the anastomosis. This ulcer was
excised, and as there was no evidence of active ulcer present, the openings in the stomach and the intestine were closed by chromic catgut suture.

The specimen showed a piece of linen thread in the serous coat, but not apparently entering into the base or edges of the ulcer.

The patient was relieved of his symptoms entirely for about two months, but recently has again suffered from epigastric discomfort. A recent radiograph shows that the stomach empties in four hours, and a test meal shows marked hyperacidity, and his further treatment has been directed to the relief of this hyperacidity.

DR. ROBERT T. MORRIS asked Doctor Douglas if he had looked up the question of elective affinity. It had been shown that certain infective agents had an elective affinity for this location, and they called out abnormal hormones followed by hyperacidity often. Antibodies also were called out to combat the toxins, and these in excess causing autolysis, might be a factor in the recurrence of ulcer. Another question was whether there was an excess of carbohydrate fermentation in the colon. Were any Welch bacilli found in the colon? Unless one took into consideration all these questions and worked them out and searched for all possible foci of infection, one was very likely to have a recurrence of ulcer at any time because the same conditions which produced the first ulcer were still in existence.

DR. A. V. MOSCHCOWITZ asked what was the location of this ulcer? Then there was some question about a linen thread in the ulcer. Was this thread in the centre of the ulcer? Also, did Doctor Douglas use linen sutures?

In answer to questions Doctor Douglas said he found the linen thread in the edge of the ulcer, not the base. It appeared as though it might have been an interrupted stitch in the serous coat. The ulcer was about one-half a centimetre away from the gastro-enterostomy. It was a jejunal, not a gastro-jejunal ulcer, as usually occurred, and was on the proximal, not on the distal side of the stoma. A supposed etiological factor in the development of jejunal ulcer was the pouring out of the acid stomach contents into the jejunum which was normally accustomed to an alkaline reaction, but in this case, as has been frequently reported in the literature, the presence of a linen suture seemed to have been a determining cause. Doctor Douglas further stated, in answer to Doctor Moschcowitz, that he had used no linen or silk sutures in stomach operations for the past five or six years.

DOCTOR MOSCHCOWITZ said he was glad that this little thread was found in the ulcer, because he believed that most gastro-jejunal ulcers were due to the fact that linen thread was used. He had been guilty of its use himself, but he liked linen thread and found it a little difficult to break the habit of using it. However, he had made up his mind never to use silk or linen threads again in the stomach. It would be interesting to know if there were any series of jejunal or gastro-jejunal ulcer cases in which chromicized catgut only had been used; he had never seen such.

MODIFIED TECHNIC FOR THE RADICAL CURE OF INGUINAL HERNIA

DR. DE WITT STETTEN, in connection with Doctor Hoguet's paper, presented some lantern slides to illustrate a modified Bassini-Andrews technic for hernioplasty, which he had been using for some time and which was particularly applicable for direct hernia. A detailed report of this procedure was published in the ANNALS OF SURGERY, June, 1920, p. 744.

He believed that it was generally conceded that any operation in which the cord was not transplanted was bad in direct hernia, and that, even in indirect cases, the percentage of recurrence was less with cord transplantation. In the typical Bassini operation the result hinges upon a frequently doubtful, solitary suture line of the internal oblique and conjoined tendon to Poupart's. In many cases this suture line was entirely inadequate. The aponeurosis of the external oblique was not used at all for the actual repair of the hernial defect, but was sutured over the cord as a superfluous covering. In the posterior Andrews and kindred modifications the upper flap of the external oblique aponeurosis was made use of and sutured to Poupart's over the Bassini suture. The lower flap was sewed over the cord where it accomplished little as far as the plastic was concerned, but tended rather to compress and angulate the cord.

The modification which Doctor Stetten had been using he said went a step further and utilized all the available material for the real hernioplasty. After the Bassini suture and the suture of the upper flap of the external oblique aponeurosis to Poupart's had been accomplished, the rather liberal lower flap was divided up to Poupart's with a scissors, perpendicularly to its fibres at a point opposite the ring. These two portions of the lower flap were now overlapped on and sutured directly to the upper flap. The cord emerged between the two portions of the lower flap, and the medial portion lay beneath the cord. The cord was left subcutaneous. This subcutaneous position of the cord, in my experience, had never been the source of any trouble.

The advantages of the proposed plan were:

First. A triple layer of tissue was used for the actual closure of the hernial orifice. The typical Bassini suture was reinforced by a double suture line overlapping the aponeurosis beneath the cord.

Second. Danger of kinking the cord was eliminated.

Third. Should there be oozing from the cord, the hæmatoma would be merely under the skin, instead of submuscular or subaponeurotic. It would be easily accessible and it would not interfere with the suture lines.

The method, Doctor Stetten felt, was particularly serviceable in direct and recurrent herniæ, especially in old, large, and difficult ones, in sliding herniæ, and in cases where the development of the internal oblique and conjoined tendon was poor and where Poupart's ligament was thin or tears easily.

In a fair-sized series of cases of almost every variety of inguinal hernia, he had, as yet, seen no recurrences in the cases which he had been able to follow up. Further, he had found the formation of a flap from the rectus muscle or the anterior rectus sheath unnecessary, even in the most unfavorable cases.

DIRECT HERNIA

Dr. P. J. Hoguet read a paper with the above title.

Dr. Wm. A. Downes said the problem of inguinal hernia had resolved itself into the management of the direct variety. Many surgeons recognized the futility of the usual technic for indirect hernia when applied to the direct type, and various modifications of recognized procedures had been devised to correct the inherent anatomical defects which gave rise to this form of rupture. Up to the present time none of these modifications had proved satisfactory in all cases. The difficulty lay in selecting the cases suitable for operation, and he for one had reached the conclusion that a certain number of direct hernias could not be cured by operation. There was a small but definite group of patients, usually thin men with poorly-developed muscles in both lower quadrants, in whom it was not wise to operate for this condition, as recurrence was almost certain to follow. Therefore, the results obtained in the operative treatment of hernia depend in a large measure upon the selection of cases. Having decided that a case was suitable for operation the next step was the selection of the proper operation. If the muscles were well developed any one of the recognized procedures might give a perfect result. On the other hand, if the muscles were thinned out and poorly developed, and the sac large, its base extending almost from the epigastric artery to the pubic bone, an entirely different operation was necessary if a satisfactory outcome was to be expected. In 1909 Doctor Downes stated that he began the use of the transplanted, or, more properly speaking, transposed rectus muscle in conjunction with the Bassini operation in the treatment of this class of patients. So many recurrences were taking place in his patients as well as those of other surgeons with whom he was associated that it became quite evident that the Bassini operation alone did not meet the indications. He therefore adopted the following method which had been modified from time to time, and which he illustrated by lantern slides: The usual skin incision was made carrying the lower angle down to the pubic bone, the aponeurosis of the external oblique was divided well over towards the edge of the rectus muscle, and both flaps were retracted. The sharp edge of Poupart's ligament was then exposed down to the pubic spine. By blunt dissection the fibres of the cremaster muscle were separated and the cord gently lifted from its bed. A small retractor was now placed under the arched fibres of the internal oblique and transversalis exposing the internal ring. By gentle traction on the cord the peritoneal reflection at the internal ring was brought into view and the presence or absence of an oblique hernia quickly determined. This step was absolutely essential and should be carried out before attempting to isolate the direct hernial sac, irrespective of its size or location, for in no other way could the error of overlooking the indirect portion of a combined sac be avoided. Personally, Doctor Downes said he believed the sac should be opened in every hernia that was of sufficient size to warrant operation. With the finger inserted through the neck of the sac for support the fat was gently stripped from its surface, and if the obliterated hypogastric artery interfered with proper dissection it should be cut. After the sac wall had been satisfactorily exposed, its base should be drawn flush with the opening in the fascia and transfixed, or, better still, if of large size sutured in the manner of closing the peritoneum in laparotomy wounds. For this purpose he used No. 1 chromicized catgut. In the cases of combined direct and indirect hernia the two portions of the sac should be converted into one, by drawing one or the other above or below the deep epigastric artery, being guided by their relative size as to whether it was best to convert the direct into an indirect or *vice versa*. Doctor Downes stated that he had formerly advised dividing the artery in this type of hernia, but was now of the opinion that the sac could be removed in most instances just as thoroughly without sacrificing this vessel. After the sac had been disposed of the rent in the transversalis fascia should be closed, if possible, using a continuous suture of chromic gut for the purpose. A second retractor was now placed low down under the continuation of the internal oblique and transversalis and the sharp margin of the rectus muscle located with the finger. The sheath of the rectus was then opened along its anterior border, and the muscle exposed from about the level of the internal ring down to its pubic attachment. Three or four sutures of kangaroo tendon were introduced between the outer portion of the rectus muscle and the deepest part of Poupart's ligament. If the transversalis fascia had not been closed satisfactorily as a separate layer it should be included with these structures. The sutures should be placed from one-half to three-quarters of an inch apart from below up—the lowest one passing from just above the insertion of the rectus muscle to the terminal portion of the ligament. After being properly placed, gentle traction should be made on the sutures, drawing muscle and ligament well together, and while thus held they should be tied in the order of their insertion. The usual Bassini operation was now performed from above downward, the sutures picking up a small bit of the rectus muscle and catching Poupart's ligament just superficial to and between those of the first row. Excessive fat should be removed from the cord, but the veins should not be excised. By making use of the rectus muscle an additional layer was added to the weakened posterior wall of the canal. It was not claimed that the fibres of this muscle formed a true union with Poupart's ligament or that they always remained permanently in the new position, but they did aid greatly in the formation of new connective tissue at the point where every bit of additional support was of value in the prevention of recurrence. By the use of this method recurrences in their hands had been reduced one-half. However, they felt that there was still room for improvement, and with this in view Dr. R. W. Bolling and the speaker had recently decided to combine transplantation of the rectus muscle with the Andrews operation instead of the Bassini. The mattress sutures were placed as recommended by Andrews for his posterior operation, with the addition of a continuous suture between the margin of the external oblique flap and Poupart's ligament. The lower flap of the external oblique was then sutured over the cord in the usual way. If there seemed to be tension in the upper flap of the external oblique a free liberating incision might be made through the sheath of the rectus well back over the belly of the muscle and parallel with its fibres. It might be stated that sutures placed under tension were of little or no value, as they soon came out. Kangaroo tendon or chromic catgut was used for all deep sutures up to the time of changing methods, but they were now trying celluloid linen in one series and absorbable sutures in another.

Dr. A. V. Moschcowitz said he fully agreed with those gentlemen who believed that an important element in a hernia operation was the union of the aponeurosis to Poupart's ligament, and not the union of the muscle to Poupart's ligament. He believed that that had been proved over and over again, and he had done a number of operations without attaching the internal oblique and transversalis muscles to Poupart's ligament. In Doctor Hoguet's operation, while it was true that the stitch was carried through the external oblique, the illustration did not show the attachment of this structure to Poupart's ligament. Doctor Moschcowitz thought that therein lies the weakness of the operation.

Of course it was well known that it was much more difficult to cure direct than indirect hernia. The difficulty of curing direct hernia was recognized in the army; for the existence and recognition of a direct hernia was considered sufficient reason for discharge. On the other hand, cases of indirect hernia were operated upon in large numbers. Doctor Moschcowitz said he had made it a rule in all his operations for direct hernia to dissect the sac up at least to the obliterated hypogastric artery. If one analyzed the underlying causes of recurrence they would be found to be various. One was that an insufficient part of the sac had been removed, or that a small sac had been overlooked. In discussing this subject some time ago he had been asked the cause of recurrences, and he wished to repeat the statement he then made; namely, that the causes of recurrence were three: (1) When a proper operation was improperly done; (2) if an improper operation was properly done, and (3) the most frequent cause, when an improper operation was improperly done. Success depended on but one contingency, namely, a proper operation properly done.

DR. FRANZ TOREK said that Doctor Hoguet had described an interesting observation, that the peritoneum of a direct hernia could be drawn up into a coexisting indirect hernia by drawing the sac of the latter outward and upward. They had probably all made that observation, but they should be thankful to Doctor Hoguet for bringing it out as a special point. In operating for combined direct and indirect hernia, he had frequently noted that after the indirect sac had been properly mobilized and pulled out the bulging of the direct hernia disappeared, and that no treatment of the direct sac was necessary.

The method of closure of the abdominal wall, as Doctor Hoguet mentioned, differed according to the development of the internal oblique and transversus muscles. When these were strong their attachment to Poupart's ligament would suffice. If they were weak and short the attachment of the rectus to Poupart's ligament was necessary. Doctor Torek said this was brought out in an article he had read before the Society last year, in which he had also called attention to the fact that in direct hernia one must always look out for the bladder, and that it was necessary to lay bare the wound right down to the pubis and to close it down to the pubis. In fact, he agreed with Doctor Hoguet in everything except, perhaps, one point, *viz.*, the slight objection the reader expressed to attaching the rectus to Poupart's, as compared with his recommendation of attaching the reduplicated external oblique to Poupart's. As to the former he mentioned that the muscle was drawn out of place and will tend, by contraction, to be drawn away from its new attachments. If this was true it would be just as much true as an objection to attaching the reduplicated external oblique, because that aponeurosis, inasmuch as it forms part of the rectus sheath, naturally followed the motion of the rectus on contraction of that muscle. Therefore, if the rectus tended to be drawn away from Poupart's, the aponeurosis would likewise tend to be drawn away, especially if there was a reduplication which made the tension greater than it was before. However, the proof of the pudding was the eating, and thus far he had yet to learn of an operation that equalled his own in its results.

DR. WILLIAM C. LUSK said an important consideration in direct inguinal hernia was what to do when the conjoined tendon was deficient. Applicable to repair in the presence of this condition was the use of the Halsted triangular flap from the anterior layer of the rectus sheath. He had illustrated this flap in connection with transplantation of the rectus muscle (ANNALS OF SURGERY, November, 1913, p. 677), and subsequently had observed that a proper cutting of the same would free the restraint exercised upon those of the arched fibres which were inserted into the rectus sheath below the upper limit of the flap, so that they could be brought down and sutured to Poupart's ligament in continuity with the flap. The flap, shaped like a right-angled triangle, was formed by two incisions meeting at a right angle, one transverse, about 1¼ to 1¾ inches above the pubic spine, located just a little above the insertion of the lowermost of the arched fibres directly into the rectus sheath, which should cut the anterior layer of the sheath outward through its outer limit, being careful not to cut through the underlying deep fascia where the layers meet, the other incision vertical, downward to the pubic spine. The carrying of the transverse arm of the incision outward until the last fibre of aponeurotic structure of the anterior layer of the rectus sheath had been severed, was a step which was essential in order to gain relaxation, and the carrying of the vertical arm of the incision downward close against the pubic spine was essential to secure the proper eversion of the flap. He had found that, while there was no slack in the anterior layer of the rectus sheath, there was considerable slack in the posterior layer, and the carving of this triangular opening in the unyielding anterior layer of the sheath gave full play to the slack in the portion of the posterior layer of the sheath behind it, so that the fibres of the internal oblique and transversalis muscles in continuity with the latter portion of the sheath, were thereby released from their tension. Thus the everted triangular flap united to Poupart's ligament and arched fibres attached to the base of the flap, now mobilized, brought down to Poupart's ligament, reconstructed the posterior wall of the inguinal canal. Why not utilize more generally this expedient of Halsted in reconstructing the deep layer of the abdominal wall in the repair of direct inguinal hernia?

Dr. H. H. M. Lyle called the Society's attention to the value of position in the treatment of inguinal hernia. Recently much has been said about the value of the physiological balance of muscles in the treatment of fractures. The same principles can also be applied in the operative treatment of inguinal hernia.

The fibres of the internal oblique and transversalis that united to form the conjoint tendon arose respectively from the outer half and outer third of Poupart's ligament. Now, if Poupart's ligament was relaxed by flexion and inversion of the limb the conjoint tendon was automatically relaxed; this relaxation of the conjoint tendon in turn relaxed the related fibres of the rectus. The rectus, the external, internal, and transversalis could be further relaxed by raising the shoulder. For a long time Doctor Lyle has been taking accurate caliper measurements of the distances between Poupart's ligament and the conjoint tendon. A comparison of this distance in the extended and the relaxed position shows that it could be reduced from 20 per cent. to 70 per cent., the average being 35 per cent.

In order to insure firm union all tension must be avoided. Tight suturing means tissue tension, impairment of nutrition, and the possibility of tissue fibrosis. In the operative treatment of inguinal hernia this elementary procedure of placing the parts in a position of muscular rest simplifies the closure, aids union, and assures a comfortable convalescence. In difficult herniæ done under local anæsthesia it is almost indispensable.

Since adopting it as a routine method Doctor Lyle had done fewer and fewer rectus transplantations. It is essential that the position be maintained for at least seven to ten days after the operation.

DOCTOR WOOLSEY said he had employed for over twenty years an operation a great deal like Doctor Stetten's, except that he did not split the outer layer of the external oblique. When the lower flap of the external oblique was brought up, overlapping the upper flap, the cord was turned upward so that it passed with a certain obliquity through the abdominal wall, just as it did in the normal inguinal canal. One could not cure a hernia, direct or indirect, unless the posterior wall of the inguinal canal was made strong. Therefore, he used all layers in fortifying this point and transplanted the cord. Doctor Woolsey said he did not see any need of putting the external oblique in front of the cord. The only trouble that could happen with the cord transplanted beneath the fatty layer was that if there was a recurrence and the man who operated did not know that the cord was left in this position he might cut it by a careless incision. If one sutured the fatty layer separately so the cord would not become adherent in the cutaneous scar, there would not be the difficulty that the cord would become so adherent that it could not be dissected out, as mentioned in the discussion.

Another point that might be mentioned was that of the suture lines for the muscle and upper layer of the aponeurosis. There was not much use in putting in a separate suture line in the muscle, for this could bear little strain without fraying out in the line with the fibres. If the muscle and aponeurosis were sutured together the latter would take the strain off of the muscle.

DR. WILLIAM B. COLEY said that excellent results were apparently obtained from each of the three methods described, and it perhaps required fine judgment to choose which operation was the best. He believed that Doctor Hoguet's operation had some advantages over the others, and that in certain cases the others, doubtless, had some advantages over Doctor Hoguet's. Doctor Coley stated that, for the past thirty years, since 1890, in all operations for inguinal hernia he had placed the lowermost suture through the reflected double layer of the aponeurosis external oblique. In Doctor Hoguet's operation he had used the same suture not only for the lowermost suture, but for all of the sutures, 3 to 4 below the cord. The greatest difficulty in obtaining a cure in direct hernia consisted in completely and firmly closing the lower portion of the inguinal canal. In certain cases the tension might be too great to permit bringing the reflected portion of the aponeurosis in apposition with Poupart's ligament all the way to the cord, according to Doctor Hoguet's method. In such cases it might be better to use the technic just described by Doctor Downes for bringing the rectus muscle in apposition with Poupart's ligament. In certain cases Doctor Coley believed it was a distinct advantage to employ the Andrews overlapping method as described by Doctor

Downes. Doctor Coley expressed the opinion that it was a great disadvantage to bring the cord out superficial to the aponeurosis and covered only by the skin, either by the method just described by one of the speakers or by the typical Halsted method. The disadvantages of the Halsted method had been the recurrences at the site where the cord came through the opening in the aponeurosis. Anyone who had been obliged to operate for a recurrence following the Halsted method must have recognized the great difficulty in separating the cord from the firm adhesions to the overlying and underlying structures. Doctor Coley believed it was far better that the cord should be covered with the aponeurosis as in the typical Bassini operation or in the overlapping Andrews method. He thought it would require at least two years before we could pass final judgment as to the value of any technic in the operation for the radical cure of hernia. It should be remembered, however, that the great majority of recurrences in hernia took place within the first year; that the direct recurrences were earlier than the indirect; that about 80 to 90 per cent. of the recurrences in direct hernia occurred in the first year (the majority of these in the first six months), so that if a patient remained free from recurrence in direct hernia for the first six months, the probability was that he would remain cured.

Dr. A. V. Moschcowitz said he thought Doctor Coley's statement that the internal oblique muscle united to Poupart's ligament was rather important; there was no doubt of that, but it was also certain that the union between two homogeneous structures like the external oblique and Poupart's ligament was much stronger and safer. He would take this occasion to repeat a story he had told before. A number of years ago a member of his family was operated on for a hernia by a most prominent surgeon. Bassini's operation was done absolutely *secundum artem*. Within six weeks there was a recurrence. At the second operation, with the exception of the cutaneous cicatrix, it was difficult to tell that any operation had been performed. The internal oblique and the transversalis were back in their old position. Doctor Moschcowitz said he was convinced that this case alone proved the flimsiness of the union between heterogeneous structures.

Doctor Downes said in regard to recurrences he did not wish anyone to get the impression that he had no recurrences. He thought he had about 6 per cent. recurrences in cases that went over one year. He cited the case of one man upon whom he had operated for hernia and who later came to him for some other trouble. In examining him he found that he had a slight recurrence of the hernia of which he was not conscious. Cases of this kind impressed him with the fact that statistics based on correspondence with the patient in regard to recurrence were not reliable, as patients frequently had a slight bulging or recurrence and did not know it. He thought recurrences were nearer 10 per cent. rather than 2 or 5 per cent. in the cases he had had in his own personal experience.

NEW YORK SURGICAL SOCIETY

Doctor Hoguet, in closing the discussion, said there were several points he wished to make clear. First, on account of the anatomical peculiarities, the more direct hernias he did the less inclined he felt to follow any set operation. He was convinced that one often found large-sized direct hernias which could be cured by the Bassini where the bulk of the internal oblique and transversalis muscle was large enough and where the rectus was narrow. There were a number of cases that could be cured by the rectus transplantation. If there was not enough conjoined tendon to suture down and the rectus narrow and tight, and if the aponeurosis was strong and firm and loose enough, it could be brought down and sutured to Poupart's ligament.

Doctor Hoguet said he wanted to correct Doctor Moschcowitz's impression. If there was any question as to whether muscle united to fascia, then this ought to be an ideal operation, for muscle was not only sutured to fascia but also aponeurosis to fascia. As one sutured one found the reflected edge of the external oblique came absolutely down to and hugged Poupart's ligament. As to the conjoined tendon he imagined it was pushed to the back and down and Poupart's ligament united to the posterior surface of the fascia lata as it came down to Poupart's ligament.

As to the objection that Doctor Torek made that it pulled the aponeurosis of the external oblique out of line, Doctor Hoguet said he would not use the operation where the aponeurosis was not loose. In many large hernias he had found the aponeurosis of the external oblique such that it could be pulled down to Poupart's ligament without any tension whatsoever.

To Contributors and Subscribers:

All contributions for Publication, Books for Review, and Exchanges should be sent to the Editorial Office, 145 Gates Ave., Brooklyn, N. Y.

Remittances for Subscriptions and Advertising and all business communications should be addressed to the

ANNALS of SURGERY
227-231 S. 6th Street
Philadelphia, Penna.

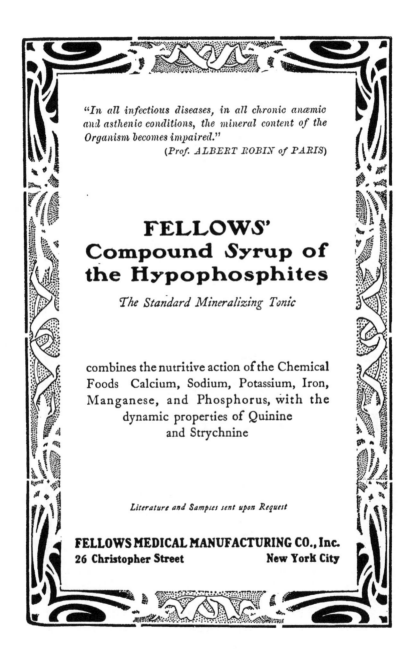

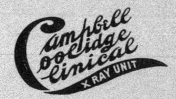

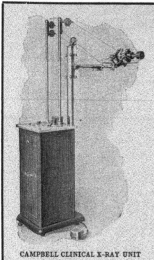
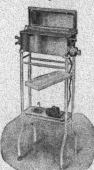
2

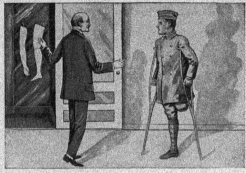
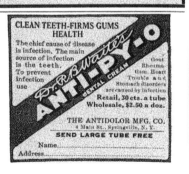

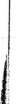
The

4

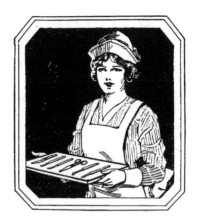

STELLITE

The master metal for surgical instruments

STELLITE is the only known metal possessing every quality that surgery demands in instruments.

Stellite is rustless. Moisture cannot affect it.

Stellite is untarnishable. Its silvery white lustre is permanent—never requires polishing.

Stellite is non-corrosive. It is proof against the chemicals used in sterilizing processes.

Stellite is the hardest known metal for edged tools and instruments. Its hardness is inherent—not tempered—therefore permanent.

Stellite surgical instruments take and hold a keener edge through longer periods of use and abuse than instruments of any other metal.

HAYNES STELLITE COMPANY

Kokomo, Indiana

Carbide and Carbon Building, 30 East 42nd Street, New York

Peoples Gas Building, Chicago, Ill.

RADIUM

Radium salts of the highest purity for use in surgery and gynecology. Deliveries on the basis of U. S. Bureau of Standards measurement.

We guarantee that the radiations of our Radium salts are due solely to Radium element and its own decomposition products.

Our Medical Staff will give instruction in the physics and therapeutics of Radium.

"The National Radium Bank" instituted by this corporation.

We manufacture improved applicators, screens and other special equipment made with alloys of our own development, also apparatus for the purification and concentration of Radium emanation.

Information on request

THE RADIO CHEMICAL CORPORATION

58 Pine Street, New York   Plants and Laboratories: Orange, N. J.
Telephone, John 3141   Mines: Colorado, Utah

6

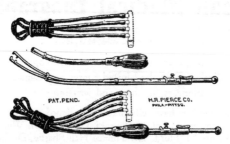

DAVIS & GECK, INC.

PHYSIOLOGICAL CHEMISTS

Sterile Surgical Sutures

217-221 Duffield Street   ᵥ   Brooklyn, N.Y., U.S.A.

Claustro-Thermal Catgut

Boilable

CLAUSTRO-THERMAL, meaning *enclosed heat*, is descriptive of the improved method of heat sterilization. The principle of the method consists in applying the heat after closure of the tubes, thus avoiding all the chances of accidental contamination.

The sealed tubes are submerged in a bath of cumol—the high boiling hydrocarbon. The temperature of the cumol bath is gradually elevated until at the end of six hours the maximum of 165° C. (329° F.) is reached. This temperature is maintained for five hours, and is then allowed to slowly decline. The temperature curve is graphically represented by the chart shown below.

It is obvious, therefore, that sterility is absolutely assured. The sutures, being stored in their original tubing fluid and reaching the surgeon's hands sealed within the tubes in which they were sterilized, are removed from all the chances of contamination incident to the customary method of sterilizing the strands in open tubes.

Sterilization by this integral method is made feasible through the use of toluol as the tubing fluid. The discovery of the value of toluol for this purpose was the outcome of an investigation aimed at finding a suitable fluid to replace chloroform. The latter was formerly in general use, but was unsatisfactory because it was found to break down into chemical products which not only exerted an extremely harmful action on the collagen of the sutures but which were responsible for considerable wound irritation.

No other mode of sterilization so completely fulfills the exacting requirements for the production of ideal sutures as does the Claustro-Thermal method. Through its use the natural physical characteristics of the strands are preserved, while the destruction of all bacterial life is absolutely assured.

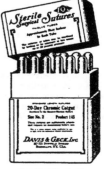

THE NEW PACKAGE
Containing One Dozen Tubes
of a Kind and Size

Claustro-Thermal sutures are not impregnated with any germicidal substance, and consequently they exert no bactericidal influence in the tissues.

This product embodies all the essentials of the perfect suture, such as compatibility with tissues, accuracy of size, maximum tensile strength, perfect and dependable absorbability, and absolute sterility.

Reprints of original articles relating to the Claustro-Thermal method will be sent upon request.

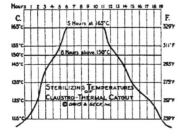

List of Claustro-Thermal Catgut

Approximately Sixty Inches in Each Tube

Plain Catgut	Product No. 105
10-Day Chromic Catgut	Product No. 125
20-Day Chromic Catgut	Product No. 145
40-Day Chromic Catgut	Product No. 185

SIZES: 000...00...0...1...2...3...4

Claustro-Thermal sutures are unaffected by age, light, or extremes of climatic temperatures

Price in U.S.A.

Per dozen tubes (subject to a fixed discount on quantities)......$3.60

Please specify clearly the PRODUCT NUMBERS and SIZES desired

CONTINUED—

Kalmerid Catgut

An Improved Germicidal Suture
Superseding Iodized Catgut

KALMERID CATGUT is not only sterile, but, being impregnated with potassium-mercuric-iodide—*a double iodine compound*—the sutures exert a local bactericidal action in the tissues.

The older practise of impregnating catgut with the ordinary crystalline iodine for this purpose was at best an unsatisfactory method, since the antiseptic power was but slight and transient. The most serious deficiencies of such iodized sutures, however, were their instability and weakness arising from exposure to light; the deterioration resulting from the continuous and unpreventable oxidizing action of the iodine; and the disintegration of the sutures when heated. Moreover, the decomposition products of iodine caused such sutures to be irritating.

These serious disadvantages of iodized catgut have been overcome through the use of potassium-mercuric-iodide instead of iodine. This double salt of iodine and mercury, the chemical formula of which is $HgI_2.2KI$, is one of the most active germicides known, exerting a killing action on bacteria about ten times greater than that of iodine. It does not break down under the influence of light or heat, it is chemically stable, and, in the proportions used, is neither toxic nor irritating to the tissues. It interferes in no way with the absorption of the sutures, and is not precipitated by the proteins of the body fluids.

Kalmerid catgut, in addition to its bactericidal attribute, embodies all the essentials of the perfect suture. It is perfectly compatible with the tissues, its absorbability is dependable, and its tensile strength is particularly good.

TWO VARIETIES—To meet the requirements of different surgeons two kinds of Kalmerid catgut are prepared—the boilable, and non-boilable.

BOILABLE GRADE—This variety is prepared for surgeons who prefer a boilable suture, such as the Claustro-Thermal product, but possessing bactericidal properties in addition. The boilable grade, therefore, besides being impregnated with potassium-mercuric-iodide, embodies the desirable physical characteristics of the Claustro-Thermal sutures. It has the same moderate degree of flexibility; it is the same in appearance; it is tubed in the same improved storing fluid—toluol; and, after impregnation with potassium-mercuric-iodide, it further receives the Claustro-Thermal sterilization—that is, heat sterilization after closure of the tubes.

NON-BOILABLE GRADE—This variety is extremely pliable as it comes from the tubes. It is made for those surgeons who have been accustomed to the flexibility of iodized catgut.

Reprints of original articles relating to Kalmerid sutures will be sent upon request.

List of Kalmerid Catgut

Approximately Sixty Inches in Each Tube

Boilable Grade	Non-Boilable Grade
Plain Catgut.............Product No. 1205	Plain Catgut.............Product No. 1405
10-Day Chromic.........Product No. 1225	10-Day Chromic.........Product No. 1425
20-Day Chromic.........Product No. 1245	20-Day Chromic.........Product No. 1445
40-Day Chromic.........Product No. 1285	40-Day Chromic.........Product No. 1485

SIZES: 000...00...0...1...2...3...4

Please specify clearly the PRODUCT NUMBERS and SIZES desired

Kalmerid sutures are unaffected by age or light, or by the extremes of climatic temperatures

Price in U. S. A.

Per dozen tubes (subject to a fixed discount on quantities).........................$3.60

In packages of twelve tubes of a kind and size as illustrated on first page

DAVIS & GECK,INC. 217-231 Duffield Street, Brooklyn, N.Y., U.S.A.

Kalmerid Kangaroo Tendons

Two Varieties — Boilable and Non-Boilable

THESE are the sutures *par excellence* for those procedures in which post-operative tension is excessive, or long continued apposition necessary, such as in herniotomy, and in tendon and bone suturing. Kalmerid kangaroo tendons are not only sterile, but, in addition, they are impregnated with potassium-mercuric-iodide, which enables them to exert a local bactericidal action in the tissues. The impregnating and sterilizing methods are the same as practised in the preparation of Kalmerid catgut, and described on the preceding page.

They are genuine kangaroo tendons; they are round, smooth, straight, of uniform contour, and possess a tensile strength about twice that of the best catgut of equivalent size.

Because of their greater strength some surgeons prefer these tendons to catgut, particularly in the finer sizes, for general intestinal, muscle, fascia, and skin suturing.

ABSORPTION TIME—The tendons are chromicized, and so accurately is the chromicizing process regulated that each size, whether it be the finest or the coarsest, will maintain apposition in fascia or in tendon for approximately thirty days. Shortly after that period the sutures, with their knots, will be completely absorbed.

TWO VARIETIES—Kalmerid kangaroo tendons are prepared in two grades—boilable and non-boilable.

The NON-BOILABLE tendons are extremely pliable and consequently require no moistening.

The BOILABLE tendons are quite stiff as they come from the tubes, but may be rendered pliable by moistening in sterile water preliminary to use. The smaller sizes will be sufficiently softened by fifteen minutes immersion, while the larger sizes should be immersed for about thirty minutes. Either sterile water, or an aqueous bactericidal solution made with Kalmerid tablets—1:5000—should be used.

Before immersion, the toluol, which is very volatile, should be allowed to evaporate so that the water may have access to the sutures.

Reprints of original articles relating to Kalmerid sutures will be sent upon request.

List of Kalmerid Kangaroo Tendons

Each Tube Contains One Tendon • Lengths Vary From 12 to 20 Inches

The Non-Boilable Grade is *Product. No. 370*

Boilable Grade is *Product No. 380*

• Sizes •

Tendon Sizes:	Ex. Fine	Fine	Medium	Coarse	Ex. Coarse
Catgut Sizes:	0	2	4	6	8

Please specify clearly the PRODUCT NUMBERS and SIZES desired

Kalmerid kangaroo tendons are unaffected by age or light, or by the extremes of climatic temperatures

Price in U. S. A.

Per dozen tubes (subject to a fixed discount on quantities).........................$3.60

In packages of twelve tubes of a kind and size as illustrated on first page

---

Actual Sizes

```
000 ————————————————
 00 ————————————————
  0 ————————————————
  1 ————————————————
  2 ————————————————
  3 ————————————————
  4 ————————————————
  6 ————————————————
  8 ————————————————
```

Standardized Sizes

The Established Metric System of Catgut Sizes is Now Used For All Sutures

IN conformity with the long recognized need for a unified system of sizes, the standard metric catgut scale has been extended to embrace all sutures, including kangaroo tendons, silk, horsehair, silkworm gut, and celluloid-linen thread.

The advantage of this standardized system is obvious.

Miscellaneous Sutures
Boilable
Sterilized by Heat After Closure of the Tubes

Product No.	Material	Approximate Quantity in Each Tube	Catgut Size
350	Celluloid-Linen Thread	60 Inches	000, 00, 0
360	Horsehair	Four 28-inch Sutures	00
390	Plain Silkworm Gut	Four 14-inch Sutures	00, 0, 1
400	Black Silkworm Gut	Four 14-inch Sutures	00, 0, 1
450	White Twisted Silk	60 Inches	000, 00, 0, 1, 2, 3
460	Black Twisted Silk	60 Inches	000, 0, 2
480	White Braided Silk	60 Inches	00, 0, 2, 4
490	Black Braided Silk	60 Inches	00, 1, 4
600	Catgut Circumcision Suture	30 Inches With Needle	00

Price in U. S. A.—Per dozen tubes (subject to a fixed discount on quantities)...................$3.60

In packages of twelve tubes of a kind and size as illustrated on first page

Minor Sutures
Short Length ▪ Without Needles
Sterilized by Heat After Closure of the Tubes

Product No.	Material	Approximate Quantity App in Each Tube	Catgut Sizes
802	Plain Catgut	20 Inches	00, 0, 1, 2, 3
812	10-Day Chromic Catgut	20 Inches	00, 0, 1, 2, 3
822	20-Day Chromic Catgut	20 Inches	00, 0, 1, 2, 3
862	Horsehair	Two 28-inch Sutures	00
872	Plain Silkworm Gut	Two 14-inch Sutures	0
882	White Twisted Silk	20 Inches	000, 0, 2
892	Umbilical Tape	Two 12-inch Ligatures	

Price in U. S. A.—Per dozen tubes (subject to a fixed discount on quantities)....................$1.80

In packages of twelve tubes of a kind and size as illustrated on first page

Emergency Sutures
With Needles
Sterilized by Heat After Closure of the Tubes

Product No.	Material	Approximate Quantity in Each Tube	Catgut Sizes
904	Plain Catgut	20 Inches	00, 0, 1, 2, 3
914	10-Day Chromic Catgut	20 Inches	00, 0, 1, 2, 3
924	20-Day Chromic Catgut	20 Inches	00, 0, 1, 2, 3
964	Horsehair	Two 28-inch Sutures	00
974	Plain Silkworm Gut	Two 14-inch Sutures	0
984	White Twisted Silk	20 Inches	000, 0, 2

Price in U. S. A.

Per dozen tubes (subject to a fixed discount on quantities)...............$3.60

In packages of twelve tubes of a kind and size as illustrated on first page

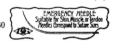

EMERGENCY NEEDLE
Suitable for Skin, Muscle, or Tendon
Needles Correspond to Suture Sizes

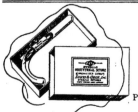

Obstetrical Sutures
Product No. 650
For the Immediate Repair of Perineal Lacerations

Each tube contains *two* 28-inch sutures of 40-day chromic catgut
one of which is threaded upon a large full-curved needle

Price in U. S. A.

Per tube (subject to a fixed discount on quantities)................$ .35

Each tube in a package as illustrated

DAVIS & GECK, INC. 217-221 Duffield Street, Brooklyn, N.Y., U.S.A.

A HELPFUL DEPARTMENT FOR SURGEONS

THE AMERICAN INSTITUTE OF MEDICINE, through its Department of Surgery, aids the progressive surgeon by keeping him informed of new developments in his field. It also performs for him many special services that conserve his time and energy, and increase his professional efficiency.

A Staff of Surgical Specialists

is maintained by the Institute at its headquarters in New York. Expert editors, abstractors, translators, research workers, investigators and consultants render the following services:

LITERATURE—Leading American and foreign journals read each month, and indexes and complete set of abstracts of all important articles relating to surgery, supplied.

RESEARCH—Investigations on surgical subjects made by trained research workers. Bibliographies compiled. Questions arising in surgical practice answered.

SPECIAL SERVICE—Special service given to meet the particular requirements of individual surgeons.

SURGICAL INFORMATION—Information furnished about important surgical developments, notices of meetings, and other matters of interest.

Conducted on Co-operative Plan

The Department of Surgery is conducted on a co-operative basis in the interest of the surgeon members of the Institute who use the department. Each member pays a moderate annual fee and in return receives the complete service provided by the staff.

Surgeons who are interested in learning more about the work done by this Department are invited to send in the inquiry coupon attached. Literature containing more detailed information and membership application blank will be forwarded. No obligation is created by this request.

AMERICAN INSTITUTE OF MEDICINE
13 East 47th Street
NEW YORK CITY

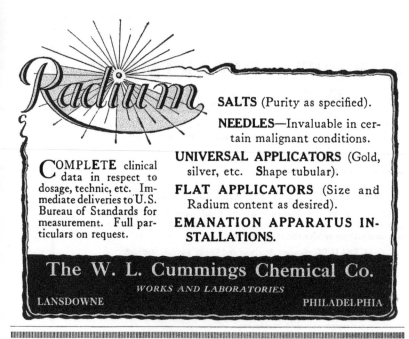
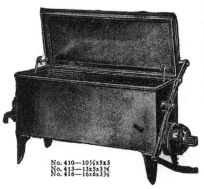

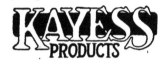

Adrenalin in Medicine

3—Treatment of Shock and Collapse

THE therapeutic importance of Adrenalin in shock and collapse is suggested by their most obvious and constant phenomenon—a loss in blood pressure.

The cause and essential nature of shock and collapse have not been satisfactorily explained by any of the theories that have been advanced, but all observers are agreed that the most striking characteristic of these conditions is that the peripheral arteries and capillaries are depleted of blood and that the veins, especially those of the splanchnic region, are congested. All the other symptoms—the cardiac, respiratory and nervous manifestations—are secondary to this rude impairment of the circulation.

The term collapse usually designates a profound degree of shock induced by functional inhibition or depression of the vasomotor center resulting from some cause other than physical injury, such as cardiac or respiratory failure.

Treatment aims to raise the blood pressure by increasing peripheral resistance. As a rapidly acting medical agent for the certain accomplishment of this object Adrenalin is without a peer. In cases of ordinary shock it is best administered by intravenous infusion of high dilutions in saline solution. Five drops of the 1:1000 Adrenalin Chloride Solution to an ounce of normal salt solution dilutes the Adrenalin to approximately 1:100,000, which is the proper strength to employ intravenously. A slow, steady and continuous stream should be maintained by feeding the solution from a buret to which is attached a stop-cock for the regulation of the rate of flow.

In those cases marked by extremely profound and dangerous shock or collapse the intravenous method may prove too slow or ineffective. Recourse should then be had to the procedure described by Crile and called centripetal arterial transfusion. Briefly it consists in the insertion into an artery of a cannula directed *toward* the heart. Into the rubber tubing which is attached to the cannula 15 to 30 minims of Adrenalin 1:1000 is injected as soon as the saline infusion begins.

The effect of this is to bring the Adrenalin immediately into contact with the larger arteries and the heart. Sometimes, even in apparent death, the heart will resume its contractions, thereby distributing the Adrenalin through the arterial system and accomplishing the object of this heroic measure—resuscitation and elevation of the blood pressure.

PARKE, DAVIS & COMPANY

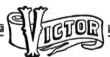

Announcement of Merging of Victor Electric Corporation with X-Ray Interests of General Electric Company

An arrangement has been completed which took effect October 1, 1920, under which the entire business of the Victor Electric Corporation and X-Ray interests of the General Electric Company have been merged in a new corporation formed for the purpose and known as the VICTOR X-RAY CORPORATION. The new company, has exchanged its capital stock for the X-Ray patents and good will of General Electric Company and for the assets and business of the old Victor Electric Corporation.

The formation of the new company will result in full manufacturing, engineering and research co-operation between Victor X-Ray Corporation and General Electric Company with respect to X-Ray problems. It will extend further the usefulness of the two companies and consequently, present needs for Coolidge tubes and other X-Ray devices will be adequately met.

The executive, administrative, engineering and sales staff of the old Victor Electric Corporation will remain practically unchanged. Mr. C. F. Samms becomes President and General Manager. Mr. J. B. Wantz retains full charge of manufacturing and designing. It is contemplated to bring about a complete co-ordination of the entire Victor Corporation organization with the research and engineering organization of General Electric Company with as little disturbance of the old relationships as possible.

Dr. W. D. Coolidge of the research laboratory of General Electric Company becomes Consulting Engineer of the Victor X-Ray Corporation. Mr. C. C. Darnell of the research laboratory of General Electric Company becomes the Commercial Engineer of the Victor X-Ray Corporation. Mr. W. S. Kendrick, who for many years had charge of the commercial sale of the Coolidge tube, will be General Sales Manager. Mr. L. B. Miller remains General Manager of Agency Sales.

The Victor X-Ray Corporation will continue to carry out the same liberal policies and practices toward the X-Ray trade that have already been established by the General Electric Company.

The primary purpose of this merger was to co-ordinate the efforts of the best and most constructive elements in the research, engineering and commercial divisions of the X-Ray field to the end that users of X-Ray equipment might be served in the best possible manner, and assurances are given by the officers of the new corporation that the ideal toward which they intend to strive is 100% service.

VICTOR X-RAY CORPORATION

C. F. Samms, President

ANNALS *of* SURGERY

| Vol. LXXII | DECEMBER, 1920 | No. 6. |

MULTIPLE POLYPOSIS OF THE INTESTINAL TRACT

By John Edmund Struthers, M.D.

OF ROCHESTER, MINN.

SCHOLAR IN SURGERY, MAYO FOUNDATION

FROM a clinical point of view intestinal polyposis is considered a comparatively rare disease occurring in young and middle-aged persons. Excrescences and polypoid projections of the mucosa in various parts of the alimentary tract are nevertheless frequently found at necropsy. The association of the excrescences or polypoid growths with inflammation of the intestines, or at least with a clinical history of dysentery, is quite common.

The earliest case reported in the literature was probably that of Menzel, in 1721, whose patient was a boy aged fifteen, with dysentery. At post-mortem it was observed that the mucous membrane of the large intestines had great numbers of wart-like excrescences. There is no further mention of the condition until 1832, when Wagner, in describing the end-results of ulceration of the colon, stated that " sometimes on the margins of scars and on the smooth cicatrices of healed ulcers, tiny polypoid excrescences were found." In 1839 Rokitansky confirmed Wagner's findings and added, " These small excrescences had their origin from islands of the mucous membrane that remained after the ulcerative process had ceased." In 1861 Lebert reported the case of a woman, aged thirty-two years, who had suffered from obstinate diarrhœa for years. At necropsy, examination of the mucous membrane of the colon showed hundreds of little polypi varying in size from 0.5 by 0.5 cm. to 0.5 by 1.5 cm.; some of these were pedunculated, others sessile. Lebert's account contains the first description of the polypi themselves. They are described as consisting of fibrous tissue containing ramifying blood-vessels but no glands. Glandular tubules, however, surrounded the base of the polypi. The same year, 1861, Luschka described his findings in a case in which the polypi covered the mucous membrane from the ileocæcal valve to the anus. These polypi were found to consist of glands resembling the glands of Lieberkühn, except that they were longer, many of them more or less branched, and some of them dilated into cyst-like spaces.

Virchow, about this time, gave the microscopic findings on the case of a boy, aged fifteen, who had dysentery. The polypi were vesicular, fluctuating prominences, and many of them had scattered over their surfaces small openings from which gelatinous material protruded and could be expressed. Under the microscope these vesicles were found to be dilated crypts of the glands of Lieberkühn filled with a mucous material. This case and the cases of Lebert and Luschka, Virchow called colitis polyposa cystica. Woodward, in 1861, reported a case similar to that of Lebert. All these early cases were associated with dysentery. Collier reported a case of multiple polypi of the stomach and intestine similar to the case of Carroll.

In 1907 Doering reported fifty-two cases; fifty he had collected from the literature; two were his own. In 1916 Soper collected eight additional cases from the literature and reported one of his own. Seven of these last nine patients were operated on, three of whom died. Doering observed from his collected cases that the greatest number of cancers developed in the cases of polyposis which occurred in early adult life; namely, between the ages of fifteen and thirty-five years. The distribution of the cases was as follows:

Between 15 and 25 years	7 cases
Between 25 and 35 years	7 cases
After 35 years	3 cases
Information lacking	6 cases

Doering also observed that intestinal polyposis occurred twice as frequently in males as in females.

On the basis of the facts presented in the sixty-one cases reviewed by Doering and Soper, the following is apparent:

1. Polypi are most frequent in children and in young adults.

2. Twenty-six (43 per cent.) showed the presence of adenocarcinoma.

3. The most frequent sites of the lesion are the rectum, sigmoid, and the splenic flexure.

4. The small intestine seems to be involved rarely; the ileum in five cases, the jejunum and duodenum each in four.

5. The polypi tend to occur in members of the same family.[9]

Ten other cases of intestinal polyposis are reported in the literature. Bratrud, Watson, Norbury, Edwards, Drummond, Furnivall, Newbolt and John B. Murphy each reported one case. Hewitt and Howard report two cases. In this series there were seven males and three females. One case occurred in a child of thirteen years. The predominating symptoms were bleeding from the rectum in three cases, blood-tinged stools in three cases, prolapse associated with bleeding in two cases, and obstinate constipation in one case. All the cases were treated surgically: cauterization with forceps removal of some of the polypi in four cases, in the remaining cases colotomy, colostomy, colectomy, appendicostomy, resection of the rectum, and end-to-end anastomosis were performed.

From röntgen and operative findings it was learned that the rectum and sigmoid were involved in eight cases; the rectum and transverse colon in one; advanced carcinoma of the sigmoid with multiple polypi above and below the growth in one.

MULTIPLE POLYPOSIS OF THE INTESTINAL TRACT

In reporting these cases five were designated as polypi; four as adenomas; and one as an adenomatous polypus. Pathologic reports on the case of carcinoma of the sigmoid and one of the other cases showed them to be papillary and tubular columnar-cell carcinoma.

Three of the ten patients are reported to have completely recovered, in two of these cauterization was done, two were reported as markedly improved; two died, and the condition of three has not been ascertained. The length of time after operation when these reports were obtained was not specified. The mortality with three cases unaccounted for is 20 per cent.

With an increasing number of cases of polypi reported in the literature there was apparent confusion in the differentiation of adenoma and the polyp type of growth. Hauser uses the term "polyposis intestinalis." Verse simply admits the difficulty of discrimination. Adami speaks of polypoid tumors of the intestinal tract which have the general structure of adenoma. Hertzler refers to intestinal polyposis as hyperplasia of the mucous membrane; Kaufmann speaks of adenomas, both polypoid and papillary. Kassemeyer reported 224 cases of intussusception caused by tumors, of which 116 were benign; 73 of these benign growths were polypi and adenomas. Watts, Hartmann, and Karajan all reported cases in which operations had been done several times for intussusception caused by polypoid adenomas and polypoid tumors. Hewitt and Howard liken their first case to that of Rokitansky and their second to that of Luschka, considering the second case but an advanced stage of the first.

The series of thirty-nine cases in this study were observed in the Mayo Clinic from January, 1911, to February, 1920. Carroll's case, which was reported by Soper, is also included, since it came within this period.

AGE AND SEX OF PATIENTS
```
19 to 30 years ............................................... 15
31 to 40 years ...............................................  9
41 to 50 years ...............................................  7
51 to 60 years ...............................................  5
61 to 68 years ...............................................  3
Males ........................................................ 29
Females ...................................................... 10
```

DURATION OF SYMPTOMS
```
Less than 1 year .............................................  4
1 to  2 years ................................................  9
3 to  4 years ................................................  4
5 to  6 years ................................................ 11
7 to 34 years ................................................ 11
Shortest period of symptoms 3 weeks; longest 34 years.
```

TYPE OF ONSET
```
Mild diarrhœa followed by pus and blood ....................  8
General abdominal distress ..................................  8
    1 marked nausea and vomiting
    1 marked constipation
```

651

1 food relief (duodenal ulcer)
Sudden onset, diarrhœa, pus and blood 6
   1 of these alternated with constipation
Constipation 3
Pain in left lower quadrant 3
   Constipation marked in 1 of these
Bleeding from the rectum 3
Marked abdominal colics with sudden diarrhœa 2
Rectal pain with diarrhœa 2
Bleeding with hemorrhoids 2
Mild symptomless diarrhœa 2

With the exception of five patients, all had periods of diarrhœa[18] later; these included two patients with constipation, two with abdominal distress, and one with diagnosis of duodenal ulcer.

Constipation, although the chief complaint on admission in but one case, was marked in one patient with general abdominal pain, in one with marked rectal pain, and in the patient with frequency of urination who was in a uræmic condition when he entered the Clinic. His case may belong to the group of cases discussed by Preble. At some time during the course of the disease thirty-one of the thirty-nine patients had abdominal pain, eight only giving a negative history. The patient with the ribbon-like stools had carcinoma of the sigmoid with multiple polypi below the growth.

Fifteen of the patients had some rectal complaint, although it was an early symptom in but eight. Four complained of absolute inability to control the bowels, the others of bleeding from the rectum, in two instances marked; the degree of bleeding in the other patients was variable.

In the more severe cases in which the colon and rectum were extensively involved by polyposis, the onset of the disease was gradual, with but few exceptions becoming progressively worse over a period of many years. The exceptions were the cases in which there was a history of diarrhœa of less than five years.

COMPLAINT ON ADMISSION TO THE CLINIC

Diarrhœa with pus and blood 17
General abdominal distress 5
Abdominal pain with nausea and vomiting 3
Hemorrhoids 3
Mild diarrhœa 3
Bleeding from the rectum 3
Rectal pain 2
Passage of ribbon-like stools, constipation slight 1
Constipation 1
Frequency of urination 1

LOSS OF WEIGHT

The loss of weight varied markedly with the severity of the disease. In two cases patients with a mild constant diarrhœa gained weight, each less than ten pounds.

BLOOD

The duration of the disease and the degree of bleeding has a marked effect on the degree of anæmia. The blood counts were made in twenty-nine patients; the eosinophile count in six cases showed an eosinophilia in one (7.3 per cent.). The lowest erythrocyte count was 2,700,000; the lowest leucocyte count was 4800; the highest leucocyte count was 17,000.

Hæmoglobin between 90 and 80 5
Hæmoglobin between 79 and 70 7
Hæmoglobin between 69 and 60 9
Hæmoglobin between 59 and 50 1
Hæmoglobin between 49 and 40 4
Hæmoglobin between 39 and 30 3

EXAMINATION OF STOOLS

Stool examinations were made in twenty-seven cases:
Stools reported negative for parasites, but containing pus and
  blood 12
Stools reported negative for parasites, pus and blood 7
Nonmotile amœba with trichomonades 3
Endamœba histolytica 2
Trichomonades 2
Cercomonades 1

PROCTOSCOPIC EXAMINATION

Multiple polyposis of the rectum and sigmoid 19
Chronic ulcerative colitis with multiple polypi 4
Probable carcinoma of the sigmoid with multiple polypi, all
  below the growth 3
Granular polyposis 2

Thirty cases were diagnosed multiple polyposis. In twenty-eight there were positive proctoscopic findings, two by means of the X-ray, one a case of gastric polyposis, and one a case of multiple polypi of the descending colon with filling defect. In three of the remaining cases a probable clinical diagnosis of multiple polypi was made.

Nineteen specimens were removed at proctoscopic examination; in two instances a second specimen. The primary diagnosis in each was carcinoma and the secondary was negative for carcinoma. The second specimens, however, were not from the same site. One of the patients came to operation and the specimen removed at operation was reported a polypus. Reports on specimens removed were:

Polypi—negative for carcinoma 8
Adenoma 6
Carcinoma 2

Inflammatory tissue 1
Papilloma 1
Mucous polypus 1

19

OPERATIONS

Twenty-two of the thirty-nine patients came to operation.

The Brown was the primary operation in ten cases. In one other case it was secondary to a colostomy performed elsewhere; in two cases it was followed by an ileocolostomy; in two by a colectomy; in two by an ileosigmoidostomy; and in four there was no second-stage operation. There were four primary ileocolostomies; two colectomies with the exception of twelve inches of the sigmoid and rectum; one was a permanent ileostomy; one was a complete colectomy with removal of five inches of the lower ileum, and permanent ileostomy; one was a Mikulicz first- and second-stage operation; one was a Kraske, secondary to a colostomy; one was an appendicostomy; one was a Desquin-Mixter midline cautery operation, and one was a partial resection of the stomach and removal of three-fifths of the pylorus. This patient was rerayed one year later; the remaining portion of the stomach was still covered with polypi.

EXTENT OF INVOLVEMENT AT THE TIME OF OPERATION

Rectum only 2
Rectum and sigmoid 3
Rectum and transverse colon 1
Rectum, sigmoid, and descending colon 2
Rectum, sigmoid, descending and transverse colon 1
Rectum to the ileocæcal valve 5
Rectum to the ileocæcal valve, with carcinoma at the splenic
    flexure and sigmoid 1
Ileocæcal valve only 1
Ileocæcal valve extending into the transverse colon 1
Ileocæcal valve extending into the descending colon 1
Ileocæcal valve, hepatic flexure marked, colon slight involvement 2
Stomach and jejunum 1
Stomach 1

REPORTS ON SPECIMENS REMOVED AT OPERATION

Polypi 9
Papillomas 3
Carcinomas 2
Adenocarcinomas 2
Colitis 1
Inflammatory tissue 1

Both cases of adenocarcinoma (Figs. 1 and 2) were in specimens from the rectum. In one of these cases the colon was found to be covered with polypi. In each instance of carcinoma of the sigmoid the polypi were below the growth.

There were two cases of duodenal ulcer and one of gastric ulcer.

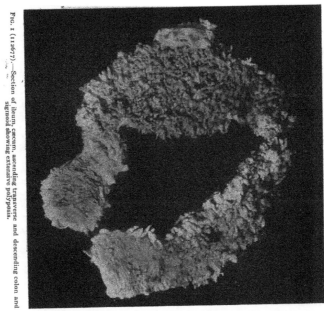

Fig. 1 (112677).—Section of ileum, caecum, ascending transverse and descending colon and sigmoid showing extensive polyposis.

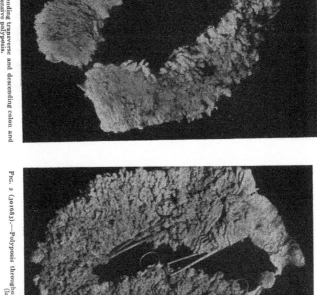

Fig. 2 (30168.3).—Polyposis throughout the colon. Numerous pedunculated polypi (largest 2.5 cm.)

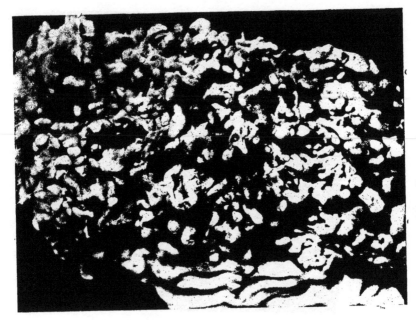

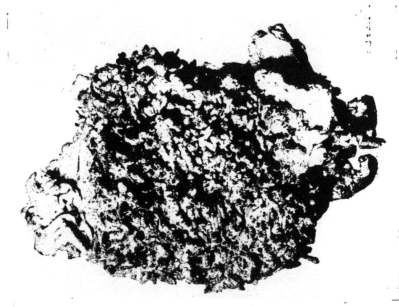

FIGS. 3 AND 4 (114349).—Section of cæcum and ascending colon showing multiple papilloma.

One case of duodenal ulcer was associated with amœbic dysentery and with a history of extensive gastric trouble; the diagnosis was confirmed by X-ray. The other duodenal ulcer and the gastric ulcer were found at operation.

RÖNTGEN EXAMINATION

Thirteen patients in the series were not rayed.

Chronic ulcerative colitis 10
Lesion of the rectosigmoid 5
Lesion of the right half of the transverse colon and hepatic
    flexure 2
Gastric polyposis 1
Multiple polypi of the descending colon with filling defect 1
Duodenal ulcer 1
Intestinal stasis with obstruction 1
Colon negative 5

Questionnaires were sent to all the patients with the exception of those who were operated on or those sent home under medical treatment, or those who had been in correspondence with the Clinic within a period of four months previous to the compilation of these statistics. Replies were received to the questionnaires from all but four.

POST-OPERATIVE DATA

Eight patients reported a decided improvement in their general health; one reported slight improvement; one made no statement as to health or general condition. Reports of death were received in two cases; diagnosis of carcinoma had been made in both of these cases and confirmed at operation. In one instance the patient died ten weeks after leaving the Clinic and came to necropsy. A report of a general carcinomatosis with metastasis to the liver was returned. The date of death of the second patient was not stated. The mortality in this group was 16.66 per cent. (Tables I and II).

Nineteen of the twenty-two cases of intestinal polyposis treated surgically are accounted for, with a mortality of nine (47.34 per cent.). If, however, Case 167383 is eliminated, the mortality falls to 42.08 per cent.

DATA CONCERNING PATIENTS NOT OPERATED ON

Questionnaires were sent to fourteen medical patients and replies were received from twelve. Four reported that they were so markedly improved that they consider themselves well; three simply reported they are improved; one is unimproved and one is growing progressively weaker. The latter was a patient with advanced nephritis and the polypi were found in our routine examination. Three patients were reported to have died, ten weeks, two years, and four years, respectively, after leaving the Clinic. The diagnosis in the case of the patient who died ten weeks after leaving the clinic was chronic ulcerative colitis of the descending and transverse colon and sigmoid with multiple polypi of the rectum. The second patient came to necropsy and the cause of death was given as

TABLE I

MULTIPLE POLYPOSIS OF THE INTESTINAL TRACT

Immediate Surgical Mortality

Date of registration	Case	Diagnosis	Operation	Date of death
Jan. 27, 1913	96200	Chronic ulcerative colitis with papillomatous colon	January 27, 1913, Brown operation;* appendectomy; July 4, 1914, ileocolostomy	August 22, 1914.
Sept. 2, 1914	114349	Chronic inflammatory mass in right lower abdomen	Resection 6 inches of ileum, all of caecum, ascending colon, one-half transverse colon; appendix involved in resection; July 12, 1915, resection of remaining one-half transverse colon, all of descending colon and sigmoid	July 27, 1915.
July 25, 1916	167383†	Papillomatous growths in rectum	July 25, 916, transfusion	August 5, 1916.
June 11, 1917	196935	Chronic ulcerative colitis with multiple polypoid growths	June 23, 19, Brown, first stage; June 25, 1917, second stage, Brown operation	June 27, 1917.
Aug. 30, 1917	206607	Chronic ulcerative colitis with multiple polypoid growths	ober 12, 1917, Brown operation	September 16, 1917.
Nov. 14, 1919	296662	Chronic ulcerative colitis	N ember 25, 1919, Brown (permanent ileostomy). Resection of caecum and ileocaecal valve. Appendectomy	December 23, 1919.
Jan. 6, 1920	301683	Polyposis of rectum and sigmoid	January 24, 1920, mplete col by with removal of 5 inches of lower ileum. Permanent ileostomy	January 26, 1920.

* The Brown operation consists of an ileostomy about 6 inches above the ileocaecal valve and bringing both ends ugh the incision, the distal end above.
† This patient was brought to the Clinic on a stretcher, markedly emaciated, haemoglobin 37 per cent., and died the sixteenth day.

656

TABLE II

MULTIPLE POLYPOSIS OF THE INTESTINAL TRACT

Surgical Cases

Date of registration	Case	Diagnosis	Operation	Data obtained from inquiries sent Feb. 2, 1920
Jan. 23, 1914	99488	Intestinal stasis with obstruction	Resection of 10 ints of jbr ap-pendix, cecum, ascending colo and hepi fleur and two-thirds of cob	Marked improvement in general condi-tion.
Aug. 12, 1914	112677	August 12, 1914, polypoid colitis; November 30, 1918, chronic ulcera-tive colitis	August 12, 1914, Brown operation* and appendectomy, January 5, 1915, complete col... y except 12 ints of the sigm	Back to normal weight, but tires easily.
May 28, 1915	131844	Chronic ulcerative colitis. Enda-moeba histolytica	Ileocolostomy	Improving steadily, gaining in weight and strength.
Mar. 24, 1916	155603	Chronic ulcerative colitis and proctitis with multiple polyps	Complete ileostomy and appende-ctomy	Marked improvement. February 5, 1920, came to the Clinic because of prolapse of the intestines. Repaired ileostomy incision. To return later.
April 10, 1916	157034	Multiple carcinoma of small and large bowel, and upper rectum	Appendicostomy	Died—date not given.
Feb. 2, 1917	184810	Granular sigmoiditis, and proctitis with multiple polypi of the sigmoid	February 20, 1917 Brown operation and appendectomy. Oct 23, 1918, ileosigmoidostomy	Marked improvement in general health.
Jan. 30, 1918	220600	Duodenal ulcer; colitis. Endamoeba histolytica	Posterior gast... pedicled, small growths extcp from jejunum into the ileum. Stomach covered with small growths	Health excellent. Gained in weight. Portion of small intestine removed elsewhere in March, 1919. Total weight gained 40 pounds.
Nov. 8, 1918	250518	Gastric polyposis	Three-fifths of stomach and pylorus reib ' . Polypa operation	No gain in weight or strength. General health slightly improved.
Feb. 22, 1919	196306	Multiple polyposis of the colon	Brown operation	Excellent.
Aug. 4, 1919	282550	Chronic ulcerative colitis with mul-tiple polyposis	First stage Brown operation	Improvement marked, though still has some ulceration in rectum.
Oct. 6, 1919	292082	Multiple polyposis of colon; filling defect transverse colon	Exploration. Extensive masses in every part of transverse colon. Diagnosis, adenocarcinoma	Died January 16, 1920. Necropsy: Gen-eral carcinomatosis. Marked involve-ment of liver.

* The Brown operation consists of an ileostomy about 6 inches above the ileocaecal valve and bringing both ends out through the incision—the distal end above.

primary carcinoma of the lower bowel with metastasis to the liver. Carcinoma had been diagnosed at the clinic. The cause of death in the third case was not stated. The mortality in this group with two patients unaccounted for was 25 per cent. (Table III).

Two of the four patients who did not reply to questionnaires were medical and two were surgical cases. One of the latter wrote that he was coming to the clinic, giving no information as to his general condition. This patient had carcinoma of the hepatic flexure and transverse colon with multiple polypi of the rectum. In 1917 he was operated on and eight inches of the ileum, together with the cæcum, ascending colon, and more than half of the transverse colon were removed, and an end-to-end anastomosis made with a Murphy button. In February, 1919, he returned to the clinic with a fecal fistula and obstruction just below the point where the ileocolostomy had been performed. There was an extensive recurrence of the polypoid growths in the transverse colon. It was thought that a Brown operation would be the best, in order to rest the colon, but no arrangement for this having been made with the patient an ileosigmoidostomy opening was made in the ileum eight inches above the point of the previous anastomosis with the transverse colon. In the second surgical case there was an extensive carcinoma of the sigmoid and rectum with multiple polypi below the growth. In the two medical cases there was extensive polyposis of the rectum as far as could be seen with a 14-inch proctoscope.

In the two groups of patients to whom questionnaires were sent there is a known mortality of two and three, respectively (20.83 per cent.). Adding to this the immediate surgical mortality of seven, and the death of one medical patient who committed suicide because of unimproved condition, the total mortality in the thirty-five cases is thirteen (37.14 per cent.).

The average age of the patients treated medically was thirty-nine years and ten months; of those treated surgically thirty-six years and six months. The average duration of symptoms in the former group was five years and eight months; in the latter, seven years. If, however, Case 167383, in which transfusion was done, is omitted, this period immediately jumps to seven years and six months. In comparing the patients age for age, the prognosis was no more favorable in the younger than in the older patients. The best prognosis can be given in those cases in which the growths are localized and can be removed surgically.

In comparing these two groups of statistics it should be remembered that the patient who came to operation had no possible chance of recovery from medical treatment, and that surgery offered him the only chance for life.

Nervous symptoms in this series were not significant enough to report.

The findings in the operative cases and in the cases that came to necropsy indicated that multiple polyposis is a diffuse condition of the

TABLE III

MULTIPLE POLYPOSIS OF THE INTESTINAL TRACT

Medical Cases

Date of registration	Case	Diagnosis	Condition of bowels, diarrhea, pus, blood	Rectal pain	Abdominal pain	General health, weight and strength
July 11, 1910	40142	Multiple polyposis of rectum, sigmoid and colon. Diagnosis of carcinoma made at Clinic	Progressively worse until death	....	....	Died January 25, 1914 post-mortem shows general carcinomatosis with marked metastasis to liver.
Jan. 25, 1912	63425	Papillomas of large bowel. Malignant	Constant passage of pus and blood with diarrhea	Slight with stools	General; localized at sigmoid	Progressively worse the last six months. Died 1916.
Mar. 14, 1912	65403	March 12, 1914, amoebic dysentery. August 17, 1914, chronic ulcerative colitis with multiple polyposis. January 10, 1918, multiple polyposis	Unchanged, 10 to 12 stools daily with pus and blood	Occasional but not severe	Slight general distress, not so severe as formerly	General health much improved, gained in weight and strength.
Feb. 18, 1914	100828	Papillomas of rectum and bowel	No diarrhea now, œ and blood	No longer present	None	Gained after leaving Clinic. Operation 1918 Type of operation not given; health good.
Sept. 5, 1914	114579	Multiple polypi of rectum and colon	No diarrhea now, occasional blood	None	None	Much stronger and does all kinds of work. Strength good; lost 15 pounds in weight.
Sept. 6, 1915	140421	Chronic diffuse papillomas with colitis	Unimproved	None	None	Weight and strength remain the same.
Jun 15, 1916	162733	Multiple polypi of rectum	No diarrhea now, occasional blood	......	Cramps entirely gone	Gain better. Weight same. Strength varies
Jan. 15, 1917	183218	Multiple polypi of rectum and colon	Periodically, less frequent	......	Some slight general pain across lower abdomen with diarrhea	Lost some weight and strength; regained.
May 7, 1917	193344	Chronic ulcerative colitis with multiple polypi	Fullness of rectum persists. Some constipation.	When cold?	Never had abdominal pain	Lost some weight and strength until past year; now stationary.
April 30, 1918	229689	Papillomas of bowel	No diarrhea now	Dull rectal pain at times, though not severe	Occasional, not sufficient to trouble patient	Weight and strength normal.
April 11, 1919	267096	April 11, 1919, chronic ulcerative colitis of descending colon and sigmoid. February 3, 1920 same plus transverse colon. Multiple polyps	Slight improvement. Pus and blood present. General colitis worse	Some dull rectal pain with stool and when tired	Never had abdominal pain	Died February 7, 1920
Oct. 4, 1919	293087	Chronic nephritis with uremia. Multiple polypi of rectum	Constipation unchanged	Slight with stool	......	Very weak; some weight loss.

colon. The findings of Hewitt and Howard, that the polypi in the rectum are situated along the side of the intestinal wall, while higher up in the colon they are situated along the line of attachment of the mesentery, have not been confirmed in the Mayo Clinic (Figs. 3 and 4). Hewitt and Howard concluded that the islands and tags of mucosa and submucosa that had been the source of polypus formation appeared to depend for their preservation on the arrangement of the blood supply. Polypi situated in these particular areas, because of the increased blood supply, could better withstand any destructive action, and necrosis would not take place. At the same time, however, it would produce active hyperplasia of the mucous glands and the submucous connective tissue and permit these particular polypi to thrive better.

One patient only had a positive Wassermann, a second a suspicious Wassermann which was to be repeated later, but the patient did not remain for complete examination (Figs. 5 and 6). There was one case of lues latens.

Nine patients gave a family history of tuberculosis, but only five of these were in the immediate family. Two gave a family history of cancer; one of these patients had a carcinoma of the rectum removed one year before coming to the clinic.

POSSIBLE ETIOLOGY AND PATHOLOGY

Schwab has advanced the theory that constipation is the cause of polyposis and that polyposis usually develops first in the rectum and then ascends the gastro-intestinal tract. This theory is hardly tenable if the prevalence of polyposis in males and of constipation in females has any significance. According to the statistics of Doering, twenty-five cases of polyposis occurred in males and seventeen in females; in nine of the cases the sex was not given. Newbolt reported thirty-seven cases, twenty-three (67.6 per cent.) of which occurred in males, fourteen (32.4 per cent.) in females. In the present series of thirty-nine cases, twenty-nine (74.3 per cent.) were in males, ten (25.7 per cent.) in females. Of the ten cases collected in the literature by me, other than those reported by Soper, seven (70.0 per cent.) occurred in males and three (30.00 per cent.) in females. Although constipation may have some bearing on the etiology of polyposis, it cannot be considered the principal etiologic factor. Rokitansky, on the other hand, believed that intestinal polypi arise from the margins of dysenteric ulcers. According to the proctoscopic examination of patients and the microscopic examination of specimens removed at operation in cases observed in the Clinic, the frequency of ulceration associated with the frequency of polyposis tends to confirm this theory. In the present series there were eleven cases of chronic ulcerative colitis and eight cases of intestinal infections. Meyer considers the entire epithelial process secondary and states that polypus formation can only be explained through a congenital malformation of

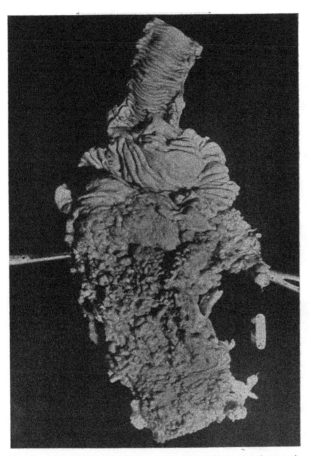

FIG. 5 (199399).—Section showing extensive polyposis at hepatic flexure, ulceration at proximal end of growth (6 by 7 cm.).

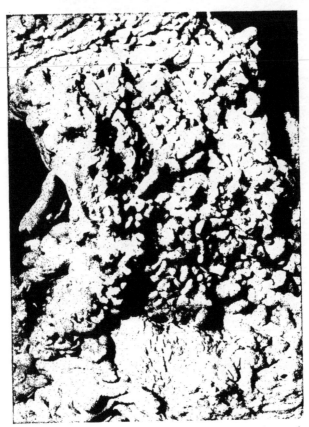

FIG. 6 (199399).—Section showing extensive polyposis at hepatic flexure, ulceration at proximal end of growth (6 by 7 cm.).

the tissue of the intestinal wall, which is primary and extends into the mucosa and submucosa. Lebert claims that a chronic irritation is the causative agent.

For the sake of convenience tumors of the intestinal tract may be divided into three groups. The papillomas are those tumors in which the surface epithelium, either cutaneous or mucous, is involved; they are usually found low down at the mucocutaneous margins. Polypi result from hypertrophy of the mucous membrane, or originate as true tumors. The adenomas form the group in which the neoplasms are derived from pre-existing glands or glandular remnants. Apparently early in this disease, in a large percentage of cases, there is a general colitis which, as it progresses, forms a number of undermining ulcers. These tend to increase in number, to fuse, and to increase in size until large areas of the colon are involved. This ulcerative process, although severe and chronic, is such that portions of the mucosa and submucosa adjacent to, and supplied by, primary arterial branches are preserved. It is these preserved portions that were seen studding the surface of the colon. As healing takes place, under favorable conditions, the irregular margins of these elevations are smoothed off and remain as rounded sessile or polypoid projections from the mucous membrane. This is the so-called multiple polyposis or colitis polyposis. As in all healing processes the proliferated fibroblasts begin to contract with resultant cicatrization, a natural result could be the occlusion of the tubules in the polypi. So long as the secreting cells in the walls of the polypi functionate they increase in size with the formation of retention cysts. Several tubules thus occluded in polypi will cause them to appear as a collection of cysts. Thus this condition, which is probably but an advanced stage of colitis polyposis, is what Virchow designated as colitis polyposis cystica.

The elevation of the thickened and altered mucosa results in increased friction and traction, which in turn stretch the surrounding adjacent mucosa and cause the formation of a pedicle. Further changes may in turn result in fibrosis and severe inflammatory conditions, the final and most important of which is carcinomatosis.[1, 11] The factors giving rise to cancer are generally accepted to be irritants, chemical, biochemical, or radio-active substances. Of these, the most common, especially in cancer of the mucous tracts, are the biochemical or the bacterial elements. Thus malignancy of adenomas, papillomas, or polypi of the intestinal tract is due to the more persistent and virulent action of the infecting organisms, or to the increased trauma which is necessarily accentuated by the passage of the fæces, and possibly by the compression of the bowel itself in its effort to pass on both fæces and polypi. This explanation of the formation of carcinomatosis, of course, assumes the condition to be due to an intestinal infection.

A natural question to ask would be, " Are all multiple polypi of the intestinal tract likely to become carcinomatous; if not, which forms are

pecially dangerous?" Because of the high rate of malignancy in dis-
ses of the colon, no tumor should be considered benign until proof to
e contrary is established. Mummery stated that "almost all recorded
ses of multiple polypi of the colon had eventually become malignant,
d this was a factor to be reckoned with in treating these cases." If
e tumor is associated with intussusception, the safest procedure which
n be followed to prevent a recurrence is the removal of the section of
e bowel which is involved.

The confusion apparent in the classification of the polypi likewise
ists in the determination of malignancy. Polypi of the nasal passages
d of the intestinal tract are similar in structure, although the former
ry rarely, if ever, become malignant. The latter, existing under entirely
fferent circumstances, are submitted to traumatism, stress and strain,
d the action of bacteria. In the twenty-six cases of malignancy re-
rted by Doering and by Soper, adenocarcinoma was the type of cancer
und in each. In the adenomas, as in the papillomas, the stroma is the
sential part. Simple irritative and regenerative hyperplasia, adeno-
itous growth, and carcinoma are successive stages which are manifested
the same kind of tissue; the differences are those of degree of devel-
ment and not of kind. Loosely speaking, we may regard carcinoma as
adenoma or papilloma which has developed into a malignant growth.
the intestinal tract the adenomatous type of growth certainly predomi-
tes, according to the statistics of Soper, 43 per cent.

INTUSSUSCEPTION

In this series of thirty-nine cases there was but one of obstruction and
ne of intussusception. Only pedicled tumors can be held responsible
intussusception. If the tumors are intramural they tend to strengthen
: wall of the bowel and to prevent its invagination. The contention
it the mere weight and pulling of the tumor will produce the invagina-
n is undoubtedly incorrect. Were this true, the tumor mass would
vays be found at the tip of the invagination, which is not the case.
e pedicled growth is most common in children, and the fact that there
re no cases of children in this series may account for the absence of
es of intussusception.

SYMPTOMS

Symptoms vary with the size, position, and number of the polypi.
nerally, patients in whom the polypi are localized in the rectum and
moid have a sense of weight, a loaded feeling in the rectum, and occa-
nally tenesmus with or without bleeding. If the polypi are pedicled
d low, they may protrude from the rectum, as in the case of Edwards;
inusually large numbers of polypi are present, prolapse of the rectum
y occur as in the case of Norbury. Diarrhœa is practically always pres-
. Diarrhœa and extensive involvement of the colon are usually asso-
ted with pus and blood. Involvement of the colon often causes a

vague abdominal pain which may be localized at the seat of the involvement. A complete or partial obstruction of the bowel will result in stasis and the formation of toxins which have an inhibitory action on the proximal section and cause distention. If this is progressive, symptoms other than those at the original site of involvement may mask the real condition. Frequently the symptoms of colonic lesions resemble those of gastric or duodenal ulcers because of the effect of food on the stomach.[13] A large percentage of painful lesions of the colon give pain in the ascending colon, around the cæcum and the appendix. Sooner or later there is loss of weight; the anæmia which develops varies with the degree of bleeding. The so-called essential hemorrhage occurred in but three of our series of cases. Repeated attacks of colic with obscure etiology and symptoms pointing to obstruction suggest polyposis.

TREATMENT

Since no specific etiologic factor is known, the treatment of intestinal polyposis varies with the individual case. If the polypi are localized in the rectum, cauterization may be practised. The patients should be kept under observation and if any signs of malignancy develop, resection of the rectum should be performed. If operation is indicated, it undoubtedly offers the best results.

CONCLUSIONS

1. Multiple polyposis of the intestinal tract is a serious disease from the standpoint of morbidity and mortality.

2. The etiology of the intestinal polypus is not known, although chronic ulcerative colitis and intestinal infections appear to be factors.

3. There is no specific medical treatment and operation undoubtedly offers the best results in the more advanced cases.

4. The rectum, the sigmoid, and the splenic and hepatic flexures are most frequently involved. The small intestines are rarely involved.

5. The predominant symptoms are diarrhœa, with the passage of pus and blood, vague abdominal pain, and rectal tenesmus. The so-called essential hemorrhage, if present, is almost pathognomonic.

6. Proctoscopic examination[6,7] should be done routinely in all cases of dysentery.

7. Adenomas do not seem to become malignant more often than polypi and papillomas.

8. In cases in which polypi were associated with carcinoma, they were usually found below the cancerous growth farther along in the intestinal tract.

9. Most marked involvement of the colon is found in the cases which begin as a mild diarrhœa and later become chronic. The more sudden and severe the onset the more localized the condition in the colon.

10. Multiple polyposis of the intestinal tract is more frequent in males than in females, a proportion of 2 to 1.

JOHN EDMUND STRUTHERS

BIBLIOGRAPHY

[1] Back, I.: Case and Specimen of Multiple Polypi of the Colon Becoming Carcinomatous. Proc. Roy. Soc. Lond., 1913–1914, vii, Surg. Sect., 193.

[2] Bratrud, T.: Intestinal Polyposis With Report of Case with Three Intussusceptions. Surg., Gynec. and Obst., 1914, xix.

[3] Carroll, W. C.: Intestinal Polyposis. Surg., Gynec. and Obst., 1915, xx, 412–414.

[4] Collier, W.: Multiple Polypi of the Stomach and Intestine. Brit. Med. Jour., 1895, ii, 973.

[5] Doering, H.: Die Polyposis intestini und ihre Beziehung zur carcinomatösen Degeneration. Arch. f. klin. Chir., 1907, lxxxiii, 194–227.

[6] Drueck, C. J.: How to Examine the Rectum and Interpret its Findings. Internat. Clinics, 1916, 26 s., iii, 242–254.

[7] Drueck, C. J.: Applied Anatomy of the Terminal Bowel. Interst. Med. Jour., 1919, xxvi, 92–100.

[8] Furnivall, P.: Three Cases of Multiple Polypi of the Rectum and Large Intestine. Proc. Roy. Soc. Lond., 1913–1914, vii, Surg. Sect., 245–246.

[9] Hertz, A. F.: Four Cases of Rectal Polypus Occurring in One Family. Proc. Roy. Soc. Lond., 1913–1914, vii, Surg. Sect., 255–256.

[10] Hewitt, J. H., and Howard, W. T.: Chronic Ulcerative Colitis With Polyps. A Consideration of the So-called colitis polyposa (Virchow). Arch. Int. Med., 1915, xv, 714–723.

[11] Kanthack, A. A., and Furnivall, P.: Multiple Polypi of the Small Intestines. Tr. Path. Soc. Lond., 1897, xlviii, 83–85.

[12] Logan, A. H.: Chronic Ulcerative Colitis, a Review of One Hundred and Seventeen Cases. Northwest Med., 1919, xviii, 1.

[13] Mallory, W. J.: Colon Lesions. Virginia Med., 1917, xxii, 137.

[14] Murphy, J. B.: Polyposis of the Sigmoid. Surg. Clinics of Chicago, 1916, 477–481.

[15] Newbolt, G. P.: Case of Multiple Adenomata of the Colon and Rectum. Proc. Roy. Soc. Lond., 1913–1914, vii, Surg. Sect., 272–274.

[16] Norbury, L. E. C.: Case of Multiple Polypi of Rectum and Colon. Proc. Roy. Soc. Lond., 1913–1914, vii, Surg. Sect., 195–196.

[17] Oden, R. J. E.: Intussusception of the Jejunum Associated With Two Pedicled Fibro-Adenomata. Surg., Gynec. and Obst., 1919, xxix, 489–492.

[18] Orth, J.: Ueber Colitis cystica und ihre Beziehung zur Ruhr. Berl. klin. Wchnschr., 1918, lv, 681–687.

[19] Preble, W. E.: Intestinal Uræmia and Sequelæ. Boston Med. and Surg. Jour., 1917, clxxvi, 296–307.

[20] Soper, H. W.: Polyposis of the Colon. Am. Jour. Med. Sc., 1916, cli, 405–409.

[21] Watson, C. G.: Case of Multple Adenomata, Associated Wth Columnar Carcinoma of the Pelvic Colon. Proc. Roy. Soc. Lond., 1913–1914, vii, Surg. Sect., 194–195.

A CASE OF DIAPHRAGMATIC HERNIA OBSERVED POST-MORTEM

By Lyman Foster Huffman, M.D.

of Cleveland, Ohio

FROM THE ANATOMICAL LABORATORY OF THE WESTERN RESERVE UNIVERSITY MEDICAL SCHOOL

Diaphragmatic hernia is not as uncommon as was formerly supposed and recently the number of cases has been considerably augmented by war wounds of the diaphragm. Nevertheless it seems advisable to report this case because of some unusual anatomical relations.

The great majority of cases of diaphragmatic hernia occur on the left side. The right lobe of the liver aids in the closure of the right side of the diaphragm and reinforces it so that hernia is prevented from occurring at weak places or defects in this part of the diaphragm.

Diaphragmatic hernia is commonly classified as to whether the case is congenital or acquired and whether it is true or false, a false hernia being one in which there is no sac.

In the acquired form a direct injury to the diaphragm by stab or bullet wound is frequently the etiological factor. In many others there is a history of trauma to the abdominal wall, such as a sudden forcible bending of the body. In such cases a rupture of the diaphragm presumably occurs at its weakest point. This weak point is frequently the hiatus of the diaphragm where the lumbar and costal portions meet. It may also be the anterior part of the muscle at the junction of the costal and sternal portions. Less frequently it is at one of the normal openings of the diaphragm—the œsophageal opening.

That part of the diaphragm in the region of the œsophageal opening develops from the mesentery of the foregut. It is always in intimate contact with the œsophagus and there is no " opening " at the œsophageal opening in the literal sense of the term. There is a weak place where the diaphragm has developed about the œsophagus. If the stomach were to develop at a higher level than normal, or the diaphragm at a lower level, the opening in the diaphragm for the passage of the alimentary canal would be larger in order to accommodate the stomach. The stomach would require more space than the œsophagus, and the space would not always be completely utilized. It would be closed by loose connective tissue instead of the muscular elements normally fitting snugly about the œsophagus. The probability of hernia occurring in the location would be increased. A case of development of the stomach within the thorax has been recently reported and indicates that the level at which the stomach develops with respect to the diaphragm may be variable and may have a bearing on the production of diaphragmatic

---

[1] Baily, P.: A Case of Thoracic Stomach. Anat. Rec., xvii, 2, p. 107, Oct., 1919.

.hernia in this locality. In this case [1] the œsophagus ended at the level of the third costal cartilage, and the stomach was situated within a sac in the posterior mediastinum. The sac was lined with serous membrane continuous with the peritoneum. The explanation offered for this condition was that the anlage of the stomach had been situated too far cephalad in the foregut.

The case which I wish to report was found on the dissecting table and no clinical history was obtainable beyond the fact that the subject was a woman fifty years old, who died a few hours after her admission to a hospital with symptoms indicating a myocardial insufficiency.

When the abdomen was opened the great omentum was seen to be drawn up into the left upper quadrant. The proximal part of the omentum and the pyloric portion of the stomach passed from the thorax into the abdomen through an opening in the diaphragm corresponding to the œsophageal opening. This opening was located opposite the twelfth thoracic vertebra and admitted three fingers.

The anterior aspect of the opened thorax was perfectly normal. The appearance of the thoracic contents from behind is shown in Fig. 1. The sac containing the stomach was in the posterior mediastium directly behind the heart. It straddled the aorta and bodies of the vertebræ, being a little more on the left than on the right side, and extended from the lower border of the eighth to the lower border of the eleventh thoracic vertebræ. The lining membrane of the sac was continuous with the peritoneum and there were no communications with or adhesions to the pleural or pericardial cavities.

The appearance with the sac opened is shown in Fig. 2. The stomach is seen to form a loop with its convexity, corresponding to the greater curvature, directed upward. The anterior aspect of the stomach, which in this case corresponded to the lesser curvature and part of the cardia, was firmly adherent to the anterior wall of the sac, so that the stomach could not be dislodged and drawn downward into the abdomen.

The blood supply is indicated in the accompanying diagram. (Fig. 3.) The right and left gastroepiploic arteries arose normally from the gastroduodenal and splenic arteries respectively. The hepatic and splenic arteries were the only branches of the cœliac axis, the coronary or left gastric arising directly from the aorta at a higher level. Near its origin the left gastric gave off the right and left phrenic arteries and then took a tortuous course between the anterior wall of the stomach and the sac. The aorta had the appearance of being twisted to the left, as its intercostal arteries arose from the right instead of from the dorsal aspect.

The œsophagus passed behind the root of the left lung and in the lower part of its course was closely applied to the right lateral aspect of the sac between it and the mesial aspect of the right lung.

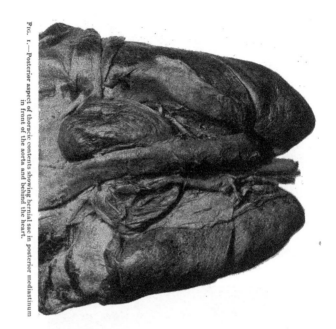

FIG. 1.—Posterior aspect of thoracic contents showing hernial sac in posterior mediastinum in front of the aorta and behind the heart.

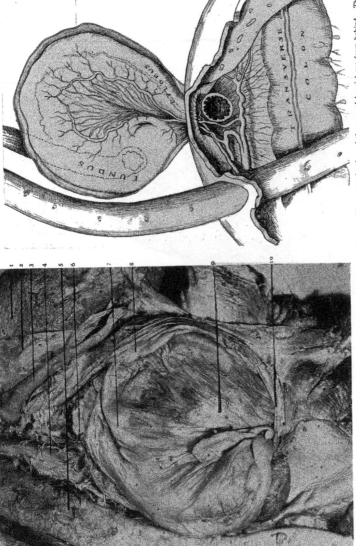

FIG. 2.—The thoracic contents viewed from behind. The aorta is drawn to the left. The hernial sac is opened. 1. Right lung. 2. Right parietal pleura. 3. Azygos vein. 4. Œsophagus. 5. Aorta. 6. Right vagus nerve. 7. Greater curvature of stomach. 8. Reflected hernial sac. 9. Great omentum. 10. Hernial opening in diaphragm, corresponding to the œsophageal opening, transmitting pylorus and great omentum.

FIG. 3.—Diagrammatic view of the opened hernial sac from behind. The aorta is drawn to one side. We are looking forward at the greater curvature of the stomach arching upward. The lesser curvature is incorporated with the anterior wall of the sac, and in this location runs the coronary (left gastric) artery represented by dotted lines. The course of the œsophagus in front of the stomach with its point of entrance into the stomach is also indicated by dotted lines. The right and left gastro-epiploic arteries, take their customary course along the free border of the great omentum. It is seen that the left gastric arises independently from the attachment of the great omentum. The cœliac axis arises independently from the aorta above the cœliac axis. The cœliac axis has two branches, the hepatic running to the right giving off the gastroduodenal from which the right gastro-epiploic arises, and the splenic giving rise to the left gastro-epiploic.

It penetrated the sac to enter the stomach 3 cm. above the opening in the diaphragm.

The course of the left vagus was normal. The right vagus passed from the œsophageal plexus along the external aspect of the right side of the sac to about its middle, where it penetrated the sac, turned backward and could be traced for only a short distance in the region where the anterior aspect of the stomach was incorporated with the anterior wall of the sac. As this normally would be gastrohepatic omentum, it probably passed on to enter into the formation of the hepatic plexus.

The origins of the diaphragm were normal and there was nothing noteworthy about this muscle except the large œsophageal opening through which the pylorus entered the abdomen and the occurrence of a well-marked hiatus on the right side.

It is interesting to note that in addition to the diaphragmatic hernia this subject had a right labial and left interstitial hernia. The foramen ovale was patent. There were only eleven thoracic vertebræ and eleven ribs. The fifth lumbar vertebra was fused with the first sacral on the left side (lumbosacral vertebra).

This case is one of true diaphragmatic hernia occurring through a congenitally weak œsophageal opening. Possibly the diaphragm was weak at this point because the stomach developed more cephalad than usual and required more space in the "œsophageal opening" than would have been needed by the œsophagus itself. This explanation is suggested by the fact that the œsophagus ended above the "œsophageal opening" in the diaphragm. The case reported by Bailey, referred to above, suggests the plausibility of this explanation and its applicability to other cases of diaphragmatic hernia at the œsophageal opening.

The gastrohepatic omentum, lesser curvature, cardia and finally all of the stomach except the pylorus were herniated into the chest. That the gastrohepatic omentum was first drawn into the thorax is indicated by the firm incorporation of its normal attachment, the lesser curvature, with the anterior wall of the sac. The peculiar relationship of the right vagus to the hernia is also explained by the assumption that the gastrohepatic omentum through which the right vagus courses on its way to the hepatic plexus was drawn into the thorax first and entered into the formation of the hernial sac.

HERNIA OF THE DIAPHRAGM*

By Frank S. Mathews, M.D.
AND
H. M. Imboden, M.D.
OF NEW YORK, N. Y.

In view of the considerable number of recent papers dealing with the subject of hernia of the diaphragm, it will only be necessary in this article to describe a case with the X-ray findings, and call attention to some of the points of interest.

Mrs. W. P., aged fifty-five years, multiparous, at the time of operation was a woman in apparently good health and stout, rather than muscular, with a history of recent increase in weight. The symptoms relating to the present difficulty date back through ten years.

First, almost daily, after eating a meal, she would put her finger down her throat to encourage the expulsion of gas, which gave her a feeling of oppression in the chest.

Second, during the entire ten years, at intervals of from a day to three months, but without any regularity, she had attacks of pain following eating. The pain was severe, epigastric or higher and largely referred to the heart. She became pale and pulse was said to become weak. To onlookers she appeared to be strangling. She would make efforts to belch gas and if she succeeded the pain was immediately relieved. In some cases it required an hour or two before any gas was evacuated.

Third, by degrees she learned to modify her diet so as to limit the distress after meals, though she could not prevent the acute, severe attacks. The type of meal that gave her least discomfort was one of concentrated food and small bulk—that is, meat, potatoes and eggs, with no soups, desserts or green vegetables. These attacks began abruptly ten years ago and have continued without any noticeable change in the character, severity, or frequency of the attacks.

Three years ago a series of X-ray pictures was made on which was based the diagnosis of diaphragmatic hernia. The patient was referred for operation by Dr. W. A. Bestedo, who confirmed the presence of the stomach in the chest by physical examination. The X-ray report made November, 1916, by Dr. H. M. Imboden is as follows:

The stomach is entirely above the diaphragm and is in the right lower portion of the thorax, extending about two inches to the left of the left sternal line. The upper border of the stomach is about eight inches above the right diaphragm. The stomach and the colon are posterior to the heart. The opening into the sac is in the posterior portion of the diaphragm near the midline. The pylorus pro-

---

* Read before the American Surgical Association, May 5, 1920.

668

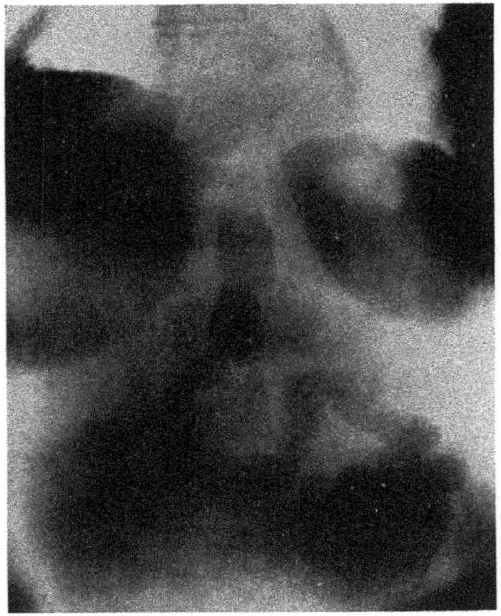

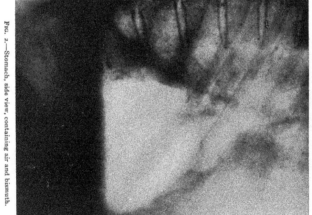

FIG. 1.—Stomach in thorax, behind and right of heart.

FIG. 2.—Stomach, side view, containing air and bismuth.

668ª

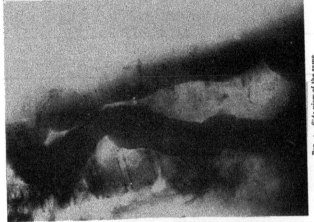

Fig. 3.—Distended colon, mainly in right chest.

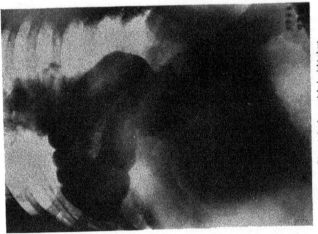

Fig. 4.—Side view of the same.

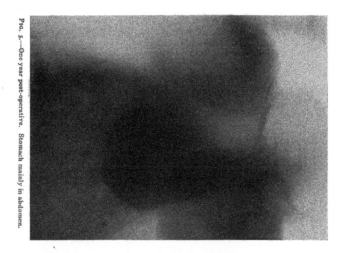

Fig. 5.—One year post-operative. Stomach mainly in abdomen.

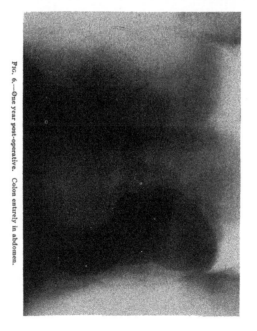

Fig. 6.—One year post-operative. Colon entirely in abdomen.

668

jects down toward the pelvis, parallel to the spine. The duodenum is also directed downward. The second portion of the duodenum is directed down. The third portion is transverse and the fourth portion is directed upward but joining the jejunum at the level of the third lumbar vertebra on the left side.

There is no evidence of disease about the pylorus or the first portion of the duodenum, but at no time were we able to get a satisfactory shadow of that portion of the stomach passing through the ring.

The stomach empties itself rather slowly. Seven hours p. c. there is a slight residue in the stomach.

The meal passes rapidly through the small intestine.

Three hours p. c. some of it is already in the hepatic flexure region.

Thirty-six hours p. c. most of it was discharged with the exception of a quantity in the descending colon, sigmoid and rectum.

An opaque enema revealed an unusually long transverse colon, most of which is in the hernial sac. We found no evidence of obstruction or occlusion of the colon, though where the two limbs pass each other in the ring, they are in rather close apposition.

Some of the plates of the colon indicated that a portion of it occasionally slips out of the sac.

The only explanation we can give to account for the patient's discomfort is the enormous gas bag in the stomach, which lies above the œsophageal opening. We fail to find any evidence of disease in any portion of the alimentary tract.

Operation (Mathews) was performed December 17, 1918, under intratracheal anæsthesia. Incision eight or nine inches in length in the left mid-rectus line from the costal margin downward. The patient was put in the position of a reversed Trendelenburg. No part of the colon was in the hernial sac. More or less of the stomach was, and it was drawn downward entirely out of the hernia without great difficulty. Its wall was thick and leathery. The hernial opening was the enlarged œsophageal one. Because of the depth of the abdomen due to the patient's large size and obesity, it was not easy to expose the orifice to sight. Two mattress sutures of heavy chromic gut were with difficulty placed at the anterior margin of the ring. The ring was at least two inches in diameter and by means of the stitches seemed to be considerably narrowed. The stomach was then sutured to the whole length of the abdominal incision. It was drawn downward as far as possible, and the first suture was inserted through the post-rectus sheath and peritoneum, and included a bite of the stomach wall just in front of the lesser curvature high up toward the cardia. The suturing was continued down obliquely across the front of the stomach for a distance of about eight inches. Sutures were placed about one-half inch apart and took a firm hold on the stomach wall. The remaining layers of the abdominal wall were closed with silkworm and catgut. Patient was kept in bed two weeks with the head of the bed elevated, and on discharge from the hospital was advised to restrict diet and encourage catharsis in order to keep down intra-abdominal tension.

At the present date, May 1, 1920, the patient has been entirely free from attacks, has abandoned her diet of small bulk, is not compelled to belch after eating, and now eats anything. Her weight is considerably increased. X-rays taken after bismuth meal a few days ago by Doctor Imboden show that the stomach stands almost vertically as though still adherent to the abdominal wall for the length of the suture line. A small portion, possibly the upper fourth, is in the chest. Bismuth enema shows that the long splenic flexure and transverse colon which formerly entered the thorax now lie to her left and entirely below the diaphragm.

Comment.—The case is interesting from a number of standpoints—not the least being that the distressing symptoms of ten years' duration have been completely relieved by an operation of no great severity and which did not remove the sac nor could it close the ring, both because of technical difficulties and because it was the normal opening for the passage of the œsophagus. The patient's milder attacks or discomfort were evidently due to an air-filled stomach occupying space intended for the lungs. The more severe attacks would seem to have been due to a greater distention of the stomach with food and air and not unlikely a mild sort of strangulation. In entering the sac the stomach seems, according to X-ray evidence, to have turned over on a transverse axis, so that the greater curvature lay higher in the chest than the œsophageal opening and so kinked the entrance of the stomach that emptying itself of air through the œsophagus became difficult or for a time impossible.

In the literature these hernias are usually recorded as occurring through the left diaphragm and usually occupying the left part of the chest, pushing the heart to the right. In this case the heart was not displaced and nearly all of the sac was in the right chest. A hand could be inserted a short distance into the hernial sac, but obtained no evidence of communication with the pleura, as is at times found, especially in congenital cases.

Intratracheal anæsthesia was very satisfactorily employed and is highly desirable because of a possible communication between peritoneum and pleura. The positive pressure in conjunction with the reversed Trendelenburg position was a great aid in keeping the contents of the sac reduced. Even then, there was quite a tug upon the stomach with each inspiration. It is worthy of comment that this hernia of at least ten years' duration was without adhesions, though the stomach wall showed very noticeable departure from the normal, and it is rather remarkable that the colon should have been able to enter the chest to such an extent through a rigid ring and not have given rise to any symptoms. In entering the chest it would seem to have passed up in front of the stomach, and the purpose in suturing the stomach to the abdominal wall was as much to keep the colon as the stomach from entering the hernia.

DIRECT INGUINAL HERNIA *

By J. Pierre Hoguet, M.D.

of New York, N. Y.

A great deal has been written about the etiology and treatment of most forms of hernia in recent years, and yet when one considers the frequency of this condition, the amount of literature on the subject is small in proportion to that of even less common diseases. And this is even more noticeable when one attempts to review the literature of the very important subject of direct inguinal hernia, for except for the papers of Schley and of Downes on this subject, practically nothing has been written. It would seem as though surgeons were satisfied with the operative treatment of direct hernia and that they considered the average results so good that they need not be improved upon. And yet, unfortunately, this is not the case; the percentage of recurrence after operation for all kinds of hernia is yet much too great, and this is especially true after the ordinary operations that are done for direct hernia. It is with the idea of renewing interest in the subject of direct hernia that this matter is again brought up, and an operation, that has been tried out for the last two years and seems to promise good results, is presented.

As a general rule, it is in the middle-aged male that direct hernia occurs, although it is occasionally found in women and in children. There is no question but that indirect and direct hernia very often coexist in the same patient, and in the very large hernias there is most often a good-sized direct and an indirect sac. In the massive ones, such as are shown in the accompanying figures, the deep epigastric vessels are indistinguishable, so that the two sacs become one. It is impossible, in these cases, to say whether the hernia started internal or external to the deep epigastric vessels, but in either case, the result is the same, that is, a giving way of the whole inguinal canal. As will be mentioned later, even when the direct hernia is of only moderate size, an indirect sac always exists, either as a definite sac or as a small protrusion of peritoneum external to the deep epigastric vessels. Another point, which although recognized, is not regarded seriously enough, is that of the presence of the urinary bladder in the direct sac. This naturally becomes of the greatest importance in the operative treatment, and it is the conviction of the writer that a portion of the bladder is practically always present in the inner part of the direct sac.

* Read before the New York Surgical Society, May 12, 1920.

The question of operative treatment of direct inguinal hernia is of the greatest interest, and here it should be stated that, in some of these cases, there is no doubt that permanent cures can be obtained from the simple Bassini operation. These are the cases one occasionally sees where the direct sac is not very large and where there is enough bulk of internal oblique and transversalis muscle, so that when these are sutured to Poupart's ligament, there is a posterior wall for the canal of enough thickness from the internal ring to the spine of the pubis. It is probable, however, that these cases are in the minority, and in the usual direct hernia one finds a good-sized sac internal to the deep epigastric vessels and an internal oblique and transversalis muscle that is represented by a few small bundles of muscle tissue only loosely connected together. It is with the idea of reinforcing these insufficient muscles that other operations have been proposed, the best, of course, being that of reinforcing the posterior wall of the canal by suturing the lower portion of the rectus muscle to Poupart's ligament. There are certain cases where this is a very good operation, and as can be seen from the writer's cases, it has given fairly satisfactory results, but it would seem that suturing the rectus muscle, with or without its sheath, to Poupart's ligament pulls the muscle out of its normal anatomical line and that the constant tendency would be for it to pull away from its new attachment when it contracts. Then again, the conjoined tendon must be sutured to Poupart's ligament as well as the rectus, and sometimes when a large number of sutures are introduced into the ligament, it splits and separates into a number of strands which really afford little support for the muscle.

Schley, in his paper on direct hernia, unfortunately, gives no figures as to recurrence in his cases. He simply states that he knows of no recurrences, although admitting that his cases have not been traced. Downes is of the opinion that there is usually about ten per cent. of recurrences after direct hernia operations, and in a paper published by Dr. W. B. Coley and the writer, in the ANNALS OF SURGERY for September, 1918, which was a review of 8589 cases of hernia that had been operated upon, the statement was made, that if patients who had been operated upon for direct hernia could be followed up for a period of at least two years, a percentage of recurrence of from ten to fifteen would be found. This statement seems to be substantiated by the results seen in some of our larger hospitals since the follow-up systems have been inaugurated.

About two years ago, when it was realized that the results of operations on direct hernias were so bad, an endeavor was made to improve upon them by reinforcing the posterior wall of the canal by the use of the aponeurosis of the external oblique, so that there would be in the repair of the hernia three distinct layers instead of two, as in the ordinary

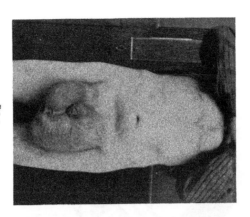

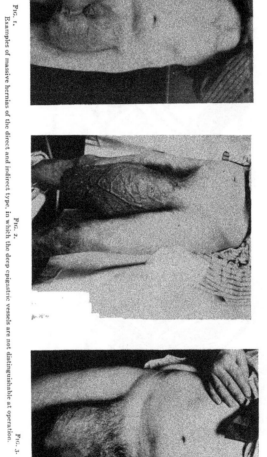

FIG. 1.

FIG. 2.

Examples of massive hernias of the direct and indirect type, in which the deep epigastric vessels are not distinguishable at operation.

FIG. 3.

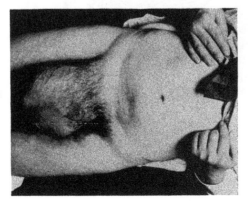

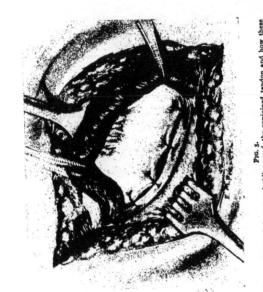

FIG. 5.

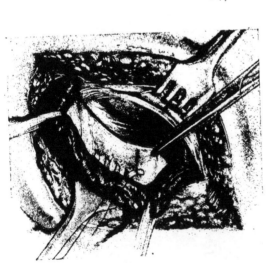

FIG. 4.

Showing how the sutures are introduced through both the reflected portion of the aponeurosis of the external oblique and the conjoined tendon and how these structures are sutured to Poupart's ligament.

Bassini operation. But the principle was always borne in mind that the same operation could not be made to fit every patient, so that in some cases the simple Bassini was done, in others the Bassini with transplantation of the rectus, and in the others the Bassini with the suture of the reduplicated aponeurosis of the external oblique. This operation, which was found to be particularly useful in those cases where the internal oblique and transversalis were very weak or where the rectus was very narrow, is done as follows: The usual skin incision was made and the aponeurosis of the external oblique split from the external ring upwards in the line of its fibres. As mentioned before, an indirect sac always can be found in these cases, although it may be very small. This sac is separated from the elements of the cord and opened. It has not been found necessary to divide the deep epigastric vessels, but by traction outwards on the indirect sac, all of the peritoneum of the direct sac may be pulled external to the vessels and the two sacs converted into one. By this proceeding, all possibility of injuring the bladder is eliminated, for as the peritoneum of the direct sac is pulled outwards under the epigastrics, if the bladder folds are adherent to the under surface of the sac, they can be clearly seen. This redundant peritoneum of indirect and direct sac is then transfixed with a suture and cut away. The steps up to this point are applicable to all cases of direct hernia, but the actual repair of the deficiency must depend upon the bulk of the internal oblique and transversalis. When the latter muscles are strong, there can be no objection to doing the ordinary Bassini which will probably give a permanent cure. In the majority of cases of direct hernia, these muscles are weak, and it then becomes necessary to reinforce them. As a double reinforcement, the reduplicated aponeurosis of the external oblique is used in the following way: The upper edge of the aponeurosis is pulled upwards and toward the midline with a sharp retractor, thus making a folded edge of fascia, lying parallel to Poupart's ligament and about one-half inch above the lower border of the internal oblique muscle. The sutures, preferably of kangaroo tendon, are then introduced through this folded edge of aponeurosis, the internal oblique and transversalis, and then through Poupart's ligament from behind forwards, posterior to the cord. It has been found very useful to use a blunt retractor in the lower angle of the wound in order to expose the lowermost portion of the canal which is essentially the weakest and which should be completely visible when the most internal suture is introduced. One suture should be inserted above the exit of the cord, making a new external pillar to the new internal ring, either in the way described above or simply through the internal oblique and transversalis, if these are strong enough at this point. The upper leaf of the aponeurosis is then brought over the cord and sutured to the lower leaf and the skin and subcutaneous tissue then closed.

The results of operation in 142 cases of direct hernia are given below in tabular form, and it can be seen that the percentage of recurrence from the simple Bassini is 7.3 per cent., from the Bassini with rectus transplantation 2.8 per cent., and from the Bassini with suture of the reduplicated aponeurosis 2.5 per cent.

	Cases	M.	F.	Adults	Children	R. E. C.	Known to be well	Not traced	Died
Bassini	68	65	3	65	3	5	41	21	1
Bassini, with rectus transplantation	35	33	2	34	1	1	16	18	
Bassini, with suture of reflected aponeurosis.	39	38	1	39	0	1	29	8	1
Total	142	136	6	138	4	7	86	42	2

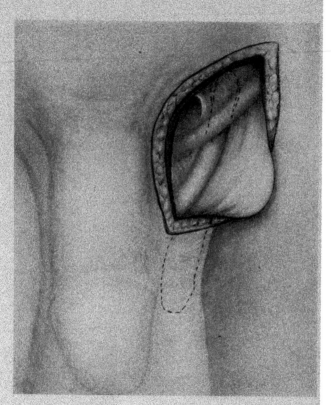

FIG. 1.—Showing protrusion of sac of inguinal hernia through the femoral ring.

DEVELOPMENT OF AN INGUINAL HERNIA THROUGH THE FEMORAL RING FOLLOWING DESCENT OF THE TESTICLE BY THE SAME ROUTE

By A. M. Fauntleroy, M.D.

Captain, Med. Corps, U. S. Navy

This case is reported on account of the fact that there is apparently no recorded instance in surgical literature where the testicle has descended through the femoral canal and into the scrotum.

C. E. R. A young man, aged twenty-two years, admitted to the surgical service, U. S. Naval Hospital, New York, N. Y., on October 22, 1919, with a diagnosis of complete left indirect inguinal hernia. The ward officer saw him on admission and at that time there was a distinct enlargement in the left inguinal region, extending into the scrotum.

The next day I examined this man, as a routine measure preliminary to operation, but no enlargement was visible in the inguinal region or scrotum, nor could any impulse be felt with the index finger in the external ring. Several other members of the surgical staff examined this man with the same result. In view of the fact that the ward officer had personally noted the inguinal and scrotal enlargement an operation was decided upon.

Operation (October 24, 1919).—Ether. The left inguinal region was exposed in the usual manner. When the aponeurosis of the external oblique muscle was divided the astounding fact was at first apparent that no cord was visible, although a testicle could be distinctly palpated in the scrotum.

After careful separation of Poupart's ligament from the internal oblique muscle the cord came into view descending vertically, passing through the femoral ring and *thence into the scrotum.* This anatomical arrangement explained why the impulse could not be elicited at the external ring. Once the anomaly was discovered the cord was lifted up and the sac dissected away, ligated at the internal ring and removed. The cord was buried, the internal oblique muscle sutured to Poupart's ligament in the usual manner, except that an effort was made to close the femoral opening (except for cord) from the inside by suturing the under side of Poupart's ligament to Cooper's ligament. The patient made an uneventful recovery and was discharged to duty in thirty days.

As a result of normal demobilization this man was discharged to civil life shortly after leaving this hospital. Several letters have been written to him at the address he gave for his parents in his health record, with the idea of following up his case, but these letters have remained unanswered.

My assistant at this operation was Lieutenant Samuel B. Burk, M.C., U. S. N. R. F., who has since been demobilized and is now practicing in New York, N. Y.

AN OPERATION TO FORM A NEW ANAL SPHINCTER AFTER OPERATIONS ON THE LOWER RECTUM

By Alfred J. Brown, M.D.

of Omaha, Neb.

One of the principal objections, if not the principal objection to the operation of perineal proctectomy devised by Quenu, is that this operation destroys the anal sphincter and leaves the patient with an incontinent bowel at the site of the anal orifice. There is no doubt that such a condition is far more disagreeable to the patient than an inguinal colostomy which can be protected and kept clean.

Attempts made to work above the sphincter, as in the Kraske operation and its various modifications, including the resection through the posterior vaginal wall, are not infrequently unsuccessful because of the tendency of stricture to follow the operation in low cancer and also owing to the inability to save the sphincter and at the same time excise the entire growth.

There are certain cases, rarely found, in which perineal proctectomy can be performed with comparative ease and the entire growth resected from below in which the patient can be spared the combined abdominal and perineal operation with attendant high mortality, provided sphincter control can be retained.

The statement has been made that with resection of the lower part of the rectum, incontinence results because of the removal of that part of the bowel supplied with sensory nerves and consequent loss of that sensation which notifies the patient of the desire for a bowel movement. In an experience of the two cases reported here this has not been the case. Both patients knew when the bowels were going to move and were able to control the bowel movement.

With the facts above in mind the operation described here has been employed in two cases, the only cases seen in which a low proctectomy seemed indicated and in each the new sphincter functioned almost from the time of operation; in the first case for a period of ten years, until the patient succumbed apparently from a recurrence of the cancer, and in the second case until recurrence of the growth formed a mechanical block to the passage of fæces and made a left inguinal colostomy necessary to prevent death from intestinal obstruction. The patients were both women and the operation will be described as performed in the two instances. The technic in the male would be but little different from the description here given.

The first steps of the operation are identical with the Quenu resection. The anus is cauterized and sutured. An incision beginning in front at the posterior commissure of the vagina passes backward to the anus, encircles it, and passes backward to just behind the tip of the coccyx. The incision is deepened, excising the sphincter ani and exposing the rectum up to the levator ani muscle of either side. The rectum is separated from the vaginal wall in front by dividing the central tendon and from the coccyx behind. It was not found necessary to remove the coccyx in either of the cases. The inner margins of the levator ani on either side are separated from the rectal wall and the recto-vesical covering the upper surface of the muscles divided also. The rectum can then be drawn downward and backward through the incision and with the finger the rectum stripped away from the posterior vaginal wall as far up as the lower part of Douglas' cul-de-sac. The middle hemorrhoidal vessels will be found surrounded by a fibrous sheath lying internal to the levator ani and recto-vesical fascia. These are tied as they appear when the rectum is drawn down and divided between ligatures. The rectum is then forward and with the finger in contact with the sacrum the tissues behind the rectum, including the lymphatic glands, are separated from the sacrum as far up as the promontory and remain in contact with the rectum, thus making a block dissection of the rectum containing the growth and the glands situated in the hollow of the sacrum. Traction downward will now bring $4\frac{1}{2}$ to $5\frac{1}{2}$ inches of the rectum below the perineum. If this is sufficient to bring the healthy bowel above the growth down to the posterior margin of the perineal wound without strain it will not be necessary to open the peritoneum. If, however, enough of the bowel cannot be drawn down because of its peritoneal attachments and the mesorectum, the peritoneum is opened and the bowel drawn down a sufficient distance (Fig. 2). The cut edge of peritoneum is immediately sutured to the wall of the gut and the peritoneal cavity closed off after the bowel has been drawn down to its final position.

Thus far the operation has followed the technic of Quenu, but from this point on it differs. The margins of the levator ani are outlined and a strip of muscle is separated from each (Fig. 3). One of the strips is left attached anteriorly, the other posteriorly. The strips are approximately 1 inch wide and as long as the muscle allows. The incisions freeing these strips pass entirely through the muscle, but do not include the rectovaginal fascia. The muscle strips are then changed from side to side (Fig. 4), so that the one originally on the right side now lies on the left and *vice versa*, and are sutured in place with interrupted sutures of chromic catgut. The rectum is amputated and its cut edge sutured to the cut edge of the circular skin incision, a gauze wick is inserted in the hollow of the sacrum and protrudes through the posterior incision, and the skin incision is closed with interrupted sutures (Fig. 5). In the illustrations the bowel is shown amputated before the muscle strips are separated. This was done for clarity of illustration. During the operation the amputation is not performed until after all deep work has been done and the superficial suture is being performed.

In the two cases which I have had, the post-operative shock has been very slight and the patients have been allowed up on the tenth day. The drainage was removed at the end of forty-eight hours, and the bowels moved by enema on the fifth day. After that there was slight incontinence for a week to ten days, and then the patients were continent and accidents did not occur.

CASE I.—Mrs. B. S., aged sixty-four years. Married, housewife. Referred by Doctor Middleditch, of New London, New York. About six months ago she first noticed small amounts of blood in her stools and slight pain on defecation. There has been no obstruction to the passage of fæces and no change in size has been noted. The bleeding has become more marked and for the past two weeks she has noticed a foul odor to the stools. She has noticed no discharge between movements. Appetite is good. She has not lost weight. Has had no fever and aside from the local condition feels well.

Physical Examination.—The patient is a large fleshy woman with negative physical findings except for the local condition. There is no enlargement of the glands in the femoral or inguinal regions. Rectal examination (digital) reveals an ulcer of the anterior wall of the rectum. Its base is hard and nodular. Its edges are everted and also hard. The mass occupies the anterior wall of the rectum and its upper margin can be felt by the examining finger—its lower margin lies about 2 inches above the anal ring. It does not apparently involve the entire rectal wall and the rectum is movable on the posterior vaginal wall.

Operation was performed February 28, 1907, according to the above technic. After a short and uneventful convalescence the patient was well and completely relieved of her symptoms. Was able to do her housework and had no trouble with lack of bowel control. Examination one year after operation showed an anal opening which looked almost normal. Rectal examination revealed a sphincteric action to the levator ani muscles which could be tightened or relaxed at will. After this time the patient did not return for examination but reported through her daughter from time to time that she was well. Finally, ten years after operation, September 28, 1907, her death was noted in the paper and inquiry elicited the following information by letter:

" About two years ago she passed some blood and pus; it was so slight it could hardly be said to show a return of the old trouble. There was no pain with it at any time. For about two years she suffered with hardening of the arteries, so that the heart was affected. Also the respiration. She was able to be about the house until two weeks before her death, when she was taken ill with bowel troubles and vomiting. This (the vomiting) subsided in about three days before they were able to check the bowels. Until she passed away the discharge was nearly all blood and pus, it was almost a constant flow, she would have a sharp pain and the blood and pus would follow. There seemed to be no pain after the first

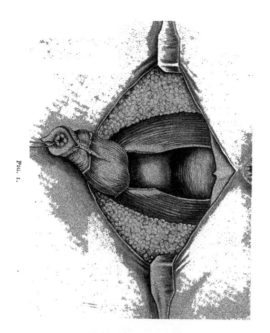

FIG. 1.

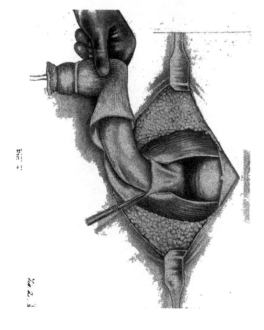

FIG. 2.

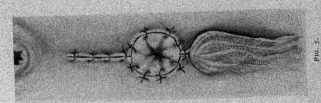

FIG. 5.

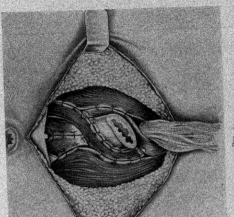

FIG. 4.

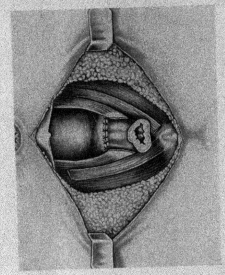

FIG. 3.

three days, but the discharge continued until the end. There was a very offensive odor."

It seems fair to assume that this is the story of the recurrence of a rectal carcinoma eight years after operation with death from intestinal obstruction two years later. Another instance of the necessity of following carcinoma for many years before cures can be reported.

CASE II.—Mrs. K. O., aged twenty-eight years, housewife. For three months has noticed slight bleeding and some pain occurring with bowel movements. There has been no change in size or shape of the stool, and so far as she knows there has been no change in her general health. Has not noticed any offensive odor. The bleeding has increased slightly. Has lost little, if any, flesh. Appetite good. Sleeps well. Bowels are constipated.

Physical Examination.—The patient is a thin, wiry woman, but fairly well nourished. Physical examination fails to reveal any abnormality save the local condition.

Rectal Examination (Digital).—Shows an irregularly rounded, hard ulcer with everted hard edges in the anterior wall of the rectum. It is movable on the vaginal wall and the entire rectum is movable. No glandular enlargement can be felt. The ulcer is approximately 1 inch by 1½ inches in size and the examining finger can be passed beyond its upper border.

Operation was performed in June, 1917. Apparently the growth was resected as completely as in the preceding case. The glands in the hollow of the sacrum did not feel enlarged and nothing could be felt above. The operation was performed according to the technic outlined, the lower 6 inches of the rectum removed, and the plastic operation on the levator ani muscles performed. Convalescence was uneventful and the patient was allowed up at the end of twelve days. Bowels were moved by enema and thereafter the patient had control of her bowel movements.

The report of Dr. J. E. MacWhorter, pathologist to the First Surgical Division of Bellevue Hospital, stated that the growth was an extremely virulent carcinoma with microscopic infiltration of all the tissue, even up to the point of removal. This could not be determined by macroscopic examination of the specimen which at the time of operation was presumed to be no more malignant than that of the previous case.

The patient returned every two weeks for examination and for three months did well. The bowels functioned normally and without loss of control. At the end of that time a recurrence occurred at the new anal orifice which rapidly increased in size and caused a stricture of the anus. At approximately the same time the patient complained of gastric symptoms and pain in the chest with dyspnœa. X-ray examination gave findings of pyloric obstruction with a doubtful shadow in the mediastinum.

The patient was again admitted to the hospital and as symptoms of chronic intestinal obstruction had appeared a left inguinal colostomy was performed. At this operation the left ovary was found

ALFRED J. BROWN

markedly enlarged, hard, and of a peculiar translucent appearance, so it was removed and upon examination proved to be a Krunkenberg tumor of the ovary.

The patient gradually failed and died less than six months after the primary operation. An autopsy was refused, so definite information as to the condition of the stomach and thorax could not be obtained. It seems fair to assume, because of the close association between carcinoma of the upper intestinal tract and the ovarian tumor first described by Krunkenberg as primary in the ovary, that the gastric condition was probably a carcinoma secondary to that in the rectum. There was no evidence of gastric involvement previous to the rectal operation and all the indications are that the rectal tumor was the primary growth. From examination of the microscopic sections it is not probable that this patient could have been saved by a combined operation. All of the perirectal tissues were invaded in every direction, though nothing could be seen or felt macroscopically—and there is no doubt that the growth had progressed beyond any possible hope of removal.

By the operation above described the lower 6 inches of the rectum can be removed by the perineal route and a new sphincter which will function can be formed from the levator ani muscles. Cases of carcinoma suitable for operation by this route can be relieved with less danger to life than by the combined operation, and subsequently live in comparative comfort.

TECHNIC OF PARTIAL COLECTOMY BY THE MIKULICZ TWO-STAGE METHOD

By Charles N. Dowd, M.D.

of New York, N. Y.

SURGEON TO THE ROOSEVELT HOSPITAL

In the ANNALS OF SURGERY for February, 1920, the writer published an article on "The Advantages of the Mikulicz Two-stage Operation of Partial Colectomy." The references to this article have been mainly of two varieties: one, communications from a number of experienced sur-

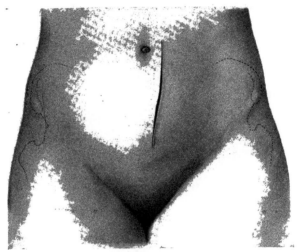

FIG. 1.—Primary incision. Used for exploration, mobilization of intestine and for removal or mobilization of enlarged lymphatics.

geons acknowledging the advantages of the principle of "exteriorizing" the growth before the intestine is opened; the other, requests for information about various details of operative technic.

There have been so many inquiries of the latter type that it seems advisable to publish a further description of this technic by giving the details of a single illustrative case of partial colectomy for cancer at the sigmoid. This is done in the hope of further popularizing an operation which diminishes the dangers of patients with cancers of the large intestine between the hepatic flexure and the lower sigmoid or with other lesions which call for partial colectomy in this region.

44   681

In the previous article, sixteen cases of partial colectomy were re-ported, with one death. Since that time the writer has successfully oper-ated upon three additional cases; one for cancer of the transverse colon, one for Hirschsprung's disease, and one for cancer of the sigmoid. This low mortality rate in a short series of cases indicates the comparative safety of the procedure, but it should not mislead the reader. Individual operators continually have short series of cases which give better results than can be maintained in long series.

History of Patient.—Mrs. D. C., a rather thin woman, aged thirty-two years, came to the Roosevelt Hospital March 13, 1920, suffering from long-continued intestinal obstruction.

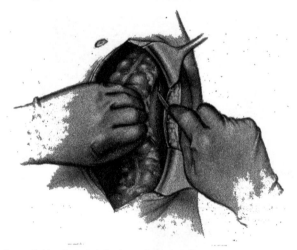

FIG. 2.—Incision of outer leaf of peritoneum beside descending colon so as to secure suitable mobility of that part of colon.

She stated that she had been in excellent health until two months ago when she had cramp-like pains across the abdomen, especially in the lower left side. These were severe and were accom-panied by constipation. She went for two weeks with very slight fecal passage. Large quantities of fæces then passed and she was relieved. For more than two weeks she then had suitable bowel movements.

On admission she stated that the last bowel movement had occurred twenty-six days ago. During that time she had eaten very little, but had taken various forms of broth. She had suffered much from abdominal pain; but had vomited very little, excepting after taking castor oil. Occasionally the return from the enemas had been blood-tinged. Just before coming to the hospital severe vomiting had begun and hence she sought immediate relief. She was in reasonably good general condition. Heart and lungs, sound; abdomen distended; visible peristalsis; no tumor palpable either by examination or by rectum.

Description of Operation.—The details of the operation for this patient are shown in the accompanying plates. They give a fair indication of the average procedure.

1. *Primary Incision.*—A low, five- or six-inch incision, near the median line, gives opportunity for suitably exploring the abdomen,

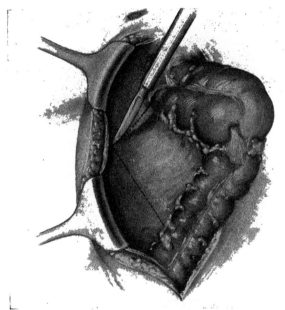

Fig. 3.—Exposure and removal or mobilization of enlarged lymphatics and part of meso-sigmoid.

learning the site and character of the primary lesion, and searching for metastases and lymphatic enlargement. With or without enlargement, it also permits the mobilization of the growth in operable cases. Figs. 2, 3, and 4 indicate the portion of work which was done through this incision in this case.

2. *The incision of the outer leaf of the peritoneum of the descending colon,* as advocated by Moynihan and others and as indicated in Fig. 2, is easily accomplished and secures wonderful mobility of the corresponding portion of the intestine. When carried upward sufficiently, it permits the mobilization of the splenic flexure.

3. *Removal of Lymphatics.*—It is desirable to examine the lymphatic areas which are liable to infection. Jameson and Dobson[1] have carefully investigated the anatomy of these areas. It is not always practicable to completely remove them, nor is it always necessary. Numerous observers have shown that cancer of the colon may long remain a local disease. Clogg[2] made post-mortem examinations in eighteen patients with cancer of the pelvic colon. Enlarged lymph-nodes were noted in seventeen instances, but only

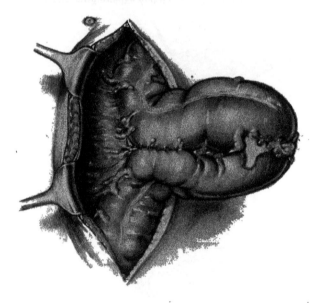

FIG. 4.—Stitching of afferent and efferent legs of intestine so as to form a septum which is suitable for later clamping.

in six were they at a distance from the colon. He found that enlarged lymph-nodes did not show cancer cells in one-third of the cases examined. The judgment of the individual surgeon must determine the extent of the lymphatic area which is to be removed.

In this instance the small intestines were retracted to the right and the mesocolon was exposed as far as the spine, the peritoneum was incised, and the lymph-nodes were mobilized and either removed at once or pushed toward the sigmoid. Branches of the left colic and inferior mesenteric arteries were clamped, tied, and cut, but the

[1] Proceedings of Royal Society of Medicine, 23, 1908–1909, Surgical Section, p. 149.
[2] H. S. Clogg: Cancer of the Colon. Lancet, 1908, vol. ii, p. 1007.

main trunks of both of these arteries were preserved. A sector of the peritoneum, with apex at inferior mesenteric artery and base at the sigmoid, together with the adjacent lymphatics, was mobilized

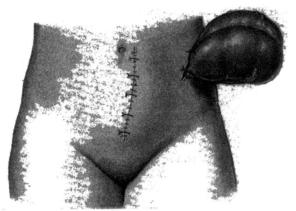

FIG. 5.—Primary wound closed. Diseased intestine delivered through small secondary intramuscular wound. (In this instance it was distended by pressure of gas from above.)

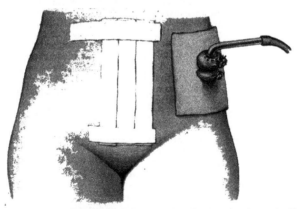

FIG. 6.—Primary wound covered by aseptic dressing. Secondary wound smeared with ointment and protected by gauze. Protruding parts of afferent and efferent intestine ligated. Diseased portion of intestine ablated. Paul's tube inserted in protruding part of afferent intestine so as to secure and temporarily control drainage.

and pushed to the sigmoid. The breadth of this sector must vary somewhat with the individual case. Since the lymphatics extend along the intestinal wall to the next afferent arterial branch, it is desirable to remove a corresponding portion of the intestine, with its adjacent arterial loops, and the incision in the mesosigmoid should be large enough to permit this.

The real point at issue is that in the two-stage operation the extent of lymphatic dissection and the length of the removed portion of intestine may be as great as in the one-stage anastomosis. Tension is to be avoided in any instance, but the danger of moderate tension is not so great in the two-stage procedure as in the one-stage procedure. Unless the abdominal wall is unusually thick, patients who give suitable facilities for one-stage anastomosis are likely to give equally good opportunity for two-stage procedure.

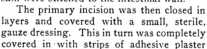

4. *Stitching of Afferent and Efferent Legs of Intestine so as to Secure a Good " Spur."*—Sound portions of the afferent and efferent legs of intestine were selected at safe distance from the cancer and stitched together with fine catgut for a distance of two inches or more. This secured suitable apposition between these portions of intestine. A good septum was thus formed to which a clamp was safely applied at a later time.

5. *Exteriorization of Cancerous Portion of Colon.*—This is best accomplished through a small separate incision at a convenient site. In this instance finger pressure was made from within the abdomen a little above and internal to the anterior superior spine of the ilium and a small intramuscular incision of the McBurney type was made there. The diseased loop of intestine was then drawn through this incision. In this instance there was so much gas pressure from above that the extruded intestine " ballooned up " like an inflated rubber bag. The edges of the skin were stitched to the intestinal wall.

FIG. 7.—Clamp for dividing the "spur" by pressure. At first the pressure was secured by a rubber band applied to the handles; afterward the ratchet is used for progressive tightening of the clamp.

The primary incision was then closed in layers and covered with a small, sterile, gauze dressing. This in turn was completely covered in with strips of adhesive plaster which extended onto the surrounding skin. In this way healing of the primary wound by first intention was secured.

The small size of the new incision and the undisturbed condition of the tissues about it leave little likelihood of mural abscess about the stoma.

6. *Treatment of Excluded Portion of Colon.*—After the skin and adjacent portion of colon have been well smeared with a 10 per cent. boric acid ointment, gauze is laid about them.

We now have the abdomen shut off. Since the intestine has not been opened, there has been little likelihood of infection. In

Mikulicz' early cases the loop of cancerous intestine was permitted
to slough in the dressing. This, however, was not done in his later
cases and is unnecessary. A ligature can be placed about each loop
of intestine outside the gauze dressing. The cancerous loop of gut
can be ablated. The·time for opening the protruding intestine depends upon the condition of the patient. In some instances it may
be deferred for forty-eight or even seventy-two hours. In this instance, owing to the pressure of gas from above, an immediate opening was desirable, therefore a purse-string was placed in the upper
leg of intestine between the ligature and the gauze dressing, a
Paul's tube was inserted and held fast by a tightening of the purse-
string. This permitted gas and fæces to escape without soiling the

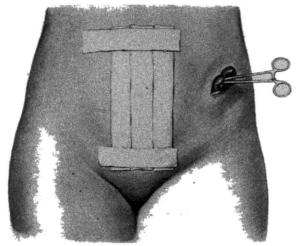

Fig. 8.—Clamp applied to septum.

dressing. The purse-string joint held for twenty-four hours, which
was sufficient to permit a reasonably good union between the abdominal wall and the intestine and thus prevent infection at that point.

7 and 8. *Clamping of the Spur.*—The ligatures about the ends of
the intestine were removed after forty-eight hours. A "double-
barrelled" intestinal stoma was thus established which provided
an exit for the intestinal contents. After nine days the union of
the abdominal wall was firm. There was no evidence of surrounding
inflammation there and the crushing of the spur between the two
legs of intestine was begun. Various clamps have been used for this
purpose. The one which bears the name of Mikulicz is believed to
be a very efficient one. We have tried various forms of clamps and,
at the present time, use an ordinary Kocher clamp (Fig. 7). or a

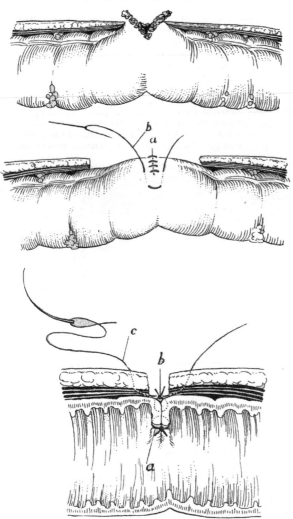

FIG. 9.—Closure of stoma. The intestine is separated from its attachment to the abdominal wall so as to expose its peritoneal surface. The lower leg is then pulled upward and the upper leg downward. Interrupted chromicized gut stitches (a) are taken through the entire intestinal wall at the upper and lower edges of the stoma and tied with their knots inside the intestinal lumen. This row is then reinforced by Lembert stitches (b). The edges of the abdominal wall are then approximated by silkworm-gut stitches (c), leaving provision for possible leakage.

similar clamp without teeth at its end. After inserting fingers on each side of the septum so as to determine the relationship of the parts, the clamp is applied and an elastic band applied about the handle so as to make firm pressure. At the end of one or two days the first notch of the ratchet was fastened. On successive days, additional pressure was applied (Fig. 8) and the clamp came away on the fifth day. In this instance the artificial anus discharged intestinal contents regularly and the mouth of the stoma contracted moderately.

9. *Closure of Stoma.*—On the twenty-fifth day an effort was made to close the stoma. The skin was dissected away from the margin of the intestine. The upper leg was pulled downward from above (Fig. 9) and the lower leg was pulled upward from below, thus securing enough intestine for good serous apposition of the ends. The peritoneum was slightly opened for this procedure, and the edges of the peritoneal opening were easily secured by a few catgut stitches. The first row of stitches was then taken between the intestinal ends. They were interrupted, chromic gut included the entire intestinal wall, and the knots were tied inside the lumen. A second row of Lembert stitches of chromic gut was then taken to secure apposition outside of the first row. The edges of the abdominal wound were then drawn together with silkworm gut, leaving a very small opening for the escape of leakage. In this instance the closure was not complete and after two weeks a clamp was applied to a portion of the spur which remained. After this clamp came away the stoma was again closed by two rows of stitches and the suture line was supported by loose, silkworm gut stitching through the overlying abdominal wall. The wound then closed satisfactorily and the patient left the hospital May 26th. The period of her operation and after-treatment was, therefore, ten and five-sevenths weeks. This was longer than a successful one-stage operation would have taken. A one-stage operation, however, was not to be considered for this case. The intestine was too greatly distended and contained too much foul fecal material. A preliminary colostomy and later one-stage operation would probably have taken longer and would have been much more dangerous.

PRIMARY CARCINOMA OF THE VERMIFORM APPENDIX IN SISTERS SUFFERING FROM TUBERCULOSIS*

BY ALEXANDER PRIMROSE, C.B., M.B., C.M., EDIN.

OF TORONTO, CANADA

PROFESSOR OF CLINICAL SURGERY IN THE UNIVERSITY OF TORONTO

THE ileocæcal region in man's anatomy is of great interest not only to the surgeon who, in recent years, operates more frequently for disease of the appendix than for trouble in any other part of the body, but also for the morphologist and physiologist. Huntington in his delightful book on " The Anatomy of the Human Peritoneum and Abdominal Cavity " presents a wealth of material in his study of the comparative anatomy and embryology of this region and its phylogenetic significance. He refers to the human vermiform appendix as a rudimentary and vestigial structure, and with this view most authorities agree. On the other hand, Keith in his book on " Human Embryology and Morphology " presents a different view. He tells us that " in all vertebrates the submucous coat of the cæcal colon is rich in lymphocytes which in mammals collect in the form of solitary follicles more or less closely crowded together. In primates Berry found a tendency for the lymphoid tissue to be aggregated in the apex of the cæcum. In man, in anthropoids and a few other forms, the lymphoid tissue becomes richly developed in the distal part of the cæcum, which has a narrow lumen, strong muscular coat, and is of great functional activity during digestion. This highly specialized part of the cæcum is the appendix; it is well developed in man and is certainly not a vestigial structure." Berry described the appendix as a lymphoid diverticulum of the cæcal apex, and Keith insists that it must be regarded as a lymphoid structure, and although it can be dispensed with, is not, therefore, to be regarded as vestigial in nature any more than the tonsil. I present this view because there has been a tendency to account for the occurrence of carcinoma in the appendix by considering it as a vestigial organ. Thus Elting favors this theory, endeavoring to explain the occurrence of cancer in this region, by stating that fetal remains as well as atrophying organs appear to be more prone to the development of carcinoma.

Primary carcinoma of the appendix is now a recognized entity. Boyer recently reviewed 300 cases from the literature. In spite of the fact that many observations have been made, we are still in the dark as to its nature and true significance. We find reference to it as a " benign carcinoma," a new term in medical literature, and yet perhaps justified by

---

* Read before the Alumni Association, Medical Department, University of Buffalo, June 10, 1920.

the course run in nearly all the cases recorded. As a rule, there is nothing to lead to a diagnosis of cancer by the gross appearance, and it is only because of the histological picture that we classify our cases as such. In recent years a routine histological examination of all tissue removed at operation is carried out in every properly-organized surgical clinic. As a result we have made many discoveries of conditions hitherto unsuspected, among others the occurrence of primary cancer in the appendix. When we depended largely on observation of gross anatomy such tumors were no doubt overlooked. Zaaijer quotes an observation of Roger Williams made in 1893 to the effect that, " In an examination of the records of 15,481 neoplasms, met with at St. Bartholomew's, Middlesex, University College and St. Thomas Hospitals, he could find no mention of any neoplasms involving the vermiform appendix." As a matter of fact, in nearly all the cases of primary carcinoma of the appendix on record there was no evidence of malignancy in the gross appearances and evidence of cancer was only demonstrated by microscopic examination. The tumor when found at operation is usually small in size, varying from that of a pea to a pigeon's egg; it presents a smooth, regular surface, and rarely shows any tendency to the formation of metastases. It is usually situated at or near the tip of the appendix. In one of my cases it was at the distal end and in the other at the extreme proximal end. In many instances there is no gross tumor and the condition is only recognized on opening the appendix or in the examination of appendices which have been the seat of an inflammation causing obliteration of the lumen with the formation of scar tissue. In certain rare exceptions, however, the evidences of malignancy are present, both gross and microscopic.

My object in reporting two cases of primary carcinoma of the appendix is because they occurred in sisters, both of whom suffered from tuberculosis. In one case the patient had pulmonary tuberculosis and the other had primary tuberculosis of the Fallopian tubes. Both patients made good recoveries from the operations performed. The histories of these cases are as follows:

CASE I.—M. H., female, aged twenty-one years. Admitted to hospital June 20, 1919, with symptoms of acute appendicitis; she had a history of pain and vomiting and on admission had a temperature of 101° F. She had had two previous attacks. She was operated upon the same day. The appendix was swollen and congested and tied down in an acute kink by firm scar tissue. At the base of the appendix was a hard, smooth nodule the size of a small pea. It was so close to the cæcum that I had to remove part of the cæcal wall in order to cut wide of the tumor. The tumor, however, was confined to the appendix and did not involve the cæcum. The uterus, ovaries, and Fallopian tubes were examined and found normal. Subsequent to operation she showed a persistent high evening temperature, and on examining the chest evidence of congestion was

691

found in the right lung; 10 c.c. of clear straw-colored fluid, withdrawn from the pleural cavity, was found to be sterile. A diagnosis of pulmonary tuberculosis was subsequently made, and she was transferred on July 12th to a sanitarium.

The report of the histology of the tumor found at the base of the appendix was made by Dr. W. L. Robinson as follows (Fig. 1):

> The lumen, mucosa and part of the submucosa are replaced by a tumor growth made up of large cells which are more or less spherical in shape.
> The nuclei are large, oval-shaped and hyperchromatic, a few of which are undergoing mitoses. These cells show a marked tendency to an alveolar arrangement. In the centre of the growth the cells are grouped in large masses, with very little stroma. Towards the periphery they are squeezed out into cords and are associated with a great deal of fibrous-tissue stroma. They are also infiltrating the muscle layers, and again appear in the subperitoneal coat as large masses, with a small amount of stroma. There are a few lymph follicles still in the submucosa. Another section of the appendix shows the lumen to be completely obliterated with fibrous tissue infiltrated with a large number of lymphocytes, and also containing a few small masses of epithelial cells similar to those described above.

CASE II.—I. H., female, aged twenty-nine years. Admitted to hospital February 14, 1920. Five or six years previously, while a nurse in training, she suffered from continued abdominal distress and was laid up for eight or ten weeks. During this time she was examined under anæsthesia and is said to have had " Endometritis." About a week before admission she developed abdominal pain which was more or less continued and persistent. On digital examination, by the rectum, pain was produced on pressure such as might be accounted for by an inflamed appendix lying low in the pelvis. The temperature did not arise above 99° F., but her blood showed a white-cell count of 19,000 per cubic mm. An operation was performed on February 17, 1920. Through a right rectus incision I was able to inspect the gall-bladder which was small, normal in appearance, and free from adhesions. The cæcum was pendulous and lay, along with the appendix, in the pelvis. The appendix was firmly adherent: it was separated from its adhesions and removed. The tip of the appendix was converted into a hard nodule, oval in shape, with a smooth surface and in bulk about twice the size of a pea. I at once remarked upon the fact that it resembled closely the nodule found in the appendix of her sister, which I had removed eight months previously, and suggested, from the gross appearance, that we again had primary carcinoma of the appendix. On exploring the pelvis I found the uterus drawn well to the left and bound down to a mass which existed in the left broad ligament. In this mass one was unable to distinguish tube or ovary until I had separated the adhesions along natural lines of cleavage: in doing so a small particle of caseous material, about the size of a grain of rice, escaped. The suggestion was made that the deeply-congested Fallopian tube, which we thus isolated, was tuberculous. The tube was removed, but not the ovary. One found similar conditions in the right broad ligament,

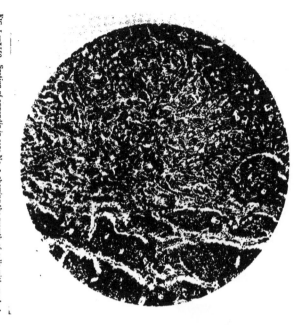

FIG. 1.—×150. Section of appendix in case No. 1, showing the growth of cells with marked tendency to alveolar arrangement.

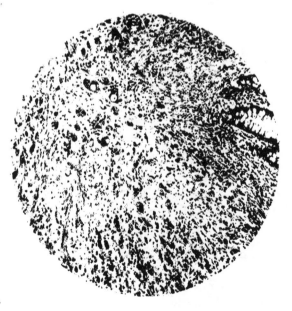

FIG. 2.—×150. Section of wall of the appendix in case No. 2, showing the cords of epithelial cells with fibrous tissue stroma.

692 a.

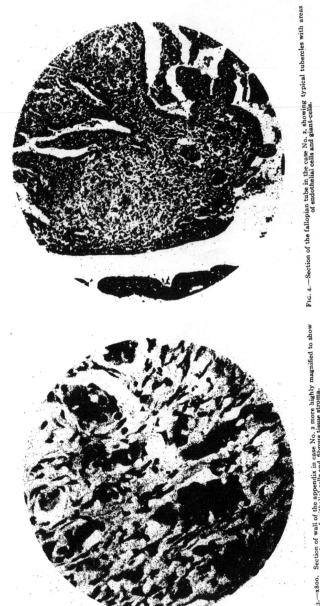

Fig. 4.—Section of the fallopian tube in the case No. 2, showing typical tubercles with areas of endothelial cells and giant-cells.

Fig. 3.—×800. Section of wall of the appendix in case No. 2 more highly magnified to show columns of epithelial cells and fibrous tissue stroma.

but the ovary was so involved in the process I removed both tube and ovary in one mass. There was no evidence of tubercle on the serosa or in lymph-glands.

Doctor Robinson's report on the histology of the tumor of the appendix and of the Fallopian tube is as follows (Figs. 2, 3, and 4).

Microscopic Report on Appendix.—The tumor growth is made up of solid cords of epithelial cells, with a considerable amount of a dense fibrous-tissue stroma. A few small masses of these cells can be seen in the mucosa, apparently extending from it and infiltrating the submucosa and muscle coats and growing out into the peritoneum. The epithelial cells are very irregular in size and shape. The nuclei are hyperchromatic. Many cells are very large and multinucleated. There are a few mitotic figures present. The mucous membrane of the appendix is intact and apparently normal apart from the tumor cells present.

Fallopian Tube.—The wall of the tube shows an increase of fibrous tissue, with a slight diffuse lymphocytic infiltration. Scattered through the mucous membrane are a large number of areas of endothelial cells, with giant-cells forming typical tubercles, some of which show a slight amount of caseation in the centre.

There are apparently two main types of so-called primary carcinoma of the appendix. In one type the histological picture shows numerous nests of small spherical or polygonal cells with a considerable development of interstitial connective tissue surrounding the individual cell nests. The marked degree of fibrosis which exists in these cases is worthy of note. The second type consists of cylindrical or columnar cells presenting an adenoid structure and comparable in its histological structure to the adeno-carcinoma found in other parts of the intestine. In both instances the tumor growth may be confined to the submucosa or may infiltrate the muscular coat and extend to the serous coat. In some instances the serosa has been penetrated and neighboring coils of intestine have been implicated. Colloid cancer has also been described, one such was reported by Elting in a man eighty-one years of age.

The frequency of occurrence in appendices removed at operation or examined at autopsy indicates that it may be looked for in about 0.4 per cent. (MacCarty, .44 per cent. in 8039 specimens; McWilliams, 0.4 per cent. in 6505 specimens.) The age of the individual indicates its occurrence at an earlier age than is usual for intestinal carcinoma: in 300 cases reported by Boyer most of the cases occurred between the ages of twenty and forty years; the youngest patient reported was five years of age, the oldest eighty-one; some interesting facts are brought out by McWilliams in his analysis of 90 cases: the spheroidal-cell cancers are 30 per cent. more frequent than the columnar type, and moreover, the average age for the spheroidal type was twenty-three years and for the columnar type forty-three years. In the small intestine and large intestine adeno-carcinoma occurs in almost three-fourths of all cases, while in the appendix adeno-carcinoma constitutes only about one-fourth of the cases. Again, according to McWilliams' statistics, if the stomach and intestines are considered together, the spheroidal-cell type of cancer occurs in only one-fifth of the cases, while they constitute three-fourths of the cases occurring in the appendix.

It would appear that from 60 to 70 per cent. of the cases are in females (Boyer). Reiman places the percentage in females as high as 65 to 75 per cent. This finding may in part be accounted for by the fact that the appendix is so frequently removed during gynæcological operations, coupled with the further fact that practically all cases of carcinoma of the appendix are discovered accidentally. Child has called attention to disease of the pelvic organs in women as an important exciting cause of appendicitis. In one of my cases there was a double tuberculous salpingitis with the carcinomatous appendix adherent to the mass in the right side of the pelvis.

A striking characteristic in these tumors is the fact that they are benign. There is no recorded instance of recurrence after removal. Metastasis is a very rare event. LeConte and Elting each describe a case with metastasis in the ileocolic lymph-glands. In only one case out of ninety in McWilliams' series was there positive demonstration of metastasis in lymph-glands. Oberndorfer reports two cases with metastasis. Local malignancy, as evidence by infiltration by the primary growth of structures beyond the appendix, is recorded in a few instances (Ross, LeConte, Coley, Elting, and Neugebauer). Batzdorff states that the disease extends beyond the appendix in 6 per cent. of the cases recorded.

All observers have recognized the association of primary cancer of the appendix with a chronic inflammation which usually leads to an obliteration of the lumen by a process of fibrosis. The etiological relationship between chronic inflammation and cancer in the appendix has been emphasized by Mayo. This was apparent in the cases recorded by the writer. Moreover, the tumor possesses a fibrous tissue stroma which is usually dense and considerable in amount. So marked is this characteristic that some authorities refer to the tumor as a scirrhous cancer (Adami and McCrae), and indeed, the histological picture in one of my cases closely resembled that of a scirrhous cancer of the breast.

Brewer narrates a case of carcinoma of the appendix in which a careful study of the specimen revealed the fact that it occurred at the site of a healed perforation, and in that perforation a little curtain of mucous membrane prolapsed through the opening. Healing had taken place and the epithelial cells of the mucous membrane were embedded in the tissue: this suggests for some cases a possible etiological factor in the displaced epithelial cells.

There is still some confusion in the attempt to determine the true nature of this interesting tumor. Aschoff compares it to tumors of somewhat similar character occurring in the small intestine first described by Lubarsch. Adami and McCrae call attention to the fact that the rare carcinomas of the lower end of the ileum are of the same benign type.

Aschoff and Mallory note the resemblance of the histological structure to the epithelial formation which occurs in connection with nævi in the skin, and the suggestion is that they should be regarded as analogous to such congenital anomalies. The cells resemble somewhat the basal cells of cutis tumors. Then there is a tendency to regard the cells, at all events those of the spheroidal type, as endothelium: Glazebrook reported a case in 1895 which he called " endothelial sarcoma of the appendix " (quoted by Elting). Ewing states that in some cases " the structure resembles that of endothelioma arising from the lymph-spaces of inflammatory connective tissue." Oberndorfer, in discussing Winkler's paper before the Deutschen Pathologischen Gesellschaft, 1910, described the spheroidal type as a growth of lymph-vascular endothelium and not a cancer. Milner also speaks of this type as a product of an inflammatory growth chiefly of the adenoid tissue of the mucosa and the lymph-vascular endothelium.

Whatever be the genesis of this interesting tumor one fact is established, namely, its association with a chronic inflammatory process. We wish, however, in this communication to emphasize its relation to tuberculosis. It is remarkable in reviewing the literature to note how frequently this association exists. In individual cases reported we find tuberculosis mentioned as an accompaniment, *e.g.*, by Lubarsch, Kelly, Letulle and Weinberg, Winkler, and others. Each of the two cases reported in the present paper exhibited tuberculous lesions. This relationship between tuberculosis and cancer is not commonly commented upon. It is conceivable, as Lubarsch points out, that tuberculous infection can, even as a local trauma, lead to the development of carcinoma. Milner, writing in 1910, in the investigation of fourteen cases of what he calls " pseudo-carcinoma " of the appendix, speaks of these tumors as reminding one of what is seen in tuberculous cases, and concludes that " the tumors are the product of a chronic hyperplastic inflammation, chiefly a hyperplastic lymphangitis, and their parenchymal cells are endothelium and not epithelium."

Tuberculous invasion of the Fallopian tube may simulate carcinoma in its histological picture: thus Barbour and Watson in studying tuberculous pyosalpinx found that while the tubercle nodules were confined to the mucous membrane, there had been a hypertrophy of the epithelium which penetrated deeply into the muscular layer together with the formation of strands and masses of epithelial cells in the substance of the mucosa. This produced " an appearance very like carcinoma." Further at the extreme ends of the tubes they found the mucous membrane free from tubercles, but there existed marked hyperplasia of the epithelial covering and a deeper extension into the muscular wall. Embedded in the muscle were gland-like spaces lined by epithelium at a considerable distance from the lumen. The condition found by these authors in the Fallopian tube, infected by tubercle, bears a striking resemblance to the histological characteristics of the so-called primary carcinoma of the appendix.

The ileocæcal region is frequently the seat of tuberculosis. It is common experience to find evidence of healed tuberculosis when operating for appendicitis, the ileocolic lymph-glands are not infrequently enlarged and caseous. Fenwick and Dodwell (quoted by Kelly) in 2000 autopsies of persons dying from tuberculosis found that the intestinal lesion was limited to the appendix in seventeen cases. Further, the appendix is often invaded by tuberculosis through direct contact with a tubercular tube or ovary. Kelly reports four such cases in his own experience. The striking feature exhibited in Case II, recorded in the present paper, was the remarkable combination of an appendix, the seat of a primary carcinoma, being adherent to a tube, the seat of primary tuberculosis.

The writer does not feel competent to enter into a controversy as to the nature of the cell growth in these tumors, but in view of the doubt which obviously exists at present as to their true nature he would urge from the clinical side that tuberculosis is too frequently an accompaniment to be a mere coincidence and must be of some significance. Furthermore, it becomes obvious that many authorities regard these cells as endothelial: this, together with the marked tendency to fibrosis, cannot but remind one of the characteristic features noted in the development of tubercle.

In conclusion one may call attention to heredity as an etiological factor. Harte reports a case in a patient forty-one years of age whose mother suffered from advanced scirrhus of the breast; this may have been a mere coincidence, but the interesting feature in my cases is that in addition to the double history of tuberculosis my two patients were sisters. As far as I am aware, this is the first time that members of the same family are reported to have suffered from primary carcinoma of the appendix; yet, hitherto, the number of cases reported are comparatively few in number, and it might well be that this specific instance may point to heredity as a factor, both in the production of the tuberculosis and of the tumor growth, with possibly some connecting link between the two pathological conditions exhibited.

BIBLIOGRAPHY

Adami, J. G., and McCrae: A Text-book of Pathology, 1914, p. 658.

Aschoff, L.: Pathologische Anatomie, 1911, Bd. 2, p. 798.

Barbour, A. H. F., and Watson, B. P.: Tuberculous Pyosalpinx, Jour. of Obstetrics and Gynæcology of the British Empire, September, 1911.

Batzdorff, E.: Ein Beiträge zur Frage des Primären Appendixcarcinoms. Langenbeck's Archiv für klinische Chirurgie, 1912, xcviii, p. 76.

Beger, A.: Ein Fall von Krebs des Wurmfortsatzes, Berliner klin. Wochenschrift, 1882, xli, s. 616.

Boyer, E. E. H.: Primary Carcinoma of the Vermiform Appendix: A Review of the Literature With a Report of Two New Cases, Amer Jour. of Med. Sciences, 1919, clvii, p. 775.

Brewer, G. E.: Discussion on LeConte's Paper, Trans. Am. Surg. Assoc., 1908, xxvi, p. 454.

CARCINOMA OF THE VERMIFORM APPENDIX

Child, C. G.: Coexistent Diseases of the Appendix and Pelvic Organs in the Female, Amer. Jour. of Obstetrics, 1919, lxxx, p. 31.

Coley, W. B.: Discussion on LeConte's Paper, Trans. Amer. Surg. Assoc., 1908, xxvi, p. 454.

Elting, A. W.: Primary Carcinoma of the Vermiform Appendix, ANNALS OF SURGERY, 1903, xxxvii, p. 549.

Ewing, James: Neoplastic Diseases, 1919, p. 644.

Harte, R. H.: Primary Carcinoma and Sarcoma of the Appendix Vermiformis, Trans. Am. Surg. Assoc., 1908, xxvi, p. 399.

Huntington, G. S.: The Anatomy of the Human Peritoneum and Abdominal Cavity, 1903, p. 218.

Kelly, A. O. J.: Primary Carcinoma and Endothelioma of the Vermiform Appendix, Amer. Jour. Med. Sciences, 1908, xxxv, p. 851.

Kelly, Howard A.: Appendicitis and Other Diseases of the Vermiform Appendix, 1909.

LeConte, R. G.: Carcinoma of the Appendix, With Metastasis to the Ileo-colic Glands, Trans. Amer. Surg. Assoc., 1908, xxvi, p. 445.

Letulle and Weinberg: Bulletin de la Société Anatomique de Paris, 1897, lxii, p. 747 and p. 814.

Lubarsch, Otto: Ueber den Primären Krebs des Ileum Nebst Bemerkungen Über das Gleichzeitige Vorkommen von Krebs und Tuberculose, Virchow's Archiv, 1888, Bd. cxi, s. 281.

Mallory, F. B.: The Principles of Pathologic Histology, 1914, p. 487.

Mayo, W. J.: The Prophylaxis of Cancer, Trans. Am. Surg. Assoc., 1914, xxxii, p. 1.

Milner, R.: Die Entzündlichen Pseudo-Karzinome des Wurmfortsatzes, Deutsche medicinische Wochenschrift, No. 25, 1910, xxxvi, p. 1191.

Moschcowitz, A. V.: Primary Carcinoma of the Appendix, ANNALS OF SURGERY, 1903, xxxvii, p. 891.

MacCarty, W. C., and McGrath, B. F.: The Frequency of Carcinoma of the Appendix, ANNALS OF SURGERY, 1914, lix, p. 675.

McWilliams, C. A.: Primary Carcinoma of the Vermiform Appendix, Amer. Jour. Med. Sciences, 1908, xxxv, p. 822.

Neugebauer, F.: Ueber Gutartige Geschwülste, Carcinome und Sogenannte Carcinome des Wurmfortsatzes, Beiträge zur klinischen Chirurgie, 1910, Bd. 67, s. 328.

Oberndorfer: Discussion of Winkler's paper, vide infra.

Reiman, S. P.: Primary Carcinoma of the Vermiform Appendix, Amer. Jour. of Med. Sciences, 1918, clvi, p. 190.

Ross, G. G.: Carcinoma of the Appendix, ANNALS OF SURGERY, 1911, liv, p. 277.

Winkler: Krebs des Wurmfortsatzes, Centralblatt für allgemeine Pathologie und pathologische Anatomie, 1910, Bd. xxi, s. 167.

Zaaijer, J. H.: Primäres Carcinom des Wurmfortsatzes, Beiträge zur Klinische Chirurgie, 1907, Bd. 54, s. 239.

RADICAL OPERATION IN CASES OF ADVANCED CANCER

By John W. Churchman
of New York, N. Y.

No problem which the surgeon has to face presents greater difficulties than the decision, in a given case, as to the operability of a malignant growth. In the very early cases the duty to intervene is clear enough; and in the very late cases attendant circumstances, like metastasis at a distance, may, in equally definite fashion, indicate the wisdom of conservatism. Many cases, however, lie between these two extremes; the growth is large, or neighboring lymphatic involvement is extensive, or there are adhesions to adjacent organs; shall one take the infinitely small chance which radical removal offers, or allow Nature to take her course?

The answer to this question, which is in part determined by the temperament of the surgeon concerned—whether conservative or bold—indicates that surgeons are divided into two camps on this point. Many men, and among them are those whose experience is limited and whose nerve is more noteworthy than their judgment, will attempt to remove any growth, and not infrequently delude themselves with the notion that an operation of the most incomplete sort has been a "radical resection." Fearful of the disrepute into which this sort of thing brings surgery, other surgeons refuse to operate at all unless there is good chance of expecting a cure. Some men have even been known to go so far as to refuse the relief of a gastrostomy to a patient suffering from cardiac cancer, because the reputation for failure which surgery may get when operation is undertaken and cure does not result, prejudices the public mind and prevents patients from presenting themselves at a time when cure might be effected.

There can be no question that as one's experience in the surgery of cancer increases one tends to draw away from the extremely radical, and approach the conservative camp. Repeated disappointment—in cases in which, hoping somewhat against hope, an extremely extensive removal has been done only to be followed by fairly prompt recurrence—is sure in time to dim one's ardor as to the value of surgery in any, save the early cases of cancer.

It is extremely easy to get into this state of mind, particularly in a hospital, where all sorts of cases, even the most desperate, must be handled; for it relieves one of the disagreeable burden of undertaking large operations when the chance of cure is slim. There are three reasons why it is a dangerous point of view.

1. Once this attitude is taken it will be found that the kind of case regarded as hopeless will be more and more frequent. At first only cases *really* hopeless will be refused operation; then cases with a bad prognosis;

698

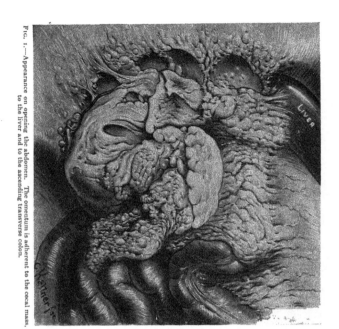

FIG. 1.—Appearance on opening the abdomen. The omentum is adherent to the cæcal mass, to the liver and to the ascending transverse colon.

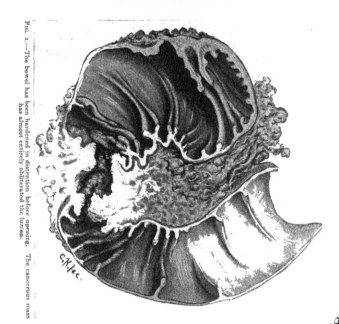

FIG. 2.—The bowel has been hardened in distention before opening. The cancerous mass has almost entirely obliterated the lumen.

869

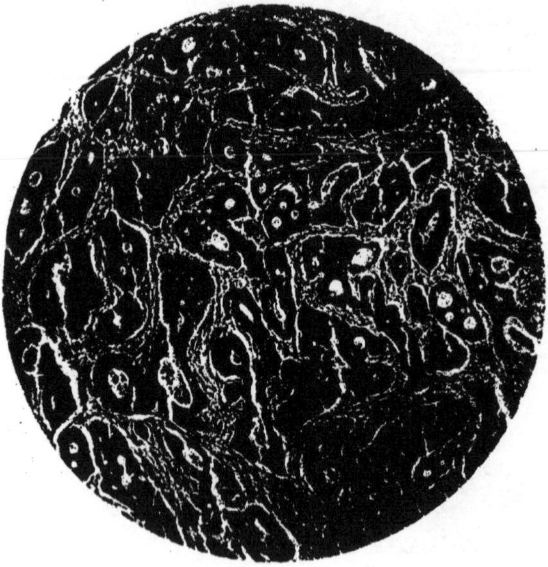

FIG. 3.—Microphotograph of tumor.

and finally even exploration will be avoided unless there is every indication that a curative operation can certainly be done.

2. Surgeons are under obligation to relieve as well as to cure; yet there is danger, if exploration in possibly inoperable cases is refused, of missing a chance to give relief. " *Guèrir quelquefois, soulager souvent, consoler toujours* " is a good rule for surgery as well as for medicine.

3. There is no way to determine accurately the prognosis in a given case. All the criteria of relative malignancy we have, though some of them are of value, are of a rough kind. Occasional cases do well even when the pathological picture, both gross and microscopic, is unfavorable. It is this occasional case which obligates the surgeon to offer operative relief wherever removal, that can in any sense be regarded as complete, is possible.

I wish to report a case which belongs in the group of " clinically inoperable cancer," but in which an extremely satisfactory result has followed radical operation. The patient was referred to me by Dr. C. P. Lindsley, of New Haven, Conn. He was a man sixty years of age who for several months had been suffering from attacks of partial intestinal obstruction. The pain, nausea, and obstinate constipation had in each instance been finally relieved by catharsis and enemas; but with each subsequent attack the difficulty of relief was becoming greater. Meanwhile the appetite was becoming poor and the patient was rapidly losing weight. When I first saw him, the clinical picture was typical of nearly complete obstruction of the large bowel, and the presence of a large mass in the right side of the abdomen at about the level of the umbilicus made only too clear what the nature of the obstruction was. At this time the patient was about sixty pounds under weight.

The obstruction, of course, demanded immediate relief, but it was feared, on account of the fixity of the tumor, and its size, that an enterostomy, or at best a short-circuiting operation, would have to be done. On opening the abdomen, the condition found seemed to justify this fear (Fig. 1). The abdomen was full of serous fluid, the omentum glued to the transverse colon, liver, cæcum, and intestinal coils, the cæcum fixed to the lateral and posterior abdominal walls. The small bowel was moderately distended, the transverse colon collapsed. A carcinomatous mass was felt on the posterior wall of the cæcum, near the ileocæcal valve, and many enlarged glands were palpable in the neighborhood. The adhesions of cæcum and omentum proved not very firm, and without much difficulty or hemorrhage the entire mass could be freed by slowly sweeping the hand about it. A resection was determined upon as the most satisfactory palliative measure; the hope of a cure was hardly entertained. A lateral anastomosis was done.

For the operation an incision across the rectus was used. This, in my opinion, is the incision of choice in all extensive abdominal operations. It provides abundant room, without dragging at re-

JOHN W. CHURCHMAN

tractors, and not only makes the procedure easier, shorter, and safer, but makes possible a really intelligent opinion as to the possibilities of the case by giving room to see and feel. If the rectus fascia is neatly divided and is overlapped in the closure, the abdominal wall is stronger after the operation than before.

The post-operative course was without event. The drainage tract closed promptly and the patient was at home, with the wound entirely healed, in four weeks.

The lumen of the bowel had been nearly obliterated by the growth (Fig. 2) which microscopic section showed to be an adenocarcinoma (Fig. 3).

The operation was done in December, 1917. The patient gained sixty pounds in the first year and is at the present time to all appearances well. There is no sign of recurrence. That recurrence will ultimately appear seems more than likely, but the several years of good health and complete comfort which the patient will have enjoyed justifies the wisdom of the decision to resect.

It seems quite probable that if the obstruction in this case had not presented an emergency demanding relief the appearance on opening the abdomen would have justified the belief that the case was hopeless and nothing would have been done. Occasional successes of this sort should act as a stimulus to do all that can be done for patients with extensive cancer, though one must, of course, be prepared for failure in a large proportion of cases.

RADIUM IN THE TREATMENT OF CARCINOMA OF THE CERVIX UTERI

A DISCUSSION OF THE PROBLEMS CONNECTED WITH THE OPERATIVE AND RADIUM TREATMENT

BY EDWARD H. RISLEY, M.D.

OF BOSTON, MASS.

IT is desired to present a paper on the treatment of carcinoma of the cervix which shall be more in the nature of a discussion of several important factors relative to operability, selection of cases for operation, precancerous conditions, results to be expected from operation, other purely palliative methods and the present status of radium—than a presentation of cases and reporting of end-results.

This is a subject in which the author has been much interested for the past six years and to which much thought and time have been devoted. A discussion of this kind seems particularly in point at the present time, because the subject is one about which our ideas just now are undergoing considerable revolution.

We stand more or less at a parting of the ways in regard to the treatment—no longer of the inoperable cases—but now of those that are unquestionably recognized to be operable. The advocates of the extended or Wertheim operation are beginning to weaken in their belief that this is the procedure *sine qua non* for operable carcinoma of the cervix, in the face of the accumulative evidence from many clinics the world over, that operation is not the only means of actually curing cancer in this region.

Such a profound change is apparently taking place at the present time in the minds of many of the foremost surgeons of the world in regard to the treatment of this disease that it behooves us to try to get at the facts as they really are and to carefully weigh the evidence at hand.

For the sake of later discussion we shall endeavor to present:

1. The essential facts in regard to surgery and the operative end-results, and

2. As nearly a correct statement as we can in regard to what is to be expected from radium alone.

In this paper statistics in regard to our own end-results are purposely avoided for the following reasons:

1. We have been using the technic outlined below in the treatment of the borderline case only about three and one-half years, and as we use the five-year period as a standard for estimating probable clinical cures our series is yet too young to be reported as end-results.

2. Our technic in the application of radium is now entirely different from our former method, the new method only being in use since July; 1919; therefore, end-results in these cases are not yet available.

On the other hand, putting statistics aside, we are strongly of the feeling that certain impressions gained from the examination and careful following up and experience with several hundreds of cases each year gives a sound basis of knowledge, which, in many instances, is of as great value in forming a final judgment about cases as are masses of figures. These will be referred to more in detail later.

Success in the treatment of carcinoma of the cervix depends, of course, as in carcinoma elsewhere, on the earliest possible diagnosis. And in this connection it would seem wise to call attention to a phase of this subject which has received scant attention in the past, which we now more and more realize is of greatest importance. I refer to the early recognition and diagnosis of the so-called pre-cancerous conditions, which must be recognized both by the general practitioner and the surgeon if our end-results are to be improved and our cases brought to earlier operation and our percentage of cures increased. We have the impression that to the average practitioner the term " pre-cancerous " is not entirely clearly defined. The following enumeration indicates the type of lesion under this heading which should be looked upon invariably with suspicion, whether they occur in the young woman of child-bearing age or in those of a more likely cancerous period.

Further and further acquaintance with malignancy of all types impresses one with the great frequency with which it occurs, not alone in those of middle life, but also in the young, in whom it is practically always of a more virulent nature than in older subjects. Malignancy as known to-day should no longer be considered a disease of old age.

The following are the commonest pre-cancerous conditions in the cervix: Lacerations of the cervix. Erosions of the cervix. Ulceration of the cervix. Cystic disease of the cervix. Polyps of the cervix. Any hypertrophy of the cervix.

All of these in any stage of development may be the forerunner of malignant degeneration and should be looked upon with suspicion.

Of course, it is to be understood that this does not apply to the recent laceration or eversion-erosion after labor, but only to those which do not tend to heal readily and which become more or less chronic in character, as evidenced by more or less discharge, œdema, sluggish ulceration, and failure to heal under appropriate treatment.

So important is it to rule out these conditions as possible precursors of malignancy, that it is believed that every such case that comes for operative relief—and many others—should be subjected to removal of a specimen for microscopical diagnosis. Only by going to this seeming extreme can we hope to get our cases early enough for a probable cure by the extended operation. It would seem wise to urge that it be made a routine practice in all hospital clinics to submit for microscopical study a specimen from every case operated on for laceration, ulceration, erosion, hypertrophy, or polyp of the cervix. In this way many cases of malignancy will undoubtedly be discovered, an early radical operation done, and a surgical cure made, while other clinically suspicious cases will be proved benign and saved from the dangers of the major operative procedure.

Cures in carcinoma of the cervix depend, first, on the earliest possible diagnosis and earliest possible resort to operation, and secondly, on the careful selection of cases, with the avoidance of possible borderline cases (defined later), and thirdly, on the type of operation used. It is now recognized that no half-hearted or palliative surgery is justifiable in the early operable case. Vaginal, supravaginal hysterectomy, amputation or cauterization of the cervix alone are never radical enough proceedings in the operable case and should be reserved solely for palliation in the distinctly inoperable case.

It is contended by some that anything short of an extensive procedure like the Wertheim operation is almost criminal negligence and should neither be contemplated nor practiced, while other surgeons feel that, because of the diffuse extent of lymphatic involvement in the deep pelvis and the probable impossibility of getting rid of all involved lymphatics even with the most extensive dissection, the cases cured by the Wertheim operation are probably only those cases that would have been cured anyway by a less extensive procedure, such as the ordinary total hysterectomy which extirpates the cervix and body of the uterus and a certain amount of parametrium. In view of the success which often follows cautery or radium alone, this latter expression of opinion probably has a sound basis of fact.

In a discussion of this kind it is necessary to have in mind the essential facts in regard to the Wertheim or extended operation, the kind of case suitable for this operation and the end-results to be expected from this and from other procedures.

Our results are largely dependent on the types of case with which we have to deal, and it is, therefore, believed that greater precision in the description of the type of case dealt with should be used in order that we may get clearer ideas of result to be expected.

One must recognize definite groups, namely, (1) early and definitely localized growths involving the cervix only (the definitely operable cases); (2) cases of borderline operability (defined later); (3) cases of extensive involvement of the cervix, but operable because confined entirely to this organ, and (4) definitely and unquestionably inoperable cases.

The question of operability is one of the greatest importance and one also which we are reluctant to say we fear depends to a too great extent on the personal equation, ability and experience of the surgeon consulted. Perhaps this is necessarily so, because no one man has at hand statistics enough of physical and operative findings and end-results by which to be accurately guided in his decision.

A review of the cases seen at such a clinic as the Huntington Memorial Hospital in Boston, while it does not furnish large masses of figures, yet gives an impression of cases which we feel is of distinct value in forming an estimate of operability, prognosis, value of certain lines of treatment, etc.

Many cases are sent to us for diagnosis and advice as to the best form of treatment, while others are those of recurrence after various operative procedures. From these two groups of cases, especially, a very definite idea of operability has been formed, and is further confirmed by an analysis of the results of large series of cases presented by such men as Wertheim, Kelly, Clark, Jacobson, Janeway and many other men of less extensive experience.

We would, therefore, define the different degrees of operability and follow this by a discussion of the forms of treatment which seem most productive of good results in cases not suited for the extended operation.

It is true that the further the lay public and the physician are educated into making early diagnosis and the percentage of operability increases in this way, it is also found to be true that the more the surgeon analyzes his cases and his own and other end-results there will be found an increasing number of cases that are not suited for operation by the extended method, but which must be treated by methods which, while only palliative, are as they are perfected giving increasingly good results.

We would define the operable case as that in which there was no contra-indication in the general condition of the patient, in which the disease is diagnosed early, in its incipiency, is definitely localized in the cervix without encroachment on the vaginal wall, and in which there is no induration in the broad ligaments or fixation or enlargement of the uterus and no evidence of metastases or extension to iliac or inguinal glands, liver or elsewhere. And we would define the borderline case as one in which the disease was not sharply localized on the cervix, in which there was some encroachment of the disease into the vaginal wall or in which any amount of fixation was present as evidenced by a slight amount of thickening in the broad ligament; especially as detected by rectal examination, which always gives a much more definite estimate of the amount of pericervical involvement than can be obtained by vaginal examination.

This is the type of case in which it is believed the greatest number of errors of judgment are made in advising operation rather than more conservative methods.

The borderline case is rarely the operative case, and this statement is based upon the large number of cases seen at our clinic in which rapid recurrence has followed attempts at removal in this class of case.

The cases in which pericervical thickening and fixation are due to chronic inflammation of the appendages and not to carcinomatous infiltration are very rare, and the fact of the existence of the above two signs or of vaginal wall encroachment or induration of the broad ligaments, practically always means that the surgeon, in trying to effect a wide excision of the diseased area, of necessity is forced to cut through tissue already invaded or so lowered in resistance from its close proximity to an area from which it absorbs toxic material that rapid recurrence or extension of the disease follows operation. Even the widest dissection in this type of case but rarely gives a cure.

Recurrence here is met with in the stump of the broad ligament more frequently than elsewhere, and in this situation is less accessible for treatment than almost anywhere else.

Thus, from observation of the frequency and situation of recurrences after attempts at the extended operation in the borderline case, we hesitate to recommend for the radical procedure even patients who are otherwise in good condition, but whose disease places them in this category, knowing, almost to a certainty, that because they fall into this group they will have early recurrence.

This would seem a pessimistic view for the surgeon to take, but it is based on observation of a considerable number of cases seen in a clinic where all varieties of cases are carefully studied and where many end-results are seen. It is believed that the importance of avoiding the radical operation in the borderline case cannot be too strongly emphasized. The more cases one sees in which attempts at extirpation in this class of case are promptly followed by rapid recurrence, the stronger is the belief that operation should be carefully avoided in this particular group.

There is another group of cases about which we have so far been unable to form a definite decision as to their chances of recurrence after panhysterectomy, but which we are inclined to believe are more operable than the borderline case. It is that group in which there is rather extensive involvement of the cervix or destruction of tissue at the cervix, but which shows no tendency to extend or to encroach on surrounding tissues. This is more liable to be the adeno than the squamous cell type.

Therefore, it is believed that the cases selected for the radical operation should be restricted to those rather few cases in which the surgeon is practically certain that he can get all around the disease with a wide margin, and in which there is absence of induration of the broad ligaments or fixation.

All cases in which the surgeon is in doubt as to his ability completely to extirpate the disease with a wide margin should be operated not by the radical method, carrying its high primary mortality, but should be reserved for the simpler procedures outlined below. With the publication in 1898 of the Wertheim operation and its adoption by the leading gynæcological clinics of the world, it was thought that a step forward had been taken in the war against uterine cancer, but now after two decades we find this operation still on trial.

The reasons for this are: (1) The very low percentage of operability by this method. In ten years Clark operated on 60 patients and found during that same period over 300 who were inoperable. An operability of only 15 per cent. In Jacobson's collection of 5027 cases only 1720, or a little

r 31 per cent., were considered operable. (2) The high primary mor-
ty. In Jacobson's large series primary mortality was 18.25 per cent.,
I in other European and American series it is found to range from 11
28 per cent. These results are the reports from the largest gynæco-
ical clinics and represent the efforts of the most skilled surgeons, which
ws how unsatisfactory they really are.

Janeway grouped and classified all the reliable, available statistics
I finds that cases with early diagnosis and early operation in the hands
skilled men should present only about a 15 to 30 per cent. operability,
to 18 per cent. immediate mortality, and 11 to 19 per cent. cures (five-
ar period) of those surviving operation.

Even this percentage of cures carries with it a 7 to 40 per cent. evi-
ice of incurable vesico-vaginal fistulæ, incontinence, necrosis of the
dder, injury to the rectum, and other distressing and disabling sequelæ
n in the hands of the most experienced men.

These results are evidently far from ideal. I might here quote Clark,
o says: "If an operation or other therapeutic procedure is to have a
manent place in our armamentarium it must be sufficiently easy to
ke it available, not for a few skilled specialists, but for the great body
urgeons working in every quarter of this and other countries. In these days
low mortality percentages attending nearly all of the major operations, no
ration can possibly gain headway which combines with it a shockingly high
mary mortality and a large number of distressing sequelæ."

However, so far, in the absence of a known, proved method which
i give better end-results, the Wertheim operation is still the method of
ice with the majority of American surgeons, but probably not any
ger with the greatest of the continental gynæcologists. As far back as
4 Dobbert concluded, after an experience with 24 cases, 18 inoperable
I 6 operable, that it was justifiable to use radium in the treatment of
operable case. Cheron used radium in an inoperable case and two
rs later, the patient dying of an intercurrent disease, autopsy showed
trace of cancer. In 1915 Döderlein advocated the use of radium in in-
erable cases and Pozzi that same year gave up the Wertheim operation
borderline cases and treated them with radium alone.

A careful consideration of the results to be expected from the Percy
d cautery method would lead one to believe that this procedure, fol-
ved, as it is, by a high percentage of recto- and vesico-vaginal fistulæ,
vic peritonitides and other operative and post-operative accidents, and
ures to cure, should be definitely ruled out in the treatment of the
erable case.

Such are the facts regarding the present status of the treatment of the
erative case—and the trend of thought in regard to radium.

Now let us turn to the treatment of the borderline case.

For this type of case when there is either some encroachment on the
ginal wall or more or less induration in one or other broad ligament,

the hope of complete extirpation, even with the widest dissection, is small.

It, of course, may be contended that induration of the broad ligament does not necessarily mean extension of the actual disease to this region, but may be the result simply of the œdema surrounding any well-developed malignant process. Nevertheless, there is no way of ascertaining beforehand—nor always even at operation—whether this induration is due to œdema only, and a careful study of the location of recurrence and knowledge of the areas where disease is most commonly cut through in trying to do a radical dissection, makes it certain that in the majority of cases broad ligament induration, with its accompanying fixation of the lower segments of the uterus—no matter how slight it may be—means inoperablity.

Also from the point of view of the actual pathology of such cases the presence of œdema means dilated and hence easily traversed lymph channels, by which cancer infection probably will later spread if it has not already done so.

Therefore, for the borderline case two methods of procedure are open. (1) Cautery plus radium, if there is enough protruding disease at the cervix to warrant the preliminary use of the cautery to get rid of mass, or (2) radium alone.

The technic which we have employed when the cautery is used is as follows and applies also to the extensive inoperable case as well as to the borderline case.

Using the water-cooled speculum and the electric cautery, a thorough cauterization is done with the actual cautery of all accessible diseased tissue; a cauterization which shall burn away and destroy all nodular or protruding growth and which shall convert the diseased cervix into a definite cavity from which all macroscopic disease has been removed. It is customary to slowly cook the diseased area until all accessible tissue can be easily removed by gentle curettage, to reapply the cautery still further, follow this by further curettage, and so on, repeating each step over and over until all disease is removed as far as can be discovered. To do this thoroughly requires much time and patience. If done in this way there is very little danger of dissemination of the disease by the curette, and a smooth-walled cavity, lined with an eschar, surrounded by presumably healthy tissue, is left into which radium is immediately placed in doses of from 75 to 200 cm. and left in for twelve hours to sixteen hours.

Post-operative Treatment.—This should be followed by further radium treatment given at intervals of about three or four weeks until all signs of disease have disappeared. And after this the patient should report for observation every month for at least six months and then every three to six months for at least three years.

There is no objection to repeated cauterization of a rapidly growing localized disease, and good results and much prolongation of life with alleviation of suffering have resulted from this procedure. Cauterization has also been successfully applied to local recurrences in the vault after panhysterectomy previous to giving of radium, with reduction in the size of the area to be treated, and with much local improvement, and apparent shortening of the radium treatment.

This is a procedure which we have found of greatest service in the inoperable cases, in many of which the disease has all but been destroyed —and certainly so delayed in its progress that patients with pain, hemorrhage, and foul discharge have been given complete relief for many months at a time, and a miserable, hopeless existence converted into a comfortable and happy one. With proper handling and enough attention to detail the inoperable case is one for whom much that is worth while can be done.

These are not the words of the enthusiast, but the gratifying experience resulting from the treatment of large groups of inoperable and seemingly hopeless cases.

The rationale of the combined cautery-radium treatment in the borderline case is based on four factors. (1) Failure of the extended operation to cure in a reasonable percentage of cases—and rapid recurrence in this type of case. (2) The high primary mortality and definite disability incidence in the operated case as against the total absence of immediate mortality and distressing sequence with our method. (3) The considerable percentage of cures or freedom from disease for long periods resulting from cauterization alone. (4) Recent improvement in results with radium alone.

At the present time, because of the relatively poor results from operation, even in the hands of the most skilled, the question of radium treatment and what can assuredly be expected from it is of greatest importance to determine.

In this connection the author believes that a conservative statement taken from the point of view of the clinical surgeon and not from that of the radium specialist will be of value.

For the past six years we have been especially interested in carcinoma of the cervix and also in its treatment in the inoperable and recurrent form by radium. We have had under our direct supervision all of the cervix cases at the Huntington Memorial Hospital during this time, where large numbers of cases are seen each year. We have undertaken this work with no preconceived faith in radium, but have been trying to find out for ourselves—unprejudiced by outside (generally enthusiastic) reports—just what radium can or cannot do.

We have struggled along for several years utterly discouraged with end-results. Temporary results and palliation were often encouraging, but end-results were apparently hopeless.

Not until within a year, when an entirely different technic of application has been adopted, have results begun to be at all promising. The old method used to be that of placing radium—in altogether inadequate doses—in variously modelled applicators *against* the outside of the cervical disease. Small areas were destroyed and symptoms largely relieved, but the great mass of the disease remained intact.

But now all cases are treated by direct insertion of three times the former dose, in unscreened steel-jacketed needles, directly into the cervical canal or other mass of disease. In this way large masses of disease are destroyed at one sitting, treatments can be given at greater intervals, and a marked change has been noted.

All of our cases treated by the new method are under a year, and we therefore refrain from making any report of results, no matter how promising some of the immediate effects seem to be. It seems evident, however, that failures in the past have possibly been due to faults in the technic of applying radium. Coincident with our own work the results obtained by Janeway, Ransohoff and others would indicate that increasingly encouraging effects were being secured by greater attention to the details of radium application.

That radium has a definite place in the treatment of the inoperable and border-line cases, I think there is now undisputed evidence.

Our feeling about early discovered and well-localized carcinoma of the cervix in the patient who is a good surgical risk is that it should always be treated by the most thorough operative removal consistent with the safety of the patient, and we would not like to be misunderstood, from any remarks on other forms of treatment, as advocating any other less radical method in the unquestionably operable case. It is only in the borderline or inoperable case that we would urge against attempts at radical surgery—and for the intelligent use of now well-tried out and proved conservative methods.

This statement does not agree with the conclusions reached by Janeway or Ransohoff—the latter of whom comes out with the flat-footed statement that he no longer hesitates to state it as his opinion that radium treatment should entirely supplant operation, not only in the treatment of inoperable cases, but also in the treatment of the operable cases as well. This, I believe, is rapidly becoming the conviction of many more surgeons each year, as operative results show little or no improvement, but radium workers are more and more positively able to demonstrate what radium can do when properly handled.

It is believed that we are in a transition stage and that within two or three years the matter of the exact place of radium and operation in the operable cases will be definitely settled. Meanwhile, because of the proved value of radium in the inoperable and borderline cases and in the locally operable cases which have some definite general contra-indication to operation, it is hoped that more and more of this latter type of case may be sent for radium treatment and in this way convincing statistics accumulated which will soon settle the question once for all.

The treatment of the borderline case, we believe, is now a settled one. It is with radium, or with cautery and radium, according to the character of the growth, and not by operation, for which this type of case has been proven to be unsuited.

It is now also pretty definitely settled that these cases are not made operable by preliminary radium treatment. Every surgeon who has attempted to do a panhysterectomy after preliminary radium treatment knows the great difficulty encountered from persistent oozing due to increased blood supply, and difficult dissection due to increase in fibrous tissue obliterating lines of cleavage at the very sites where the most delicate dissection is necessary in order to avoid important structures and the cutting into presumably diseased areas.

It is probably true that the borderline case that does well under radium treatment better continue to be treated with radium rather than to run the very definite risk in operation of stirring up semi-latent foci of disease and possibly causing rapid dissemination of the disease instead of obtaining an operative cure.

The treatment of the definitely inoperable case is also now standardized. It should be with cautery and radium if the mass is large or protruding, or with radium alone when the cautery is not indicated.

The recurrent case is best treated with radium should the recurrence be confined to the vaginal walls or vault, and by the combined use of radium to the vault and deep cross-fire X-ray in multiple areas to the sacral region and deep pelvis should there be involvement of the pelvis.

With greater efforts in the way of educational campaigns among the laity, with earlier diagnosis from more frequent removal of specimens for pathological diagnoses of suspicious pre-cancerous conditions, with earlier operation in the small percentage of operable cases, with improved methods of technic in the application of radium in the borderline and inoperable cases, with the combined use of X-ray and radium in the extensive cases and with a more perfect system of following up all cases in all classes, we believe that the percentage of actual cures in carcinoma of the cervix is going to be materially increased in the next few years.

It is evident from a review of recent literature that the trend of thought in regard to the treatment of operable carcinoma of the cervix is less and less sanguine as regards the extended operation, but more and more towards the use of radium.

Convincing statistics are rapidly accumulating which emphasize, on the one hand, the failure of operation to cure in a large enough percentage of cases to warrant placing it as the only means of curing the operable case, and, on the other hand, the increasingly good results to be obtained from and expected of radium when given by a proper technic and in sufficiently large doses.

We are unwilling at the present time to state definitely that we believe that radium will eventually supplant operation in the treatment of all operable cases, but, on the other hand, we cannot deny the convincing evidence of the real advances made in radium technic and the highly satisfactory results obtained with radium alone.

It seems probable that with greater familiarity with the disease, with a more careful selection of cases—avoiding the acceptance for operation of any cases of the borderline type—that operation will soon be confined to a very small per cent. of distinctly operable cases, and that the remainder will be treated with increasingly greater success with radium alone.

Certainly radium has very definitely established its place firmly in our armamentarium as an agent which in the inoperable case can accomplish such a praiseworthy and definite diminution and often almost complete cessation of distressing symptoms that it must be looked upon as one of the greatest therapeutic advances of the age, especially when applied to carcinoma of the cervix.

BONE TUMORS. MYXOMA, CENTRAL AND PERIOSTEAL

THEIR RECURRENCE AFTER EXPLORATORY EXCISION AND PIECEMEAL REMOVAL

By Joseph Colt Bloodgood, M.D.

OF BALTIMORE, MD.

IN 1906 I observed a recurrence in the soft-part scar left by the removal one year previously of a small periosteal myxoma of the humerus. At the original operation the tumor was explored and removed piecemeal. This patient died in 1915, ten years after the operation, with metastasis to the chest and scalp. During these ten years there had been numerous operations for local recurrence in the soft parts and in the bone, until finally in 1912, seven years after the first operation, amputation was done at the shoulder-joint.

In this case both the original and all of the recurrent tumors retained the microscopic picture of a myxoma.

This was a very impressive experience, that a tumor considered histologically benign could recur by what appeared to be definite transplantation of tumor tissue at the operation, and finally lead to death from metastasis. (Case I, Figs. 1 and 2.)

Not until 1919, fourteen years later, did another similar case come under my observation, which so impressively indicated the danger of recurrence in myxoma when the tumor is explored and removed piecemeal. In this instance the original tumor was central in the astragalus. In March, 1918, the astragalus was removed piecemeal. One year later I saw the patient with recurrence of the tumor in the scar and amputated the leg above the ankle. Six months later he returned with a tumor of the same character involving the tubercle of the tibia of the stump. Then the thigh was amputated; at the present time (October, 1920) the patient is apparently well. Case II.

Between 1906 and 1919 I had this myxoma of bone constantly in mind, and in reading some old textbooks on surgery written from 1840 to 1880, I found quite frequently the statement by the older surgeons who had large experience with tumors: " The myxoma of bone is a benign tumor, but it usually recurs." In more recent textbooks and literature this pretty definite knowledge has been lost, and none of the recent authors seem familiar with this characteristic feature of the myxoma of bone.

In the ANNALS OF SURGERY for April, 1919 (page 357), in a contribution on Central Giant-cell Tumors, I discussed briefly Recurrence After Operation for Benign Connective-tissue Tumors, *and emphasized the danger of enucleating, or peeling out, or removing piecemeal, such tumors as the mixed tumor of the parotid, the intracanalicular myxoma of the breast, the fibromyxoma of nerve-sheaths, the epulis of the lower jaw, and especially the central and periosteal myxoma of bone.*

712

When the tumor must be removed by this method, chiefly indicated in the central giant-cell tumor of bone and in the epulis, one should thoroughly cauterize the wound with pure carbolic followed by alcohol, or with a piece of gauze saturated in 50 per cent. solution of zinc chloride, or, when possible, employ the electric cautery for the removal of the tumor. Of all the neoplasms mentioned, recurrence seems most dangerous in the pure myxoma of bone, as it usually leads to amputation because of the recurrence and in some instances to death from metastasis.

Since the experience with Case II in 1919, I have gone over all of our records in the Surgical Pathological Laboratory of the Johns Hopkins Hospital and find that in every case of periosteal and central myxoma in which the original tumor has been explored and removed piecemeal, there has been recurrence, while in every case resected or amputated without such exploratory incision the patients have remained well, both from recurrence and metastasis.

I do not include in this group myxosarcoma.

I have as yet no experience of what will happen when we explore myxomas and, after making the diagnosis, locally remove the tumor with the precaution noted. In Case II, when I explored the upper end of the tibia and exposed a myxomatous area destroying the tubercle, I explored with the cautery, packed the wound with a piece of gauze saturated with zinc chloride, and three days later amputated above the knee-joint. I did this, because I feared there might be other areas of myxoma in the stump of the first amputation, and amputation above the knee-joint would give almost as good function with the artificial limb the patient already had.

Myxomas of bone are rare tumors. They occur both as periosteal and central tumors. In the beginning they may be small and can be removed without sacrificing the limb by amputation. In some cases resection and bone transplantation will be indicated. But as in the cases about to be reported, I do not see how a diagnosis can be made without an exploratory incision. Therefore, it is of the utmost importance to have in mind a technic which will allow the conservative operation without this danger of recurrence by transplantation of tumor tissue into the uninvolved wound of exploration.

I have not been able to get evidence that either X-rays or radium will destroy a myxomatous tumor of bone. Perhaps in these cases it might be worth while to try radium and the X-rays before operation under X-ray control.

The myxomas occur as periosteal and central growths unmixed with any other tissue, they may frequently be found combined with chondroma, rarely with exostosis. I will report here (Case III) a tumor that had the X-ray picture of a benign exostosis; it was removed piecemeal; there was recurrence and death. When I studied the tissues removed from this case, I found areas of myxoma. Up to the present this is the only exostosis, among 110 cases, with areas of myxoma, and the only one in which the recurrence led to death.

Although the problem is yet unsettled, it seems important to publish these three very instructive observations, in order to call attention for the first time in recent literature, in a separate article, to this very serious result when central or periosteal myxomas are explored and removed piecemeal.

One gets the impression, at least from these three cases, that the patients might have lived longer and in greater comfort if they had been left alone; or if amputation had been done without exploratory incision, but there was nothing in the X-ray picture to justify such an amputation.

For this reason, when a bone tumor is explored, one should always have in mind the possibility of myxomatous tissue, whether central or periosteal, and especially so in all cartilage tumors.

The differential diagnosis between young, soft cartilage tissue and myxoma, can only be made by an immediate frozen section. To make this diagnosis one must be familiar with the histology of pure myxoma and young cartilage.

The pure chondromas are a separate group and must be discussed in a second article.

The danger of recurrence, when a pure chondroma is explored and removed piecemeal, is distinctly less than in the myxoma, but my recent studies have demonstrated that recurrence due to transplantation of pieces of the cartilage tumor is also possible. One recent experience seems to show that radium may inhibit or even destroy a small cartilage growth.[1]

I have called attention to the danger of recurrence in the pure myxoma in my reviews in *Progressive Medicine* and in the reference already given, and in an article about to be published in the *Journal of Radiology*. But this is the first time that I have made a contribution devoted exclusively to myxoma of bone, and this contribution is made possible by the most careful restudy of the three cases described in detail in this paper, and a short summary of our entire experience with myxomas of bone.

CASE I (Pathol. No. 6773).—Figs. 1 and 2. (Previously reported in *Progressive Medicine*, December, 1906, page 222, Fig. 19.) *Periosteal Myxoma of Shaft of Humerus.*

This patient, a white female, aged fifty-three years, was admitted to Johns Hopkins Hospital in May, 1905, because of local pain and a small tumor in the middle of the shaft of the left humerus. She was quite positive that she had had a tender spot in the region

[1] A second recent case of recurrent chondroma of the knee-joint did not react to radium (October, 1920).

of the present tumor for twenty years, but the little nodule had been felt only nine months; she remembers an injury to this arm, but was not certain whether this occurred before or after she experienced pain. The little lump has not grown rapidly, but since its appearance there has been more pain, and the area has become distinctly tender when struck. The X-ray (Fig. 1) shows a distinct periosteal growth resting on the shaft of the humerus, surrounded and almost encapsulated by a collar of bone. There is no evidence of bone destruction of the shaft beneath the lighter area.

In view of a pretty distinct history of syphilis twenty-six years ago, the condition was diagnosed as lues, and the patient was given mixed treatment for several months. On examination nothing could be made out but a small palpable nodule fixed to the shaft of the bone. It felt smoother than the usual exostosis, and the X-ray demonstrated that the larger part of the growth was not bone. The chief indication for operation was the pain, increasing tenderness and apparently the increase in the size of the growth.

At the exploration it had the appearance of a benign myxoma. The danger of exploring a myxoma at that time was not known. After demonstrating the apparently benign character of the growth, it was separated from the surrounding soft parts and chiseled off from the shaft of the humerus. The exposed shaft showed no evidence of infiltration.

The microscopic study made by me at that time (Fig. 2) showed a pure myxoma.

It is not necessary to describe in detail the history of the frequent recurrences, but the first one, one year later, was in the soft parts, and between the original operation in 1905 and 1910—a period of five years—there were five operations for either recurrence in the soft parts or in the shaft. Finally in 1910, so much bone of the shaft had been removed that fracture took place. Later, when this fracture was plated, there was no evidence of recurrence, and there was an interval of more than one year apparently free from recurrence, and finally in 1912, seven years after the first operation, the recurrence in the remaining shaft and soft parts was so extensive that the arm was amputated at the shoulder-joint. There was then a free interval of about eighteen months, when the patient returned with metastasis to the scalp and mediastinum. Death took place in 1915, ten years after the first operation. There was no autopsy, and no opportunity to study microscopically the scalp and mediastinal tumor.

As mentioned before, all the recurrent tumors, whether in bone or soft parts, retained the picture of a pure myxoma with no sarcomatous areas.

CASE II (Pathol. No. 22929).—*Central Myxoma of Astragalus.*
This patient came under my observation April 5, 1919. The first operation was performed by a colleague in March, 1918, when the astragalus was completely removed piecemeal. The history was somewhat confusing: In the first place, for two years

there had been pain in the wrist, elbow and ankle, a history of tonsillitis and gonorrhœa. His tonsils had been removed and the gonorrhœa treated. Even at this time he had some pain and swelling of the right ankle, but up to January, 1918, the ankle apparently gave the patient no more trouble than the other joints. In March, 1918, he returned again, because the right ankle was giving him more trouble and was more swollen. For this reason an X-ray was taken and was diagnosed by the röntgenologist infectious arthritis. The movements of the foot and the ankle were limited and painful, and the chief pain was referred to the head of the astragalus. The pain and swelling of the other joints had disappeared and not recurred.

The X-ray (Fig. 3) should not have been interpreted as infectious arthritis, as the chief lesion is central. The anterior portion of the astragalus contains a definite light shadow, but there are no changes in any of its joint surfaces. The anterior surface of the astragalus between the tibia and the scaphoid shows partial destruction of the thin outer table and a slight bulging of bone— a picture we frequently see in bone cysts and giant-cell tumors. In my opinion this should have been interpreted as a central lesion of the astragalus of a neoplastic and not inflammatory type, including the bone cyst in the neoplastic group.

Central Tumors of the Astragalus.—Up to the present time I have records of two other central tumors of this bone—one a bone cyst in a male, aged twenty, in which there had been pain after trauma one year ago, and swelling four months; the other, a giant-cell tumor in a colored female aged thirty-three, in which there had been pain and swelling five months. These two patients have remained well after curetting, leaving the bone shell.

In the central myxoma of the astragalus under discussion the operator explored. The subcutaneous tissue over that portion of the astragalus which, in the X-ray, shows changes in the bone shell, was œdematous, and irregular new bone formation was found. It is to be remembered that the operator had in mind an infectious arthritis. In attempting to remove this irregular bone he exposed the cancellous bone of the astragalus and found it largely replaced by a softened myxomatous tissue with, here and there, reddish currant-jelly areas. The entire astragalus was then removed piecemeal, and the tissue sent to the laboratory is shown in Fig. 4. The larger pieces are the inner surfaces of the bone shell attached to which are the remains of cancellous bone, and the smaller pieces are myxomatous tissue containing no bone.

The wound was closed without attempt at chemical or electric cauterization.

Microscopic Diagnosis.—Fig. 5 illustrates a typical myxomatous area. The irregular darker areas are minute particles of bone. There are no cellular suggestions of sarcoma, and no evidence of ostitis fibrosa. This picture is a definite pathological entity and can be recognized by the stellate and lymphoid cells imbedded in an unstaining intercellular substance. Fig. 6 is from one of the

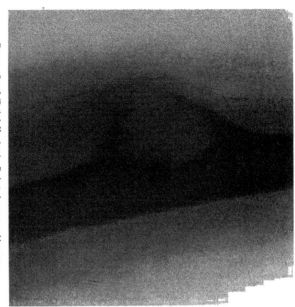

FIG. 1.—Case I (Pathol. No. 6773). Periosteal myxoma of humerus.

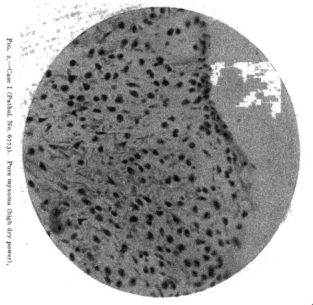

FIG. 2.—Case I (Pathol. No. 6773). Pure myxoma (high dry power).

7 6 ᵃ

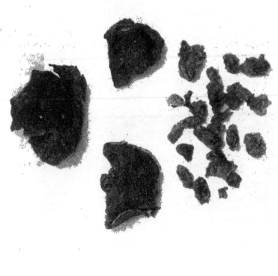

FIG. 4.—Case II (Pathol. No. 2929). Photograph of pieces of astragalus removed at the first operation. The larger pieces are the bone shell, the smaller pieces the myxoma.

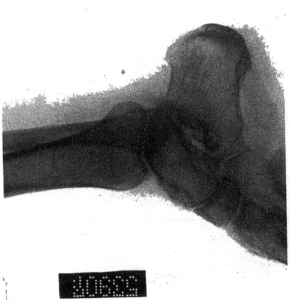

FIG. 3.—Case II (Pathol. No. 2929). Central myxoma of astragalus. X-ray before first operation.

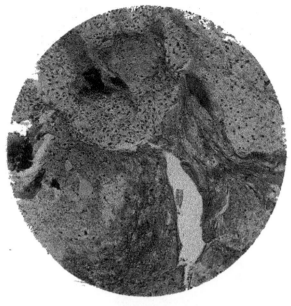

FIG. 5.—Case II (Pathol. No. 27929). Microscopic picture (low power) showing the pure myxoma, a few islands of bone, and the eosin-staining fibrous tissue which separates the myxomatous tissue into smaller and larger islands.

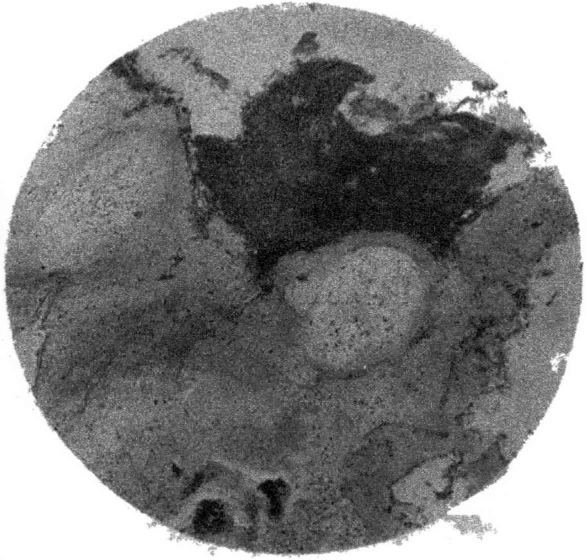

FIG. 6.—Case II (Pathol. No. 27929). Microscopic picture (low power) from another myxomatous area showing a cellular area. For the high power of this see Fig. 7.

716

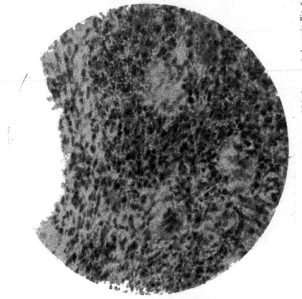

FIG. 7.—Case II (Pathol. No. 29929). Cellular area (high dry power) shown in Fig. 6. This shows giant-cells, cells resembling osteoblasts, and granulation tissue. Areas similar to this were not found in the first and second recurrent tumor.

currant-jelly areas. Here we see the same myxomatous tissue surrounding a cellular area. This cellular area (Fig. 7) contains giant-cells imbedded in stroma not unlike that of the giant-cell tumor. The first pathologist who examined these sections diagnosed the tumor as giant-cell, although he gave a clear description of the myxomatous area.

In January, 1919—about ten months after this operation, the patient returned to the first operator because of recurrence of the swelling and pain in the ankle and inability to walk without crutches. At that time an exploration was made, but no tumor tissue was sent to the laboratory.

Examination (April 5, 1919).—It is now one year since the first operation and about three months since the last incision. The region of the ankle is intensely swollen and œdematous. Below the position of both malleoli one can palpate what appears to be bulging tumor tissue. There is no œdema above the ankle and none of the toe.

The X-rays (Fig. 8), lateral and anteroposterior views, show that the astragalus has been removed and that there is some bone destruction of the articular surface of the tibia, but it does not picture the extent of the soft-part tumor.

Operation (April 10, 1919).—Amputation of lower third of leg without exploratory incision.

I performed this amputation because of my knowledge that the original tumor was a myxoma. I amputated in the lower third, because the X-ray of the shaft of the tibia showed no involvement above its articular surface.

Gross Pathology.—Fig. 9 is the outer surface of the dissected mass in the region of the ankle, and in the lower portion, corresponding to the area below the internal malleolus, I have made a section to picture the fresh appearance of the myxoma. You will note that it corresponds with the description of the first operator—myxomatous tissue with red currant-jelly areas. The tumor is confined by a distinct capsule.

Fig. 10 is a longitudinal section through the tibia and bones of the ankle. The myxomatous tumor with its current-jelly areas is seen to occupy the space of the astragalus and to extend in all directions around the lower end of the tibia. One will also observe that the articular surface of the tibia is partially destroyed and tumor tissue is invading the cancellous bone. Invasion of the os calcis and scaphoid is distinctly less.

The *microscopic appearance of this tumor tissue* is identical with that shown in Figs. 5, 6 and 7. The tumor had, therefore, not changed into a sarcoma.

Currant-Jelly Areas.—From my experience these small currant-jelly areas which usually contain giant-cells imbedded in very cellular stroma are not diagnostic. I have observed them in ostitis fibrosa, in the giant-cell tumor, in myxoma, and in chondroma. Their true significance is still unsettled.

Results.—Before this patient left the hospital X-rays were taken of the stump to ascertain again whether we had overlooked any possible involvement in the remaining shaft of the tibia or fibula. Careful inspection was negative. It is not out of place here to state that before my amputation X-rays were made of the chest and other bones also with negative findings. The urine contained no Bence-Jones bodies, and the blood was negative for Wassermann. There was no evidence of the patient's old polyarthritis.

In October, 1919, the patient returned because of pain and tenderness in the beak-shaped process of the tibia which he attributed to the pressure of the artificial limb. It is now six months since the amputation. An X-ray (Fig. 11) now shows an area of bone destruction in the tubercle of the tibia.

On October 14, 1919, I explored this area with the cautery, demonstrated the myxomatous tumor, removed it with the cautery with a good margin of cancellous bone and soft parts and packed the wound with a piece of gauze saturated with zinc chloride solution. Frozen sections showed a myxoma similar to that removed in the two previous operations.

The amputation above the condyles of the femur was not done until three days later, because until then the patient's consent could not be obtained.

At the present time (October, 1920), one year since operation, the patient is free from pain and walks well on his artificial limb.

CASE III (Pathol. No. 10150). *Periosteal Exostosis of Lower Third of Shaft of Femur with Myxomatous Areas.*—In this case the large exostosis was removed piecemeal by a colleague in December, 1909. There was nothing in the clinical picture, in the X-ray, nor at the operation to suggest a malignant tumor. The microscopic diagnosis made in the laboratory was *benign exostosis.*

Recently when I restudied some 110 cases of exostosis, this patient was the only one reported dead. We were informed that he died four years after operation with recurrence of the tumor in the region of the knee and symptoms of metastasis to the lung.

On reëxamination of the tissue in the laboratory I found definite areas of myxoma between the cancellous bone in this exostosis— a microscopic finding not present in any other case of this group.

Clinical History.—The patient is a white male aged fifty-five. There is no history of injury. Six years before operation he observed stiffness of the left knee, then a definite hard lump in the popliteal area, later some interference with flexion.

X-ray (Fig. 12).—This shows a large bony growth springing from the posterior surface of the lower third of the femur above the condyle. In some places it shows lighter areas. There is no definite change in the shaft of the bone. The appearance is that of a benign exostosis.

The *examination* was negative, except for the palpation of the tumor.

At the *operation* the tumor had a capsule and was composed

chiefly of bone. It was chiseled from the shaft of the femur, but no note was made of the condition of the shaft. The patient left the hospital in apparently good condition.

Gross Pathology.—The tissue received in the laboratory consists of two pieces of bone 2x3x5 cm. and fourteen smaller pieces. The surface of the tumor shows a connective-tissue capsule and what appears to be definite periosteum. Beneath this periosteum in places there is cartilage, in other places there is no cartilage. The tumor beneath is composed of rather soft cancellous bone which can be cut with the knife. In my experience this is unusual in the benign exostosis, and such a finding should be regarded as suspicious.

Microscopic Study.—The greater part of the tumor is composed of cancellous bone. The soft tissue between the bone lamellæ is the seat of an inflammatory reaction; lymphoid cells predominate; there are no giant-cells, but many osteoblasts. In a second section (Fig. 13) we observe the cartilage covering and the cancellous bone beneath, but here between the lamellæ of bone there is definite myxomatous tissue. Here and there, between the cartilage and bone, a giant-cell.

Fig. 14 is from an area in which the tissue between the bone lamellæ shows lymphoid-cell reaction. I am unable to interpret this picture—whether this is an inflammatory reaction, or young myxomatous tissue.

I think there can be no question that there is myxoma in this exostosis, and the recurrence and death four years later are pretty good evidence that the lesion was not a benign exostosis.

What would be our procedure in these cases to-day?

In Case I, the periosteal lesion of the shaft of the humerus, we could be quite positive that we were not dealing with a growth composed entirely of bone, because the centre contained no bone. The possibilities are: cartilage (chondroma), myxoma and a cyst. I have an example of each. In this case one could have removed the tumor without exposing the tumor tissue; the soft parts could have been divided down to the shaft of the bone, the periosteum divided some distance from the pedicle, and a piece of the shaft chiseled away giving the tumor a good margin. I would then swab the exposed chiseled bone with pure carbolic acid followed by alcohol, pack the wound with a piece of gauze saturated with a solution of zinc chloride. Then I would divide the removed tumor, make frozen sections of the centre, and study the zone of bone removed from beneath the tumor for possible infiltration.

CASE IV (Pathol. No. 10693).—Fig. 15 is the X-ray of a tumor which somewhat resembled that in Case I (Fig. 1). I removed it after the method just described. Fig. 16 shows the result after operation, and Fig. 17 (*a* and *b*) the removed tumor, which proved to be a bone cyst with a definite connective-tissue lining of ostitis fibrosa. This patient is well (July, 1920) ten years after operation.

In Case II, the central myxoma of the astragalus, I think it would be justifiable to try X-ray or radium first. If signs of ossification did not present themselves quickly, I should explore under an Esmarch with the Paquelin cautery. If it proved to be a bone cyst, I should curette, leave the bone shell, and close without drainage. If it were found to be a giant-cell tumor, I should curette thoroughly, swab with pure carbolic acid followed by alcohol and close without drainage. I have already noted that we have had examples of each one of these types who remained free from recurrence after curetting.

If the tumor proved to be an chondroma without myxomatous areas, I would employ the same method as for the giant-cell tumor, but use radium afterwards, placing the radium in the wound and closing later.

If the tumor proved to be a myxoma, I would curette with the cautery, followed by carbolic acid and alcohol; I then would pack the wound with zinc chloride gauze and leave it in for twenty-four hours. I would then close the wound and watch the case most carefully.

There is, however, no case to prove the efficacy of this treatment in myxoma, but as the myxoma recurs first locally, the amputation could be done later if there was a recurrence.

In the third case, the exostosis of the femur with myxomatous areas, I should attempt to remove the tumor as in Case I, without exposing tumor tissue. In this case, as in the majority of exostoses, the growth can be isolated and chiseled from the shaft without exposing tumor tissue. Should the exostosis be of such size that removal *en-bloc* would be impossible, I would advise immediate frozen sections of the soft areas, and if myxoma were found I should immediately employ the electric cautery and chemical cauterization.

As I have noted before, one will frequently find in exostosis cartilage, and in the cartilage there may be soft areas which resemble in the gross myxomatous tissue. The differentiation can be made only in the frozen section.

I have recently had such an observation in an exostosis composed largely of cartilage in which there were soft gelatinous areas suggesting myxoma.

I emphasize again here the possibility of implanting even cartilage in a piecemeal operation. For this reason chemical destruction or the cautery should be employed as a means to prevent recurrence. I have a case to prove the point: The original tumor was apparently a cartilaginous exostosis of a metacarpal bone; it was first removed with a knife by a colleague; the tumor recurred. I then exposed and removed the recurrent tumor with the cautery, preserving part of the metacarpal bone. Before operation I was rather inclined to the view that it was

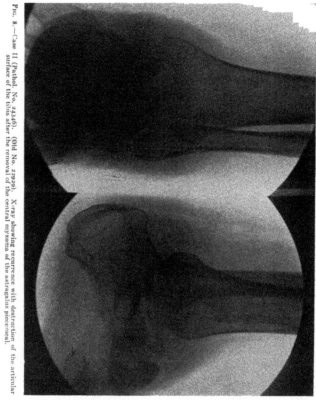

Fig. 8.—Case II (Pathol. No. 24346). (Old No. 29339). X-ray showing recurrence with destruction of the articular surface of the tibia after the removal of the central myxoma of the astragalus piecemeal.

720

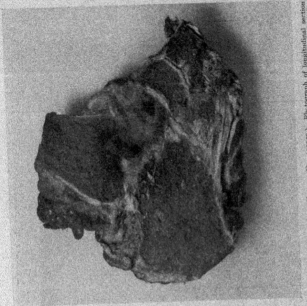

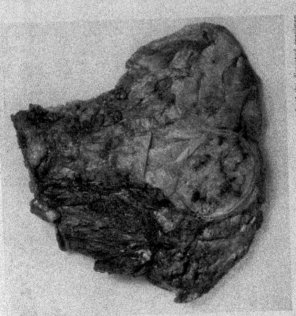

Fig. 9.—Case II (Pathol. No. 21346). (23919.) Photograph of the dissected specimen after amputation. In the lower mid-area a cut has been made exposing the myxomatous tumor. The light, lobular areas are characteristic of myxoma, the red currant-jelly areas tumor. But is ostitis fibrosa, and they predominate in have been observed not only in this tumor, but is ostitis fibrosa, and they predominate in the giant-cell tumors.

Fig. 10.—Case II (Pathol. No. 21346). (23929.) Photograph of longitudinal section through ankle-joint, showing the recurrent myxoma surrounding and invading the lower end of the tibia.

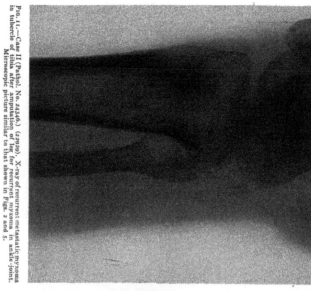

FIG. 11.—Case II (Pathol. No. 24346.) (2929). X-ray of recurrent metastatic myxoma in tubercle of tibia after amputation of leg for recurrent myxoma in ankle-joint. Microscopic picture similar to that shown in Figs. 2 and 5.

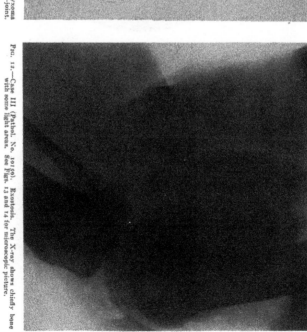

FIG. 12.—Case III (Pathol. No. 101569). Exostosis. The X-ray shows chiefly bone with some light areas. See Figs. 13 and 14 for microscopic picture.

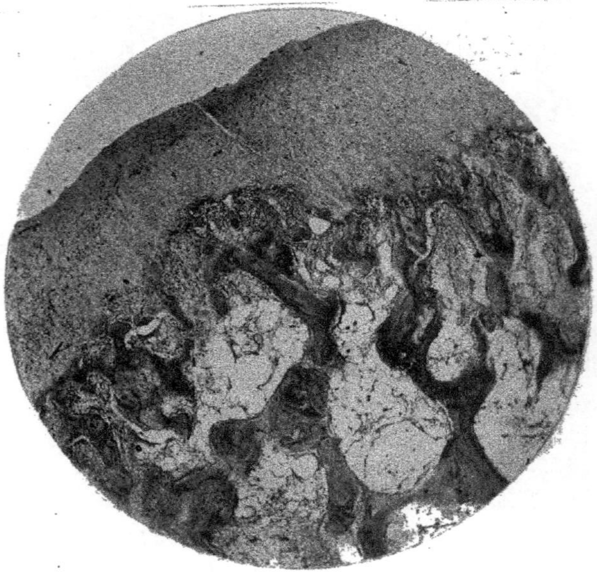

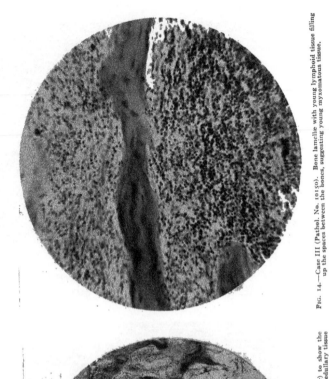

Fig. 13.—Case III (Pathol. No. 10150). Microscopic picture (low power) to show the cartilage capsule of the exostosis, the bone lamellæ of its framework, the medullary tissue and myxoma between the bone lamellæ.

Fig. 14.—Case III (Pathol. No. 10150). Bone lamellæ with young lymphoid tissue filling up the spaces between the bones, suggesting young myxomatous tissue.

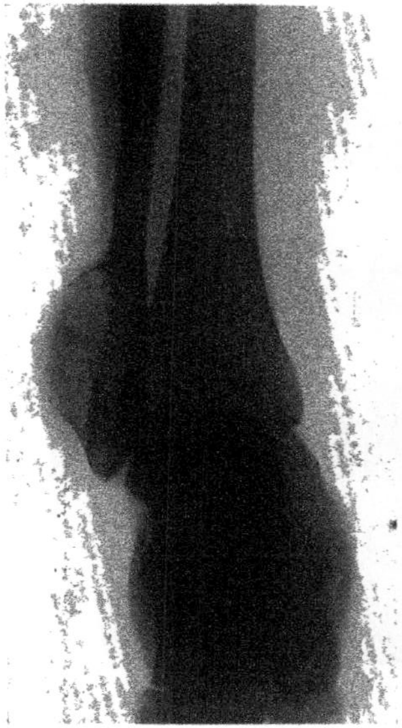

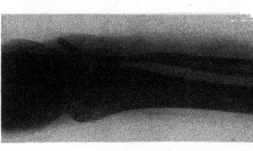

FIG. 15.
FIG. 15 AND 16.—Case IV (Pathol. No. 10693). X-ray of a benign bone cyst before and
after operation. Compare this with X-ray shown in Fig. 1, a pure myxoma.

FIG. 16.

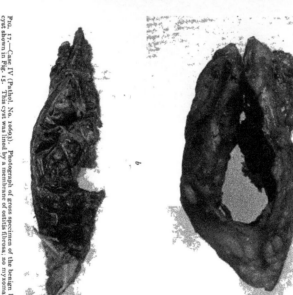

FIG. 17.—Case IV (Pathol. No. 10693). Photograph of gross specimen of the benign bone
cyst shown in Fig. 15. This cyst was lined by a membrane of ostitis fibrosa; no myxomatous
tissue.

720

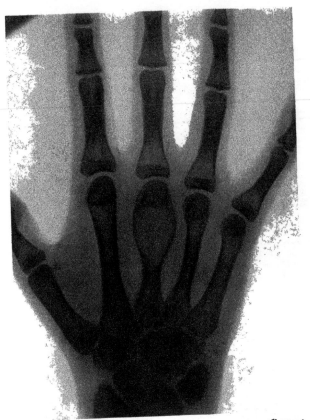

FIG. 18.—Case V (Pathol. No. 14552). Central myxoma of metacarpal bone. X-ray and tissue sent me by Doctor Kimpton of Boston. Compare this X-ray with Figs. 1, 3, 11 and 15.

a periosteal myxoma because of the recurrence, but the sections showed only cartilage. This patient is now well for a longer interval after the second operation than after the first.

BRIEF SUMMARY OF MYXOMA AND CHONDROMYXOMA OF BONE

Among about 270 bone tumors which I have studied, 12 may be classed as myxoma; 9 of these are pure myxomas, and 3 are chondro-myxomas. Of the pure myxomas, 2 were periosteal tumors and 7 central. Of the chondromyxomas, 1 was periosteal, 2 central. The myxoma, therefore, is more frequently a central tumor of bone.

The combination of myxoma and cartilage is relatively infrequent—only 3 examples of chondromyxoma as compared with 14 pure chon-dromas, 7 periosteal and 7 central.

Nevertheless, when one exposes a tumor resembling cartilage there is always a possibility of myxoma, and its presence should be deter-mined at once by a frozen section.

Results in Myxoma and Myxochondroma.—Three cases are apparently cured. At the operation in each instance the tumor was not exposed. In one a central myxochondroma of the humerus was removed by amputation at the shoulder-joint (Johns Hopkins Hospital, 1894), and this patient died thirteen years later at the age of eighty-three of other causes. In the remaining two cases the tumor was a pure myxoma, involving the central cavity of a phalanx; in one, the lesion was removed by amputation (by Rhodes, Roanoke, Va.), in the other by resection (Codman, *Boston Med. and Surg. Jour.*, Feb. 25, 1904). These patients have been followed only two and three years respectively.

Unfortunately, for scientific purposes, the two examples of central myxoma of the phalanx of the finger subjected to curetting only, were not followed by the operators.

Up to the present time there is not a single case of myxoma or myxo-chondroma which has remained well and free from recurrence after an operation consisting of curetting only.

In addition to the three cases reported here, one of which recurred after curetting and the remaining two after piecemeal operations, there are two other cases which recurred and were subjected to second opera-tions, and which at the present time are apparently well. This would make three cases of myxoma which have been apparently cured in spite of recurrence: *viz.:* the following:

Case II, reported here (Pathol. No. 22929), well October, 1920. one year since the last operation, amputation of the femur for a recurrence in the upper end of the tibia.

Pathol. No. 14552, Central Myxoma of Shaft of Metacarpal Bone (Fig. 18). In this case, in May, 1912, Doctor Kimpton, of Boston, removed the tumor by resec-tion. but he is of the opinion that during the resection tumor tissue was exposed and that some of it may have been left in the wound. On account of recurrence ·

he operated again one year later, and this patient was free from recurrence two years after the second operation. I have studied the sections in this case, and it is an example of pure myxoma. The patient at the time of operation was fifteen years of age; the central tumor was found accidentally in taking an X-ray because of a recent injury, and this showed both a fracture and the tumor. The X-ray shown in Fig. 18 was taken one year later and illustrates that if there had been a fracture it has healed, and there is no evidence that myxomatous tissue infiltrated outside through the crevice of the fracture. I have been unable to get the first X-ray, but this is a very interesting observation, demonstrating that the fracture may heal even if the central tumor is a myxoma.

. ' *Pathol. No. 19545. Central Myxochondroma of the Os Calcis.*—I have recently restudied the section in this case. There is chiefly cartilage, with small islands of myxoma in the cartilage. When this patient was admitted to Johns Hopkins Hospital in 1916 he was twenty-three years of age; there had been pain in the os calcis for one year; there had also been an operation on the os calcis three months ago, but apparently the operator did not expose the disease in the centre of the bone. The X-ray diagnosis was ostitis and periostitis of the os calcis. Doctor Dandy, who operated, describes a small opening in the bone from which there exuded gelatinous material. This at once would suggest myxoma, although in some instances softened cartilage may also produce this gelatinous material. On removing a shell of bone there was exposed a cavity, the size of a lemon, filled with tissue resembling cartilage, with here and there gelatinous, myxomatous areas and a few areas resembling the giant-cell tumor. After thoroughly curetting, Doctor Dandy disinfected with carbolic and alcohol. There was local recurrence followed by amputation one year later, and the patient was reported well two years later (September, 1919).

Here the pure carbolic and alcohol did not prevent recurrence. From a study of the sections of the bony shell I am confident that in this case the entire shell is infiltrated with myxoma, so that the disease was not completely removed.

Five patients are dead: Cases I and III, already reported here, and the following:

Pathol. No. 2331.—Here the myxoma was periosteal, involving the sacrum and the lower lumbar vertebræ, with infiltration of the soft parts. At the exploratory operation the tumor could not be removed. The patient died five months later.

Pathol. No. 8475.—Central Myxoma of the Shaft of the Humerus.—Here curetting was done, as the patient refused amputation. There followed a local recurrence in seven months and death from the disease in four years.

Pathol. No. 18554.—This case is of interest chiefly because it was a small periosteal tumor springing from the body of the seventh dorsal vertebra and bringing the patient under observation because of pressure on the spinal cord. The tumor was the size of a ten-cent piece and was composed chiefly of cartilage, with myxomatous areas. The patient died ten months after operation. The pressure symptoms were not relieved. The question as to recurrence could not be decided.

Literature on Myxoma of Bone.—In 1904 (*Progressive Medicine,* December, 1904, p. 185), in the discussion of bone cysts due to ostitis fibrosa, I reviewed the case reported by Codman (*Boston Med. and Surg. Jour.,* Feb. 25, 1904, p. 211). The tumor was central in the second phalanx of a finger, Codman reported this case as the only cyst in that situation. Doctor Whitney, the pathologist, was of the opinion from the gross appearance that it was a myxochondroma, but unfortunately the sections have been lost. The probabilities are that this was either a myxoma or a chondroma.

In describing the gross appearance of the tumor after resection, Doctor Codman writes that within the bone shell there was a small cavity, and between the bone shell and the cavity fine trabeculæ lined with soft myxomatous tissue.

In ANNALS OF SURGERY (vol. lii, August, 1910, p. 150) I isolate from bone cysts due to ostitis fibrosa in which the central lesion was composed of myxomatous tissue. At that time I had Codman's case, one case sent to my laboratory by my colleague Doctor Baer, and three cases from the literature (Dreesmann, Blake and Bostrom, for references, see my article just quoted). Since then I have in my own collection up to date, ten cases of central lesions of the phalanx of the finger, five of which are myxomas and three chondromas. There is therefore up to the present time no reported case of ostitis fibrosa of the phalanx of the finger in which the diagnosis has been confirmed by a microscopic study of the lining of the cyst.

In *Progressive Medicine* (December, 1906, p. 221) I reviewed the first article on pure myxoma of bone which had come under my attention. Soubeyran (*Revue de Chir.*, 1904, xxix, p. 239) in reporting his single observation gives but six references to the literature. The case reported by this surgeon was apparently a periosteal growth from the lower third to the shaft of the tibia. The mass was 8 cm. long and 2 cm. wide. At the exploratory operation after dividing a connective-tissue capsule in which in places there was thin shell of bone, there exuded a gelatinous material, and this material was confined to a space circumscribed by this capsule and shell of bone in the shaft of the tibia. Between the gelatinous material there were small spicules of bone. The treatment was curetting. In a few months there was recurrence, and at the second operation cortical bone was chiseled away with the recurrent tumor. One year after operation there was no recurrence.

Soubeyran makes this interesting remark: " In these myxomas there is no definite line of demarcation." I infer that he means that the myxomatous tissue may infiltrate the cortical bone without sufficient bone destruction to be seen either in the X-ray or in the fresh tissue. This is an important point to remember when dealing with myxoma. In spite of this, Soubeyran advocates conservative methods.

In the same number of *Progressive Medicine* I reported for the first time Case I (Pathol. No. 6773) described in this paper.

It is interesting to note in confirmation of Soubeyran's remarks that I have just reëxamined a bit of the bone shell removed with the chisel beneath the periosteal myxomatous growth in Pathol. No. 6773 and find it infiltrated with myxomatous tissue without much bone absorption.

Up to the end of 1914, the literature on bone tumors was most carefully followed without finding any references to this rare lesion. Within the past year William H. Fisher, of Toledo (ANNALS OF SURGERY, 1919, vol. lxix, p. 596) makes a most interesting contribution to pure myxoma, but his tumor involved the soft parts of the labium majus. He gives a very interesting summary of the views of pathologists up to date on myxoma, but does not discuss myxoma of bone. He refers to the case of pure myxoma of the phalanx reported by me and to one reported by Cotton (*Amer. Jour. of Röntgenology*, 1918) in which the myxomatous tumor involved the whole shaft of the femur from neck to condyles.

The best description of myxoma from a histological standpoint is in Ewing's recent book (" Neoplastic Diseases," 1919, p. 166), but he does not mention myxoma of bone.

In the excellent article on Bone Tumors written by Channing Simmons of Boston, for the " American Practice of Surgery ' by Bryant and Buck in 1907, (vol. 888, p. 394) myxomas of bone are not mentioned, nor are they referred to in a short article on bone tumors by Nichols of Boston in 1907 (" Keen's Surgery," vol. II).

Referring back to Senn in 1895, we find no mention of myxoma of bone in his book on the " Pathology and Surgical Treatment of Tumors." The chapter on pure myxoma, about eight pages, does not mention this tumor as involving bone. This is good evidence of the rarity of the lesion, because he was most familiar with surgical literature, especially on tumors.

HYPOPHYSEAL DUCT TUMORS

A REPORT OF THREE CASES AND A FOURTH CASE OF CYST OF RATHKE'S POUCH

By William C. Duffy, M.D.

OF NEW HAVEN, CONN.

ASSISTANT IN SURGICAL PATHOLOGY, DEPARTMENT OF SURGERY, YALE UNIVERSITY

(*Continued from page 552*)

THE following case *intra vitam* was briefly referred to from the röntgenographic viewpoint by Heuer and Dandy (Case IV) in 1916 in their study of röntgenography in the localization of brain tumor.

CASE III.—*Suprasellar cystic squamous epithelial tumor of infundibulum, with metaplastic and extensive degenerative changes, developing from an inclusion of the hypophyseal duct. Bitemporal hemianopsia. General pressure and neighborhood symptoms for two years. Amenorrhœa (the first symptom) for three years with increase in weight (dystrophia adiposo-genitalis); atrophy of endometrium. Calcified area above sella (X-ray). Lateral intracranial operation with temporary relief. Exitus subsequent to second operation. Autopsy.*

Abstract of J. H. H. (Surgical Histories Nos. 32604 and 34653). A young white woman, twenty years old, was transferred from the medical to the surgical service May 25, 1914, *complaining* of blindness (on account of which she had previously been admitted to the medical service). Her family history was negative. She was the wife of a farmer to whom she had been married for a year and a half. Beginning at twelve years of age she had suffered with poor general health and occasional headaches. At fourteen years of age there was a severe attack of tonsillitis, and about a year later a slight attack of catarrhal jaundice lasting a week. Her menstrual periods, at first regular, after lengthening intervals, gradually ceased three years ago. At that time she weighed 100 pounds. Since then her weight has rapidly increased to 130 pounds. *Two years ago* she had her first episode of severe nocturnal headache, lasting a few minutes, followed next day by partial right-sided hemianopsia with dimness of vision persisting for two days. There was no other attack until eight months ago, when a more severe attack occurred. Sick in bed; headache with roaring in ears and spots before eyes. At the end of one week she was unable to count fingers held before her eyes. Flashes of color and imaginary objects were seen. Vomited once. Dimness of vision for three weeks, thence normal; polyuria and dysuria one week. Polydipsia. Rapid improvement. The last attack occurred two months before admission. There was gradually increasing dimness of vision in both eyes for two weeks, followed by severe headache with tinnitus. *En route* to another clinic she vomited once, but attributed this to "car sickness." The severe headache continued for one week. The diagnosis of tumor near the

725

optic chiasm was made, and X-ray treatment was employed for three weeks without benefit. From time to time the vision seems better, then worse again, and so on until admission here.

Examination.—A rather juvenile looking young woman, rather well nourished. Axillary and pubic hair a little less than normal. Head: Normal in appearance. Eyes: Left eye does not converge, vision dim in both eyes, almost *nil* on left, right 16/100, counts fingers at three feet. Nose: Negative. General neurological examination: Negative. No general glandular or thyroid enlargement. Thorax, heart, and abdomen negative.

Blood examination: Red blood count, 4,300,000; white blood count, 8000; hæmoglobin, 85 per cent.

Wassermann: Negative.

Urine: Sp. gr. 1005–1012, no sugar or albumin.

Carbohydrate tolerance: After taking 200 grams of glucose no glycosuria in subsequent twenty-four hours.

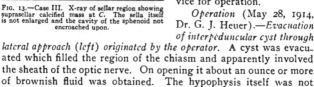

Ophthalmoscopic: P o s t - neurotic atrophy, more advanced on left.

X-ray report: No. 23351 (Dr. F. H. Baetjer).

Small calcified area in top of sella (Fig. 13).

Transferred to surgical service for operation.

Operation (May 28, 1914, Dr. G. J. Heuer).—*Evacuation of interpeduncular cyst through lateral approach (left) originated by the operator.* A cyst was evacuated which filled the region of the chiasm and apparently involved the sheath of the optic nerve. On opening it about an ounce or more of brownish fluid was obtained. The hypophysis itself was not seen at any time. Usual closure.

Fig. 13.—Case III. X-ray of sellar region showing suprasellar calcified mass at C. The sella itself is not enlarged and the cavity of the sphenoid not encroached upon.

Uneventful recovery from operation. On July 22, 1914, she wrote: " Enjoying best of health. No change in vision " (or amenorrhœa).

Second Admission.—March 22, 1915.

Present Illness.—The patient was well for three months after discharge from the hospital nine months ago. Then she noticed vision was becoming dimmer. Now she cannot read the largest print and is only able to recognize familiar persons within a range of three feet. She has put on considerable fat since last operation. Appetite good, is always hungry, likes vegetables, especially. Does not care for sweets. No other symptoms—no headaches, vomiting, change in mentality or irritability. No relief of amenorrhœa; she has not menstruated in four years. Does not void unusual amounts. Occasional nycturia.

Examination.—A very well-nourished young woman, skin somewhat dry, subcutaneous layer everywhere rather thick and shows slight painful sensitiveness to pressure. Hands, wrists, feet and ankles small. Fingers tapering. Temperature, 99°. Pulse, 92.

Fundi: Bitemporal hemianopsia.

Operation (March 27, 1915, Doctor Heuer).—*Evacuation of infundibular cyst.* (At the previous operation the left side was operated on.)

A large flap was turned back on the right. The interchiasmal space was filled with a cystic tumor having the same appearance as at first operation. The cyst was opened with a knife over the left optic tract, producing a " gush of yellowish-white fluid with most beautiful shimmering golden crystals. They were found to be cholesterin crystals. At first they were taken for minute globules of fat." Probably 1 or 1½ ounces of fluid escaped.

" At this time looking still farther back a second cyst with translucent wall was evident." Passing a clamp into this a gush of fluid even larger in amount than the first occurred, which contained similar substances. This fluid in a test-tube was of a yellowish-brown color and quite turbid. It was felt that the direction of this second cyst was both upward and downward, into the third ventricle and into the chiasm. In attempting to remove the lining of the cyst a considerable amount of hemorrhage occurred. As soon as this was controlled by silver clips on the anterior communicating cerebral artery, closure of the wound was made.

The patient succumbed twelve hours after operation. Temperature reached 106°.

Autopsy.—No. 4315. (Dr. Thornton Stearns.)

Anatomical Diagnosis.—Parahypophyseal cyst, arising from Rathke's pouch.

Body.—Is that of a young, very well nourished and well-developed white woman. Head has been entirely shaved, and there is a surgical wound on the right side extending from behind the ear almost to the sagittal median line, forward down on the forehead and extending down to the outer edge of the right orbit. The recent incision is in excellent condition. On the opposite side is a similar but well-healed linear scar.

The body was that of a fairly well-developed female. There is a good deal of fat throughout the body. The breasts are not very large and are not well developed. The hair in the axillæ and over the pubis is present, but not of luxuriant growth; otherwise there are no external abnormalities.

Partial autopsy was obtained, median section through the abdomen, through which the pelvic organs were examined, and the uterus, tubes and ovaries were removed. The uterus was small, was retroverted and retroflexed; the ovaries were small and the tubes were perfectly normal. On cutting into the uterus it showed a normal cavity with some mucus in it. The *adrenals* were removed and were both perfectly normal, showing a brownish centre, with a yellowish-white cortex. They were of normal size.

Brain.—After formalin fixation *in situ* was removed in the usual manner. The surface of the hemispheres showed slight flattening of the convolutions. The hypophyseal region, which was removed by Doctor Heuer, showed a small amount of bloody ooze of the operation two days ago. The floor of the cranial cavity was normal.

The sella turcica was normal and the hypophysis located in a perfectly normal manner, and on being removed was found to be of normal size. The infundibulum of the hypophysis was not seen and was thought to be involved in the tumor mass. Situated at the base of the brain in the interpeduncular region was the remains of the cyst which was opened and partly removed at operation. After sagittal hemisection of the brain the cyst wall is seen to involve the suprasellar (infundibular) region and the lower part of the third ventricle.

The brain was cut sagittally. It showed a cyst occupying the lower portion of the third ventricle. The wall of the cyst was quite thin, about 1 mm. in thickness. It was rather rough and granular on its inner surface. Small yellow granules which appear to be calcified were present. These were probably little crystals of cholesterin.

At the base of the cyst there was a crystallized granular mass about the size of a pea. On being cut through it was very hard, cartilaginous

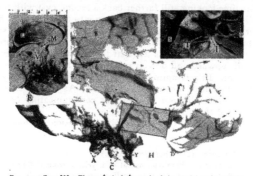

FIG. 14.—Case III. The central photograph of the mesial surface of the right half of the brain shows the calcified mass (C) which produced the shadow in the X-ray. At A is a second mass of tumor tissue. The squared area is shown enlarged in the right upper insert. The cystic tumor has extended above, displacing the floor of the third ventricle (R) upward, almost obliterating the space of the ventricle, which is reduced to the area between R and N. Posteriorly the wall of the cyst (T) has encroached upon the aqueduct of Sylvius (I). Anteriorly the floor of the third ventricle becomes deficient at (A). In the left half of the brain (left upper insert) the wall (V) of the cyst is deficient above and the widely dilated foramen of Monro (M) is seen leading into the dilated lateral ventricle (L). The extent of solid tumor (most of which has been removed) is shown at E. Blocks taken at S. P=pineal. H=pons. D=fourth ventricle. (Y)=basilar artery.

almost, but was probably made up of the same crystals. They were of yellowish color. There was some blood clot present here. There was no very definite tumor tissue seen anywhere.

Further Description and Microscopic Study by the Writer.—The roof of the cyst has been displaced upwards and corresponds with the floor (Fig. 14, *a*, *R*) of the third ventricle. The cavity of the latter is clearly separate from the cyst cavity and is continuous with the space of the aqueduct of Sylvius (Fig. 14, *I*). The foramen of Monro (Fig. 14, *M*) is present on each side, and the moderate dilatation of the lateral ventricles is probably accounted for by pressure of the distended cyst wall posteriorly (Fig. 14, *T*) upon the aqueduct. The cyst measures 3.4 cm. anteriorly. Its vertical measurement is difficult to estimate on account of the destruction of much of the base of the cyst. The upper part of the cyst wall is about 1 mm. thick, the lower much thicker. In addition to the larger masses of tissue at the base smaller yellow granules are present higher up.

The masses of material at the base of the cyst constitute the major residuum of tumor tissue. They are blood-stained a slate brown color, but on section, or after removing clotted blood, show yellowish to chalky areas, which blend with light yellow to orange-colored zones, resulting in a marbled effect. The chalky areas are the result of calcium salts deposit or bone formation. On cutting through this partly decalcified tissue a gritty sensation is felt. In the protocol these masses were attributed to the presence of cholesterin crystals.

Blocks for microscopic study included ones: through the upper limit of cyst wall and adjacent third ventricle wall, the above-mentioned granular or yellow plaque areas; and the larger masses of tissue, containing calcified material which project into the cyst cavity lower down at the base of the tumor mass. In addition the sections made at the time of the autopsy (Doctor Stearns) are available.

Microscopic Examination.—The cyst wall is composed of a varyingly thick fibrous wall carrying a lining of squamous epithelium, which shows certain interesting hyperplastic, metaplastic and degenerative phenomena.

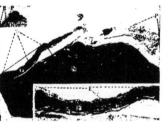

The simpler structure of the cyst wall is seen where the roof of the cyst bulged upward into the space of the third ventricle. A block (Fig. 15, upper insert) taken through the upper extremity of the right lateral half of the cyst wall, underlying brain substances, and adjacent choroid plexus (Fig. 15, P) of the third ventricle shows at the lower part of the section, extending upward into the third ventricle, a segment of the roof of the cyst composed of squamous epithelium (Fig. 15, E), underlaid by fairly dense fibrous tissue. Beneath the latter lies brain tissue (Fig. 15, N), to which the fibrous wall is adherent.

FIG. 15.—Case III. The left upper insert shows the gross block of tissue which is composed of a fragment (E) of the roof of the cyst extending high into the space of the third ventricle. At P is seen a tuft of choroid plexus. The central cut is a low power photomicrograph of the same tissue. At E the squamous epithelial lining may be seen, but is shown more distinctly in the lower insert which is a slightly higher magnification. F = fibrous wall of the cyst. N = nervous tissue.

The intermediate zone shows a slight proliferation of neuroglial elements, which bind the tumor wall to brain substance. Between the two are several small cyst-like spaces, with a lining of one layer of flattened or cuboidal epithelial cells closely resembling the ependymal cells lining the third ventricle above. These cystic spaces apparently were formed from ependymal cells isolated during the fusion of the cyst wall with the wall of the ventricle. This intimate relation between brain substance and tumor wall is present only in a small area, above which the union becomes interrupted progressively, until finally the tip of epithelial-covered fibrous wall is seen projecting free into the cavity of the ventricle. Beneath this tip of cyst wall which lies free, the ependymal lining of the ventricle extends downward until the zone of adhesion between cyst wall and brain substance is reached. This squamous epithelial-lined process tapers toward its upper extremity, and near the tip of the latter one sees villous-like branches of choroid plexus (Fig. 15, P). The epithelium covering this extension of the cyst wall is atypical squamous epithelium, with a well-preserved cylindrical basal layer; intercellular bridges are present, but there is no horny layer.

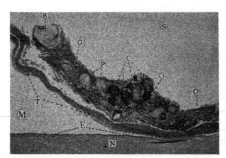

FIG. 16.—Case III. Lower-power magnification of a similar area which shows a segment of the roof of the cyst curving away from the ependymal (*E*) lining of the brain substance (*N*). The epithelium covering the fibrous wall (*T*) has undergone degenerative changes. At *P* one sees epithelial pearls. Calcified masses of keratinized stratified epithelium at *C*. Necrotic mass of epithelium at (*R*). Extensive round cell infiltration at (*O*). The cyst cavity=*S*. The third ventricle cavity = *M*. At *G*, under a higher-power foreign body giant cell reaction could be seen about disintegrating necrotic fragments of epithelium.

Its cells show rather marked reticulation, apparently a hydropic change, which will be referred to more fully below. For the most part, this stratified epithelium is composed of only a few layers; in places down-extending processes are present. Beneath the epithelium in such regions are atypical epithelial pearls composed of pink-staining keratinized cells, one of which is isolated in the fibrous tissue at a depth of .4 mm. below the squamous epithelial zone. The underlying brain substance shows no obvious changes. The choroid plexus present in this section is normal and there are no hyperplastic changes in the ependymal epithelium.

Sections of a block from a similar locality taken vertically through the upper limit of cyst wall and wall of third ventricle, show again the overhanging roof (Fig. 16) of the cyst, which is also lined on its surface bordering the cyst cavity (Fig. 16, *S*) with squamous epithelium. The adjacent ependymal lining (Fig. 16, *E*) of the third ventricle is even better preserved, the zone of separation between brain substance and overlying tumor wall is sharp in this preparation, no small ependymal cysts such as are mentioned in the preceding block are present. The epithelium covering this portion of the cyst wall, which in the gross had the appearance of a yellow, slightly raised, granular patch, shows interesting histological changes, however. Numerous necrotic, keratinized, concentric, epithelial cell nests (Fig. 16, *P*) are present, and several of these show marked peripheral calcification (Fig. 16, *C*). At the base of the section where the tumor wall is attached to the underlying brain substance the squamous epithelium is in places thinned

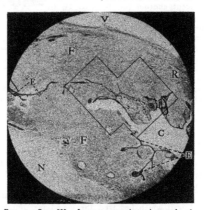

FIG. 17.—Case III. Lower-power photomicrograph of section through wall of cyst high up where the fibrous wall (*F*) is reflected to form the roof (*R*) of the cyst. The squamous epithelial lining (*E*) of the cyst sends processes into the fibrous zone. Note the epithelial area (*S*) projecting into the cyst cavity (*C*). *V*=cavity of third ventricle; the roof of the cyst is devoid of ependymal covering (*cf.* Fig. 16, *E*). *N* = cerebral nervous tissue.

to only a few cell layers. There is a slight reticulation of the epithelial cells in a few areas. A very marked lymphoid infiltration (Fig. 16, *O*) is present toward the tip of the process, which has broken up the epithelial continuity. Here there is a tendency to invasion by granulation tissue from beneath the epithelial zone. Nearer the tip the epithelium has lost entirely its regular appearance. Its stratification has disappeared and the individual cells are irregular in size, shape, and staining affinities, resulting in a slight hyperplastic picture. No mitoses are seen. In this area, particularly about the peripheries of the calcified epithelial processes, occasional small foreign-body giant cells are present. A moderate number of polymorphonuclear leucocytes are present in the areas of lymphoid infiltration and epithelial hyperplasia, and at the extreme tip, scattered through the necrotic hyalinized mass (Fig. 16, *R*), which has lost practically all traces of the outlines of its original epithelial cells.

Sections of another block show the cyst wall (Fig. 17, *F*) partly underlaid by adherent, but sharply demarcated, brain substance (Fig. 17, *N*). Near one end of the section the fibrous wall is sharply kinked on itself to form the roof (Fig. 17, *R*) of the cyst (Fig. 17, *C*). Close to the angle of the kink the epithelial surface shows an island of epithelium (Fig. 17, *S*) composed of large clear cells, with dark-staining, comparatively small, irregularly polyhedral nuclei. The almost clear, but faintly staining, apparently lipoid, cytoplasm of these cells contains a delicate net-like reticulum (Fig. 18, *S*). Morphologically they resemble sebaceous-gland epithelial cells. The periphery of this area is partly outlined by a double layer of flat or cubical epi-

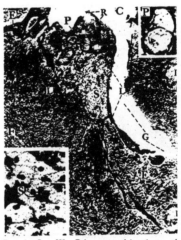

Fig. 18.—Case III. Enlargement of boxed area of Fig. 17. Note the appearance of the epithelium at *S* which under still further enlargement in the left lower corner is seen (*S*) to be made up of cells resembling epithelium. This mass of degenerated or metaplastic epithelium (*S*) is surrounded by a thin layer of modified squamous epithelium (*L*) directly continuous with the epithelial lining (*E*) of the cyst. (*cf.* preceding figure.) Part of this mass bordering the cyst is composed of keratinized epithelium (*R*) with pearl formation (*P*) (enlarged in the right upper insert). Other groups of keratinized cells at *I*. At *G* the section is broken. Cavity of cyst at *C*.

thelium (Fig. 18, *L*), but on one side several epithelial pearls (Fig. 18, *P*) are present, the apex of this zone showing a curious excavation (apparently artifact) of a mass of hyaline necrotic epithelium. A second smaller area of this lipoid epithelium is present in the same section, and in sections from another block a third is found which is less sharply demarcated and less well preserved. Shaft-like clear spaces within the area evidence the formation of cholesterin crystals, which have been dissolved out. Between the lipoid epithelium and the lining epithelium is a dense zone of lymphoid infiltration, in places .1 mm. in width. This zone extends over a considerable extent in the section, and its relation to the sebaceous-like epithelium is not apparent. The lining of squamous epithelium shows atrophy in places; in other places slight hyperplastic changes, consisting of a loss of the characteristic basal layer of cells

WILLIAM C. DUFFY

and irregularity in size and shape of the epithelium. In the same section
isolated islands of stratified epithelium are found lying 1 mm. deep in the
fibrous wall, but it seems probable that such islands are due to transection
of down-extending processes.

In sections from a mass of tissue at the base of the cyst, scattered
through a fairly loosely meshed stroma very rich in lymphocytes (Fig. 19, R)
and plasma cells are a number of lipoid epithelial cells (Fig. 19, S) undergoing further degenerative changes. Often where several lie together
the cell borders are obscure. In many cases the delicate cytoplasmic reticulum has largely disappeared, leaving a large, nearly clear cell, with a very
faintly staining cytoplasm, from which the nucleus often has disappeared.
In a few cases a globular clear space presents apparent evidence of a fatty

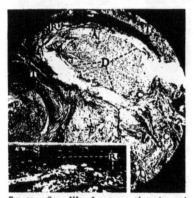

transformation. In the same
locality a number of foreign-
body giant-cells have ar-
ranged themselves around
shaft-like clear spaces (Fig.
19, C) in the tissue. It seems
obvious that transformation
of material from the lipoid
cells into cholesterin crystals has taken place, and that
the latter are responsible for
the foreign-body giant-cell
reaction. Near by (Fig. 19,
D) there is a large cystic area
filled with amorphous pink-
staining detritus, through
which a few crystalloid clear
spaces are scattered. This
material resembles histologically that of a sebaceous cyst,
and the presence of so much
degenerating lipoid epithelium
in the wall points pretty
clearly to its origin. As to
the origin of this lipoid epithelium, it is difficult to determine definitely whether it

FIG. 19.—Case III. Low-power photomicrograph
through tissue at base of cyst. Keratinized stratified
epithelial masses at E. The fibrous stroma (T) shows
round-cell infiltration (R) in some places, in others the
occurrence of numerous crystals (C). The latter occur
also in the debris (D) filling the cyst-like space. The
insert below is an enlargement of the squared area (A)
at the edge of the mass of amorphous debris (D). In the
insert numbers of degenerating sebaceous epithelial cells
(S) (cf. Fig. 18, S) are seen. It seems likely that the
area (D) is composed of the broken-down material of
these cells. The presence of cholesterin crystals supports
this possibility.

it is the result of metaplastic or degenerative changes. The epithelial nature
seems indicated by the presence of such areas (Fig. 17, S) entirely within
the squamous epithelial lining of the cyst. In favor of a degenerative process
are the absence of typical arrangement as sebaceous epithelial glands, association of other degenerative changes, and the fact that such lipoid degenerative changes are not uncommonly found elsewhere, particularly in association with chronic inflammatory conditions.

In sections of all the blocks taken from the larger masses of tissue
present at the base of the cyst the structure is more complex. Here (at the
base of the cyst) hyperplastic and degenerative processes involving both
epithelium and stroma had resulted in the production of masses or excrescences the size of a pea or larger, which projected into the cavity of the cyst.
Macroscopically these were seen to contain calcified material, and in the
protocol macroscopically they were attributed to the presence of cholesterin

crystals. Microscopically these masses are seen to be composed largely of areas of necrotic keratinized or hyalinized epithelium (Fig. 20), much of which has undergone calcification (Figs. 23 and 26, C). Under the low power one sees the fibrous wall of the tumor lined by irregular squamous epithelium. The necrotic epithelium is contiguous to the latter, and tends to become more prominent as the cavity of the cyst is approached. The tissue bordering the cyst cavity is ragged in outline and composed almost en-

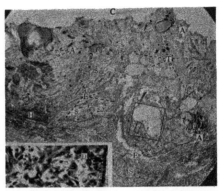

FIG. 20.—Case III. Low-power photomicrograph through one of the masses at the base of the cyst. Necrotic keratinized masses (T) may be seen, some of which (A) are partly calcified. The stroma (S) becomes scanty toward the cyst cavity (C) into which the necrotic tissue is desquamating. Hyperplastic atypical squamous epithelium (E) has invaded the stroma (S). The small squared area is enlarged in the insert. At B is seen the atypical basal layer. Irregularly formed epithelial cells are seen with heavily chromatinized cells at D. H is an area of recent hemorrhage.

tirely of necrotic masses, which show evidences of desquamation into the cyst cavity (Fig. 20, C). One mass, 3 x 2 mm. in size, composed entirely of keratinized and hyalinized necrotic epithelium, was noted in the gross as a bit of chalky material. As to the nature of the necrotic change, there is little doubt that keratinization plays a large part. In a number of epithelial processes, or " pearls," in which the outer layers are not completely necrotic, keratohyalin granules are present in abundance (Fig. 22, L). These stain intensely with hæmatoxylin in the usual preparations, and it was not found necessary to employ Heidenhain's method or the Gram-Weigert stain for their demonstration. They appear as discrete fine or coarse, deep blue granules, scattered through the cytoplasm. In such cells as they occur the nucleus has lost its staining affinity to a varying degree, some completely. Occasionally these granules are seen in completely keratinized cells in the centre of a nest of dead epithelium, but usually, and much more abundantly, they occur at the periphery of such masses (Fig. 22, E), often in half-moon or sickle-shaped cells (Fig. 22, G).

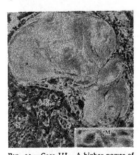

FIG. 21.—Case III. A higher power of the larger squared area of the preceding figure. The refractile completely hyalinized area shows scarcely any evidence of its epithelial origin. It is a further degenerative stage than the keratinized masses in which the outlines of the dead epithelial cells may still be seen (cf. E, Fig. 27). Note the atypical squamous epithelial hyperplasia (E) with a mitotic figure (M) in the insert (enlarged from a similar area). There is a moderate degree of round-cell infiltration of the stroma (S).

At the base of the cyst the epithelial lining itself is frequently composed of keratinized stratified epithelium, viable squamous epithelium being scanty and fragmentary. A fragment of viable, modified, squamous epithelium from the base of the cyst is shown in Fig. 24, at " T " projecting into the cyst cavity. This area is interesting histologically, as it shows well-defined *adamantinoma* characters. At the periphery (Fig. 24, *G*) is a layer of deeply staining cylindrical cells (Fig. 24, *L*), placed at right angles to the underlying cells. The cells of the peripheral layer where well differentiated show a distal cytoplasmic zone, with long, oval, dark-staining nucleus occupying the proximal two-thirds of the cell. The nuclei of the underlying cells are often larger and more vesicular, the cells themselves lying at right angles to the columnar layer, and have a well-marked spindle-cell appearance (Fig. 24, *S*), with definite intercellular bridges. These cells also show an occasional arrangement into concentric whorls, with flattened peripheral layers, but no keratinization. The same zone shows several small cysts (Fig. 24, *C*) lined by cubical or columnar epithelium. One of the smaller of these cysts contains a calcified lamellated concretion (Fig. 24, *I*). That such concretions may

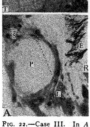

FIG. 22.—Case III. In *A* at *P* is a necrotic keratinized epithelial "pearl" in which the cell outlines are indistinguishable. This area is surrounded by concentric layers of cells which contain larger (*L*) and smaller (*S*) keratohyalin granules. In the insert (*R*) at the right may be seen more densely staining granules (*E*). In the insert (*T*) above, under oil immersion magnification discrete sharply outlined keratohyalin granules (*G*) are present in a sickle-shaped cell which partly encircles the periphery of a keratinized cell. The necrotic nuclei of two keratinized cells at *N*.

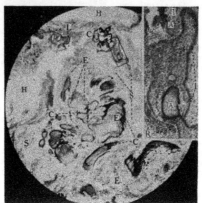

FIG. 23.—Case III. Lower-power photomicrograph showing masses of keratinized (necrosed) epithelium (*E*), calcified (*C*) to a varying extent, scattered through the sparse stroma (*S*). The squared area at a higher magnification, in the insert, shows the characteristic cylindrical cell peripheral layer (*I*) of the adamantinoma epithelium. Keratinized partly calcified epithelial groups at *A*. Note the round cell infiltration of the stroma at *R*. At *L* is seen a second bit of viable epithelium bordering the cavity (*H*) of the cyst.

be a secretory rather than a degenerative product seems probable, since the presence of small amounts of mucoid débris appears to be an evidence of the secretory nature of the columnar epithelial cells. In the third or central zone reticulation is a very striking feature and tends to increase as the centre is approached. The nuclei of the reticulated cells are shrunken and atrophic, frequently having disappeared entirely. The cytoplasm is reduced to wisp-like strands, often in its radiate arrangement resulting in the appearance of the so-called *stellate* cells (Fig. 24, *Y*). Occasionally both cytoplasm and nuclei of several cells have disappeared, leaving a clear space (Fig. 24, *O*). This reticulation is usually interpreted as a hydropic phenomenon. Its appearance is somewhat similar to that of a markedly œdematous tissue. The small clear spaces do not have the rounded contour of fat globules. Elsewhere viable squamous epithelium, which lines the cyst cavity, shows such reticular changes in varying degrees.

In places hyperplastic changes have occurred in the epithelium which surrounds the keratinized stratified masses. Such epithelium lies in the stroma as strands (Fig. 20, E) or irregular collections of atypical squamous epithelial cells (Fig. 21, E), or separates the masses of dead epithelium from the underlying fibrous zone. The individual cells are much larger and tend to stain more pinkly. The nuclei are likewise large and very vesicular (Fig. 21, insert), taking the stain lightly. A number of hyperchromatinized cells are found and a few atypical mitoses (Fig. 21, M). These atypical cells are continuous, with characteristic modified squamous epithelium, and also show occasional intercellular bridges. Frequently single or small numbers of such cells have undergone keratinization. These cells are of many shapes; large round or polygonal cells are present, but a tendency to an irregular spindle shape is more frequent. It is interesting that these hyperplastic epithelial cells occur only between the fibrous zone of the wall and the edge of the cyst cavity. Nowhere do they compose the invasive processes which have penetrated the fibrous zone of the wall. Despite this, one must attribute to them a local malignant nature on account of their cytological features and invasion of the stroma. The cells individually resemble cells of spindle-cell carcinoma rather than the less malignant basal-cell type.

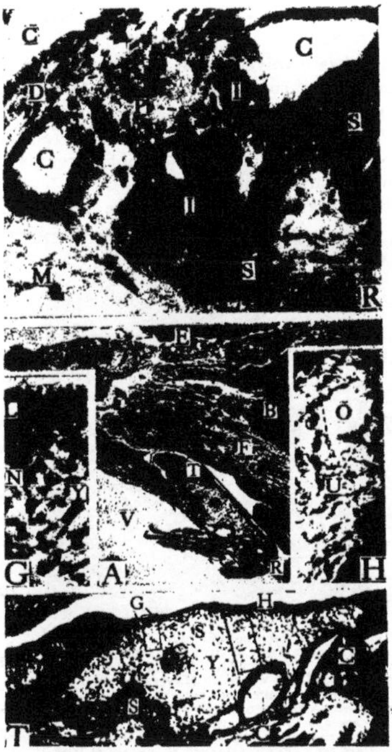

Keratinization has involved groups of cells varying from a few cells concentrically arranged, resembling epithelial pearls (Fig. 18, P), to large stratified masses Fig. 23, E), which may be so numerous as to fill the lower-power field of the microscope.

Fig. 24.—Case III. The central area (A) is a low-power photomicrograph of tissue from the base of the cyst. The enclosed area (T), enlarged slightly in the insert below, shows typical adamantinoma characters. The enlarged squared area (G), left central insert, shows the typical palisaded peripheral layer of columnar epithelium (L). At S and N one sees the spindle-shaped epithelial cells of the subperipheral, and at Y the reticulated star-shaped cells of the central zone. The process of reticulation with atrophy of the cells leads to an occasional hiatus (O, insert H), surrounded by shrunken nuclei (U). The presence of cystic spaces (C) is better shown in the insert above: an enlargement of the small boxed area (R). The cystic spaces (C) are lined with cuboidal epithelium (D). At I are calcified masses filling spaces in which a trace of an original epithelial lining (P) may be seen. These masses (I) are probably a calcified secretory product. At E are other traces of reticulated epithelial lining in which calcific concretions may be seen. At F the fibrous wall. B = area of hemorrhage, V = central cavity of the large cyst.

These large areas may be completely deprived of blood supply, and isolated small vessels plugged with calcific concretions are found occasionally in the surrounding stroma. The cell and nuclear outlines (Fig. 25, R, E and n) may usually be recognized, the nucleus appearing as a round, almost colorless, space in the pink cytoplasm. Occasionally, however, the cell outlines have largely disappeared, the cell bodies having fused into a homogeneous, shining, hyalinized mass, in which traces of the original cell outlines may be seen very indistinctly (Fig. 21). The degenerative changes in the epithelial masses apparently have no definite relation to the vascularity of the adjacent stroma.

Calcification has involved the dead epithelium to an extent varying from a light *dusting* of amorphous blue staining material, often involving only the exterior of a necrotic mass (Fig. 20, *A*), to a diffuse, deep blue staining of an entire group of cells (Fig. 29, *I*). Sometimes the calcium salts are present in granular form, but such granules are not as regular in outline, discrete, or densely staining as the keratohyalin granules.

Foreign-body giant-cell reaction is an interesting phenomenon in its relation to the keratinized and calcified epithelium. This foreign-body reaction seems somewhat greater where the stroma is young and vascular in appearance. These giant-cells are formed in the stroma possibly owing to the presence of calcium salts. It appears that they are engaged in dissolving out the calcium salts and in phagocytozing the necrotic epithelium. Evidence of this is seen in a number of places. Instances are noted where the stratified masses of dead epithelium have retained the calcium salts save where foreign-body giant-cells lie closely applied to the periphery

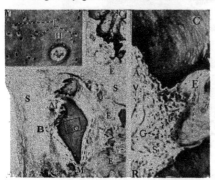

FIG. 25.—Case III. A low-power photomicrograph showing the presence of an island of osseous tissue at *B*, closely associated with adjacent areas of dead epithelium (*A*). The squared area is enlarged above in the insert (*Y*) where an Haversian canal (*H*) is plainly shown; near by are a number of bone cells (*I*). Below at *M* are Vascular spaces. A cluster of partly calcified keratinized stratified epithelial masses at *C*. Non-calcified similar epithelium at *E*. Stroma=*S*. In the insert (*R*) at the right two foreign-body giant cells (*G*) are seen closely attached to a mass of keratinized stratified epithelial cells (*E*). The outlines and some of the nuclear shadows (*n*) of these necrotic cells are shown. At *C* is a similar mass but calcified at its periphery (*A*). Blood-Vessels =*V*. Stroma=*S*.

(Fig. 25, *G*). Regarding the phagocytic action, it is sufficient to note that in a number of instances fragments of dead epithelium are seen partially encircled (*cf.* Fig. 12, *G*) or engulfed by foreign-body giant-cells. Other instances are observed of isolated small nests of dead epithelium which are rimmed, invaded, and partially absorbed by these giant-cells.

True bone, with Haversian canals (Fig. 25, *B*, *H*) and viable bone corpuscles (Fig. 25, *I*), is present in the tumor. The osseous processes stain a deep lavender to blue color, and often have a peripheral zone of pink-colored bony matrix (osteoid tissue), which contains immature bone corpuscles. All areas in which bone formation is taking place seem to be associated with surrounding or adjacent zones of vascular stroma (Fig. 25, *V*, *S*), which often are somewhat myxomatous in appearance, and show a scattering of lymphocytes and plasma cells. At the periphery of calcified epithelial masses foreign-body giant cells (acting as phagocytes) are often present (Fig. 29, *G*), and where bone is being laid down osteoblasts are to be seen

(Fig. 28, O). Thus a process is present which finds its analogy in normal ossification of the long bones, viz., there is a substitution of osseous tissue for the calcified tissue, and never a direct conversion of the pre-existing tissue (calcified epithelium, or in the case of the long bones, calcified cartilage matrix or degenerating cartilage cells) into bone.

The processes of ossification is taking place at the periphery of keratinized epithelial processes (Figs. 26 and 27). In the interior areas of such processes as are almost completely ossified at the periphery (Fig. 27) substitution of bone for dead epithelium proceeds without the intermediation of extraneous

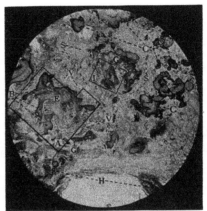

FIG. 26.—Case III. A low-power photomicrograph showing the close relation between the masses of keratinized (necrosed) epithelium and the newly formed bone tissue. At E is a mass of keratinized epithelium which is being replaced by bone tissue growing in from the periphery. An enlargement of this squared area (A) is shown in the next figure. Smaller masses of dead (keratinized) epithelium are shown at C, all of which are partly calcified, the calcium slats in most instances being deposited at the periphery. Other areas of bone formation are shown at G. These islands of tissue lie strewn through a young fibrous stroma (S) which is unusually vascular (V) near the areas of bone formation. The squared area (I) is enlarged in a subsequent figure. Hemorrhagic areas at H.

phagocytes (foreign-body giant-cells) or of stroma (Fig. 27, N), the growing bone cells apparently possessing the property of absorption of dead

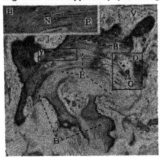

FIG. 27.—Case III. An enlargement of the squared area (A) of Fig. 26. The layers of stratified dead epithelium (E) are more clearly visible. This is almost surrounded by bone (B) which is growing into and replacing the dead tissue: a *substitutive* and not a "*metaplastic*" process. The small squared area (Y) is shown in the insert above further enlarged. Here one sees the nuclei (N) of bone cells which are extending into the keratinized epithelium (E). At I is the most peripheral zone of uncalcified newly formed bone. V = blood-vessels. The larges squared area containing an island of bone (D) and two prominent giant cells (G) is further enlarged in Fig. 28.

epithelium and calcium salts and of proliferating. Here the advancing line of ossification is irregular, single, newly formed bone cells lying somewhat in advance of their fellows (Fig. 27, N). Such newly formed bone cells have the calcium content (as denoted by their dark staining) of adult bone cells, apparently having directly appropriated the calcium content of the necrotic epithelium. The newly formed bone tissue follows closely the lines of stratification (often curvilinear) of the dead tissues which is being replaced. Not always is the internal limit of osseous advance irregular; sometimes it is sharply delimited (Fig. 28, D, E).

Hypophysis. — The hypophyseal sections are grossly of normal size, although somewhat flattened. The sections contain both anterior and posterior lobes. There seems to be

48   737

WILLIAM C. DUFFY

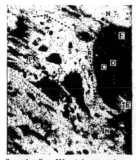

FIG. 28.—Case III. A further enlargement of the area (D, G) squared in Fig.
27. At G are foreign body giant-cells
which are phagocytozing hyalinized
strands (N) of dead epithelium. At the
right is an area of newly formed bone
(D). R is the zone of newly formed bone
matrix, incompletely calcified, closely
applied to the periphery of which are two
osteoblasts (O). Two of the latter have
been enclosed in the bone and become
mature bone corpuscles (C). Also
growth of bone is shown into the dead
epithelium, the outlines of several adjacent keratinized cells with faintly visible
nuclear spaces being apparent at E.
Stroma = S.

possibly a slight increase in eosinophilic
elements throughout the anterior lobe.
Chromophobe and basophile cells are relatively very few in number. There is a
small (150µ) area found in which the neu-
trophile elements are hyperplastic and the
stroma decreased in amount; the area is
circumscribed, but not encapsulated, resembling somewhat a miliary adenoma.
The pars intermedia shows only a few
rather small tubules filled with colloid; no
large colloid cysts are present.

Thyroid.—The picture is essentially a
normal one. Practically all of the vesicles
are filled with colloid. There is no tendency to hyperplasia.

Adrenal.—Shows nothing abnormal
save perhaps a slightly increased vacuoli-
zation of the cells of the zona fasciculata.
Perhaps a slight diminution in size of
the gland.

Ovaries.—Grossly were noted as small.
In the microscopic preparations they seem
slightly smaller than normal. No corpus
luteum is found. Numerous cysts are
present, from 2 to 4 millimetres in diam-
eter. These are filled with a finely granular, pink-staining, homogeneous
material, which represents the gelatinous material seen macroscopically in
the formalin-fixed specimen. These cysts (Fig. 30, O) are lined by young
connective-tissue elements, which show occasional mitoses, apparently a
growth acceleration in an effort to fill in the cavities. Numerous primordial
and a few developing follicles in
the cortex, but no nearly mature follicles.

Salpinges.—Sections from one
of the Fallopian tubes show a
definite, rather early miliary
tuberculosis (Fig. 30, S), which
in the gross was at first unsuspected. The lumen on reëxamination of the gross specimen is
seen to be occluded near the
fimbria for a distance of 1 cm.
by opaque-looking material. The
other tube is patent throughout.

Uterus.—Macroscopically was
slightly below normal size, measuring 5.5 cm. in length, and of
normal relative thickness.

Microscopically the endometrium shows an atrophy (Fig.
30, U), which closely approaches
that of the senile type. The sur-

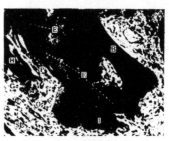

FIG. 29.—Case III. An enlargement of the squared
area I of Fig. 26. The dead epithelium (E) is being
replaced by bone. At B is a large mass of bone
containing mature bone cells. Part of the periphery
of E is invested by a layer of newly deposited bony
matrix (P) which is in turn approximated by a
number of osteoblasts (O). Two of the latter at e
are seen entering the osseous matrix (P) to take up
the rôle of bone cells. Note the greater activity of
the stroma cells (S) in the left lower corner than
above near X (vascular spaces) where bone formation has ceased. Giant cell formation at G near a
spine of dead epithelium (H) with calcified periphery. At I a mass of solidly calcified epithelium.

738

face epithelium has retrogressed to a flatter type or is desquamated entirely in places. The endometrium is greatly diminished in thickness, and the uterine glands very few in number, small and atrophic in appearance. The interglandular tissue is greatly increased in amount, and near the surface in places is of a definite fibrous character. The atrophy of the glandular tissue is present also in the cervical region to an equal extent.

Pancreas.—Certainly no increase in number or size of the islands. No fibrosis.

Kidney.—Normal.

No other tissues available (partial autopsy).

Summary of Case III.—In a young married woman, twenty years old, the first symptom of intracranial tumor was the establishment of persistent amenorrhœa at seventeen years of age. A year later there was a transient attack of hemianopsia associated with severe headache; this was not followed by other severer attacks until over a year afterwards, when failing vision and general pressure symptoms supervened. The

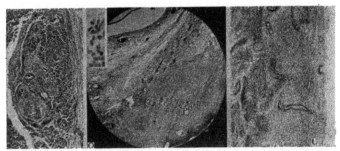

Fig. 30.—Case III. At *S* a conglomerate tubercle without caseation from the unilateral early tuberculous salpingitis. At *O* a photomicrograph of the ovarian cortex showing (above) the edge of one of the large cysts and below (P) numerous primordial follicles. The small upper insert shows a mitosis from the wall of one of the cysts, which, however, are not malignant. At the right is shown the endometrium (*U*) which presents practically a senile picture. The individual was twenty years old but had had amenorrhœa for four years.

röntgenogram showed a calcified area just above the sella, and the *fundi* showed a marked post-neuritic atrophy. Following evacuation of the suprasellar cyst by means of a lateral craniotomy there was relief of pressure symptoms for three months, followed by a gradual return of the old *status*. After the second operation (partial extirpation of lining of cyst) the patient succumbed.

The autopsy studies demonstrate the presence of a partly calcified suprasellar cyst, apparently developed from a squamous epithelial inclusion of the hypophyseal duct, which had compressed the third ventricle above and was separated from it only by a thin membrane (Figs. 15 and 16). Histologically, the cyst showed a squamous epithelial lining with the so-called adamantinoma structure, associated with small areas of localized malignant epithelial hyperplasia, and other areas of interesting calcification of masses of dead keratinized epithelium which showed partial replacement by osseous tissue growing into the dead epithelium from the stroma. Involved in the process of absorption and replacement of the keratinized and calcified epithelium was a marked foreign-body giant-cell reaction (see photomicrographs) and other cellular changes apparently analogous with the normal skeletal process of ossification. The ovaries of this twenty-year-old girl showed a cessation of ovulation with absence of corpora lutei. The endometrium showed histologically a marked atrophy resembling the senile type. The hypophysis, thyroid, adrenals, and pancreas showed no apparently important histological alteration. The anatomical diagnosis of this case may be rewritten as follows: Suprasellar calcifying cystic squamous epithelial tumor of infundibulum (developed from an inclusion of the hypophyseal duct), with adamantinoma characters, localized malignant epithelial hyperplasia, degenerative and osseous regenerative changes; compression of aqueduct of Sylvius; internal hydrocephalus (slight); atrophy of endometrium; adiposity (slight). Operations: (1) Lateral craniotomy, evacuation of cyst; (2) partial extirpation of lining of cyst wall; cerebral œdema. Subsidiary: Early unilateral tuberculous salpingitis (primary (?)—incomplete autopsy).

A histological study is presented in the next case of a true Rathke pouch cyst, which is strikingly different from, although sometimes confused with, hypophyseal duct cystic tumors such as those presented above.

CASE IV.—*Ciliated columnar epithelial-lined cyst developing from an inclusion of Rathke's pouch, associated with a huge adenoma, in an elderly negro man. Intracranial and subsellar extension of tumor with displacement of Rathke cyst into sphenoidal cavity. Primary optic atrophy. Operation. Death. Autopsy.*

Abstract of J. H. H. Surgical History No. 40428½, a negro male laborer fifty years old, was transferred August 14, 1916, to the Surgical Service of the Johns Hopkins Hospital from the medical service, to which he had been previously admitted complaining of "blindness."

The history is negative save for an injury (struck by a rock) to the left eye at the age of twenty-five, following which dimness of vision of the left eye resulted permanently. He continued to work as a day laborer handicapped by the practical loss of one eye until November, 1915, when failing vision in the other eye compelled him to stop work.

Apparently there had been no vomiting, headache, ataxia or convulsive episodes.

Examination.—A well-nourished, well-developed elderly negro of short stature. General examination quite negative except for complete blindness due to double optic atrophy (ophthalmoscopic), immobile pupils, and moderate impairment of hearing in both ears. Röntgenographic report (Dr. F. H. Baetjer): Destruction of sella, suggesting tumor. Wassermann: Negative. Urine: Negative.

Operation (August 15, 1916, Doctor W. E. Dandy).—Through the left lateral approach a tumor in the hypophyseal region about the size of an orange was removed which weighed 77 grams. The tumor

740

was firmer than most adenomas, and save for its attachment at the sella shelled out much like a dural endothelioma.

The patient died about nine hours after the operation.

For the pathological material I am indebted to Dr. Montrose T. Burrows who made the autopsy.

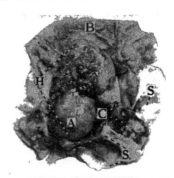

FIG. 31.—Case IV. Shows the under surface (H) of the portion of the adenomatous tumor of case IV which has expanded the sella and broken into the sphenoid. The sphenoid walls (S) and the basilar process (B) have been reflected and the distended pear-shaped cyst (C) attached to the capsule of the adenoma is shown. The histology of this cyst is shown in Figs. 32 and 33.

Autopsy (No. 4787).—*Anatomical Diagnosis.* Adenoma of anterior lobe of hypophysis. Destruction of sella turcica. Infiltration of basilar process of occipital bone. Operation: Enucleation of extension of tumor under frontal lobe. Bronchopneumonia. Encapsulated apical tuberculosis (bilateral); fibrous pleurisy, pericarditis, and perisplenitis.

Body.—Height 5 ft. 5 2/3 in. (163 cm.). A well-nourished dark mulatto. Musculature well developed. Genitalia of normal size; testes of normal consistency.

Head.—The skin flap on the left side measures 15 x 10 cm. in diameter; the opening in the skull measures 12 x 8.5 cm.

After injection *in situ* with 10 per cent. formalin the brain was removed, and the sella, together with adjacent parts of the base of the skull, removed *en masse*.

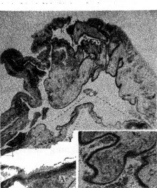

FIG. 32.—Case IV. Low power (10 diams.) photomicrograph of collapsed wall of cyst shown in Fig. 31. The wall is ruptured at R. The proximal wall (Y) of the cyst has been stripped away from the capsule covering the adenoma (A). C = cavity of collapsed cyst. The convoluted character of the cyst wall is shown above. The squared area (V) is shown enlarged in the insert at the lower right. F = connective-tissue stroma of one of the convoluted projections. E = tall ciliated columnar epithelial lining. G = desquamated epithelial cells.

Doctor Burrows kindly gave me the autopsy material for further study. His thorough autopsy is only partly abstracted above. (The lesions of the other organs—see anatomical diagnosis—being irrelative.) A study of the large hypophyseal adenoma may be included in a subsequent publication.

Description of Cyst.—The sella (Fig. 31) is filled with solid tumor, the cut surface of which at the top is level with what is left of the eroded clinoids. The sella measured 2.5 cm. antero-posteriorly, 2.4 transversely, and 1.7 cm. vertically.

On dissecting away the bone fragments adherent to the under surface of the intrasellar portion of tumor, the sphenoidal cavities were seen to be filled by solid growth and two small cysts, the larger of which (Fig. 31, C) measured 1.5 cm.

WILLIAM C. DUFFY

in diameter, and was attached by a narrow pedicle to the capsule of the solid growth. On puncture of the larger cyst a few drops of fluid escaped. There was no cystic change in the solid tumor in the vicinity of the pedicle of the cyst.

Microscopic Examination.—The cyst wall is composed of fibrous tissue, with occasional myxomatous and hyaline areas. Extending into the cyst cavity are numerous thick convoluted, papillary infoldings of fibrous tissue (Fig. 32). Both wall proper and papillary projections are lined with a single layer of very tall, ciliated, columnar epithelium (Fig. 33, *E*), which shows occasional goblet cells (mucous secretory). In the wall of the cyst one sees groups of numerous gland-like structures, such as often are seen in the region of the cleft between the anterior and posterior lobes. Some of these glands contain a colloid-like material. A few groups of cells are seen composed of large polygonal cells, which are larger in the centre of the group. Here one sees occasional intercellular bridges. The wall of the cyst is directly continuous with the capsule of the solid tumor at either extremity of the section. Throughout the wall there is a scattering of polymorphonuclears, plasma, and mast cells. Large numbers of desquamated, ciliated, columnar, epithelial cells (Fig. 32, *G*) lie in places in the cavity of the cyst.

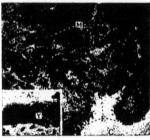

FIG. 33.—Case IV. A somewhat higher magnification showing groups of glands (*M*) in the wall of the cyst similar to ones which occur commonly in the pars intermedia in the vicinity of Rathke's cleft between the anterior and posterior lobes of the hypophysis. *R* = round cell infiltration. At *E* the columnar epithelial lining with ciliated periphery is seen. In the insert *Y* = the layer of palisaded cells, with ciliated zone at *A*. *P* = leucocyte.

Summary of Case IV.—This case is presented so briefly above that a summary is hardly necessary. The case is included solely on account of the presence of the small cyst which is an example of those which it is desired to show are distinctly different from the squamous-cell cysts detailed above. Lined with a single layer of ciliated columnar epithelium the wall contained a number of gland-like colloid-containing structures easily recognizable as constituents of pars intermedia. These furnish additional proof of the origin of the cyst from the vicinity of Rathke's cleft, probably either from the cleft itself or from a persistent embryonic diverticulum thereof. The location of the cyst in the sphenoid cavity is readily explained by pressure of the superimposed enormous hypophyseal adenoma, weighing nearly 100 grams, which had destroyed the floor of the sella.

DISCUSSION

Etiology.—Although the inciting factor or factors in the etiology of hypophyseal duct tumors remains obscure, some light has been thrown on the probable circumstances of origin. The demonstration of Erdheim of persistent fetal inclusions of squamous epithelium in the precise position of origin of these tumors in a large percentage of normal hypophyses points clearly to the significance of the embryonal (Cohnheim) theory in these tumors. The early age at which a number of these tumors have become large enough to cause symptoms is also a fact favoring the congenital nature of the tumor anlage. One case has been reported (Erdheim, 1906) in which the individual succumbed when only five years old, and a large malignant squamous epithelial tumor ("hypophysengang carcinom") was found. Among other cases occurring in later infancy or early youth are those of: Zenker (1857), aged nine years; Walker (1902), nine and one-half years; Erdheim's (1904) Case III, eleven years; Case II of the writer, eleven years. Three other cases of Erdheim (1904) were sixteen, twenty, and twenty-one years old, respectively, in which adolescent group belong the Case III of the writer, the case reported by Jackson and Kanavel, and a number of others. Jackson (1916), from a study of 38 cases in the literature, stated that 33 per cent. occur under twenty years of age, 42 per cent. between twenty and forty years, and 25 per cent. over forty years. As to sex the cases were about equally divided. Trauma has been only rarely associated as a possible factor.

CASES COLLECTED FROM THE LITERATURE

JACKSON (1916) reported an hypophyseal duct tumor and assembled thirty-seven others from the literature. To these thirty-eight should be added the following seventeen cases, many of which were apparently overlooked by Jackson. Possibly there are a number of other reports I have been unable to find, particularly in Teutonic periodicals of the war period, which are not yet fully available. Also there are a number of disputable cases, such as that of Ehlers (1910), which I will not list. The older cases collected by Erdheim of Boyce and Beadles, not confirmed histologically, are not included. However, a number of undoubted additional reported tumors belong in this group, and of these I have found the following: (1) Gotzl and Erdheim (1905) in a chiefly clinical study reported the pathology of a tumor apparently similar to that reported by Saxer (1902). (2) Erdheim (1906) reported an additional tumor, a solid and cystic, "*hypophysenganggeschwulste*," in a five-year-old child. (3) Fahr (1918). (4) Schwab (1913). (5) Guiseppe Masera (1910), and (6) Mensinga (1897), reported very malignant spinal-cell carcinomas of this group, in which has been placed also the case of (7) Rothmann (1893). (8) Case II of Strada (1911), "a benign, multilocular, cystic, papillary, squamous, epithelial tumor of the hypophyseal duct," previously reported by Buhecker in a Strassburg (1893) dissertation simply as, "a cystic tumor of the hypophysis," is not contained in Jackson's table under either Buhecker's or Strada's name, and should be included. (9) The "papillary tumor of the hypophysis" of Gut (1899) apparently was overlooked by both Erdheim and Jackson. (10) The case of Makay and Bruce (1909), of "epithelioma of the hypophyseal duct" belongs and is apparently the best example of the resemblance which these tumors may have for the basal-cell epithelioma of skin. (11) Farnell (1911) recorded a typical tumor. (12) Teutschlaender (1914) described a "cystic, carcinomatous, hypophyseal-duct adamantinoma." (13) Harms in the same year added one, and (14) Warthin in 1916 described an adamantinomatous tumor. These, with the three examples (Cases I, II and III) of the writer, when compiled with the thirty-eight cases tabulated by Jackson in 1916, bring the total number of cases assembled from the literature to fifty-five.

WILLIAM C. DUFFY

Nomenclature.—The differentiation of the squamous equithelial tumors of hypophyseal duct origin from the majority of " cholesteatomas " and " dermoids " of the subdural space was indicated by Erdheim (1904) and has been emphasized more recently by Teutschlaender (1914; p. 243). It is believed that the squamous cell rests from which most dermoids and cholesteatomas arise are carried into the cranium coincidently with the closure of the cerebral vesicles. It was pointed out that basal cholesteatomas rarely lie in the midline and are often situated below the tentorium, whereas hypophyseal duct tumors are found just behind (or below) the optic chiasm, or fill the sella, and a connection with the infundibulum or hypophysis is always demonstrable when the growth is small or of moderate size.

In the smaller field of tumors whose location pointed to an origin either from the hypophysis, infundibulum or from the third ventricle or its choroid plexus there are a number of squamous epithelial tumors in the literature attributed to ependymal or choroid plexus origin. There is the " Ependymal Papilloma " of. Selke (1892); the Papilloma of the choroid plexus " of Fahr (1903); the " Epithelioma of the plexus choroideus " of Ziegler (1902); and the " Epithelial (carcinomatous ?) tumor of the infundibulum and the third ventricle " of Saxer (1902). In most of these cases the tumor had closely involved or broken into the ventricle. Ingermann (1889) described a tumor arising in the sella containing cysts, epithelial pearls, intercellular bridges, and calcified material, and diagnosed " Hypertrophy of the hypophysis with cystic degeneration of the stroma." Erdheim's Case VII appears to have been first referred to by Rokitansky (1856) in his text-book and later (Erdheim, 1904, p. 674) correctly diagnosed as an hypophyseal duct tumor. Bregman and Steinhaus (1907) called their tumor a " Squamous cell epithelioma of the hypophysis." Höhl (1903) considered an origin from the pia mater: " Cystic pial-endothelioma.' '

Onanoff (1892) was the first to note the resemblance to adamantinomata of the jaw, and designated his tumor as an " Epithelioma of the anterior lobe of the hypophysis," stating that its structure was strong evidence of its ectodermal origin. Contrariwise, Walker (1902), finding calcified material with spongy bone in a tumor which apparently developed in the infundibulum, diagnosed a " Primary Osteoma of the Brain," and, concerning other osseous tumors of the brain described in the literature, decried " the looseness of description of the earlier writers " which " render their cases worthless when an attempt is made to collect examples of this form of growth."

. From this veritable melting pot of terms have emerged a few which may be correctly and expressively used in naming the majority of squamous epithelial tumors of the hypophyseal region. *"Hypophyseal duct tumor"* (*" hypophysenganggeschwulste "*), the term originating with Erdheim (1904), is in good standing, as also is the designation of nearly similar meaning "craniopharyngeal duct tumor." Bregman and Stein-haus (1907) suggested the term "squamous-cell epithelioma of the hypophysis," since "the hypophyseal duct exists for only about half the duration of fetal life." The term "adamantinoma," first applied by Onanoff (1892), indicates a tumor of the above origin with the specification of its particular histological differentiation into a structure resembling the neoplasms arising from rests of the *enamel organ* in the jaw. Since there is considerable variation in both the gross and microscopic appearance of these tumors, some of which are neither adamantinomas nor epitheliomas, the term "squamous epithelial hypophyseal duct tumor of the hypophysis and infundibulum" has suggested itself to the writer as especially applicable, indicating at once their fundamental histological and embryological derivation.

Clinical Diagnosis and Importance of Röntgenography.—The frequent association (70 per cent., according to Jackson) of the dystrophia adiposo-genitalis syndrome together with the early appearance of primary optic atrophy, in contrast with the comparatively unusual or late occurrence of choked disk, has been emphasized (D. Lewis, 1910). At variance with the statement of Jackson (1916) that röntgenography is usually negative in hypophyseal duct tumors, the röntgenograms (Dr. F. H. Baetjer) were positive in all three of the above cases. In the röntgenogram of Case I, in which the tumor developed from a squamous-cell inclusion beneath the capsule of the anterior lobe, the sella was widely dilated and the clinoids eroded. This tumor was an intracystic squamous epithelial papillary tumor of relatively simple histology. In the röntgenograms of Cases II and III there were suprasellar calcified nodules, and in neither case was the sella enlarged. In both the tumor was suprasellar and each tumor presented adamantinoma characters with extensive necrosis of epithelium and subsequent calcific deposition. In two of Erdheim's cases in which röntgenograms were made suprasellar shadows caused by calcified material were found, but it does not appear that the diagnosis was made *intra vitam*. It seems that the finding of a shadow of a suprasellar calcified nodule in the X-ray plate of an individual with symptoms of intracranial tumor is highly suggestive of a calcifying squamous epithelial adamantinomatous tumor of hypophyseal duct inclusion origin. In scarcely any other condition in the vicinity of the sella turcica does such a localized nodular calcification occur. However, Dandy and Heuer (1916, Case V) referred to a single instance of such a shadow in a tumor, verified at operation, as developing from the optic nerve sheath. In another instance (Case VI) the same writers reported an interesting case of extensive dense calcification within the sella in an individual totally blind, but there was no opportunity for certification of the lesion.

As to the probable frequency of röntgenographic shadows due to calcification in squamous epithelial tumors of hypophyseal duct origin and basing an opinion on the frequency of the adamantinomatous type which is so prone to calcification and osseous changes, it would appear that such shadows might be expected to be found in something like one-half of all squamous epithelial hypophyseal or suprasellar (infundibular) tumors, or, in other words, in the majority of tumors of the adamantinomatous type. The röntgenographic examination must be made by those specially trained. In a röntgenographic study of a hundred cases of brain tumors reported by Heuer and Dandy (1916) note is made of a certified tumor (Case III of the present paper) in which a similar shadow was present which by another observer had been considered normal; hence the röntgenologist should be familiar with the limits of normal variation in size and shape of the clinoid processes.

With regard to the question of differential röntgenographic diagnosis, another condition occurring in the vicinity of the sella may be briefly mentioned here which was also reported by Heuer and Dandy in the same monograph. The röntgenograms of a white man twenty-eight years old for four years a sufferer from intracranial pressure and ocular symptoms, showed extensive calcific concentric incompletely circular shadows indicating the periphery of a large mass above the sella. At autopsy a mass 24 cm. in diameter was found which was composed of two aneurisms, of the right and left internal carotid arteries, respectively. Heuer and Dandy in retrospect considered the ring-like shadows as rather characteristic of aneurism, as they found no similar calcification reported in the literature in any case of true tumor.

Histological Classification of Hypophyseal Duct Tumors.—Erdheim classified the tumors reported by him according to whether malignant or benign and whether the tumor had developed in the infundibulum or the hypophysis. It is doubtful that his alleged malignant tumors showed unmistakable metastases and he made no reference to the tumors with outspoken spinal-cell carcinoma characteristics, including obvious metastases.

The hypophyseal duct derived tumors may be conveniently placed in three groups arranged with regard chiefly to the microscopic morphology. The *first* is that of the simple papillary cyst, or intracystic papilloma with intracystic cauliflower papillomatous structure (Case I of the writer, cases of Selke (1891), Cornil and Ranvier (1881), Ziegler, and others). These intracystic papillary tumors are the simplest in structure and save when they have broken through the floor of the ventricle (pressure destruction) retain the simplest characters; the wall of the cyst usually shows no invasion.

The *second* group embraces the simpler and the more complicated adamantinomas, including the " autochthonous teratoids " of Ewing. Of the simpler adamantinomas the Case II of the writer is an example, while Case III is of more complex nature, simulating a teratoma, but not of true teratomatous nature. Similar cases are those of Hecht and several of Erdheim. Such tumors show local invasion or localized carcinomatous degeneration, but do not metastasize.

The *third* group consists of only five known cases, and so far as I have determined none of them have been referred to in the American literature. The tumors of this group show all the ear-marks of malignant spinal-cell carcinoma and may extensively metastasize. In the fifth case more recently reported by Fahr (1918) the first symptoms were caused by a cervical swelling. At autopsy the growth had replaced the hypophysis, grown through the base of the skull into the pharynx and produced extensive cervical metastases. The other cases referred to as belonging in this group are those of Schwab (1913), Masera (1910), Mensinga (1897), and Rothmann (1892).

From all examples of squamous epithelial tumors or cysts of the hypophyseal duct should be differentiated the *cysts* arising from *Rathke's pouch,* i.e., the *cleft* between the anterior and posterior lobes.

In the following paragraphs other exemplary cases from the literature may be cited and the cases described in this paper discussed and correlated with the classification suggested above.

1. *Benign squamous epithelial papillary cyst, or intracystic papilloma* of the hypophysis or infundibulum. Example: Case I described in detail above. Two cases briefly reported by Cushing (1912) also belong in this group. One of Cushing's cases was a walnut-sized bilocular infundibular papillary cyst filled with a gelatinous substance (after fixation *in situ* with formalin), projecting from the wall of which were numerous verrucous nodules composed of squamous epithelium. The other cyst was larger but of the same gross characters. It seems that these two cases of Cushing represent the simplest form of these tumors, since there was no real papillary growth, but only a few small verrucous excrescences. Cushing (page 289) advanced the hypothesis that " these papillary infundibular cysts " may arise, owing to " developmental aberrations," which " may occur in relation to the neurohypophysis," i.e., the posterior lobe. Cysts of the posterior lobe, however, are rare and usually result from extensions (which may later be cut off) into the posterior lobe of cysts arising from relics of Rathke's pocket, and are lined, as a rule, by ciliated columnar epithelium (*vide infra*).

Case I of this series is of a type corresponding with Cases VI and VII reported by Erdheim in 1904. The latter were Vienna museum specimens with the dates May 23, 1848, and November 28, 1868, respectively. Erdheim's tumors both arose apparently from rests in the infundibulum, the hypophysis was flattened but not destroyed or incorporated in the cyst wall and hung by its pedicle polyp-like below. Erdheim collected a number of cases from the literature in which the cystic tumor was lined with stratified squamous epithelium, but only the cases of Wagner (1861), Cornil and Ranvier (1881), Selke (1891), Langer (1892), and Fahr (1903) showed an intracystic papillary structure resembling that of the case presented above. Often in the literature the term *papillary* is applied on account of small squamous-cell excrescences. Frequently in the reported cases desquamation has occurred to such an extent that only traces of squamous epithelium remain. Neither of Erdheim's two cases showed such extensive proliferation of pedunculated intracystic papillary masses, or stratified squamous epithelium with such well-preserved characters.

The case of Selke (1891) may be briefly abstracted here because it had the same extensive intracystic papillary morphology and at the same time illustrates a source of error in the pathological diagnosis of these particular tumors.

In a forty-two-year-old woman who died following trepanation, the third ventricle was found dilated and filled with a cauliflower-like mass, which involved the floor of the ventricle and extended through the *foramina Monroi* into both lateral ventricles. The villous-like masses composing the tumor were composed of stratified, non-keratinized epithelium, seated on a strong connective-tissue framework. At the base of the brain the tumor arched forward, dragging the chiasm, and was overlaid with pia. The latter also extended directly into the connective-tissue framework of the papilloma. Selke diagnosed "a papilloma arising from the ependyma of the third ventricle floor," and decided that the squamous epithelial rest from which it arose entered the third ventricle during fetal life, when the infundibular region was in intimate relation with the buccal cavity. Erdheim pointed out the thinness of the roof of the cyst in one of his own cases (Case II), and attributed the ventricular involvement in Selke's case to a breaking through of the papilloma mass into the already highly raised third ventricle. That such a mechanism is easily possible may be appreciated from a study of Case III (*vide supra*), and a glance at the photographs in Figs. 14 and 15.

2. *Benign or locally malignant adamantinomatous cystic or solid tumors, of the hypophysis or infundibulum*, often with calcification, not infrequently of "autochthonous teratoid" character, occasionally with basal-cell epithelioma differentiation.

The largest number of hypophyseal duct tumors fall in this group. Cases II and III reported above belong here. The structure shown in the tumor of Case II may be taken as characteristic of the simpler forms of adamantinomata, although the histological possibilities of this tumor should not be considered exhausted by the examination of the fragment of the cyst wall removed at operation.

The resemblance of these tumors to the adamantinomata of the jaw was first noted by Onanoff in 1892, who had in mind the classical work of Melassez (1885). Adamantinomata of whatever location produce a structure which tends to reproduce the essential features of the *enamel organ*. In the histological description above (Cases II and III) the columnar peripheral layer of the neoplastic epithelial processes corresponds with the so-called *inner layer* (of *adamantoblasts*) of the enamel organ, the sub-columnar transitional zone of vesicular epithelial cells with the *intermediate zone*, and the reticulated hydropic central zone of *stellate* epithelial cells with the enamel pulp or middle zone of the enamel organ, respectively. (That such a tumor may develop elsewhere is possible. Ewing (1919, p. 694) quotes B. Fischer as describing an adamantinoma involving the cortex of the shaft of the tibia. For the origin of this tumor a down-

748

growth of embryonal ectoderm was assumed to have penetrated the tibia and differentiated as enamel organ, just as the gingival epithelium does after penetrating the maxilla.) Mallassez demonstrated larger numbers of squamous epithelial-cell " rests " of the enamel organ in the normal mandible, and to these rests, which he designated " *débris epitheliaux paradentaires*," assigned the origin of the mandibular adamantinomas. Furthermore, he interpreted the presence of these cell groups as analogous with the rich dental apparatus of some lower vertebrates and as giving rise to the supernumerary teeth of the so-called third dentitions in the human.

In view of the probable origin of at least some of the *dentigerous* cysts of the jaw (Hildebrand, quoted by Ewing) from structures resembling the enamel organ, it is interesting to note the hypophyseal tumor of suggestive adamantinomatous histology in a seventy-seven-year-old woman reported by Beck (1883) in which a number of actual teeth were present. Thus oncologically one might consider every adamantinoma as a potential producer of teeth. The reader is referred to Beck's article for a collection of cases of true teratomas of the hypophysis. Many of these were associated with epignathi.

The hypophyseal duct adamantinoma produces masses of dead stratified epithelium varyingly calcified. These necrotic cell masses by some (Farnell and Lambert) have been compared to abortive enamel prisms. In unusual instances (Case IV of Erdheim and Case III of the writer) this dead epithelium may be partially replaced by bone.

The not infrequent resemblance of hypophyseal duct tumors to various cutaneous epitheliomas is interesting. The case of Bruce and MacKay (1909) bears a striking resemblance to the frequent basal-cell epithelioma of skin, as also do certain areas of the tumor of Case II described above. It was noted by Erdheim that a rarer epidermoid derived tumor which is located subcutaneously, the so-called calcified epithelioma of the skin, is interestingly similar to the hypophyseal duct tumors which undergo calcific and osseous changes.

Case III is a typical example of the adamantinoma-like tumors arising from squamous-cell inclusions, in which, however, degenerative and regenerative biological processes are active. Consequently, it exhibits a structure more complex and worthy of more careful study than the tumor of Case II. Possibly some pathologists might at once designate such a tumor a " teratoma." However, it consists entirely of squamous epithelium and its associated stroma which have undergone progressive and regressive changes. The epithelium has by degenerative or metaplastic changes produced a sebaceous-like epithelium, but no sweat glands or hair follicles. In a small localized area there was some hyperplasia of squamous epithelium showing malignant characteristics which, however, could scarcely have any general malignant significance. Extensive areas of dead, keratinized, partly calcified epithelium were present as a result

749

of regressive (degenerative) changes. In places these had excited a foreign body reaction on the part of the stroma with production of osteoclasts and osteoblasts and resultant actual bone formation about the partly calcified masses of dead epithelium which were being absorbed. The presence of such osseous tissue where the successive stages of its production can be followed as above indicated with no suggestion of attempted formation of skeletal bony structures does not suggest a congenital osseous anlage. Neither do the connective tissue elements seem present in other than the rôle of stroma. No smooth or striated muscle was found or reproduction of the histology of any somatic glandular elements. A tridermal composition cannot be demonstrated.

Recently an interesting study concerning the formation of bone in calcified epithelial tumors was made by G. W. Nicholson (1917), who studied the formation of bone in a calcified subcutaneous epithelioma (the socalled calcified epithelioma of skin) which had undergone osseous changes. Nicholson was concerned with interpretation of the conversion of pavement epithelium into bone. He was able to show that this took place not by " metaplasia," which is a direct substitution of the cells of one tissue for those of another, but by an indirect process involving several steps, essentially as follows: (1) Death and calcification of the epithelium; (2) proliferation of granulation tissue; (3) formation of foreign body giant cells; (4) a dissolving out of the calcium salts of the epithelium (solvent action of CO_2 as correlated with the hypothesis of Hofmeister (1910) : oxidation in the case of the giant cell being rapid) ; (5) formation of osteoblasts from the fibroblasts of the granulation tissue, stimulated by the concentrated solution of lime salts which has been diffused out of the giant cells; (6) formation of the bony matrix by hyalinization and calcification of the connective tissue fibres. The all-essential factor in this series of steps is the presence of lime salts. The phenomenon is shown clearly to be similar to the normal process of ossification in cartilage (skeletal), the calcified epithelium being comparable with cartilage, the stroma with the bone marrow. In Nicholson's epithelioma of skin the stroma in places somewhat resembled normal bone marrow.

Another interesting histological feature of the tumor of Case III was the finding of typical keratohyalin granules. These were thought by Erdheim to be absent in hypophyseal duct tumors and present only in cholesteatomas. In the tumor of Case III they were found in relatively limited areas in a few of a large number of sections of many different blocks, so that if only a small bit of tissue was available they might not be found. They have been demonstrated before in the cases of Bartels (1906) and Strada (1911), although Jackson (1916) without reference to their findings states that they do not occur in hypophyseal duct tumors. Some weight was attached by Erdheim to the presence or absence of keratohyalin granules in the differential diagnosis between cholesteatomas and tumors of hypophyseal duct origin. That these granules were not demonstrated in some of Erdheim's cases possibly is related to the age and preservation of the specimens, several of which had rested on the museum shelves of the Vienna University for decades.

Cysts of Rathke's Cleft.—A type of cyst (*cf.* Case IV) which should be differentiated from those of squamous epithelial origin arises from Rathke's cleft or residual diverticuli of Rathke's pouch, and is lined by cylindrical (often ciliated) epithelium. Similar cysts may, indeed, arise from traces (*ependymal*) of the formerly existing canal of the posterior hypophyseal lobe. A third origin suggested for these cysts is from " colloid containing glandular epithelial tubules " (Weichselbaum, 1879) in the region of Rathke's cleft, but in this case the lining is not of ciliated epithelium. These cysts are usually " colloid containing," although this can scarcely be of much differential value, and microscopically the lining cells may show colloid droplets. Such cysts are usually small, up to that of a cherry seed, and usually intrasellar. In general, one may say that unless there is strong reason to suspect an ependymal or colloid glandular (*i.e.*, from acini of the pars anterior) origin for such cysts (Case IV) lined with a single layer of ciliated columnar epithelium they may properly be attributed to an origin from the cleft or from a diverticulum of the pouch of Rathke. It is a mistake, on the other hand, to designate to squamous epithelial-lined cysts an origin from Rathke's cleft, since the latter in the fully developed hypophysis is lined only with a single layer of columnar or cubical epithelium. It may be borne in mind that in intracystic papillary squamous epithelial cysts where much desquamation has occurred a cylindrical change may rarely be present (Erdheim), but in fresh or well-preserved specimens this is usually of limited occurrence and associated with other areas of typical squamous epithelium. An origin from Rathke's pouch was erroneously ascribed to the tumors of Cases I and III (above) by other observers.

SURGICAL CONSIDERATIONS

Prognosis.—There is an important surgical consideration directly dependent upon the correct recognition of hypophyseal duct tumors. In the past at operation the neurological surgeon who has explored a suprasellar growth in intimate relation with the third ventricle above, has often thought it derived from the third ventricle. Hereafter on microscopic examination of tissue from the base of a suprasellar cyst (at operation or between operations) the surgeon, after ascertaining the squamous epithelial cell nature of the cystic tumor, may be certain that it is of extra-ventricular origin, and this will guide him in subsequent operative procedures, in the course of which it will be of great importance to him to realize the delicate character of the cyst wall in the neighborhood of the third ventricle floor (*cf.* Figs. 14, 15, and 16), which may otherwise be ruptured in attempts at removal of the lining of the cyst, as the wall between the cyst cavity and third ventricle cavity may consist only of a thin membrane (Case III of the writer, Cases II, III, and IV of Erdheim, and others).

The suprasellar location of the majority of hypophyseal duct tumors may be emphasized. Five out of seven of Erdheim's original series (1904) of tumors developed in the infundibulum, but the entire seven had extended above into the intracranial cavity. Two out of three of the writer's cases arose above the sella (infundibulum), the third arising in the upper part of the anterior lobe, but presenting above the sella in the course of its development. Therefore, in this group of tumors an intracranial mode of approach similar to that devised by Heuer (1918) seems particularly applicable. By no other means than an intracranial approach can the majority of them be properly attacked, and by this route the chance of destroying the hypophysis itself is obviated.

It is entirely possible that the prognosis of these cases may be entirely altered within the next decade. So far as I know at present among this group only the case of Kanavel has survived for over three years and retained his working efficiency. Kanavel's case apparently developed within the sella, since it was successfully attacked transphenoidally. Symptoms having returned after the first two operations, Kanavel applied a tampon of tincture of iodine which was left in for twenty-four hours. This vigorous treatment apparently destroyed the epithelial lining of the cyst. The subsequent history of this patient will be of great interest.

Associated Endocrinopathic Effects.—In addition to the gross somatic change of adiposity which, together with its allied concomitants of the syndrome of Fröhlich, have received the attention of numerous observers, marked histological alterations were present in the genital organs of two of the above considered individuals. Of these the senile changes in the endometrium of the adolescent (Case III) are the rarer and perhaps more interesting, although the histological picture of testicular atrophy in the individual of Case I is of striking distinctness.

Case III was a young married woman in whom amenorrhœa was established over three years before death, being in effect the first symptom. Following the establishment of amenorrhœa her weight had increased from 100 to 130 pounds. At the autopsy the ovaries contained cysts but no corpora lutea, numerous primordial follicles, but no nearly mature follicles. In one tube there was an early tuberculous lesion, the other being perfectly free. Histologically the uterus showed a striking *atrophy* of the endometrium (Fig. 30, U) comparable with that of a senile endometrium.

The endometrical atrophy seems to have been immediately dependent upon the cessation of ovulation and absence of *corpora lutea*. The latter in turn seems dependent upon the intracranial condition. Cushing (1912) has attributed such effects to a shutting off of the secretion of the posterior lobe into the cerebrospinal fluid *via* the infundibulum and third ventricle. Subsequent investigators have questioned his results in the demonstration of such a secretion in the cerebrospinal fluid. In this case the hypophysis showed gross pressure effects, but no correlative histological changes of note.

Histological changes in the thyroid, adrenal, and pancreas were not apparent.

In Case I, a white male, married, thirty-five years old, the patient had regarded his *libido sexualis* as " a little below normal," before the onset of headaches and loss of vision, but after these symptoms appeared his loss of *libido* became complete. In this instance the tumor had developed in the upper part of the anterior lobe and the latter was flattened out saucer-like below but incorporated into the wall of the cyst. The apparent displacement of anterior lobe tissue into the wall of the cyst is so striking as to suggest a glandular transplant in which the blood supply has been preserved and the transplantation gradually effected. The localized necrosis of anterior lobe cells in the wall of the cyst was limited in extent, evidently a recent occurrence, possibly related to the exploratory operation, and could have borne no causal relationship to the testicular changes of long duration.

The testes, of normal size, showed a striking atrophy of the spermatogenous epithelium and absence of spermatogenesis with persistence only of the supporting (Sertoli) cells. The interstitial cells of Leydig were reported present in normal numbers. The interstitial fibrous tissue was increased.

The other glands of internal secretion showed no striking changes. Thymus tissue (15 or 20 grams) was present, but consisted very largely of fat and histologically was evidently a regressive thymus. The origin of the testicular changes is complicated by the presence of clinical serological evidence (positive Wassermann tests on spinal fluid and serum) of syphilis. There are no miliary gummata in the testicle, but occasional small areas of round-cell infiltration. In view of the absence of luetic history (although he confessed having had a urethritis several years before), together with the coincidence of impotence and onset of his intracranial symptoms, it seems that the changes in the testes are probably dependent more upon the tumor than upon a syphilis which left no definite mark. Somewhat similarly in the papillomatous intracystic tumor of Fahr (1903) there was no evidence of other than a coincidental relationship between the tumor and an organic lues.

In Case II, a female child eleven years old, there was no necropsy, but clinically the case is interesting because there is no apparent retardation of secondary sexual characters; on the contrary, they seem slightly accelerated (Fig. 9).

CONCLUSIONS

1. Although there are embryological possibilities for growth of squamous epithelial neoplasms between the pharynx and the sella turcica, the great majority of such tumors develop from squamous epithelial em-

bryonic rests of the hypophyseal duct either in the infundibulum or beneath the upper surface of the anterior lobe of the hypophysis. *Of either
origin the tumor usually presents above the sella.*

2. In view of the fact that a majority of these tumors are suprasellar in
position from the beginning and that nearly all early assume this position, it appears that they are especially suitable surgically for an intracranial approach. In tumors which arise beneath the capsule of the
anterior lobe (*cf.* Case I) the latter becomes flattened out below and a trans-
sphenoidal approach may destroy the entire anterior lobe of the hypophysis.

3. The tumors derived from embryological remnants of the hypophyseal duct are quite different in structure from those derived from Rathke's
pouch or cleft (between the anterior and posterior hypophyseal
lobes). From the duct *reliquii* develop papillary squamous epithelial
cysts (Case I) and solid and cystic, frequently calcified squamous epithelial adamantinomatous tumors (Cases II and III); whereas, from Rathke's
pouch or the cleft develop simpler cysts lined by a single layer of ciliated
cylindrical epithelium (Case IV).

4. The hypophyseal duct tumors histologically may be divided into *three
groups*. *Group I* is that of the papillary cyst or intracystic papilloma
(Case I) which is histologically the most benign example of hypophyseal
duct tumors. *Group II* includes the uncalcified or calcified adamantinomas
(solid or cystic), the rarer tumors which closely resemble the basal
epithelioma of skin (*cf.* case of Bruce and Mackay and Case II of the
writer), and the more complicated adamantinomas (Case III), the " autochthonous teratomas " of Ewing. The tumors of this group may show
criteria of local malignancy, but do not metastasize. *Group III* comprises
a very rare group of cases which show all the ear-marks of malignant
spinal-cell carcinoma and may metastasize extensively to the cervical
lymphatics (Fahr, 1918).

5. The frequent occurrence of calcification in hypophyseal duct tumors is
an important diagnostic fact. At variance with the statement of Jackson (1916) that röntgenography is usually negative, in each adamantinomatous tumor (Cases II and III) described by the writer the röntgenograms showed a suprasellar calcified nodule. The rarity of such
calcified shadows in tumors of other types (adenomas, endotheliomas,
etc.) makes such nodular shadows almost pathognomonic.

6. The occurrence of bone in hypophyseal duct adamantinomas is not due
to the presence of a congenital osseous anlage but is a result of activity
on the part of the stroma, apparently excited by the presence of calcium
salts which have been deposited in the necrotic stratified epithelium.
The mechanism of osseous change is apparently similar to that described
by Nicholson for the same phenomenon in calcified cutaneous epitheliomas.

7. Hypophyseal duct tumors of the infundibulum not infrequently break
into the third ventricle (*cf.* Case III). To the contrary, the tumors of the
ependyma or choroid plexus of the third ventricle are very rarely present in

the suprasellar region; this is explained by spread of the growth along the intraventricular paths of least resistance.

8. During operations on suprasellar cysts in intimate contact with the floor of the third ventricle microscopic demonstration of squamous epithelium from the lining of the cyst will assure the surgeon that the cyst (or solid tumor) originated below the ventricle. A pathological fact of importance for the surgeon to appreciate is the intimate and delicate relation of such cysts with the floor of the ventricle, from which they are frequently separated only by a very thin membrane (Case III).

9. The very frequent occurrence of the clinical syndrome of *dystrophia adiposo-genitalis* (Fröhlich) in patients suffering with hypophyseal duct (squamous epithelial) tumors makes the pathological findings in the genital organs of two individuals (Cases I and III) of particular interest. In the uterus of a twenty-year-old girl (Case III) there was an *atrophic endometrium*, almost equal to that of the senile type, associated with cessation of the process of ovulation (ovaries). The testes of a thirty-five-year-old man showed a marked atrophy of the spermatogenous epithelium.

10. In my study of the literature reports of fourteen additional hypophyseal duct tumors have been found, which when added to the thirty-eight compiled by Jackson in 1916, together with the three cases reported above, bring the total number collected from the literature to fifty-five cases.

In conclusion, I wish to xpress my thanks to Professor W. G. MacCallum of the Johns Hopkins Hospital for the privileges of his laboratory, extended to me for resumption of this work upon my return from overseas. To Dr. G. J. Heuer, Dr. W. E. Dandy, and Dr. M. C. Winternitz I am indebted for the clinical histories and pathological material, and to Dr. F. H. Baetjer for the use of his excellent röntgenograms. The photomicrographs are the result of my own efforts in Professor MacCallum's laboratory.

BIBLIOGRAPHY

Arai, H.: Der Inhalt des Canalis craniopharyngius Anat. Hefte, 1907, 33, 411.

Bartels, M.: Ueber Plattenepithelgeschwülste der Hypophysengegend (des Infundibulums). Ztschr. f. Augenh., 1906, 16, 407, 530.

Beck, H.: Ueber ein Teratom in der Hypophysis cerebri Ztschr. f. Heilkunde, 1883, 4, 393.

von Bonin, G.: Classification of tumors of the pituitary body. Brit. M. J., 1913, 1, 934.

Bregman, L., and Steinhaus, J.: Zur Kenntnis der Geschwülste der Hypophysisgegend. Virchow's Arch. f. path. Anat., 1907, 188, 360.

Bruce and MacKay: Epithelioma of the Hypophyseal Duct. Rev. of Neurol. and Psychiatry, 1909, vii, 445–455.

Christeller, E.: Die Rachendachhypophyse des Menschen unter normalen und pathologischen Verhaltnissen. Virchow's Arch. f. path. Anat., 1914, 218, 185.

Cornil and Ranvier: Cited by Erdheim (1904).

Cushing, H.: The pituitary body and its disorders. Lipp., 1912.

Dandy, W. E., and Goetsch, E.: The blood supply of the pituitary body. Am. J. Anat., 1910–11, 11, 137.

WILLIAM C. DUFFY

Ehlers, H.: Ein Beitrag zur Kenntnis der Infundibularzysten des menschlichen Gehirnes. Virchow's Arch. f. path. Anat., 1910, 199, 542.

Erdheim, J.: Zur normalen und pathologische Histologie der Glandula thyreoidea, parathyreoidea und Hypophysis. Beitr. path. Anat. u. z. allg. Path., 1903, 33, 158.

Erdheim, J.: Ueber Hypophysenganggeschwülste und Hirncholesteatome. Sitzungsb. d. k. Akad. d. Wissensch. Math.-naturw. Cl., Wien., 1904, 113, 537.

Erdheim, J.: Ueber einen neuen Fall von Hypophysenganggeschwülst. Centralbl. f. allg. Path. u. path. Anat., 1906, 17, 209.

Ewing, J.: Neoplastic diseases. Phila., 1919.

Fahr, T.: Papillom an der Basis des dritten Hirnventrikels. München. med. Wchnschr., 1903, 50, 2, 1897.

Fahr, T.: Beitrag zur Pathologie der Hypophysis. Deutsch. med. Wchnschr., 1918, 44, 1, 206.

Farnell, F. J.: An extracerebral tumor in the region of the hypophysis. New York .M. J., 1911, 93, 462.

Götzl, A., and Erdheim, J.: Zur Kasuistik der trophischen Störungen bei Hirntumoren. Zeitschr. f. Heilk., 1905, 26, Abt. f. int. Med., 372.

Haberfeld, W.: Die Rachendachhypophyse, andere Hypophysengangreste und deren Bedeutung für die Pathologie. Beitr. z. path. Anat., u. z. allg. Path., 1909, 46, 133.

Harms, H.: Ueber Hypophysenganggeschwülste. Deutsch. Ztschr. f. Nervenheilk., 1914, 51, 438.

Hecht, D'O.: A teratoma of the hypophysis. J. A. M. A., 1909, 53, 1001.

Herring, P. T.: The histological appearance of the mammalian pituitary body. Quart. J. Exp. Physiol., 1908, 1, 121.

Heuer, G. J., and Dandy, W. E.: Röntgenography in the localization of brain tumor. J. H. H. Bull., 1916, 27, 311.

Heuer, G. J.: A new hypophysis operation. J. H. H. Bull., 1918, 29, 154.

Jackson, H.: Craniopharyngeal duct tumors. J. A. M. A., 1916, 66, 1083.

Jordan, D. S., and Evermann, B. W.: Fishes of North and Middle America, 1896, pt. 1, p. 8.

Kanavel, A. B., and Jackson, H.: Cysts of the hypophysis. Surg., Gyn. and Obst., 1918, 26, 61.

Kon, J.: Hypophysenstudien. I. Seltene Tumoren der Hypophysengegend (Teratom, Peritheliom, telangiectatisches Sarkom). Beitr. z. path. Anat. u. z. allg. Path., 1908, 44, 233.

Langer, L.: Ueber cystische Tumoren im Bereiche des Infundibulum cerebri. Zeitschr. f. Heilk., 1892, 13, 57.

Lewis, D. D.: A contribution to the subject of tumors of the hypophysis. J. A. M. A., 1910, 55, 1002.

Luschka, H.: Der Hirnanhang und die Steissdruse des Menschen. Berl., 1860.

Mallassez, L.: Sur le rôle des débris epitheliaux paradentaires. Arch. de Physiol., 1885, 1, 309; 2, 379.

Margulies, A.: Ueber ein Teratom der Hypophyse bei Kaninchen. Neurolog. Centralb., 1901, 20, 1026.

Masera, G.: Ueber eine interessante Geschwulst der Schadelbasis. Virchow's Arch., 1910, 199, 471.

v. Mihalkovics, V.: Wirbelsaite und Hirnanhang. Arch. f. mikrosk. Anat. u. Entw., 1875, 11, 389.

Nicholson, G. W.: The formation of bone in a calcified epithelioma of the skin. J. of Path., 1917, 21, 287.

Onanoff, J.: Sur un cas d'epithelioma. Thèse de Par., 1892.

Rathke, H.: Ueber die Entstehung der Glandula pituitaria. Arch. f. Anat., Physiol. u. wissensch. Med., 1838, 5, 482.

Rippmann, T.: Ueber einen bisher nicht beobachteten Fall multipler Intrafoetation in- und ausserhalb der Shädelhöhle. Inaug. Diss., Zurich, 1865.

Rothmann, M.: Ueber multiple Hirnnervenlahmung in Folge von Geschwulstbildung an der Schadelbasis, etc. Ztsch. f. klin. Med., 1893, 23, 326.

Salzer, H.: Zur Entwicklung der Hypophyse bei Saugern. Arch. f. mikr. Anat., u. Entw., 1898, 51, 55.

Saxer, F.: Ependymepithel, gliome und epitheliale Geschwülste des Centralnervensystems. Beitr. z. path. Anat. u. z. allg. Path., 1902, 32, 276.

Schwab, W.: Beitrag zur Kasuistik der Schadelbasistumoren. Med. Klin., 1913, 9, 291.

Teutschlaender, O. R.: Zwei seltenere tumorartige Bildungen der Gehirnbasis. Virchow's Arch., 1914, 218, 224.

Walker, J. W. T.: A case of primary osteoma of the brain. Reports of the Society for the Study of Disease in Children, 1902, 2, 172.

Warthin, A. S.: A study of the lipin content of the liver in two cases of dispituitarism. J. Lab. and Clin. Med., 1916, 2, 73.

Wegelin, Bericht ueber die Tatigkeit der St. Gallischen naturwisschaftln. Gesellsch., St. Gallen, 1860.

Ziegler, E.: Lehrbuch der speziellen pathologischen Anatomie, 1902, ed. 10, 403.

THE WAR'S CONTRIBUTION TO CIVIL SURGERY*

By BURTON JAMES LEE, M. D.

OF NEW YORK, N. Y.

PUBLISHED and oral testimony as to the soundness and efficacy of certain new lines of surgical treatment seems to have failed to make its full impress upon the majority of American surgeons. It is highly desirable, therefore, that such a group as ourselves should seriously consider various phases of the surgery of war, inquiring what, if any, application may be made of the knowledge gained, placing this society on record as to its convictions and its practice. Has surgery acquired nothing, leaving its theory and practice just where it was when the war found it? I am of those who believe that a great deal has been given by the war to surgery. This paper represents an effort to find the mind of The New York Surgical Society as to the applicability of certain of the war surgical methods to civil practice. No attempt has been made to cover the whole field, but a certain limited number of topics deemed the most fruitful for discussion have been considered. The following letter and questionnaire were sent to every active member of the Society, numbering seventy, forty-four responding:

DEAR DOCTOR:

I am conducting an inquiry in an effort to find to just what extent certain principles recognized as efficient in the War Zone are being used in civil surgery. If you would be kind enough to answer briefly the enclosed questionnaire I would be very grateful.

I am hoping to make a summary of the questionnaire answers in a paper to be read before the Society in January. Will you, therefore, respond at the earliest convenient moment.

Sincerely,

QUESTIONNAIRE

1. To what extent do you practice primary closure of compound fractures of extremities? Do you approve the principle?
2. To what extent do you use the principle of secondary closure of soft-tissue wounds? Do you approve the principle?
3. To what extent do you use the Carrel-Dakin solution and technic? Do you approve the principle?
4. To what extent do you use the principle of immediate active mobilization in post-operative joint conditions? Do you approve the principle?
5. To what extent do you use the principle of active mobilization in septic joints? Do you approve the principle?

A summary of the various replies to these questions presents the following results:

---

* Read before the New York Surgical Society, January 14, 1920.

758

1. To what extent do you practice primary closure of compound fractures of the extremities? Do you approve the principle?

Five men absolutely opposed the use of this principle. The majority favored its employment in properly chosen cases, and several successful results were reported. In general, considerable wound contamination or extensive muscle injury were considered contraindications to the use of primary suture, and when considerable time had elapsed from the receipt of the injury, caution should be exercised in deciding for primary suture. Some men favored not opening the wound where compounding was small and from within, but others seemed to feel these were above all others the cases to open, as being most favorable, and the writer agrees with the latter opinion. Careful *débridement* of all soiled and devitalized tissues was recognized as essential to a successful result, such dissection including cleaning of the bone-ends when soiled. Several preferred to always make use of Carrel-Dakin wound treatment followed by delayed primary or secondary suture. All agreed that when in doubt as to the dissection having been successful in obtaining a clean wound, primary suture had best not be employed. The more accurate one's *débridement*, however, the less doubt there will be in the surgeon's mind as to the degree of wound disinfection accomplished.

We may then fairly conclude that the practice of primary closure of compound fractures is sound and that the principle is approved, but that the cases should be carefully selected and the surgery well done to achieve success.

2. To what extent do you use the principle of secondary closure of soft-tissue wounds? Do you approve the principle?

The writer has made no attempt to differentiate sharply between delayed primary suture (six to eight days) and secondary suture (any time later) as to indications or technic, as these have been completely discussed in the war literature.

With one exception, there was absolute unanimity in favor of secondary suture and the principles underlying its use, this decision, however, being conditional upon having in hand a Carrel-Dakin supply and technic beyond criticism. The exception noted made use of the procedure "only to avoid subsequent cicatricial contraction."

The Society as a whole, therefore, places itself on record as almost unanimously favoring secondary suture.

3. To what extent do you use the Carrel-Dakin solution and technic? Do you approve the principle?

There was but one viewpoint concerning this question, and that an enthusiastic one for the principle and use of wound sterilization by the Carrel-Dakin technic. The only differences of opinion were those as to its scope, and all appreciated the difficulties of obtaining a faultless technic. The Society is apparently unanimous upon one point: only the accepted technic or none at all. Culture control and bacterial charts are essential to the proper use of the method. It was very gratifying to receive such statements of approval as the following: "As one who has witnessed the transition from antiseptic to aseptic surgery twenty-five to thirty years ago, I regard the demonstration of the fact that septic wounds can be sterilized without damage to the tissues, as the greatest contribution to surgery that the war has made. I do not understand why many able surgeons do not recognize the *new* principle involved in the Carrel-Dakin treatment"; also, "I use the Carrel-Dakin treatment in practically every case of infection." "I look upon the treatment as one of the great advances in surgery"; and, "one of the most important additions to modern surgery."

Certain special points of interest were brought out in the questionnaire.

a. Two large hospital services have practically abandoned the use of the technic because it seemed impossible to provide proper apparatus and solution, and technical difficulties seemed insurmountable. I believe that this Society should stamp any general service where the technic cannot be applied for the reasons stated as not measuring up to the standards of first-class surgery.

b. Two men whom I presume have had but limited experience with the Carrel-Dakin technic felt that surgery alone or surgery plus moist saline dressings gave equally good results. I can only say that experience with a real Carrel-Dakin technic will be the only convincing argument needed for their conversion.

c. As to its use in intra-abdominal abscess cavities, the Society's opinion was divided.

The New York Surgical Society is, therefore, almost unanimously for wound sterilization by the Carrel-Dakin method done properly, and the hospitals of this city must provide apparatus and accurately made solutions, and the surgeons must insist upon faultless technic, that the method may be really available. Following proper surgery, it may, therefore, be used in—

Compound fractures which are unsuitable for primary closure.
Lacerated wounds of soft tissues.
Acute cellulitis.
Osteomyelitis, and
Empyema.

The Carrel-Dakin technic is perhaps the greatest contribution of the war to civil surgery, and it is applicable to numerous groups of cases, both as a prophylactic against infection or to accomplish wound sterilization in the presence of established infection.

4. To what extent do you use the principle of immediate active mobilization in post-operative joint conditions? Do you approve the principle?

The writer, in September, 1918, and again in June, 1919, endeavored to bring home to American surgeons the full significance of Willem's joint surgery, and other writers have added their testimony, but many here in

America still seem ignorant of its principles. Willem's method of immediate active mobilization is thoroughly applicable in civil surgery. It may be used in most of the surgery upon clean joints, such as for movable cartilage of the knee-joint or excision of a small fractured carpal bone or after a traumatism with penetration of a joint, or even, with caution in fracture of the patella. It may also be employed successfully in intra-aritcular fractures without separation and of slight extent. Its use is contraindicated, however, when joint fractures are extensive, or with tendency to displacement, and also in tuberculous joints. The measure then should be applied with judgment.

The motion should be *active* and *immediate* and *frequently repeated.* After the treatment has been instituted, the active motion must be carried out at two-hour intervals in the presence of a nurse or doctor, and the patient is wakened two or three times during the night and encouraged to move the joint.

Two of the members favored passive, rather than active motion, but Willem and Delrez have shown that the latter traumatizes joint tissues less than the former and the degree of pain guides the patient to the limit of active mobilization. *Immediate* active motion may be interpreted to mean any time within the first six post-operative hours, for it is sometimes impracticable to begin earlier, as the patient may hardly be in condition to accomplish much that is really worth while. *No splint* is applied. The dressings over the joint should be loose and no larger than are necessary to insure wound protection and allow for drainage absorption. When feasible, the use of adhesive straps assures the least possible limitation of motion. A tight, large dressing makes any degree of active mobilization impossible. With a knee-joint operated upon for movable cartilage the patient is up and about the ward with crutch support upon the fourth post-operative day and restoration of function may be accomplished in about three weeks.

The results obtained abroad, in those hospitals where the principles were carefully followed through, gave excellent results and justified the enthusiasm of Willem, Delrez, and others for it. Some of the members seem to be wavering between doubt and disapproval as to the efficiency of the method, but experience with the measure must convince them.

It may be said, then, that the majority of the members of this Society are in favor of Willem's method, in dealing with clean joint operations.

5. To what extent do you use the principle of active mobilization in septic joints? Do you approve the principle?

When Willem's method is applied to suppurating joints we have a traditional established mode of treatment thrown rudely into the discard. Many surgeons cannot believe that moving an inflamed septic joint will help the condition and frequently cure it. Some stand aghast and will not or cannot believe. Ten of our members are absolutely opposed to the use of this principle, and a few quotations will illustrate their attitude.

"To my mind to move an active suppurating joint is to add insult to injury. Drainage, rest, and proper local treatment seem to me to be imperative."

"This does not appear to me as reasonable while the process is active nor even when the process has become subacute. After the acute infection has been brought under control and also the swelling and local heat have gone away, then I believe in limited motion every day."

"Not until activity of infection entirely subsided."

"We have had no extended opportunity to practice this type of case. I am not convinced that the principle is sound."

"No experience would doubt its general applicability."

"I confess, however, to a certain amount of fear."

"I would move the elbow in all cases, but not the hip or the knee."

Willem recognized that the only adequate drainage of a septic joint is accomplished by moving it and continuing to move it, lateral openings being the ones usually employed. Active motion will really give the best possible drainage, while immobilization, drainage tubes, and irrigation cannot accomplish this result. I have seen many men with suppurating knees walking about the wards at La Panne with normal knee-joints as regards function and perfectly painless joints, with a thin stream of pus running through the dressings covering their joint wounds and down their legs. These cases were impressive and absolutely convincing. The method is sound, and the experience in practicing it has furnished the proof. It represents a distinct advance in the treatment of septic joints, and it is thoroughly applicable to civil surgery.

The result of our inquiry, therefore, has shown that these types of treatment considered, representing a part of the war's contribution to civil practice, are heartily approved by the majority of the membership of the New York Surgical Society. Only by a thoughtful assimilation and application of such knowledge as the war has developed may the science of surgery truly progress.

SEHRT'S METAL TOURNIQUET FOR PRODUCING ARTIFICIAL ANÆMIA

By Willy Meyer, M.D.
of New York, N. Y.

In the summer of 1916, while looking over some foreign medical literature which, at that time, reached our shores rather sporadically, a brief article of Sehrt's,[1] of the University of Freiburg, entitled " A New Method of Producing Artificial Anæmia " attracted my attention. The author's description of the application of the method greatly appealed to me, and I immediately ordered the instrument through the Kny-Scheerer Company of New York City. Soon after our country entered the war, and the order was not filled.

In the fall of last year, the firm inquired whether I still wanted the tourniquet, to which I replied in the affirmative, and so the instrument reached me in December, 1919. I did not have a chance to try it until early in February of this year, first in a case of amputation of the thigh in its middle, and soon after in an operation for a twice-recurrent sarcoma of the thigh in its posterior aspect. I was so much impressed with the usefulness and simplicity of the device that I made up my mind to present it before the New York Surgical Society.[2]

Since that time I have further employed the tourniquet many times in operations on upper and lower extremities to my entire satisfaction, in no instance did it fail, in no case did it produce a pressure-paresis of one or more nerves of the brachial plexus at the arm.

The tourniquet, made of the best steel, has the appearance of a clamp. The two arms are rounded and bent up at the end; they can be separated sufficiently wide to slip over any size of extremity—thigh or arm (Figs. 1 and 2)—and cross each other when tightened; a thumb-screw, moving on a serrated rod, forces them together as tightly as desired. It can be applied as quickly as these words are spoken, and any ordinarily intelligent person can put it to use. The arms of the instrument are covered with rubber tubing—in emergency cases with cotton or gauze—before the operation, when it is sterilized with the other instruments. It can be placed in position, always within the sterile field, away up at the crotch (Fig. 3) or close to the axilla, best over a piece of gauze or a folded towel wound around the limb (Fig. 4), with the same ease as further down on the extremity. If during an operation the constriction is found too loose, a turn or two of the screw of the instrument, which is covered by the sterile drapings, will make the artificial anæmia complete. When the

---

[1] Münch. med. Wochenschr., May 25, 1916.
[2] At the meeting of March 10, 1920, see page 386, Annals of Surgery, Sept., 1920.

main vessels have been tied, the screw is loosened by turning it to the left until the vessels not yet secured begin to bleed. Should the bleeding be alarming a few turns of the screw to the right will easily and instantly tighten the grip of the limbs of the instrument upon the extremity. Before the dressing is applied the tourniquet is, of course, removed.

On looking over the latest American literature, I found that Dr. P. E. Truesdale, of Fall River, Mass., has described this same device in the *Jour. of the Am. Med. Assoc.* of January 31, 1920. He states that when the Germans had evacuated the Saint Mihiel salient this instrument was found in one of their advanced post surgical hospitals and given to him for trial. He used it many times and found it " simple to adjust, safe in its effect on the tissues, definite in its control of bleeding, and very adaptable for the purpose in operations on the upper and lower extremities."

The instrument was sent to the office of the chief surgeon, and Doctor Truesdale did not see it again. However, he recalled the principle of the design and had one made by Codman & Shurtleff, of Boston, slightly modified, with heavier arms and an oblong slot in the centre of one handle, through which passes the adjustment screw (Fig. 5). This part of t h e instrument is slightly c u r v e d, so that when the thumb-screw is firmly adjusted with the tourniquet in position, the adjustment screw may be shifted forward, re-

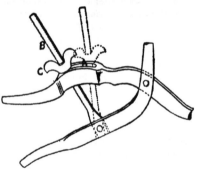

FIG. 6.—Modified handles of tourniquet. *A*, slot through which adjustment screw *B* passes; heavy lines represent adjustment screw holding clamp in position of compression with thumb-nut *C* set; broken lines represent adjustment screw shifted and compression released. (From Journ. Am. Med. Assoc., Jan. 31, 1920, p. 316.)

leasing compression, and back again for renewed control of hemorrhage should this be necessary (Fig. 6). In the original German instrument the thumb-screw itself has to be turned to the right or left in order to tighten or loosen the compression, as mentioned above.

The principle of this type of compression certainly seems to be ideal. The tourniquet, enlarged or reduced in size, according to the local needs, ought to work equally well in other parts of the body. Recently a tourniquet of larger size (abdominal clamp) was successfully applied " by a nurse " in compressing the abdominal aorta in a case of severe post-partum hemorrhage (*Centralbl. f. Gynäkol.*, No. 1, 1920).

At present I am personally engaged in constructing a number of metal tourniquets of very small size, on basis of Sehrt's principle, for the compression of the pedicle of the lobe of the lung in lobectomy, in order to get full surgical control of the pulmonary stump in this operation. With

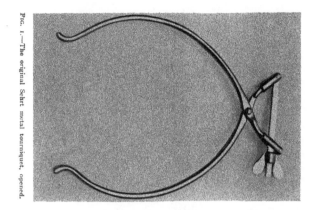

FIG. 1.—The original Sehrt metal tourniquet, opened.

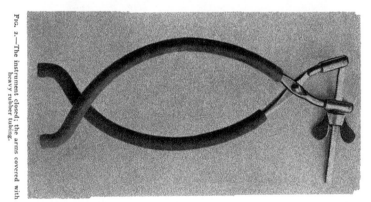

FIG. 2.—The instrument closed; the arms covered with heavy rubber tubing.

764

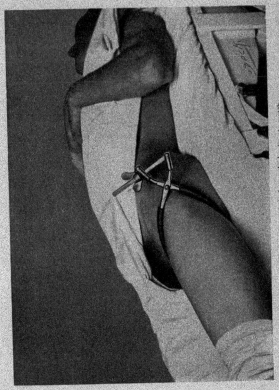

Fig. 3.—Tourniquet switched over thigh, close to crotch.

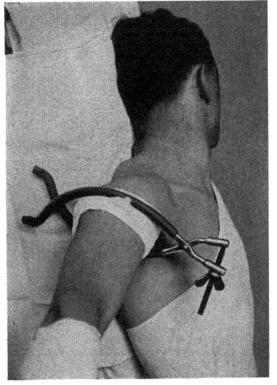

FIG. 4.—Compressing the vessels of the arm.

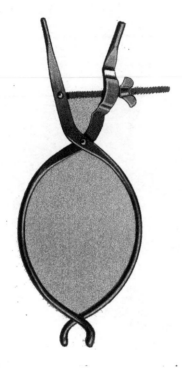

FIG. 5.—Truesdale's modification of Sehrt's tourniquet.

such a tourniquet in place we should be able to tie securely and, if desired, individually, its compressed vessels after amputation of the lobe of the lung, and also—by means of the gradual release of the compression—to find those that have not yet been secured. We should then likewise be able to deal with the stump of the bronchus as may be deemed fit. I hope that such procedure may contribute to a gradual reduction in the still high mortality of this important and often absolutely imperative operation.

At all events, there can be no doubt that Sehrt's metal tourniquet as described above represents the greatest advance made within recent years as regards effectiveness and ease of producing artificial anæmia. Whoever has experienced the annoyance of Esmarch's elastic bandage or tube, particularly on applying or loosening it near the gluteal fold before and during an amputation of the thigh, will be glad of this simple, efficient, and absolutely reliable substitute.

BOOK REVIEWS

PLASTIC SURGERY OF THE FACE. By H. D. GILLIES. Oxford University Press. London. 1920. Cloth, Quarto, pp. 408.

In this book the author presents the results of his experience in dealing with war injuries of the face, as the surgeon in charge of the department for plastic surgery in the Queens Hospital, Sidcup, during the recent World War.

The abundance of material which forms the basis of this book is very great and the skill and industry with which the various problems involved in dealing with such injuries have been met, is most striking and commendable.

A series of eight hundred and forty-four illustrations make a clear, graphic record of the work done both as regards its various steps and methods and the results obtained. The whole constitutes a most valuable contribution to the medical literature of the war and to the history of surgery. All the possibilities of plastic work evidently have been utilized in the work here recorded, although it is evident that at Sidcup the use of bone transplants and of mechanical devices were resorted to less frequently than in some of the French clinics or in similar cases among our American surgeons.

The book constitutes a storehouse of clinical records which will always merit the careful study of every surgeon who undertakes to remedy by plastic work the deformities of the face, which are often so distressing to the subject and difficult of relief to the surgeon.

LEWIS S. PILCHER.

PLASTIC SURGERY—Its Principles and Practice. By JOHN STAIGE DAVIS. Philadelphia. P. Blakiston's Son & Co. Cloth, Octavo, pp. 770.

In this book the whole field of plastic surgery is covered. For many years the author has specialized in this work at the Johns Hopkins Hospital. The author is of opinion that the time has come for the creation of the new specialty of plastic surgery and advocates the appointment of a specially trained plastic surgeon on the staff of every large general hospital.

Notwithstanding, the greater prominence which the plastic surgery of the face has hitherto occupied, the author claims that plastic surgery of the trunk and extremities is equally important.

The frequent contributions to literature during the last few years by the author has prepared the way for this book, and it should be welcomed as a full and systematic presentation of the possibilities and methods of plastic surgery in all of its departments in all portions of the body. It will be seen that such subjects as exstrophy of the bladder, skin grafting of all kinds and the tissue transplantations come fully within the scope of this work.

The book is abundantly illustrated and is sure to find a welcome place in the library of every general surgeon.

LEWIS S. PILCHER.

GRAY's ANATOMY—Descriptive and Applied. Twenty-first Edition, edited by ROBERT HOWDEN, M.A., M.B., D.Sc., Professor of Anatomy in University of Durham. Longmans, Green & Co. London and New York.

An anatomical text-book ought to be crammed full of illustrations each so clear and distinct as to speak for itself. Gray's Anatomy, always well illustrated—the first illustrations were drawn by Vandyke Carter—shows marked improvement in this respect in this latest edition. More than 80 new drawings made by Mr. Sydney Sewell have been added along with others taken from Poirier and Charpey's excellent work. Altogether there are 1215 illustrations in this new edition of which there are 568 colored. The slight coloring aids and accentuates the differentiation of the various structures and impresses their co-relation on the student's mind. The volume would have been still further enhanced in value had it included illustration of head sections, showing the relation of the brain to its external coverings and the best means of gaining access to the brain. For brain surgery such sections are necessary, and even for the student and practitioner desiring to follow localizing symptoms of cerebral lesions, such head sections would much more readily enable them to realize and understand the phenomena.

The omission of such head sections is the more remarkable as this volume gives excellent sections of the upper and lower limbs—showing the structures in a single plane, such as the surgeon would see after amputation, and are useful in many other ways. The editor has been vigilant in keeping abreast of present-day requirements, and has added to anatomical knowledge by bringing into relief points which hitherto were overlooked or considered of little practical importance, but upon which surgical advancements have necessitated accurate information, such as that of the position of the supra-meatal triangle in its relation to the mastoid antrum. The anatomical relations of inguinal and femoral herniæ ought to be improved.

Difference of opinion may certainly be held regarding the introduction of the Basle terminology. It is considered unfortunate to have changed a nomenclature when the editor himself confesses that neither the old nor the new phraseology is entirely satisfactory, and when the Anatomical Society of Great Britain and Ireland concluded that there was no reason for departing from the use of the old nomenclature. Confusion is very apt to ensue. The new terminology may, however, popularize the volume with the Americans who have generally adopted the Basle terminology.

BOOK REVIEWS

The work generally is very well done. Gray's Anatomy has ever been a favorite text-book with students and practitioners, and this twenty-first edition will assuredly greatly increase its popularity. Credit is due to the Messrs. MacLehose, who have printed this volume. It is produced in a good, clear type with differentiated headings and care has been taken with the illustrations which are remarkably clear and distinct.

WILLIAM MACEWEN.

A MANUAL OF PRACTICAL ANATOMY. By THOMAS WALMSLEY, Professor of Anatomy in Queen's University of Belfast. Longmans, Green & Co.

The present volume of some 180 pages represents the first of three parts into which the work is divided, and deals with the dissection of the upper and lower limbs, containing besides an introduction by the author. The introduction deals with the objects of dissection, the order in which the work is best done, and the nature of structures met with. It is open to question whether the anatomist's view expressed therein, that the student " in the practice of his profession will be called upon to operate on the living body, and a true preparation for this task is careful and thoughtful dissection," will meet with the approval of the teacher of surgery, who often finds the eradication of the " dissecting habit " one of the most difficult tasks in a course of practical operative work.

Each section is prefaced by an order of dissection recommended and time table, and these are followed by a short note on the surface anatomy of the part, and instructions for making the incisions and exposing the parts. The general directions are printed in a bold type and the descriptive matter in smaller type, while reference to the principle structures is facilitated by the use of thick type and an index. The instructions are commendably brief and clear, and the text is supplemented by numerous diagrams.

JOHN A. C. MACEWEN.

FRACTURES. Compound Fractures, Dislocations, and their Treatment, with a section on Amputations and Artificial Limbs. By JOHN A. C. MAC-EWEN, M.B., C.M., B.Sc., Maclehose Jackson & Coy, Glasgow, 1919.

This is a text-book for students and medical practitioners of 271 octavo pages. The author is a teacher of the subjects discussed, who has taught large classes of students in two of the largest of Scottish general hospitals; and besides his practical acquaintance with these injuries in industrial life, he has to his credit similar experience in the Army in the field during the Boer War and in military hospitals at home during the European War. The teaching inspired by so long and varied experience and practice is simple, direct, and lucid.

The first portion of the book deals with fractures, a brief discussion of fractures in general, growth of bone as affecting healing, and general considerations regarding diagnosis and treatment, being followed by a detailed account of fractures of individual bones. The text is illustrated by outline drawings indicating the sites of insertions of muscles and the directions of the displacing forces. While varieties of splints are freely illustrated and their mode of application carefully described, more recent methods of dealing with such injuries without splints have full justice done them and the cases suitable are indicated.

A similar method is followed in dealing with dislocations, the varieties of dislocation at each joint being considered in detail one after the other, and the various steps of reduction by manœuvre being precisely stated.

A section is devoted to amputations necessitated by compound fracture, and here there is a valuable summary of the newer methods of treating shock, the composition, method of preparation, and mode of giving the various saline or gum-saline solutions being carefully noted, as well as the method of blood transfusion, and the means of determining suitable donors, while the causes of persistent sepsis in the stump are discussed.

In considering the best method of amputating in each individual case, the author keeps in view throughout the necessity of providing " a stump which, when fitted with an artificial limb, will restore in varying degree the usefulness of the damaged limb." With this end in view, amputations affecting the upper and lower extremities are discussed with reference to the possibilities of adaptation of artificial limbs, and modifications as to site of election and detail of method are suggested as the result of improvements effected in the manufacture of artificial limbs, stimulated by the war. The author had abundant opportunities in the Scottish Hospital for Limbless Sailors and Soldiers at Erskine of taking part in these developments, and this text-book profits thereby.

This section of the book is specially well illustrated by plates from photographs, illustrating useful and unsuitable stumps, and various types of artificial limbs, both apart and applied, including the Erskine provisional limb.

An Appendix summarizes the scale of payments for compensation for such injuries under the Workmen's Compensation Act (1906). An unusual abundance of illustrations for a text-book of this size is obtained by full-page plates from photographs, three, four, and sometimes six subjects being combined in one plate without loss of distinctness.

Only the author's long experience in the teaching and practical handling of these subjects could have enabled him to compress so successfully, without sacrifice of needful detail, so much material into a handbook of this convenient size, which an excellent Index renders quickly available.

J. MacGregor Robertson.

X-RAY OBSERVATIONS FOR FOREIGN BODIES AND THEIR LOCALIZATION. By HAROLD C. GAGE, Conducting Radiographer to the American Red Cross Hospital, Paris. Heinemann.

This is a short practical manual which deals clearly with methods of localization, illustrated by numerous diagrams and skiagraphic reproductions. Methods of centring the tube are carefully given, and localization by screen, stereoscopic photographs and tracings, pierced screen, and geometrical localization are described in detail. Localization of foreign bodies in the eye forms a special section. The author describes with particular clearness a method of localization by means of three intersecting lines, which he has developed and perfected, to the success of which Colonel Joseph Blake pays tribute in the preface. There are also short practical dscriptions of the use of the Bergonie vibrator, telephone probe, la Baume Magnetic Finger Cot, auxiliary switch-boards and bromide paper. The book will prove of interest to all who have had practical experience of the difficulties of localizing foreign bodies during the war, and is a good practical manual for those engaged in such work.

JOHN A. C. MACEWEN.

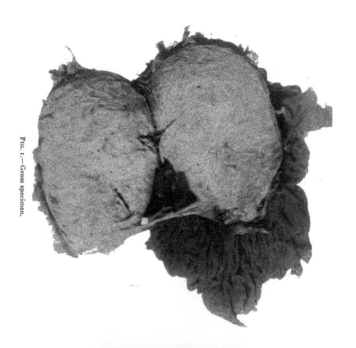

FIG. 1.—Gross specimen.

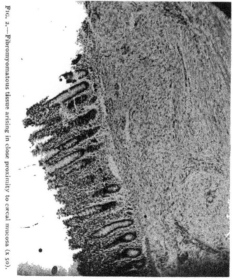

FIG. 2.—Fibromyomatous tissue arising in close proximity to caecal mucosa (× 50).

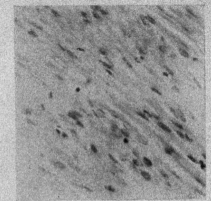

Fig. 4.—Fibroblasts and muscle cells (x 350).

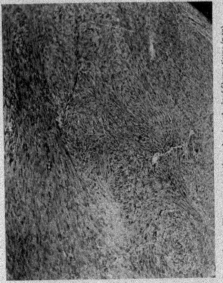

Fig. 3.—Fibromyomatous tissue showing whorls of fibrous tissue (x 50).

CORRESPONDENCE

FIBROMYOMA OF THE CÆCUM

EDITOR, ANNALS OF SURGERY:

CASE A216159. M. B., a woman aged thirty-six years, was examined in the Mayo Clinic December, 1917. She complained, chiefly, of dysmenorrhœa. During the preceding six months menstruation had been painful, necessitating the use of morphine. There had been no metrorrhagia or menorrhagia; the bowels had always been constipated. On vaginal examination a thickening of the tissues in the right tubal region was felt. At operation the appendix was found to be congested, covered by organized lymph and adherent to the right ovary and tube. The right ovary contained a hemorrhagic cyst; in the left ovary was a simple cyst about 6 cm. by 8 cm.; a right-sided salpingitis and some free fluid in the peritoneal cavity were found. The cysts were enucleated from both ovaries, a right salpingectomy was performed, the appendix was removed, and the uterus suspended.

The patient was well until April, 1920, when she noticed a small swelling in the right groin; this had not apparently increased in size. Her general health was good with the exception of constipation. On examination a mass about 10 by 12 cm. was found in the right iliac fossa. There was no abdominal rigidity and the mass seemed immovable. The urine and blood were negative, but the Röntgen-ray showed a filling defect in the cæcum. A diagnosis of carcinoma of the cæcum was made. The operation showed a hard, firmly fixed tumor about 7 by 7 cm. in the cæcum (Fig. 1). The mass together with 5 cm. of ileum and ascending colon were resected and an end-to-end anastomosis made. The mass was found to be a fibromyoma arising in the cæcal wall. A few of the mesenteric glands showed healed tuberculosis.

Pathological Report.—The specimen consists of an ovoidal, encapsulated, solid tumor situated apparently in the wall of the cæcum, the mucosa and serosa being intact. The tumor is a white fibrous neoplasm surrounded by a capsule consisting of all the layers of the cæcum. Microscopic sections (Figs. 2, 3 and 4) show the layers of the cæcum to be intact, although somewhat thinned out by pressure of the neoplasm which apparently arises in the cæcal muscularis. The neoplasm itself consists of fibroblasts and smooth-muscle cells.

J. A. H. MAGOUN, JR., M.D.,
Fellow in Surgery, The Mayo Foundation, Rochester, Minnesota.

A NEW GASTRO-ENTEROSTOMY CLAMP

EDITOR, ANNALS OF SURGERY:

THE number of clamps on the market for the purpose of gastro-enterostomy is very considerable. So many and varied types have been introduced that, perhaps, mine deserves the term " modification " rather than new "; but I have not seen one so like it as to disqualify it entirely from the latter title. From the numbers of these clamps one may infer that there is, in general, a lack of satisfaction with them; and most will agree that this inference is borne out in practice. One naturally hesitates to offer an addition to the number. I believe, however, that the clamp I shall describe has certain advantages over those in common use which justify a brief description of it here.

The objects in view in applying clamps during such an operation as gastro-enterostomy are: To prevent the escape of septic contents, to control hemorrhage, and to support the viscera to be anastomosed in a convenient position for that purpose. Thus infection risk is minimized, the advantages of a bloodless operation field secured, and ease and accuracy in suturing facilitated. In order to attain these objects satisfactorily, the clamps used must conform to certain general principles.

The blades must distribute their pressure equally on the surface grasped that no undue pressure be applied at any part, and that no bleeding or slipping shall occur.

The gripping surface must be of a texture that holds well without inflicting damage, in order that a minimum pressure for the control of contents, hemorrhage and slipping may be used.

The two clamps must be capable of easy and close attachment to each other.

Other requirements are ease of manipulation, lightness, convenience in size and form, simplicity, durability, and moderate cost.

The figures illustrate a clamp in the design of which an attempt has been made to carry these principles into effect. Fig. 1 shows the complete instrument. The two clamps are fixed together. Fig. 2 illustrates the clamps separated; one is opened.

1. The inner, rigid and fixed blade.

2. The outer flexible and moving blade. Its flexibility and curvature are so arranged that when closed it becomes straight and presses evenly at all points.

3. Spring of outer blade, by means of which it is automatically adjusted to viscera of any thickness between 0 and $\frac{1}{4}$ inch, maintaining its parallel position.

4. Hinge, of large diameter to minimize wear and side movement.

5. Screw, which can be folded down parallel to the blades for withdrawal of the clamp after the anastomosis is complete (Fig. 3).

6. Split, milled nut, and thimble. This slips freely over the thread until it is brought into contact with the blade, which the left hand is holding closed in position; the thread then engages and it is fixed with half a turn. There is thus no tedious screwing up. These split nuts and thimbles are largely used on engineers' calipers, and are very convenient for the present purpose.

7. Undercut, sliding attachment for approximation.

8. " Patent fastener " clip, such as one sees on the wrist of a glove. This completes the simple fixing mechanism.

Fig. 3 shows the clamp in use. The anastomosis is complete and the blades opened ready for withdrawal.

I should like to mention some points of comparison with clamps generally used for anastomosis operations.

With the usual " scissors action " clamps it contrasts to advantage as regards parallelism of blades and even distribution of pressure, and these points are of vital importance in securing adequate control of hemorrhage and slipping, without causing bruising at some part. The accompanying diagrams illustrate this. A thick viscus, such as hypertrophied stomach, is supposed to be grasped. A single arrow ($\downarrow$) indicates correct pressure; two arrows ($\downarrow\downarrow$) excessive pressure; O indicates insufficient pressure.

A is a simple clamp. It will be seen that the stomach is unduly crushed at the joint end of the blades, while their free ends gape and exert no control at all.

B, the free ends are fixed by a clip. This is an improvement, but, as shown, bruising is still liable to occur at the joint end or slipping and bleeding at the centre.

C shows the equality of pressure given by clamp under description. Note how the spring at X has risen to accommodate the thick stomach. It adjusts itself equally well to thin intestine, always keeping the blades parallel. It may also be mentioned here that the screw is capable of much finer adjustment than is a ratchet, as in handled clamps.

As regards the texture of the gripping surface; rubber-covered or smooth, fluted metal blades tend to slip, and injurious pressure is necessary to prevent this. Coarse serrations hold well but inflict direct damage. The optimum is a finely but sharply roughened metal surface: this has been adopted (Fig. 3).

The two clamps are entirely independent, an advantage over the three-bladed types, in using which difficulty may be experienced in securing the second viscus, and under these circumstances a distorted hold is more liable to be taken. They are fixed together by slipping in the undercut slide and pressing the " patent fastener " home.

It is capable of very rapid manipulation, and is more easily applied than clamps with handles, especially in the absence of assistance. It begins to grip at the spring end. Here one end of the selected loop is secured, one hand controlling the free end of the blade while the other spreads out the loop as the blade closes on it. Most clamps close simultaneously at the joint and distal ends, and the single free hand is unable to spread out the loop satisfactorily. The blade, having been closed, is instantly fixed by the split nut.

It weighs somewhat less than 140 gm., while the approximate weight of the commoner patterns is about 250 gm.

The working surface of the blades is 14 cm. long, as compared with 12.5 cm. of a typical gastro-enterostomy clamp. The over-all length is 20 cm. as against 34 cm. This moderate size has been found very convenient in private practice, where a large sterilizer may not be available.

The blades are curved. The convexity of the curve is directed into the abdomen, should delivery of the viscera be difficult. When this can be easily accomplished the convexity is directed outwards, and holds up the selected portions conveniently for suture (Fig. 3).

When the clamps are joined the laterally projecting screws steady the instrument and prevent its rolling.

It is, perhaps, rather more delicate than the usual instruments. The screw and joints require very thorough drying and a little oil when laid aside. It has, however, stood the severe test of four years' constant use in hospital well, and any clamp should have the above-mentioned attention.

A limitation which it shares with most other gastro-enterostomy clamps is that it can only take a lateral hold, since both ends are closed. It can, however, be applied across the stomach in gastric resections, where the curvatures of that organ have been freed from their peritoneal attachments. Hence it is a somewhat specialized instrument, its sphere of action being gastro-enterostomy, entero-anastomosis, enterotomy, gastric resection, etc.

It is made entirely of steel, and all angles and projections are rounded off. It is silver plated, and the screws are gilt: this wears much longer than does nickel plating, and adds but little to the cost.

As regards its cost relative to that of other instruments of the same class; I am told that if it were made in similar numbers its price would be approximately the same. Being made specially, to single orders, it naturally costs considerably more.

Mr. J. W. Dowden, F.R.C.S.E., Surgeon to the Royal Infirmary, Edinburgh, has used the clamp for four years. I wish to express my gratitude to him for the interest he has taken in its production.

To Mr. S. Hurford I am much indebted for his intelligent coöperation in the manufacture. The instrument is obtainable from Messrs. Hurford & Drysdale, Surgical Instrument Makers, 15 Drummond Street, Edinburgh.

NORMAN M. DOTT, M.B., Ch.B.,
Edinburgh, Scotland.

THE RELATIVE PLACE OF PLASTER DRESSING AND OF SUSPENSION APPARATUS IN THE TREATMENT OF FRACTURES

EDITOR, ANNALS OF SURGERY:

In an article entitled " The Portable Suspension Frame Employed in the Treatment of the Wounded During the European War," [1] by Dr. H.

---

[1] ANNALS OF SURGERY, June, 1920.

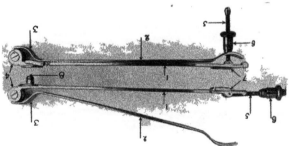

FIG. 1.—Clamp assembled.

FIG. 2.—The two elements of the clamp separated, one open, one closed.

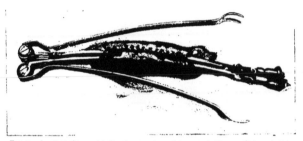

FIG. 3.—Anastomosis completed; set screws turned down to facilitate withdrawal of the clamp.

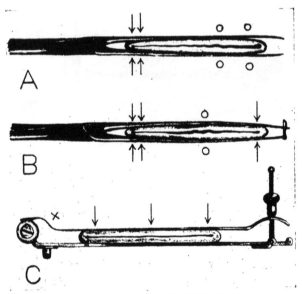

FIG. 4.—Showing the more equal impression exercised by the author's clamp as compared with the scissors action of the usual model of clamp.

H. M. Lyle, the author elaborates the description of his invention with a few remarks in connection with the treatment of fractures.

He says, " in the early period of the war the dominant note in the treatment of fractures was immobilization. The majority of cases were encased in plaster of Paris in which windows were cut, or metal arches made to give access to the wounds. The immediate results were filth, infection, and gangrene; the late results pressure sores, atrophied muscles, and ankylosed joints. So much for the so-called orthopædic treatment of fractures."

This statement is too sweeping to escape comment. What Doctor Lyle doubtless means is that the results he deplores were due to the attempt to treat compound fractures by plaster of Paris, a phrase which he condenses by the use of the shorter and uglier one, " orthopædic treatment." He then goes on to imply that the results of the treatment of fractures by plaster of Paris are " pressure sores, atrophied muscles, and ankylosed joints."

This implication is not well founded, as for years fractures have been treated with immobilization in plaster of Paris by surgeons in general as well as orthopædic surgeons with a fair degree of success. It is also inaccurate to confuse orthopædic treatment with the use of plaster of Paris. The results he criticises were those of the early days of the war, when all treatment was in a generally chaotic state. The atrophied muscles, pressure sores, and gangrene were the results of the infected wounds occurring in conjunction with the fractures, when surgeons were falling between the two stools of treating wounds and neglecting the fracture, or treating the fracture and neglecting the wounds. In the light of further experience the attempt to apply plaster of Paris in conjunction with open wounds and the possibility of extension of the suppurative process beneath the plaster appears, to say the least, ill advised. The statement may hardly be disputed that the development of the treatment of fractures by traction and suspension was due to the necessity of evolving a method of treatment which allowed primarily ready access to the wounds and the maximum comfort of the patient. The further application of traction for the treatment of fractures came next. Last of all was the general discovery that fractures so treated gave good functional results.

The enthusiastic advocacy of the treatment of all fractures by traction and suspension represents the furthest excursion of the pendulum from the pre-war practice of the almost universal use of plaster of Paris. The present extremists were forced to treat fractures as an incident in the treatment of wounds, and as a necessity in saving the lives of their patients. They were incidentally surprised to note the unexpectedly good functional and anatomic results which they obtained in the fractures. The treatment of fractures by traction and suspension is being very gen-

CORRESPONDENCE

erally spoken of as one of the great lessons of the war, in spite of the fact
that Bardenheuer had published a book upon the subject in 1907.[1]

No one will deny that the treatment is an excellent one in the hands
of certain individuals. Its disadvantages are that it confines the patient
to bed, that it requires very considerable mechanical ingenuity and skill
on the part of its applicator, and that it is largely at the mercy of the
patient and his attendants, who may easily disarrange one of its several
essential features with consequent unhappy results.

No one will deny that plaster of Paris in the hands of certain individuals is also an excellent treatment. It can rarely be used in the presence of suppuration. The danger of swelling beneath the plaster is
always present. If not properly applied no dressing is more uncomfortable,
and no dressing offers the possibility of graver complications in
unskilled hands.

The confusion of " orthopædic treatment " with the use of plaster of
Paris is difficult to understand. The consulting orthopædic surgeon to
the hospital with which Doctor Lyle is connected has been a life-long
opponent of the use of plaster of Paris. Sir Robert Jones, an orthopædic
surgeon of distinction, scarcely ever uses it, which explains the fact that
it was practically never seen throughout the British Army. The distinction between orthopædic and general surgery lies in the fact that the
former has as its constant purpose " to prevent or to correct deformity
and to preserve or restore function, a purpose which governs treatment
from the beginning and to the end." [2]

The treatment of fractures has unquestionably been greatly benefited
by the war. It is now generally appreciated that they are difficult to
treat; that they may be treated in a variety of ways; that they should be
treated by surgeons familiar with these various methods and capable of
weighing their advantages in relation to their application to a given case;
and most important of all, is the great stress now being laid upon the factor of greatest importance to the patient, the ultimate functional result.

ARMITAGE WHITMAN, M.D.

---

[1] Die Allgemeine Lehre von der Frakturen und Luxationen. B. Bardenheuer,
Stuttgart, 1907.
[2] Whitman, R.: Orthopædic Surgery. Lea & Febiger, Philadelphia, 6th Edition.

To Contributors and Subscribers :

All contributions for Publication, Books for Review, and Exchanges should be
sent to the Editorial Office, 145 Gates Ave., Brooklyn, N. Y.

Remittances for Subscriptions and Advertising and all business communications
should be addressed to the

ANNALS of SURGERY
227-231 S. 6th Street
Philadelphia, Penna.

INDEX TO VOLUME LXXII

A

Abdomino-thoracic Injuries, 370.

ADAIR, FRANK: Traumatic Fat Necrosis of the Female Breast, 188.

After-treatment of Surgical Patient, by Willard Bartlett and Others, Review of, 534.

Amberine, Effect of Healing After Burns, 633.

American Surgical Association, Presidential Address, 1.

Amputation Stump, End-bearing Condition After Forty Years, 526.

Anæsthesia, Regional, Review of, B. Sherwood-Dunn, 534.

Anal Sphincter, Operation to Form New After Operation on Rectum, 693.

Anatomy, Practical, Review of Walmsley's Manual of, 768; Gray's, Review of, 767.

Aneurism of Radial Artery, 391.—

Angio-keratoma of Scrotum, 635.

Anus, Artificial, Control of, 383.

Appendicitis, Acute, Causes of Death by, After Operation, 207.

Appendix, Vermiform, Primary Carcinoma, 685; Retrocæcal Gangrene of, 379.

ASHHURST, ASTLEY P. C.: Observations on Empyema, 12; Jacksonian Epilepsy Caused by Brain Tumor, 402; Hæmatomyelia, with Crossed Paralysis, 406; End-results of Bridging Defects in Peripheral Nerves, 408.

Astragalus, Forward Dislocation of the, 494.

B

BARTLETT, WILLARD: The After-treatment of Surgical Patients, Review of, 534.

Bladder, Large Stone in the, 520.

BLAKE, JOSEPH A.: Overhead Suspension Frame, 385.

BLOODGOOD, JOSEPH COLT: Bone Tumors, Myxoma, Central and Periosteal, 712.

BOHMANSSON, G.: The Diagnosis and Therapy of Bone Typhoid, 486.

Bone Flap, Cutting in Cranial Surgery, 511; and Joint Lesions, Syphilitic, Surgical Aspects of, 488; the Recognition of Dead, 456; the Rôle of Cancellous Tissue in Healing, 452; Tumors, 712; Typhoid, the Diagnosis and Therapy of, 486.

BOORSTEIN, SAMUEL W.: Orthopædic Treatment of Burns, 618.

Brain, Large, Removed from Child, 416; Operations, Appliance to Secure Position and Steadiness of the Head During, 591; Treatment and Results of Wounds of, 538; Tumor, Causing Jacksonian Epilepsy, 402.

Branchio-genetic and Ranular Cysts, Relationship Between, 164.

Breast, Cancer of the, Late Results of Radical Operation for, 177; Cancer of, Technic in Operations for, 181; Female, Traumatic Fat Necrosis of the, 188; Sarcoma of, 387.

Breasts, Cancer of Both, 417.

BREWER, GEO. EMERSON: Duties and Responsibilities of the Civil Surgeon When Called to Active Service, 1.

Bronchial Fistulæ, the Treatment of, 345.

BROWN, ALFRED J.: Operation to Form New Anal Sphincter, 693.

BROWN, HENRY P., JR.: Intraperitoneal Hernia of the Ileum, 516.

BUNTS, FRANK E.: Operation for Empyema in Young Adults, 66.

Burns, Orthopædic Treatment of, 618; the Surgical Treatment of, 631; X-ray, Radical Treatment of, 224.

Bursitis, Epitrochanteric, Simulating Sarcoma, 392.

C

Cancellous Tissue in Healing Bone, the Rôle of, 452.

Cancer, Advanced, Radical Operation in Case of, 698; of Both Breasts, 417; of the Breast, the Late Results of Radical Operation for, 177; of Cervix Uteri, Radium in the Treatment of, 701; of the Ovary, Invading the Sigmoid Flexure, 218; of the Rectum, 382; Technic in Operations for, 181.

Cæcum, Fibro-myoma of the, 771.

Carcinoma of the Duodenum, 602.

Cervical Ribs Simulated by Adventitious Ligaments, 497; Vertebra, Seventh and Fibrous Ankylosis of the Right Shoulder-joint, 525.

Charcot Joint, Surgical Aspects of the, 488.

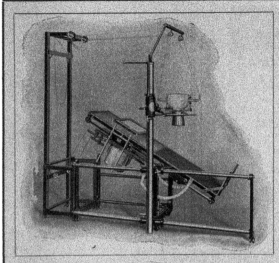

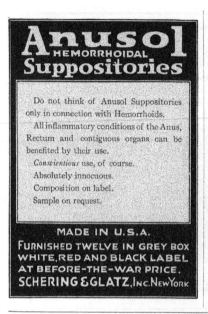
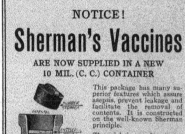
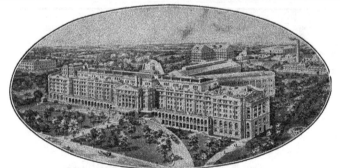
18

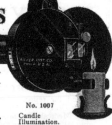
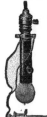
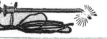
For

For

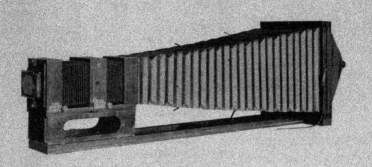

The Eastman
X-Ray Reducing Camera

For lantern slides or 5 x 7 copies

—Complete equipment—illuminator, negative holding kits,
lens and plate holder.

For general clinical photography

—A complete camera—with Kodak Anastigmat $f.7.7$ lens
and extension permitting the taking of "close-ups."

EASTMAN KODAK COMPANY
ROCHESTER, N. Y.

21

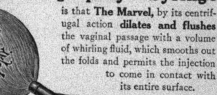
22

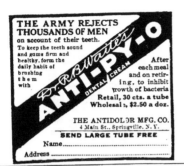
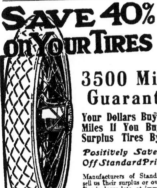
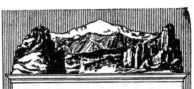

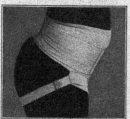
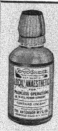
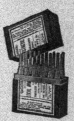